Access Videos, Fitnes... Programs, and More!

Self-Study Companion Website resources included with any new book.

Access to MyFitnessLab, including assignments and eText, sold separately.

REGISTER NOW!

Registration will let you:

- **See It!** with exercise videos, lab demos, and *ABC News* videos.

- **Hear It!** with audio case studies and audio PowerPoints.

- **Do It!** with interactive labs.

- **Live It!** with customizable fitness programs.

Registration also gives you access to multiple practice quizzes, mobile apps, web links, critical thinking exercises, and more.

www.pearsonhighered.com/hopson

TO REGISTER

1. Go to **www.pearsonhighered.com/hopson**
2. Click on your book cover.
3. Select any chapter from the drop-down menu and click "Go."
4. Click "See It" and then click one of the video options.
5. Click "Register."
6. Follow the on-screen instructions to create your login name and password.

Your Access Code is:

Note: If there is no silver foil covering the access code, it may already have been redeemed, and therefore may no longer be valid. In that case, you can purchase access online using a major credit card or PayPal account. To do so, go to www.pearsonhighered.com/hopson click on "Buy Access," and follow the on-screen instructions.

TO LOG IN

1. Go to **www.pearsonhighered.com/hopson**
2. Click on your book cover.
3. Select any chapter from the drop-down menu and click "Go."
4. Click "See It" and then click one of the video options.
5. Enter your login name and password.

Hint:
Remember to bookmark the site after you log in.

Technical Support:
http://247pearsoned.custhelp.com

Stop!

Did you register? Don't miss out!

Turn back one page to register and get help preparing for exams... whenever and wherever you need it.

www.pearsonhighered.com/hopson

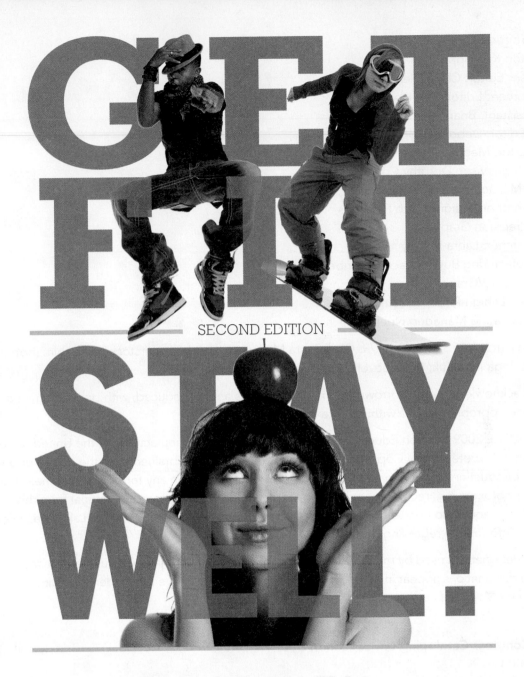

GET FIT

SECOND EDITION

STAY WELL!

Janet L. Hopson, M.A.
San Francisco State University

Rebecca J. Donatelle, Ph.D.
Oregon State University

Tanya R. Littrell, Ph.D.
Portland Community College

PEARSON

Boston   Columbus   Indianapolis   New York   San Francisco   Upper Saddle River
Amsterdam   Cape Town   Dubai   London   Madrid   Milan   Munich   Paris   Montréal   Toronto
Delhi   Mexico City   São Paulo   Sydney   Hong Kong   Seoul   Singapore   Taipei   Tokyo

Executive Editor: Sandra Lindelof
Project Editor: Kari Hopperstead
Development Editor: Claire Alexander
Art Development Editor: Kari Hopperstead
Editorial Assistant: Briana Verdugo
Managing Editor: Deborah Cogan
Assistant Editor: Meghan Zolnay
Production Supervisor: Dorothy Cox
Production Management and Compositor: PreMediaGlobal
Cover and Interior Designer: Yvo Riezebos
Illustrator: Precision Graphics
Photo Researcher: Laura Murray
Senior Manufacturing Buyer: Stacey Weinberger
Text Printer: Quad/Graphics
Cover Printer: Lehigh-Phoenix Color
Executive Marketing Manager: Neena Bali

Cover Photos: (top left) Shutterstock/R. Gino Santa Maria; (top right) Shutterstock/Samokhin; (bottom) Shutterstock/Inga Marchuk; (back cover) Shutterstock/ULKASTUDIO

Credits and acknowledgments borrowed from other sources and reproduced, with permission, in this textbook appear on the appropriate page within the text [or on p. C-1–C-2].

Library of Congress Cataloging-in-Publication Data
Hopson, Janet L.
  Get fit, stay well! / Janet L. Hopson, Donatelle, Rebecca J., Tanya R. Littrell.
  —2nd ed.
    p. cm.
  ISBN 978-0-321-75433-2
  1. Physical fitness—Textbooks. 2. Health—Textbooks.
  I. Donatelle, Rebecca J., 1950- II. Littrell, Tanya R. III. Title.
  RA781.H65 2011
  613.7—dc23   2011042231

ISBN 10: 0-321-75433-6; ISBN 13: 978-0-321-75433-2 (Student edition)
ISBN 10: 0-321-78036-1; ISBN 13: 978-0-321-78036-2 (Brief Edition)
ISBN 10: 0-321-78041-8; ISBN 13: 978-0-321-78041-6 (Exam Copy)
ISBN 10: 0-321-80229-2; ISBN 13: 978-0-321-80229-3 (a la Carte edition)

www.pearsonhighered.com   1 2 3 4 5 6 7 8 9 10—QGD—15 14 13 12 11

About the Authors

Janet L. Hopson, M.A.

A full-time author and lecturer, Janet L. Hopson has written or co-authored nine books, including two popular nonfiction books on human pheromones and human brain development, and eight textbooks on general biology and wellness for college and high school students. Ms. Hopson currently teaches science writing at San Francisco State University and the University of California at Santa Cruz. She holds B.A. and M.A. degrees from Southern Illinois University and the University of Missouri. She has won awards for magazine writing, and her articles have appeared in *Smithsonian, Psychology Today, Science Digest, Science News, Outside,* and others. She is married and enjoys golfing, swimming, reading, traveling, competitive tennis, and teaching horseback riding.

Rebecca J. Donatelle, Ph.D.

Dr. Rebecca J. Donatelle is a Professor Emeritus in Public Health at Oregon State University, having served as the Department Chair, Coordinator of the Public Health Promotion and Education Programs, and faculty member and researcher in the College of Health and Human Sciences. She has a Ph.D. in Community Health/Health Education, a M.S. in Health Education, and a B.S. with majors in both Health/Physical Education and English. Her main research and teaching focus has been on the factors that increase risk for chronic diseases and the use of incentives and social supports in developing effective interventions for high-risk women and families. Her research has been published in numerous journals, and she has been a guest speaker and presenter at professional conferences throughout the country. Dr. Donatelle is also the author of the highly successful introductory health textbooks *Access to Health* and *Health: The Basics,* as well as the new *My Health: An Outcomes Approach.*

Tanya R. Littrell, Ph.D.

Dr. Tanya R. Littrell is a full-time faculty member in Fitness Technology and Physical Education at Portland Community College in Portland, Oregon. Dr. Littrell worked as a fitness director for many years before attending graduate school at Oregon State University, where she earned both a master's degree in Human Performance/Exercise Physiology and a doctoral degree in Exercise Science/Exercise Physiology. Dr. Littrell has been teaching lifetime fitness classes for undergraduates since 1998. When she is not teaching, preparing to teach, or writing, you can find Dr. Littrell on the trails running or mountain biking, rock climbing, traveling, or spending quality time with her family.

Brief Contents

Contents

3 Conditioning Your Cardiorespiratory System 67

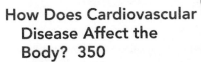

13 Avoiding Substance Use, Abuse, and Addiction 405

14 Reducing Your Risk of Sexually Transmitted Infections 433

15 Maintaining Lifelong Fitness and Wellness 453

Feature Boxes

Labs and Programs

LABS

ACTIVATE, MOTIVATE, & ADVANCE YOUR FITNESS

You may have noticed that health, fitness, and wellness are highly popular topics! Open a newspaper, turn on the TV, or surf the Internet and you will undoubtedly find articles about the benefits of exercise, the health risks associated with obesity, or the results of a recent nutritional study. At the same time, if you are a college student taking a fitness and wellness course, you may feel a sense of disconnect between those stories and your own life. You might wonder: What has any of this got to do with me?

Our primary goal in writing this textbook was simple: to get students to realize that the lifestyle choices you make now—regardless of your current age—have real and lasting effects on your lifelong wellness. We also wanted to write a textbook that takes into account the many challenges facing today's students and offers you maximum flexibility and options for creating a fitness and wellness program that you can personalize for your own goals and time demands. Finally, we wanted this textbook to address a common fact of life: the gap between knowing what we *ought* to do (for example, exercise more, eat healthier foods, quit smoking, etc.) and actually *doing it*. Throughout this textbook, we emphasize that effective behavior change is a gradual process, based on having realistic expectations and setting achievable short-term and long-term goals.

With these aims in mind, the following are some of the unique features you'll find in *Get Fit, Stay Well!*:

New to This Edition

- *The text has been revised and streamlined from 16 chapters to 15 chapters* to address the need for a book that fits easily into a 15-week semester schedule.

- *The nutrition chapter has been updated per the 2010 USDA guidelines* and the book draws upon the latest exercise recommendations from American College of Sports Medicine, American Heart Association, and U. S. Department of Health and Human Services.

- *New Activate, Motivate, & Advance sample fitness and wellness programs* placed at the ends of

Chapters 2–5, 8, and 9 are like having your own personal trainer built into the book. Each program contains guidance on 3 parts of a fitness or wellness program: getting started, motivating to continue, and taking it to the next level. The customizable "pre-fab" programs and the related tracking features and technique videos on the website make it easy to jump into a behavior change project.

- *New Learning Outcomes* replace Chapter Objectives in the chapter openers.

- *New exercise photos* expand options for alternate equipment and exercises, and replace those photos identified by reviewers as showing less than optimal form or atypical equipment.

- *New media callouts* in the chapter openers, end-of-chapter material, and throughout the text direct students to the extensive supporting electronic media, including videos, audio files, assignments, and review materials. In the eText versions, these callouts provide direct links to the media assets.

- *New Think!/Act!* questions at the end of the case studies and throughout the text are designed to encourage critical thinking and to help students reflect on how the material applies to their own lives.

Updates to the Media Program Include:

- *MyFitnessLab™* has been redesigned and now contains more assignable, gradable content for every chapter. Assigning and grading homework has never been easier! More than 180 assignments, including interactive lab worksheets, pre- and post-chapter quizzes, Case Study quizzes, video quizzes, and discussion questions are available for instructors to assign with the a click of a button.

- *New ABC News videos* with accompanying quizzes and discussion questions are available on the instructor resource DVD, MyFitnessLab, and Companion Website.

- *Revised and expanded exercise videos* include new options for stability ball exercises and demonstration videos for fitness assessment labs—over 100 videos in all!

- *New sample fitness and wellness programs* link to demonstration videos and related tracking tools for customizing and logging a behavior change project.

Other Key Features

- *Unique Case Studies presented in each chapter* introduce a "character" who reflects the concerns, questions, and thought processes that students are likely to have themselves. Think!/Act! questions at the end of the case studies encourage critical thinking and help students consider how the material applies to their own lives.

- *Labs employ a unique three-pronged approach:* 1) skill-acquisition labs, 2) self-assessment labs, and 3) action-plan labs. The labs not only measure a student's current level of fitness/wellness, but also teach practical lifelong skills and encourage real behavior change. Many additional labs are offered online on the book's website. All labs are also available online in interactive PDF format and are assignable through MyFitnessLab.

- *The most modern strength-training presentation available* includes photos of more 80 strength-training and flexibility exercises featuring actual college students, modern gym equipment, and options for students with limited access to equipment. Videos of the exercises in the book, as well as many alternate exercises, are available online at the Companion Website and MyFitnessLab—allowing students access to additional instruction on their own time.

- *A separate chapter on diabetes and other chronic diseases* makes this text a valuable reference for fitness and wellness courses, as it emphasizes one of today's national health epidemics.

- *A strong emphasis is placed on behavior change throughout the text*. Think!/Act! features provide suggestions for immediate action and Tools for Change boxes provide tools for longer-term change. The "Plan for Change" labs ask students to write out an action plan for behavior change.

- *Questions boxes* investigate common questions and concerns students may have in relation to chapter topics.

- *Diversity boxes* address topics relevant to diverse student populations, acknowledging that age, race, gender, disability, and individual life circumstances can result in specific fitness and wellness needs.

- *A running glossary* helps students easily review and master key terms.

- *End-of-chapter review questions and critical thinking questions* encourage students to evaluate material they have just learned.

- *Research citations* demonstrate the accuracy, currency, and scientific grounding for information presented in the text.

- *A pre- and post-course progress worksheet* included at the beginning of the book and available online allows students to assess their progress on key fitness/wellness assessments.

Instructor Supplements

This textbook comes with unparalleled supplemental resources to assist instructors with classroom preparation and presentation.

Teaching Tool Box

Save hours of valuable planning time with one comprehensive course planning box containing a wealth of supplements and resources that reinforce key learning from the text and suit virtually any teaching style. The Teaching Tool Box includes:

- *Instructor Resource DVD* with all art, photos, and tables from the text; PowerPoint® lecture slides; a computerized test bank; *ABC News* videos; exercise demonstration videos, Active Lecture (clicker) Questions; Quiz Show Game PowerPoint slides; interactive PDF lab worksheets; PDF transparency masters, Instructor Resource and Support Manual PDFs, and Test Bank Word files

- *Instructor Resource and Support Manual* with detailed chapter outlines incorporating IR-DVD assets, in-class discussion questions, and activities, additional resources, first-time teaching tips, sample syllabi, and tips for using MyFitnessLab

- *Test Bank* with over 1000 questions in multiple-choice, true/false, and short-essay formats

- *User's Quick Start Guide* for getting up and running using the materials in the Teaching Tool Box

- *Access to MyFitnessLab™* course management website with more than 180 separate assignments, a gradebook, and an annotatable eText

- *Great Ideas: Active Ways to Teach Health and Wellness*, a manual of ideas for classroom activities related to fitness and wellness topics, including activities that can be adapted to various topics and class sizes

- *New Teaching with Student Learning Outcomes* publication containing useful suggestions and examples for successfully incorporating outcomes into a fitness and wellness course

- *New Teaching with Web 2.0* handbook introducing popular new online tools and offering ideas for incorporating them into a fitness and wellness course

- *Behavior Change Log Book with Wellness Journal*, newly revised to include updated worksheets, nutrition information, journals, and fitness logs

- *New Food Composition Table* containing detailed nutrition information about thousands of foods

- *Live Right! Beating Stress in College and Beyond* booklet on handling life's challenges including sleep, finances, time management, academic pressure, and relationships

- *Eat Right! Healthy Eating in College and Beyond* booklet of guidelines, tips, and recipes for healthy eating

- *Take Charge of Your Health!* self-assessment worksheets

MyFitnessLab

www.pearsonhighered.com/myfitnesslab
This redesigned online course management program is loaded with valuable teaching resources that make it easy to give assignments and track student progress. The preloaded content in MyFitnessLab includes unsurpassed resources for teaching online or hybrid courses and is arranged into five learning areas.

In the Read It area:

- *New Pearson eText* gives students access to the text whenever and wherever they have access to the Internet. The powerful functionality of the eText includes the ability to create notes, highlight text in different colors, create bookmarks, zoom, click on hyperlinked words and phrases to view definitions, and view in single-page or two-page view.

- *New RSS feeds* provide students easy, online access to news and spotlights about hot fitness and wellness topics, updated daily.

- *New chapter learning outcomes* reiterate the important points in each chapter.

In the See It area:

- *More than 100 exercise videos* demonstrate strength-training and flexibility exercises with resistance bands, stability balls, free weights, and gym machines, as well as lab assessment techniques. The videos are also available for download onto iPods® or other media players, and some have related quizzing.

- *New ABC News video clips* bring fitness and wellness topics to life. Related quizzing is available for assigning and automatic grading.

In the Hear It area:

- *New audio cases studies* from the text pertain to each chapter's content. All are available for download as MP3 files and have related assignable and gradable quizzing.

- *Audio PowerPoint lectures* support classroom lectures and enhance self-study options.

In the Do It area:

- *Pre-course/Post-course assessment* lets students evaluate their own fitness and wellness status both before and after taking the course.

- *New interactive labs* automatically perform calculations on students' input. Completed labs can be submitted to instructors by digital dropbox, e-mail, or print. More than 55 labs guide students through assessing fitness and wellness levels, learning core skills, and developing behavior change plans. Additional labs available only online are designed to accommodate varying skill levels, differing access to equipment, and the specific needs of students with disabilities.

In the Review It area:

- *Multiple-choice and true/false self-study quizzes* for every chapter are automatically scored, so students can get feedback and check their understanding. Quizzes can also be assigned by instructors and feed to the gradebook.

- *Online glossary* is a quick and easy resource for definitions of key terms.
- *Interactive flashcards* allow students to build a deck of flashcards from the key terms in every chapter, review them online, print them out, or even export them to a mobile phone.

In the Live It area:

- *New Activate, Motivate, & Advance programs* from the text help students commit to and track a new fitness or wellness routine. Links to exercise demonstration and technique videos provide further guidance for students just getting started on a new fitness program.
- *Behavior Change Logbook and Wellness Journal* is provided in interactive PDF format for easy assigning and submitting.
- *Take Charge of Your Health! worksheets* in interactive PDF format offer more options for self-assessment and developing behavior change plans.

Student Supplements

A wealth of materials is available to help students review and explore course content and enact behavior change in their own lives.

MyFitnessLab

www.pearsonhighered.com/myfitnesslab
This online course management program has been redesigned for greater usability and is loaded with valuable resources. The preloaded content includes unsurpassed resources for online or hybrid courses; see the full description under Instructor Supplements above.

Companion Website

www.pearsonhighered.com/hopson
The *Get Fit, Stay Well!* companion website offers hundreds of practice quiz questions, interactive labs, 50 additional health self-assessment worksheets, web links, glossary and flashcards of key terms, audio case studies and audio PowerPoint lectures, more than 30 ABC News videos, and more than 100 exercise demonstration videos.

Behavior Change Log Book and Wellness Journal
978-0-321-80317-7 / 0-321-80317-5

This booklet helps students track their daily exercise and nutritional intake and create a personalized long-term nutrition and fitness program. It has been newly revised to include updated worksheets, nutrition information, journals, and fitness logs

Eat Right! Healthy Eating in College and Beyond
978-0-8053-8288-4 / 0-8053-8288-7

This handy, full-color booklet provides practical guidelines, tips, shopper's guides and recipes for putting healthy eating principles into action. Topics include healthy eating in the cafeteria, dorm room, and fast food restaurants; eating on a budget; weight management tips; vegetarian alternatives; and guidelines on alcohol and health.

Take Charge of Your Health! Worksheets
978-0-321-49942-4 / 0-321-49942-5

Twelve new worksheets have been added to this edition's collection of self-assessment activities, providing a total of 50 self-assessment exercises in a gummed pad that can be packaged with the text.

New Lifestyles Pedometer
978-0-321-51803-3 / 0-321-51803-9

Take strides to better health with this pedometer, a first step toward overall health and wellness. This pedometer measures steps, distance (miles), activity time, and calories, and provides a time clock.

MyDietAnalysis
Powered by ESHA Research, Inc., MyDietAnalysis features a database of nearly 20,000 foods. This easy-to-use program allows students to track their diet and activity for up to three profiles and to assess the nutritional value of their food consumption.

Food Composition Table
978-0-321-66793-9 / 0-321-66793-X

This comprehensive booklet provides detailed nutritional information on thousands of foods and is correlated with MyDietAnalysis.

Acknowledgments

From Janet Hopson

Preparing a new edition of a college program such as *Get Fit, Stay Well!*—including the book and all of its accompanying study and instructional materials—is an enormous undertaking. The authors' efforts are just part of a complex, well-integrated team effort. We would like to thank the following members of the Pearson book team: Kari Hopperstead, who so ably, tirelessly, and cheerfully coordinated and managed the second edition text and ancillary revision effort; Barbara Yien, Frank Ruggirello, Sandra Lindelof, and Deirdre Espinoza, who all championed this book in its early stages; Claire Alexander, our dedicated and very able development editor; our superb marketing manager Neena Bali; Dorothy Cox and Tracy Duff, our production coordinators; art lead Mimi Bickel and all her colleagues at Precision Graphics; the talented composition and production team at PreMediaGlobal; photo researcher Laura Murray; Yvo Riezebos and Riezebos Holzbaur Design Group, who are responsible for this book's dynamic design; permissions editor Jennifer Bevington; Sade McDougal, who managed the online supplements; ancillary production managers Miriam Adrianowicz and Megan Power; and editorial *wunderkinds* Meghan Zolnay and Briana Verdugo. Finally, and in many ways primarily, I would like to personally thank my coauthors Becky and Tanya for their years of effort and their superb knowledge and experience.

From Rebecca Donatelle

After working on several college textbooks over the years, one thing has become very clear to me: the publishing house you choose to work with is the single most important factor in producing a quality textbook that is going to be successful in the marketplace. Pearson has assembled a truly remarkable group of top-notch acquisition, editorial, production, marketing, sales, and ancillary staff to help nurture a text through its development and growth. I am fortunate to have had the opportunity to work with individuals who worry the details and possess an incredible degree of creativity and professionalism. You are truly THE BEST . . . thank you so much to each and every one of you. A special thank you to Kari Hopperstead, who, in usual fashion, exemplified all that any publisher and author would want in an outstanding project editor. Additionally, I would like to thank my co-authors, Jan and Tanya. From conceptualization to final product, this text would not have happened without your efforts.

From Tanya Littrell

I would like to first and foremost thank my family for all of their support through the long hours of creating and revising this textbook. Thank you to my co-authors, Jan and Becky, whose expertise and experience have really guided this textbook. Working with the staff at Pearson has been a great experience. Thank you to Sandra Lindelof for bringing me into this project, Barbara Yien for her unending patience on the first edition, and Kari Hopperstead for keeping me on track with the many second edition updates. I would

Acknowledgments *(continued)*

also like to thank fellow faculty members at Portland Community College who have been supportive throughout this project; in particular, Janeen Hull, a faculty peer and friend. Ms. Hull was the knowledgeable and creative mind behind the new fitness programs for this edition. My graduate work and teaching at Oregon State University really set the stage for my work on this project, and so I would like to thank Anthony Wilcox, department chair of Nutrition and Exercise Sciences, for having faith in me as an instructor and giving me teaching and supervisory experience that lead to this opportunity.

From The Publisher

For their work on the ancillary materials, we thank Denise Wright and Rebecca Hendricks of Southern Editorial and David Payne. Many thanks go to Janeen Hull of Portland Community College and Ven. Dhammadinna of Bodhiheart Sangha for their contributions to the new Activate, Motivate, & Advance programs. Special thanks go to the participants in our second edition photo shoots: photographer Elena Dorfman; C. J. Jones, Fitness Center Coordinator at De Anza College in Cupertino, California; and models Crystaldawn Bell, Manuela Cortez, Maureen Healy, Sandra Jasso, Jodece Mason, Roy Nutt, Jaehyun Park, Philip Saneski, and Janie Zapata-Wilson. In addition, we thank the participants in our second edition exercise video shoot: Dr. Stephen Ball of the University of Missouri; Dan Desloge and Tim Donsbach from Bad Dog Pictures; and models Celsi Cowan, Dakota Evans, Marshida Harris, Marcus Johnson, Erick King, and Jordan Kroell. Dr. Tom LaFontaine deserves special recognition for facilitating our filming at Optimus: The Center for Health in Columbia, Missouri (www.optimushealth.com). The mission of Optimus is to provide research-based, lifestyle interventions designed to reduce the risks for chronic diseases. Optimus strives to provide a positive, safe, and comfortable atmosphere and environment to assist clients in achieving their personal health, fitness, and wellness goals.

Reviewers

Many thanks to the the hundreds of instructors and students who reviewed and class-tested the first edition of this text, and to the following reviewers who contributed feedback for this revision:

George J. Abboud, Salem State College

Kym Y. Atwood, University of West Florida

Stephen D. Ball, University of Missouri

Diana Carey, Rockland Community College

Mandi Dupain, Millersville University

Robert Femat, El Paso Community College

Jennifer L. Gordon, Manchester Community College

Megan Granquist, University of La Verne

Carol Kennedy-Armbruster, Indiana University

Angela Baldwin Lanier, Berry College

Michelle Lesperance, Greensboro College

David Mann, Darton College

Mike Manning, Indiana Wesleyan University

Holly Molilla, Dutchess Community College

Laurie Moris, William Paterson University

Catherine R. Nolan, Moraine Valley Community College

William J. Papin, Western Carolina University

Rod Porter, San Diego Miramar College

Edgar Reed, Hardin-Simmons University

Jenifer Hudman Roberts, Northwest Vista College

Amanda Salyer Funk, Ball State University

Jay Douglas Seelbach, Anderson University

Robin Siara, Rio Hondo College

Jennifer Spry-Knutson, Des Moines Area Community College

Susan M. Tendy, United States Military Academy

Virginia L. Trummer, University of Texas at San Antonio

Michael Webster, University of Southern Mississippi

Mary Winfrey-Kovell, Ball State University

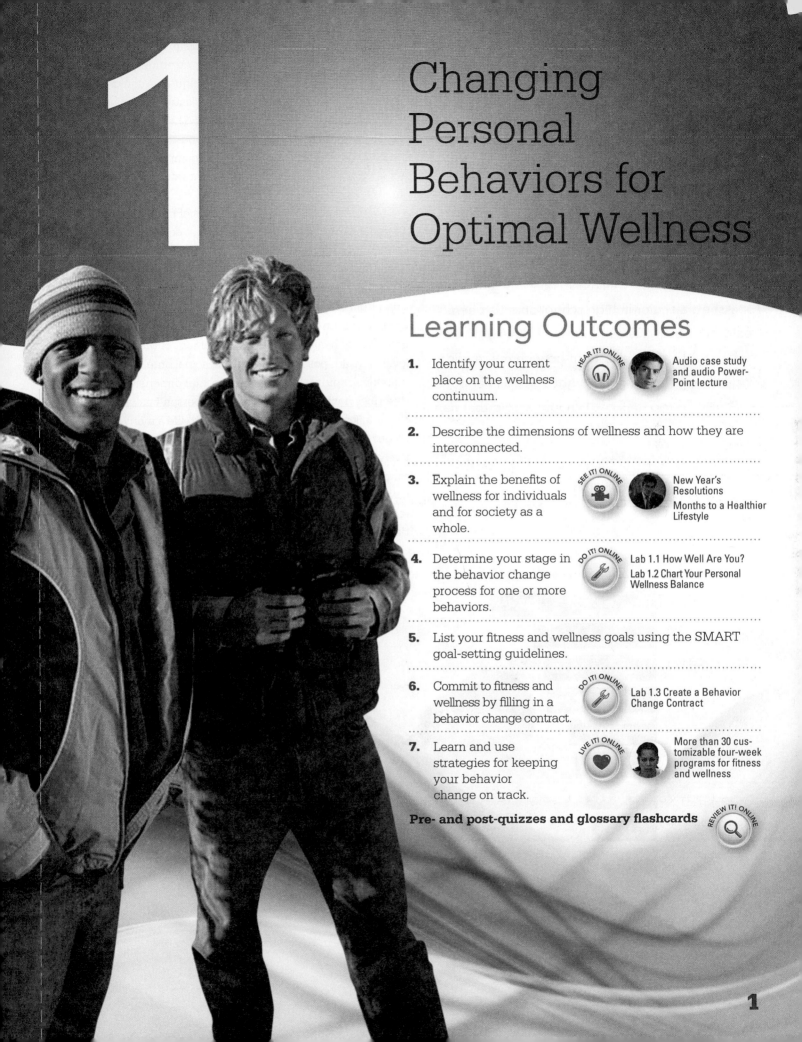

1

Changing Personal Behaviors for Optimal Wellness

Learning Outcomes

1. Identify your current place on the wellness continuum.

   HEAR IT! ONLINE — Audio case study and audio PowerPoint lecture

2. Describe the dimensions of wellness and how they are interconnected.

3. Explain the benefits of wellness for individuals and for society as a whole.

   SEE IT! ONLINE — New Year's Resolutions / Months to a Healthier Lifestyle

4. Determine your stage in the behavior change process for one or more behaviors.

   DO IT! ONLINE — Lab 1.1 How Well Are You? / Lab 1.2 Chart Your Personal Wellness Balance

5. List your fitness and wellness goals using the SMART goal-setting guidelines.

6. Commit to fitness and wellness by filling in a behavior change contract.

   DO IT! ONLINE — Lab 1.3 Create a Behavior Change Contract

7. Learn and use strategies for keeping your behavior change on track.

   LIVE IT! ONLINE — More than 30 customizable four-week programs for fitness and wellness

Pre- and post-quizzes and glossary flashcards

REVIEW IT! ONLINE

1

casestudy

CARLOS

"Hi, I'm Carlos. I just started my freshman year in college. It's my first time living away from home, and I'm getting used to lots of new things. I know my family had to sacrifice for me to be here, so I feel pressure to do well. I also miss my girlfriend, Liz—she's a senior in high school and it's been really hard being away from her. I like my classes so far, but I am never caught up with my reading, and I haven't had a good night's sleep in about a month. To top it all off, I caught a cold that has been going around, and I feel miserable! What can I do to better manage my life?"

HEAR IT! ONLINE

Can you relate to any of Carlos's problems? If so, you are not alone. Many college students report that stress, depression, inadequate sleep, frequent colds, and relationship problems negatively affect their academic performance (Figure 1.1).[1] When asked to rate their overall **wellness,** at least one-third of college students described it as only "good" compared to "very good" or "excellent." About 10 percent rated it as just "fair" or "poor."

Wellness is an optimal soundness of body and mind. To understand wellness, it helps to first consider the concept of "health." While historically the term *health* meant merely the absence of disease, experts today view it as an inclusive term that encompasses everything from environmental health to the health of populations. The term *wellness* conveys a more personalized definition of health. It is the achievement of the highest level of health possible in physical, social, intellectual, emotional, spiritual, and environmental dimensions. It describes a vibrant state in which a person enjoys life to the fullest, adapts relatively easily to life's many challenges, feels that life is meaningful, and functions effectively in society. In this book, we will sometimes use the terms *health* and *wellness* interchangeably, but *wellness* always refers to a more individualized, dynamic concept, requiring significant personal effort, but with the potential to bring great rewards.

Central to wellness is **physical fitness**, or simply *fitness*, the ability to perform moderate to vigorous levels of physical activity without undue fatigue. Fitness is just one dimension of wellness, but we give it special attention in this book because it influences so many of the other dimensions and because the tools for improving fitness are readily available while you are a college student—a period in your life when you can establish personal habits that will benefit you for a lifetime.

Impediment	Percentage
Stress	27.4%
Sleep difficulties	20.0%
Cold/flu/sore throat	18.3%
Anxiety	18.0%
Work	13.7%
Internet use/computer games	12.3%
Depression	11.7%
Concern for friend/family member	11.1%
Relationship difficulties	11.0%
Extracurricular activities	9.1%

Percentage of students reporting impediment

FIGURE **1.1** The top 10 wellness impacts on college performance.

Data from: American College Health Association, *American College Health Association—National College Health Assessment II: Reference Group Executive Summary Spring 2010* (Linthicum, Maryland: American College Health Association, 2010).

| Irreversible damage | Chronic illness | Signs of illness | Average wellness | Increased wellness | Optimum wellness |

FIGURE **1.2** The double-headed arrow depicts the continuum of wellness states.

Where Am I on the Wellness Continuum?

Improving your wellness—moving toward that vibrant multidimensional state—is an ambitious but achievable goal. The wellness patterns you establish during this course can change how you live each day and can positively affect your quality of life for years to come. However, no single college course can address every health concern or guarantee a lifetime of wellness. Your age, personal history, genetic susceptibility to medical conditions, and your physical environment all affect your wellness. So does access to high-quality medical care, nutritious food, good exercise facilities, and social support networks.

The first step in achieving optimal wellness is assessing how close you are at present to that long-term goal. We can picture wellness as a continuum of greater or lesser total soundness of body and mind (Figure 1.2). Understanding your current place on the **wellness continuum** is important for changing wellness behaviors.

What Are the Dimensions of Wellness?

We can think of wellness as consisting of six primary dimensions (physical, social, intellectual, emotional, spiritual, and environmental) (Figure 1.3). Wellness is a process, and at times you may experience faster growth in one dimension than in others. The dimensions are interconnected, however, so positive effort in one area can help you make progress in others and move you toward greater overall health and well-being.

Physical Wellness

Physical wellness encompasses all aspects of a sound body, including body size, shape, and

FIGURE **1.3** Wellness is an optimal level of health in six interconnected dimensions of human experience.

composition; sensory sharpness and responsiveness; body functioning; physical strength, flexibility, and endurance; resistance to diseases and disorders; and recuperative abilities. The physical

wellness Achieving the highest level of health possible in each of several dimensions

physical fitness The ability to perform moderate to vigorous levels of physical activity without undue fatigue

wellness continuum A spectrum of wellness states from pre-mature death to optimum wellness physical wellness A state of physical health and well-being that includes body size and shape, body functioning, measures of strength and endurance, and resistance to disease

social wellness A person's degree of social connectedness and skills, leading to satisfying interpersonal relationships

intellectual wellness The ability to think clearly, reason objectively, analyze, and use brain power to solve problems and meet life's challenges

emotional wellness The ability to control emotions and express them appropriately at the right times; includes self-esteem, self-confidence, self-efficacy, and other emotional qualities

spiritual wellness A feeling of unity or oneness with people and nature and a sense of life's purpose, meaning, or value; for some, a belief in a supreme being or religion

state we call fitness includes measures of physical wellness and allows a person to exert physical effort without undue stress, strain, or injury. Many of your day-to-day choices and habits can support or undermine your physical wellness, including your diet; amount and types of exercise; sleep patterns; level of stress; use of tobacco, drugs, or alcohol; participation in unsafe sex; observance of traffic laws and wearing helmets and seat belts; daily hygiene (e.g., flossing and brushing teeth); and access to quality medical attention (e.g., regular checkups, vaccinations, and treatment).

Social Wellness

Social wellness is the ability to have satisfying interpersonal relationships and maintain connections in a diverse range of social networks. This means you can successfully interact with others, adapt to a variety of social situations, and act appropriately in various settings. Whether you are shy and introverted or outgoing and extroverted, social wellness includes the ability to communicate clearly and effectively; the capacity to establish intimacy through trust and acceptance; a willingness to ask for and give support; the ability to maintain friendships over time; and skills for interacting within groups, such as on the job or in the community.

Intellectual Wellness

Intellectual wellness is the ability to use your brain power effectively to solve problems and meet life's challenges. It allows you to think clearly, quickly, creatively, and critically; use good reasoning and make careful decisions; continually learn from your successes and mistakes; organize and streamline your tasks; and maintain a sense of humor.

Emotional Wellness

Emotional wellness means being able to control your emotions and express them appropriately at the right times. Social and emotional concerns,—such as stress, anxiety, depression, and relationship problems—are increasingly common on college campuses and can impede academic success. Improving emotional wellness requires developing good self-esteem; gaining self-confidence; being able to cope with sadness, anger, resentment, and negativity; and developing an appropriate balance of emotional dependence and independence.

Spiritual Wellness

For some people, **spiritual wellness** may involve a belief in a supreme being or a way of life prescribed by a particular religion. For others, spiritual wellness is a feeling of unity or oneness with others and with nature, and a sense of meaning or value in life. Developing greater spiritual wellness may deepen one's understanding of life's purpose; allow a person to feel a part of a greater

casestudy

CARLOS

"I know that my life is pretty good. I'm in college, studying what interests me, and I'm excited about the future. I just constantly feel behind. I fall asleep in class sometimes, eat a lot of junk food, and I'm not exercising—who has time? Then I got this cold, partly because I have been stressed out and not sleeping much. I've made some friends in my dorm, and it helps to know that a lot of them are going through the same thing. Talking to Liz every night on the phone helps, too."

THINK! In which dimensions of wellness could Carlos be stronger? Where would you place him on the wellness continuum? How do you compare to Carlos?

ACT! Identify your strongest wellness dimensions as well as the ones you could improve. Create a wellness balance chart and plan the balance you would like to achieve **(Lab 1.2)**.

DO IT! ONLINE   HEAR IT! ONLINE

• •

spectrum of existence; and promote feelings of love, joy, peace, contentment, and wonder over life's experiences.

Environmental Wellness

Our home, work, community, and school environments can be relaxing, safe havens or toxic, threatening, and stressful places to be. **Environmental wellness** entails understanding how the environment can positively or negatively affect you; the role you play in preserving, protecting, and improving the world around you; and what you can do to conserve dwindling resources for future generations.

Related Dimensions of Wellness

Occupational and financial wellness overlap with other wellness areas, and are sometimes considered their own dimensions. Your wellness in these areas can dramatically affect your overall wellness and add to your life's balance (or lack thereof). If you ask family members and friends about their current problems, many will identify their jobs or finances as the top stressors in their lives.

Occupational Wellness Occupational wellness is the level of happiness and fulfilment you experience in

your work. An important component of occupational wellness is finding a non-toxic, hazard-free work environment that provides contact with managers and co-workers who value your skills and opinions. Contrary to what people often think, job satisfaction is not closely tied to high wages.[2] You can reach optimal occupational wellness when your personal goals align closely with those of your employer, and when you feel that you are making significant contributions to both sets of goals.

environmental wellness An appreciation of how the external environment can affect oneself, and an understanding of the role one plays in preserving, protecting, and improving it

occupational wellness A level of happiness and fulfilment in work, including harmony with personal goals, appreciation from bosses and co-workers, and a safe workplace

financial wellness The ability to balance and manage financial needs and wants with income, debts, savings, and investments

Financial Wellness Financial wellness is the ability to successfully balance and manage your financial needs and wants with your income, debts, savings, and investments. If you cannot pay your bills, it can be hard to think of much else and this dimension can overshadow and unbalance the others. People who are managing their finances but just breaking even will still need to make wise consumer choices, carefully control debt, and continually prioritize expenses (see the box How Can I Handle My Finances Better?).

Balancing Your Wellness Dimensions

You may have healthy relationships, but no fondness for exercise. Perhaps your spiritual life is rich, but you have trouble juggling academic demands. Virtually everyone is stronger in some dimensions of wellness than others. Striving for improvement in all six wellness dimensions is a lifelong process. One good approach is to concentrate on those dimensions that present the most pressing need, while working on the others in a steady but relaxed and motivated way. Over time, a balance of work on all the dimensions—one or two now, others later—will eventually promote overall wellness. Your brain and body, your thoughts and emotions, your actions and reactions, your relationship to yourself and others—all are interconnected and integrated. Likewise, the dimensions of wellness are interrelated. For example, increasing your exercise and general activity will also help you manage stress, mood, body composition, and so on.

How Can I Handle My Finances Better?

Figuring out how to manage one's money can be tough for college students—especially for traditional-age students who are living apart from their families for the first time and perhaps also learning to use credit cards. Here are some tips that can help you handle credit and finances:

Buy only the items you truly need—and pay cash when you can.

Resist the urge to buy things on impulse. Do the research, find out a reasonable price for your major purchases, and wait a day or so before buying to make sure you really need the thing.

Watch for signs you are too deep in debt.

If you are borrowing money to pay off other loans, paying bills late on purpose, or putting off health care or other important activities because you can't cover the costs, there is a good chance you are in over your head. If you think this describes you, aim to pay off your credit cards or other high-interest loans as soon as you can, even cutting up your credit card, if needed, to save yourself from adding to the problem.

Pay bills on time.

Your actions now affect your ability to get loans later. If you want to have a good financial reputation in the future, start now. Pay your credit card, loans, rent, and other commitments on time to establish your reputation as a reliable consumer.

Keep a minimum of credit cards, and use them wisely.

Carrying more than two credit cards leaves you susceptible to impulse buying and makes you look like a bad risk to creditors. Don't fall prey to tempting credit card offers; just get the one or two cards you need and ignore the rest. Before you make your purchase, think! Will you be able to pay the bill off in full when it comes? If not, interest will start to build up and you may end up paying more in interest charges than what the item originally cost.

Watch your expenses.

Whether you use an online budgeting tool or handwritten notes, keep track of what you spend and make sure it's in line with your long-term goals.

Save for your future.

Before you pay your bills each month, put away money for your future, even if it is only 25 or 50 dollars.

Avoid fees whenever you can.

To avoid costly fees, use your own financial institution's ATMs and watch your checking account balance so you don't "bounce" checks or overdraw your account with your debit card, incurring more fees.

Take responsibility for your finances.

Review your bills and bank statements as soon as possible after they are issued each month. Be sure to check for errors, unauthorized charges, or indications of identity theft. Get errors or problems corrected immediately. Remember—it's your financial reputation on the line!

Start now!

Start small, and stretch yourself a bit to pay off your credit cards and put away money for the future. Even small changes make a big difference!

Lab 1.1 and **Lab 1.2** at the end of the chapter will help you assess your wellness in each of the primary dimensions and analyze the areas that need improvement.

Why Does Wellness Matter?

Wellness has many benefits for individuals, as well as for society as a whole.

Good Wellness Habits Can Help You Live a Longer, Healthier Life

Months to a Healthier Lifestyle.

In the United States, federal health experts consider the average life expectancy at birth for males to be 76 years, and for females to be 81 years.[3] The precise numbers depend on the methods used for calculating, and some experts project a slight decline in those numbers in coming years.[4] A more important issue is average healthy life expectancy—the years a person can expect to live without disability or major illness: about 68 for males and 72 for females (Figure 1.4).[5] Maintaining good wellness habits can help extend your overall life expectancy, as well as your healthy life expectancy.

Consider the leading causes of death among Americans ages 20–24 (Figure 1.5).[6] Note that accidents kill more young adults than almost all the other causes combined. By making better wellness choices—such as wearing seat belts and bike helmets, and avoiding dangerous behaviors such as driving under the influence of drugs or alcohol—you can reduce your risk of premature death in an accident.

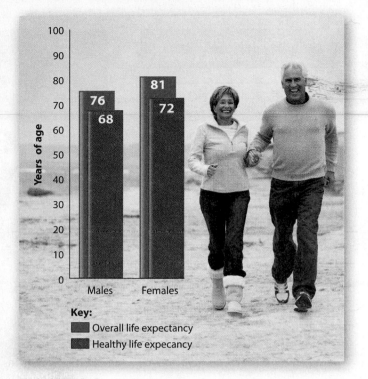

FIGURE 1.4 Healthy life expectancy is a subset of overall life expectancy. Lengthening the span of your healthy years is an important wellness goal.

Data from: World Health Organization, *World Health Statistics 2010*. www.who.int/whosis/whostat/2010/en/index.html.

The leading causes of death for Americans overall are heart disease and cancer (Figure 1.6).[7] Adults contribute greatly to their own risk for these diseases through poor diets, inactivity, and smoking.[8] *Modifiable* risk factors for heart disease and cancer—that is, *risk factors* that are within your control—include high blood pressure, tobacco use, alcohol use, high cholesterol, obesity, low fruit and vegetable intake, and physical inactivity.

Leading causes of death among Americans ages 20–24

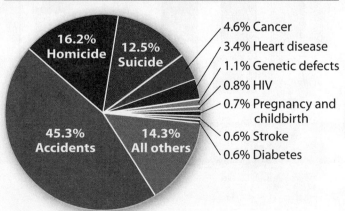

FIGURE 1.5 The leading causes of death among Americans ages 20–24.

Data from: *National Vital Statistics Reports* 58, no. 14 (March 31, 2010).

Leading causes of death among Americans overall

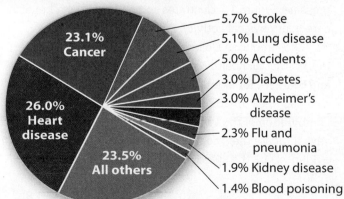

FIGURE 1.6 The leading causes of death among Americans overall.

Data from: *National Vital Statistics Reports* 58, no. 14 (March 31, 2010).

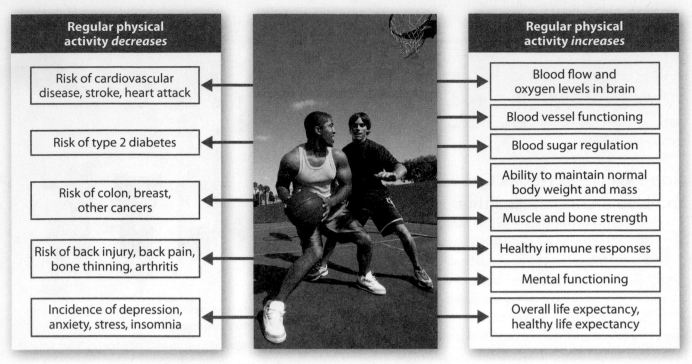

Regular physical activity *decreases*		Regular physical activity *increases*

Regular physical activity *decreases*

- Risk of cardiovascular disease, stroke, heart attack
- Risk of type 2 diabetes
- Risk of colon, breast, other cancers
- Risk of back injury, back pain, bone thinning, arthritis
- Incidence of depression, anxiety, stress, insomnia

Regular physical activity *increases*

- Blood flow and oxygen levels in brain
- Blood vessel functioning
- Blood sugar regulation
- Ability to maintain normal body weight and mass
- Muscle and bone strength
- Healthy immune responses
- Mental functioning
- Overall life expectancy, healthy life expectancy

FIGURE **1.7** Regular physical activity results in many health benefits.

Researchers have made a compelling case for the role of physical activity in decreasing the risk of chronic disease. Medical researchers have shown in hundreds of studies that the vast majority of all illnesses of middle age and later years (including heart disease, cancer, and type 2 diabetes) are related to, and exacerbated by, a lack of physical activity.[9] Living a **sedentary** life also increases the danger of *hypokinetic diseases*—conditions that can be triggered or worsened by too little movement or activity, such as obesity, back pain, arthritis, and high blood pressure. Figure 1.7 illustrates some of the health benefits of regular physical activity.

The American College of Sports Medicine recommends that all healthy adults between the ages of 18 and 65 strive for at least 150 minutes of moderate exercise per week (or 75 minutes of vigorous exercise or a combination of the two).[10] However, recent national surveys indicate that most Americans are too inactive, as evidenced by the steady climb in percentages of overweight and obese adults (Figure 1.8).[11] Indeed, we are one of the most sedentary and overweight nations on earth.[12]

sedentary Physically inactive; exerting physical effort only for required daily tasks and not for leisure-time exercise

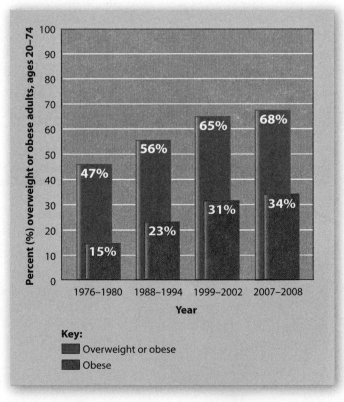

FIGURE **1.8** Overweight and obese adults are now the clear majority, with percentages rising steadily in the past 30 years.

Data from: K. Flegal and others, "Prevalence and Trends in Obesity Among US Adults, 1999–2008." *JAMA* 3003, no. 3 (2010): 235–41.

Good Wellness Habits Benefit Society as a Whole

The higher a population's levels of wellness, the happier and more productive are its people and the less money it spends on health care. Accordingly, achieving better wellness and combating today's chronic diseases are important national priorities.

National public health priorities cited by the Office of the Surgeon General of the United States are summarized in a set of objectives titled *Healthy People 2020*, which has four broad goals: 1) attain high-quality, longer lives free of preventable disease, disability, injury, and premature death; 2) achieve health equity, eliminate disparities, and improve the health of all groups; 3) create social and physical environments that promote good health for all; and 4) promote quality of life, healthy development, and healthy behaviors across all life stages.[13] In order to address some of these major public health priorities, the Surgeon General advises Americans to eat healthier, be more physically active, not smoke, limit alcohol, and avoid drugs—all of which are wellness behaviors.[14]

The high cost of health care and health insurance is a major concern for Americans. In 2009, Americans spent $2.5 trillion on health care, or 17.6 percent of the gross domestic product (GDP).[15] Employer health insurance premiums increased by 131 percent between 1999 and 2009 at four times the rate of inflation.[16] Nearly 49 million Americans lack health insurance, largely due to the high cost of coverage.[17] This makes them less likely to seek preventive care and adopt wellness behaviors early enough to prevent illness down the line. Such concerns led to sweeping new health legislation in 2010 to increase the percentage of Americans with health coverage.[18]

How Can I Change My Behavior to Increase My Wellness?

New Year's Resolutions

If you are like most people, you have made a New Year's resolution on January 1, have worked hard to adopt some new behavior until about the 10th, have started slipping back to your old habits by the 15th, and have forgotten about the whole thing by the 31st. Your resolution may well have been a new wellness behavior—lots of resolutions are. Perhaps it was an easy one, such as "eat more fruit," and you succeeded. More likely, it was a harder one—"start lifting weights three times a week," or "lose 20 pounds," or "give up junk food"—and despite your good intentions, it just didn't stick.

People often see change as a singular event instead of a process that requires preparation, has several stages, and takes time to succeed. Classic research shows that we must go through a series of mental and emotional stages over a period of months to adequately prepare ourselves for **behavior change**. The rest of this chapter takes you through a series of practical steps inspired by a blueprint for change called the *transtheoretical model of behavior change* developed by psychologists James Prochaska and Carlo DiClemente.[19]

> **behavior change** An organized, deliberate effort to alter or replace an existing habit or pattern of activity
>
> **stages of behavior change** From the transtheoretical model, a set of states most people pass through in their awareness of, determination to alter, and efforts to replace existing habits or actions

Step One: Understand the Stages of Behavior Change

The transtheoretical model of behavior change delineates six **stages of behavior change**: precontemplation, contemplation, preparation, action, maintenance, and termination. The model shows that changing behaviors usually involves a gradual process of awareness, preparation, and then action. Understanding this process can help you proceed more deliberately to identify and successfully change a problem behavior. Keep in mind that the steps of this model are general and people often backtrack as they work on them.

Precontemplation People in the precontemplation stage have no current intention of changing. They may have tried to change an old habit and given up, or they may be in denial and unaware of the problem.

Contemplation In this stage, people recognize that they have a problem and begin to contemplate the need to change within six months or so. People can languish in this stage for months or years, however, realizing that they have a negative wellness pattern, yet lacking the time, energy, or commitment to make the change.

Preparation Most people at this stage are within a month or so of taking action. They have thought about what they might do and may even have come up with a plan. Rather than thinking about why they can't begin, they have started to focus on what they can do.

Action In this stage, people begin to execute their action plans. Unfortunately, many people try to take shortcuts; they start behavior change here rather than going through the earlier stages. However, without making a plan, publicly stating the desire to change, enlisting other people's help, and setting realistic goals, they are likely to fail.

Maintenance In the maintenance stage, people work to prevent a relapse into old habits through a conscious application of wellness tools and techniques. Maintenance requires vigilance, attention to detail, and long-term commitment. You are in the maintenance stage after you have incorporated the new action and have continued it for six months or longer without relapse into old habits.

Relapse While not an original stage of behavior change, relapse is something that happens periodically for most people trying to change behaviors. Common causes of relapse include overconfidence, daily temptations, stress or emotional distractions, and putting yourself down.

Termination At the termination stage, the new behavior is ingrained; you are maintaining it and are no longer at risk for relapse. The new behavior has become a part of the way you live and thus the temptation to return to former behaviors is greatly reduced.

casestudy

CARLOS

"In an ideal world I'd reduce my stress by sleeping eight hours a night, eating healthier food, and exercising more. Maybe then I would ace my exams and still have time for a social life. But I know I can't just snap my fingers and make all of that happen. Right now, I *really* have to get more sleep—it doesn't do me any good to stay up all night studying and then fall asleep in class. Some of my friends take 'power naps' in the afternoon. I might try that! I'm also thinking of signing up for a gym class next quarter. That way I can be sure to work some exercise into my schedule. Beyond that—well, I think I should probably take things one at a time."

THINK! What are Carlos's main wellness goals? What is his current stage of behavior change for each goal?

ACT! Name a wellness behavior that you would like to change and write down your stage of behavior change for that item. Tape this up where you can see it each morning.

HEAR IT! ONLINE

Step Two: Increase Your Awareness

LIVE IT! ONLINE

Worksheet 1
Health
Behavior Self
Assessment

Wellness behaviors that are important to college students can be simple to think about but are often challenging to achieve. An important starting point is to become aware of what is required to achieve wellness in each of the following areas.

Staying Physically Fit Nowhere does the phrase "Use it or lose it" apply more fully than to your physical fitness. Much of the decline people expect with advancing age is, in fact, a reflection of inactivity and its toll on the body. Staying active every day is probably the single most important wellness behavior you can adopt.

Eating Healthy Foods The American diet tends to be light on nutrition and heavy on calories. Most Americans consume more calories than they burn off each day. We also tend to eat too much protein, salt, sugar, animal fat, and solidified vegetable oils (trans fats). We consume too little fiber and too few helpings of fruits and vegetables.[20] Good nutrition has many wellness benefits, including increased energy, greater stamina, better weight management, stronger disease resistance, and reduced risk of chronic illness.

Managing Your Weight As we saw in Figure 1.8, 68 percent of American adults have a body weight and mass (fat-to-lean ratio) above recommended ranges. Overweight and obesity are correlated with arthritis, bone and joint problems, back pain, decreased physical performance, more chronic illness, and a shorter life expectancy. Modifying your activity level, exercise habits, eating habits, and stress levels can all contribute to maintaining a healthy weight.

Managing Your Stress Most students find college stressful. Whether you are fresh out of high school or returning to school later in life (see the box Nontraditional Students and Wellness), the lifestyle changes and the competing demands of academics, work, and social life associated with college can take an emotional and physical toll. Research shows that high levels of unrelieved stress can disrupt thinking and memory, disturb sleep, increase depression, impair our immunity to infections, and even contribute to weight gain and abdominal fat.[21] Over many years, unrelieved stress may also contribute to higher blood pressure, premature aging, and increased risk for chronic illnesses.

DIVERSITY

Nontraditional Students and Wellness

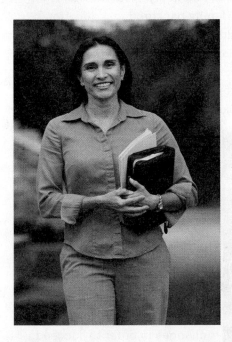

Since the 1980s, there has been a steady decline in the percentages of *traditional students* at colleges and universities—that is, 18- to 24-year-olds who go right on to college after high school with financial support from their parents.[1] During the same time period, schools have welcomed more and more *nontraditional students*—those who are 25 or older and who have spent time working, doing military service, or engaging in other activities before returning to post–high school education, full- or part-time. Nontraditional students are usually employed, self-supporting, and often married with children. They represent at least 40 percent of today's college students. And they broaden our discussion of student wellness.

The wellness needs of nontraditional students tend to differ from those of younger students for several reasons. 1) Many of them juggle work, school, and family, and thus they often derive special benefit from learning stress management skills.[2] 2) They tend to have more life experience but also to cope with more demands on their time; this can narrow their focus to educational and career goals and exclude much time for exercise. As a result, many need encouragement and creative ideas for increasing activity. 3) Nontraditional students make meals for themselves and for children more often than do traditional students and thus have broader nutritional considerations. Many also want to model good eating habits for their children, thus they tend to be receptive to nutritional improvements. 4) Many nontraditional students see themselves as unprepared for vigorous college work and are more likely to be stressed and insecure about their academic performances.[3] At the same time, most nontraditional students report having strong social support from family and friends, and thus appear to be richer in social wellness than younger students.

Sources:
1. L. G. Lunsford, "Post Secondary Education for Non-Traditional Students—The New Majority," North Carolina State University (2003).
2. J. E. Myers and A. K. Mobley, "Wellness of Undergraduates: Comparisons of Traditional and Non-traditional Students," *Journal of College Counseling* 7, no. 1 (2004): 40–49.
3. S. San Miguel Barriman and others, "Non-Traditional Student's Service Needs and Social Support Resources. A Pilot Study," *Journal of College Counseling* 7, no. 1 (2004): 13–17.

Avoiding Drugs, Smoking, and Alcohol Abuse Using drugs, smoking, and abusing alcohol are all ways of manipulating the brain chemically. Unfortunately, the use and abuse of these substances carry high risks for illness and injury and can undermine multiple dimensions of wellness.

Practicing Accident, Injury, and Disease Prevention Prevention has several practical meanings for wellness behavior. It can mean preventing injuries and the accidents that account for most deaths among young adults. It can mean self-care such as daily dental hygiene and regular prostate or breast self-exams. And it can mean preventing disease through medical checkups and vaccinations.

Step Three: Contemplate Change

Habits are usually deeply ingrained, and even minor habits can be surprisingly hard to change. As we have discussed, research has confirmed that people are more successful when they prepare for change emotionally and mentally rather than starting right in on the change itself. Contemplating change can include examining your current patterns, identifying your beliefs and attitudes, solidifying your motivation, and choosing a realistic target for your efforts to change.

Examine Current Habits and Patterns What current behavior should you work on changing? The assessment in **Lab 1.1** will help you identify habits that lower your wellness. When considering a habit, ask yourself the following:

- How long has it been going on?

- How often does it happen?

- How serious are the consequences of the habit or problem?

- What are some of your reasons for continuing this problematic behavior?

- What kinds of situations trigger the behavior?

- Are other people involved in this habit? If so, in what way?

Habits involve elements of deliberate choice but are also influenced by demographics, personal attitudes and beliefs, and many other factors. Age, sex, race, income, family background, education, and access to health care all increase or decrease the likelihood of developing certain health habits. If your parents smoke, for instance, you are 90 percent more likely to start smoking than someone whose parents don't smoke.[22] If your peers smoke, you are 80 percent more likely to smoke. Identifying factors that may encourage negative behaviors or block positive ones can help you prepare for behavior change. Analyzing the factors that reinforce your current habit pattern can also help you understand why you developed and maintained unwanted habits and where you need to make changes in order to succeed.

Assess Current Beliefs and Attitudes Your attitudes about health and wellness affect your daily choices. When reaching for another cigarette, smokers, for example, sometimes tell themselves, "I'll stop tomorrow" or "They'll have a cure for lung

What Moves You?

Like many students, you may need powerful motivation to start a fitness program and follow it through. Researchers have discovered several interesting facets of student motivation to be active and fit that you can apply to your own wellness plan.

Studies have found that college students who participated in repetitive exercises such as weight lifting, swimming laps, or jogging around the track usually had *external* motivations for their participation. Many, but not all, tended to focus on their appearance, weight, or stress management and on the improvements that exercise could promote.[1] Conversely, college students who participated in recreational sports such as tennis, softball, and rowing usually had *internal* motivations for participating. They tended to focus on enjoyment and challenge.

If you have trouble sticking with exercise programs, you might find fitness easier if you were to choose a sport—even a mildly aerobic one such as badminton, horseback riding, ping-pong, or bowling—that provides fun and social opportunities as well as physical activity. As long as you spend enough

hours at an activity each week, you will benefit. Researchers have also confirmed that the social aspect of sports and activities—a sense of belonging to a team, a gym, or simply a group of friends who like to take bike rides or play Frisbee in the park—helps people enjoy fitness activities and stick with them.

THINK! What are your main motivations for fitness and physical activity? Are they primarily external or internal? Do you participate in sports? Why or why not? Which of your activities are the most fun, and what makes them so?

ACT! If increasing your physical fitness is a goal, make a list of new activities that you could add for: a) more social contact; b) more fun and enjoyment, and c) more time willingly spent participating.

Sources:
1. M. Kilpatrick, E. Hebert, and J. Bartholomew, "College Students' Motivation for Physical Activity: Differentiating Men's and Women's Motives for Sport Participation and Exercise," *Journal of American College Health* 54, no. 2 (2005): 87–94.
2. C. J. Hale, J. W. Hannum, and D. L. Espelage, "Social Support and Physical Health: The Importance of Belonging," *Journal of American College Health* 53, no. 6 (2005): 276–84.

● ●

cancer by the time I get it." These beliefs allow them to continue smoking. One model suggests that several factors must be in place before you successfully change a habit that diminishes wellness.[23] Among these factors are the following:

• You must believe that your current pattern could lead you to a serious problem. The more severe the consequences, the more likely you are to change the behavior. For example, smoking can cause cancer and emphysema and promote heart disease. The fear of developing those diseases can help a person stop smoking.

• You must believe that you personally are quite susceptible to developing the health problem. For example, losing a parent to lung cancer could make a person work harder to stop smoking.

What beliefs underlie your current pattern of wellness habits, both positive and negative?

Assess Your Motivation What is your **motivation**, or inducement, to change a wellness behavior? For some, a rewarding result, such as looking better, can motivate change. For others, a feeling of accomplishment or just feeling better every day may do it. See the box What Moves You? to explore recent research on exercise motivation in students.

LIVE IT! ONLINE

Worksheet 3
Health Locus
of Control

Motivations can be external (come from someone or something else) or internal (come from inside yourself), but in either case are part of your sense of self. The degree to which you believe in your own abilities is your **self-efficacy**. Your conviction that you can control events and factors in your life is your **locus of control**. An *internal* locus of control usually gives you a strong belief in your

> **motivation** One's inducement to do something such as change a current behavior
>
> **self-efficacy** The degree to which one believes in his or her ability to achieve something

ability to effect change. An *external* locus of control usually leads you to see other people and things as controlling what you do and whether you can change.

A person with a strong sense of self-efficacy and a largely internal locus of control has a better chance of following through with a decision to change wellness behavior. For example, suppose you wish to bring your weight down to a healthy range. If your parents are both overweight, you may think, "My weight is controlled by my genes," and thus be resigned to being overweight. By gathering information about weight management, however; by identifying behaviors that are within your power to change (such as food choices, eating habits, and exercise); and by acknowledging their importance, you can shift to a more internalized locus of control and increase your chances of successful weight management. Likewise, you can help boost your own self-efficacy through this shift to more internalized control.

. . . .

THINK! Where is your locus of control? Are you motivated by external factors (e.g., your genes) or internal factors (e.g., your own power)?

ACT! Write down three things you can control about the behavior you want to change. For example, if you want to lose weight, one thing you can control is rerouting your walk to class so that you don't pass tempting vending machines.

. . . .

Choose a Target Behavior The last preparatory step is to choose one well-defined habit, or **target behavior**, as your initial focus for change. It is a much better strategy to start small and build on success than to try for too much and end up failing. To choose potential target behaviors, ask yourself these questions:

- *What do I want?* What is your ultimate goal? To lose weight? Exercise more? Reduce stress? Have a lasting relationship? Whatever it is, you need a clear picture of your target outcome.

- *Which change is my greatest priority at this time?* People often decide to change several

locus of control Belief that control over life events and changes comes primarily from outside of oneself (external locus of control) or from within (internal locus of control)

target behavior One well-defined habit chosen as a primary focus for change

things at once. Suppose you are gaining unwanted weight. Rather than saying, "I need to eat less and start exercising," identify one specific behavior that contributes significantly to your greatest problem and tackle that first.

- *Why is this important to me?* Think through why you want to change. Are you doing it because of your health? To improve your academic performance? To look better? To win someone else's approval? It's best to target a behavior because it's right for you rather than because you think it will help you win others' approval.

- *Fill in the details.* Rather than using a generality ("I need to eat better"), consider specific behaviors that relate to the general problem. What are your unhealthy eating habits? Do you eat too few fruits and vegetables? Do you have fast food for lunch every day? Identifying the specific behavior you would like to change will help you set clear goals.

Step Four: Prepare for Change

Once you have assessed your current status and chosen a target behavior, you are ready to make specific preparations, including observing role models, setting realistic goals, anticipating barriers, and making a commitment to change.

Observe Role Models Watching others successfully change their behavior can give you ideas and encouragement for your own changes. This process of modeling, or learning from role models, can be very helpful. Suppose you have trouble talking to strangers or new acquaintances and want to improve your communication skills. Try observing friends whose social skills you admire and note how they make conversation. What techniques help make them successful communicators? If you see behaviors that work well, separate their components so you can model your behavior change on a proven approach.

Set Realistic Goals and Objectives Your wellness goals and objectives should be both achievable for you and in line with what you truly want.[24] Achievable, truly desired goals increase motivation, and this, in turn, leads to a better chance of success at behavior change.

To set successful goals, try using the SMART system. SMART goals are *specific, measurable, action-oriented, realistic,* and *time-oriented.* A vague goal would be "Get into better shape by exercising more." A SMART goal would be

- *Specific*—"Start weight training";

- *Measurable*—"Increase the amount of weight I can safely lift";

- *Action-oriented*—"Go to the gym three times per week";

- *Realistic*—"Increase the weight I can lift by 20 percent [not 200 percent]";

- *Time-oriented*—"Try my new weight program for 8 weeks, then reassess."

Anticipate and Overcome Barriers to Change Anticipating **barriers to change**, or possible stumbling blocks, will help you prepare for behavior change. A majority of students, for example, want to lose or gain weight but have failed to do so permanently.[25] Diet failure is based on several barriers to change, including internal drives to eat high-calorie foods and external temptations such as snacks and fast foods on sale in most campus buildings. The following are a few general barriers to wellness change:

- *Overambitious goals* can derail behavior change. Most people cannot lose weight, stop smoking, and begin running three miles a day all at the same time. It tends to be equally unsuccessful to try for dramatic change within an unrealistically short time frame—such as losing 20 pounds in one month. Habits are best changed one at a time, taking small, progressive steps; rewarding successes; and being patient with yourself.

- *Self-defeating beliefs and attitudes* can impede successful change. Believing that you are too young to worry about fitness and wellness can bar you from making a solid commitment to change.

Likewise, thinking you are helpless to change your weight, smoking, or fitness habits could undermine your efforts. Greater self-efficacy and more positive expectations may help.

> **barriers to change** Stumbling blocks faced in the efforts to alter a current behavior
>
> **behavior change contract** A formal document that clarifies the goals and steps needed to change a current habit or habit pattern

- *Failing to accurately assess your current state of wellness* could block progress. You might assume that you are strong and flexible, for example, when you are actually below average for your age. Failing to gather enough data on wellness risks and benefits can also be a barrier that leaves you with weakened motivation and commitment.

- *Lack of support and guidance* can act as a barrier. Supportive friends are a good start. You should also seek guidance from your fitness and wellness instructor; from counselors and other campus resources; from up-to-date, trusted health sources on the Internet (see the box How Can I Find Reliable Wellness Information?); and from health professionals.

Make a Commitment The more strongly you state an intention to change a wellness habit, either verbally or on paper, the more likely it is you will succeed. A formal written document called the **behavior change contract** functions as a promise to yourself

- as a public declaration of intent,

- as an organized plan that lays out start and end dates and daily actions,

- as a listing of barriers or obstacles you may encounter,

- as a place to brainstorm strategies for overcoming those impediments,

- as a collected set of sources of support, and

- as a reminder of the rewards you plan to give yourself for sticking with the program.

Writing a behavior change contract will help you clarify your goals, make a commitment to change, and, if you wish, announce your intentions to supportive friends and family. In **Lab 1.3** you will create

DO IT! ONLINE

a behavior change contract as part of your fitness and wellness plan.

Step Five: Take Action to Change

Now that you've put some thought into it, and made a plan for change, it's time to take action! The following are some strategies to keep your behavior change process on track.

Visualize New Behavior Athletes often use a form of mental practice called *imagined rehearsal* or simply *visualization* to reach their performance goals. Picturing themselves accomplishing an action in their minds ahead of time helps prepare them for real competition. Visualization can help you imagine the way a current negative behavior unfolds, and then allows you to practice in advance what you will say and do to counter it.

Control Your Environment If you are trying to quit drinking, going to a bar could lead you to resume an undesired behavior. Going to dinner and a movie with a sympathetic friend, on the other hand, could help reinforce your abstinence. Think about which people and settings tend to trigger your unwanted behavior, then stay away from them as much as possible and set up supportive situations instead.

Change Your Self-Talk Your *self-talk*—that is, the way you think and talk to yourself—matters. Think about what you say to yourself when something goes badly or when something succeeds. Purposely blocking or stopping negative thoughts and replacing them with positive ones can help you change a habit.

Learn to "Counter" Countering is another term for substituting a desired behavior for an undesirable one. You may want to stop eating junk food, for example, but "cold turkey" just isn't realistic—unless the turkey is on a

countering Substituting a desired behavior for an undesirable one

journaling Keeping a written record of personal experiences, interpretations, and results

sandwich! Instead, compile a list of substitute foods and places to get them and have this ready before your mouth starts watering at the smell of burgers and fries.

Practice "Shaping" *Shaping* is a stepwise process of making a series of small changes, starting slowly and mastering one step before moving on to the next. Suppose you want to start jogging three miles every other day, but right now you get tired and winded after half a mile. Shaping would dictate a process of slow, progressive steps such as walking one hour every other day at a slow, relaxed pace for the first week; walking for an hour every other day but at a faster pace the second week; and speeding up to a slow run the third week. Regardless of the change you plan, remember that current habits did not develop overnight, and they will not change overnight, either.

Reward Yourself Setting up a system of rewards can help you keep new behavior on track. Rewards can be consumable, like cookies or gourmet meals. They can be active, like going to a concert or playing Frisbee. They can be possessional, like getting a new MP3 player or buying a new CD. A reward can be an incentive, like being taken to a special event by a friend. It can be social, like receiving praise or a hug. And it can be intrinsic, meaning a new behavior feels so enjoyable it becomes its own reward. Whatever your motivating rewards may be, build a few (but not too many) into your program.

Use Writing as a Wellness Tool Throughout the labs in this textbook, you will examine your current wellness habits and analyze them through writing. **Journaling**, or writing personal experiences, interpretations, and results in a journal or notebook, is an important skill for behavior change. Journaling can help you monitor your daily efforts, measure how much you have learned, record how you feel about your progress, and note ideas for improving your program.

LIVE IT! ONLINE

Worksheet 2
Weekly Behavior Change
Evaluation

How Can I Find Reliable Wellness Information?

Fitness and wellness are important American preoccupations—and major industries as well. It can be hard to distinguish legitimate information from thinly disguised advertising for products and services. Here are some general tips and specific sources of reliable information.

Look for organizations without a direct interest in your wallet.

Examples are health-related agencies of the state and federal government (e.g., CDC or FDA); major colleges and universities; big-name hospitals and medical centers (e.g., Mayo Clinic or Cooper Institute); and well-known nonprofit organizations (e.g., American College of Sports Medicine or American Medical Association). Cross-check any information you gather from other sources against these kinds of known and reliable sources to see whether facts and figures are consistent.

If a newspaper or magazine quotes a research report, look up the research itself.

Consider details of the study, noting whether the researcher works for a large, recognizable university, government agency, or research institute; whether the study had human subjects or inferred conclusions from lab animals; and whether the conclusions were based on dozens or hundreds of research subjects or just a few.

Take fitness advice only from experts who represent reliable sources.

Well-meaning friends often have misinformation, and promoters of products and services are usually strongly biased.

Read consumer health newsletters published by distinguished universities, research institutes, and nonprofit organizations.

Examples include Harvard Health Letter; Mayo Clinic Health Letter, and Nutrition Action Health Letter.

Finally, use approved websites such as the following to learn more about fitness and wellness topics:

CDC Wonder (wonder.cdc.gov)

Mayo Clinic (www.mayoclinic.com)

National Center for Health Statistics (www.cdc.gov/nchs)

National Health Information Center (www.health.gov/nhic)

Harvard School of Public Health, World Health News (www.worldhealthnews.harvard.edu)

American Heart Association (www.americanheart.org)

American Medical Association (www.ama-assn.org)

Healthy People 2020 (www.healthypeople.gov)

U.S. Department of Health and Human Services (www.healthfinder.gov)

American College of Sports Medicine (www.acsm.org)

President's Council on Physical Fitness and Sports (www.fitness.gov)

FDA Information for Consumers (www.fda.gov/opacom/morecons.html)

Note: Web links are always subject to change. Visit this book's website at www.pearsonhighered.com /hopson to view updated Web links for each chapter.

chapterin**review**

videos

Log on to **www.pearsonhighered.com/hopson** or MyFitnessLab to view these chapter-related videos.

New Year's Resolutions   Months to a Healthier Lifestyle

onlineresources

Log on to **www.pearsonhighered.com/hopson** or MyFitnessLab for access to these book-related resources, and for links to other useful websites.

 Audio case study
Audio PowerPoint lecture

 Customizable 4-week fitness and wellness programs
Take Charge of Your Health! Worksheets:
   Worksheet 1 Health Behavior Self-Assessment
   Worksheet 2 Weekly Behavior Change
      Evaluation
   Worksheet 3 Multidimensional Health
      Locus of Control
Behavior Change Log Book and Wellness
Journal

 Lab 1.1 How Well Are You?
Lab 1.2 Chart Your Personal Wellness Balance
Lab 1.3 Create a Behavior Change Contract

 Pre- and post-quizzes
Glossary flashcards

reviewquestions

1. How does *wellness* differ from *health*?
   a. Wellness is the absence of disease.
   b. Wellness is the achievement of the highest level of health possible in physical, social, intellectual, emotional, environmental, and spiritual dimensions.
   c. Wellness and health are equivalent.
   d. Health is a more individualized, dynamic concept than wellness.
2. Which dimension of wellness includes good organizational skills?
   a. Social
   b. Intellectual
   c. Emotional
   d. Environmental
3. Which of the following is a modifiable risk factor for disease?
   a. Age
   b. Race
   c. Genetics
   d. Tobacco use

4. The American College of Sports Medicine recommends that all healthy adults between the ages of 18 and 65 strive for
   a. at least 150 minutes of moderate exercise per week.
   b. 30 minutes of exercise once a week.
   c. 50 minutes of moderate exercise per week.
   d. 20 minutes of walking once a week.
5. Which of the following is a top cause of death among Americans 20 to 24?
   a. Accidents
   b. Heart disease
   c. Stroke
   d. Lung Disease
6. Which of the following is a stage of the transtheoretical model of behavior change?
   a. Increased wellness
   b. Preparation
   c. Social wellness
   d. Motivation

7. What is meant by the term *healthy life expectancy*?
   a. How many years a person can expect to live
   b. How many years a person can expect to live without disability or major illness
   c. A realistic attitude toward how long a person can expect to live
   d. How many years a person believes he or she has to live

8. Imagined rehearsal is a form of
   a. countering.
   b. modeling.
   c. rewarding.
   d. visualization.

9. What is "shaping"?
   a. A stepwise process of change, designed to change one small piece of a target behavior at a time
   b. A model of behavior change that uses mental imaging to reshape the brain's signals
   c. A journaling strategy
   d. A way of learning behaviors by watching others perform them

10. Which of the following would be a poor reason to incorporate journaling into your wellness program?
   a. It helps you monitor your daily efforts.
   b. It helps you measure how much you have learned.
   c. It helps you record how you feel about your progress.
   d. It provides good material for blogging or tweeting.

critical**thinking**questions

 REVIEW IT! ONLINE

1. What does it mean to be well? What are the benefits of wellness?
2. Why is it important to find your current place on the wellness continuum?
3. Describe the SMART goal-setting guidelines.
4. Name the dimensions of wellness and assign yourself a score (1 to 5) for your degree of wellness in each dimension. Identify your place on the wellness continuum in Figure 1.2.
5. Which risk-lowering choices do you incorporate into your lifestyle? Choose two or three of them and discuss the personal attitudes and beliefs that underlie your present behavior.

6. Using the stages of change (transtheoretical) model, discuss what you might do (in stages) to help a friend stop smoking. Why is it important that a person be ready to change before trying to change?
7. Which habits (wellness-related or not) have you tried to change in the past? Why do you think your efforts succeeded or failed? Using the skills for behavior change from this chapter, write a plan that will help you approach each habit more successfully.
8. Describe your current level of exercise motivation.
9. Discuss your current commitment to fitness and wellness.

references

1. American College Health Association, *American College Health Association—National College Health Assessment II (ACHA-NCHA II): Reference Group Executive Summary Spring 2010* (Linthicum, Maryland: American College Health Association, 2010).
2. G. D. A. Brown and others, "Does Wage Rank Affect Employees' Well-Being?" *Industrial Relations: A Journal of Economy and Society* 47, no. 3 (2008): 355–89.
3. World Health Organization, "World Health Statistics 2010." www.who.int/whosis/whostat/2010/en/index.html (2010).
4. Ibid.
5. Ibid.
6. M. Heron, "Deaths: Leading Causes for 2006," *National Vital Statistics Reports* 58, no. 14 (Hyattsville, MD: National Center for Health Statistics, 2010).
7. Ibid.
8. Centers for Disease Control and Prevention, "Nationwide Trend," Health-Related Quality of Life; National Center for Chronic Disease Prevention and Health Promotion,
www.cdc.gov/hrqol (accessed October 29, 2007).
9. World Health Organization, "Diet and Physical Activity: A Public Health Priority," Global Strategy on Diet, Physical Activity and Health, www.who.int/dietphysicalactivity (accessed January 31, 2011).
10. C. E. Garner and others, "American College of Sports Medicine Position Stand: Quantity and Quality of Exercise for Developing and Maintaining Cardiorespiratory, Musculoskeletal, and Neuromotor Fitness in Apparently Healthy Adults: Guidance for Prescribing Exercise," *Medicine and Science in Sports and Exercise* 43, no. 7 (2011): 1334–59.
11. K. Flegal and others, "Prevalence and Trends in Obesity Among US Adults, 1999–2008." *Journal of the American Medical Association* 3003, no. 3 (2010): 235–41.
12. C.L. Ogden and M. D. Carroll, "NCHS Health E-Stat: Prevalence of Overweight, Obesity, and Extreme Obesity Among Adults: United States, Trends 1976–1980 through 2007–2008," Centers for Disease
Control and Prevention, www.cdc.gov/nchs/data/hestat/obesity_adult_07_08/obesity_adult_07_08.htm (updated June 2011).
13. Healthy People 2020, Framework: The Vision, Mission, and Goals of Healthy People 2020, www.healthypeople.gov/2020/consortium/HP2020Framework.pdf.
14. U. S. Department of Health and Human Services, Office of the Surgeon General, "Public Health Priorities," www.surgeongeneral.gov/publichealthpriorities.html#disease (accessed January, 31 2011).
15. National Coalition on Health Care, "Health Care Facts: Costs" September 2009. http://nchc.org/sites/default/files/resources/Fact%20Sheet%20-%20Cost.pdf (accessed January 2011).
16. Ibid.
17. B. W. Ward and others, "Early Release of Selected Estimates Based on Data from the January–June 2010 National Health Interview Survey," National Center for Health Statistics, www.cdc.gov/nchs/nhis/released201012.htm (December 2010).

18. U.S. Department of Health and Human Services, "Understanding the Affordable Health Care Act: Introduction," www.healthcare.gov/law/introduction/index.html (accessed January 31, 2011).

19. J. Prochaska, C. DiClemente, and J. Norcross, "In Search of How People Change: Application to Addictive Behaviors," *American Psychologist* 47, no. 9 (1983): 1102–14.

20. U. S. Department of Agriculture, "Report of the Dietary Guidelines Advisory Committee on the Dietary Guidelines for Americans, 2010," www.cnpp.usda.gov /DGAs2010-DGACReport.htm (January 2011).

21. V. Vicennati and others, "Stress-Related Development of Obesity and Cortisol in Women," Obesity 17, no. 9 (2009): 1678–83; E. Dias-Ferreira and others, "Chronic Stress Causes Frontostriatal Reorganization and Affects Decision-Making," *Science* 325, no. 5940 (2009): 621–25.

22. M. Yanai and others, "Smoking Incidence and the Effect of Smokefree Education Programs in Juveniles," *Chest* 128, no. 4 (2005): 205S.

23. E. P. Sarafino, *Health Psychology* (New York: Wiley, 1990) 189–91.

24. University of Iowa Advising Center, "Motivation, Goal Setting, and Success," www.uiowa.edu/web/advisingcenter /motivation.htm (accessed January 31, 2011).

25. American College Health Association, *ACHA-NCHA II: Reference Group Executive Summary Spring 2010* (2010).

LAB 1.1 • HOW WELL ARE YOU?

Name: _____   Date: _____

Instructor: _____   Section: _____

Purpose: This lab will help you assess your current level of wellness in each of the six dimensions and identify which wellness areas to target for behavior change.

Directions: Complete sections I–VII. For each item, indicate how often you think the statements describe you by checking the box under the relevant score. After each section, total your scores for that section and write your score in the space provided. After completing all sections, you will summarize and analyze your results.

SECTION I: PHYSICAL WELLNESS

	Never 1	Rarely 2	Sometimes 3	Often 4	Always 5
1. I listen to my body and make adjustments or seek professional help when something is wrong.					
2. I do moderate activity every day, such as taking the stairs instead of riding the elevator.					
3. I engage in vigorous exercise three to four times per week.					
4. I do exercise for muscular strength and endurance at least two times per week.					
5. I do stretching and limbering exercises at least five times per week.					
6. I do yoga, Pilates, tai chi, or other exercises for balance and core strength two or three times per week.					
7. I feel good about the condition of my body. I have lots of energy and can get through the day without being overly tired.					
8. I get adequate rest at night and wake on most mornings feeling ready for the day ahead.					
9. My immune system is strong, and my body heals quickly when I get sick or injured.					
10. I eat nutritious foods daily and avoid junk food.					
Total for Section I: Physical Wellness = _____					

SECTION II: SOCIAL WELLNESS

	Never 1	Rarely 2	Sometimes 3	Often 4	Always 5
1. I am open, honest, and get along well with others.					
2. I participate in a wide variety of social activities and enjoy all kinds of people.					
3. I try to be a "better person" and work on behaviors that have caused friction in the past.					
4. I am open and accessible to a loving and responsible relationship.					
5. I have someone I can talk to about private feelings.					
6. When I meet people, I feel good about the impression they have of me.					
7. I get along well with members of my family.					
8. I consider the feelings of others and do not act in hurtful or selfish ways.					
9. I try to see the good in my friends and help them feel good about themselves.					
10. I am good at listening to friends and family who need to talk.					

Total for Section II: Social Wellness = _____

SECTION III: INTELLECTUAL WELLNESS

	Never 1	Rarely 2	Sometimes 3	Often 4	Always 5
1. I carefully consider options and possible consequences as I make choices.					
2. I am alert and ready to respond to life's challenges in ways that reflect thought and sound judgment.					
3. I learn from my mistakes and try to act differently the next time.					
4. I actively learn all I can about products and services before buying them.					
5. I manage my time well rather than letting time manage me.					
6. I follow directions or recommended guidelines and act in ways likely to keep myself and others safe.					
7. I consider myself to be a wise health consumer and check for reliable sources of information before making decisions.					

	Never 1	Rarely 2	Sometimes 3	Often 4	Always 5
8. I have at least one personal-growth hobby that I make time for every week.					
9. My credit card balances are low, and my finances are in good order.					
10. I examine my own perceptions and then check evidence to see whether I was correct.					

Total for Section III: Intellectual Wellness = _____

SECTION IV: EMOTIONAL WELLNESS

	Never 1	Rarely 2	Sometimes 3	Often 4	Always 5
1. I find it easy to laugh, cry, and show emotions such as love, fear, and anger and I try to express them in positive ways.					
2. I avoid using alcohol or drugs as a means to forget my problems or relieve stress.					
3. My friends regard me as a stable, well-adjusted person whom they trust and rely on for support.					
4. When I am angry, I try to resolve issues in nonhurtful ways rather than stewing about them.					
5. I try not to worry unnecessarily, and I try to talk about my feelings, fears, and concerns rather than letting them build up.					
6. I recognize when I'm stressed and take steps to relax through exercise, quiet time, or calming activities.					
7. I view challenging situations and problems as opportunities for growth.					
8. I feel good about myself and believe others like me for who I am.					
9. I try not to be too critical or judgmental of others.					
10. I am flexible and adapt to change in a positive way.					

Total for Section IV: Emotional Wellness =_____

SECTION V: SPIRITUAL WELLNESS

	Never 1	Rarely 2	Sometimes 3	Often 4	Always 5
1. I take time alone to think about life's meaning and where I fit in to the greater whole.					
2. I believe life is a gift we should cherish.					
3. I look forward to each day as an opportunity for further growth.					
4. I experience life to the fullest.					
5. I take time to enjoy nature and the beauty around me.					
6. I have faith in a greater power, nature, or the connectedness of all living things.					
7. I engage in acts of care and goodwill without expecting something in return.					
8. I look forward to each day as an opportunity to grow and be challenged in life.					
9. I work for peace in my interpersonal relationships, my community, and the world at large.					
10. I have a great love and respect for all living things and regard animals as important links in a vital living chain.					

Total for Section V: Spiritual Wellness = _____

SECTION VI: ENVIRONMENTAL WELLNESS

	Never 1	Rarely 2	Sometimes 3	Often 4	Always 5
1. I am concerned about environmental pollution and actively try to preserve and protect natural resources.					
2. I buy recycled paper and purchase biodegradable products whenever possible.					
3. I recycle my garbage, reuse containers, and try to minimize the amount of paper and plastics that I use.					
4. I try to wear my clothes for longer periods of time between washings to save on water and reduce detergent in our water sources.					
5. I try to reduce my use of gasoline and oil by limiting my driving.					
6. I write my elected leaders about environmental concerns.					

7. I turn down the heat and wear warmer clothes at home in the winter and use the air conditioner only when really necessary.					
8. I am aware of potential hazards in my area and try to reduce my exposure whenever possible.					
9. I use both sides of the paper when taking notes and doing assignments.					
10. I try not to leave the water running too long when I shower, shave, or brush my teeth.					

Total for Section VI: Environmental Wellness = _____

SECTION VII: REFLECTION—YOUR PERSONAL WELLNESS CONTINUUM

1. Enter your totals for sections I–VI below:

Physical Wellness _____

Social Wellness _____

Intellectual Wellness _____

Emotional Wellness _____

Spiritual Wellness _____

Environmental Wellness _____

2. Understanding your scores:

Scores of 35–50: Outstanding! Your answers show that you are aware of the importance of these behaviors in your overall wellness, and that you are putting your knowledge to work by practicing good habits that should reduce your overall risks.

Scores of 30–34: Your wellness practices in these areas are very good, but there is room for improvement. What changes could you make to improve your score?

Scores of 20–29: Your wellness risks are showing. Find information about the risks you face and why it is important to change these behaviors.

Scores below 20: You may be taking unnecessary risks. Identify each risk area and, whenever possible, seek additional resources, either on your campus or through your local community health resources.

LAB 1.2 • CHART YOUR PERSONAL WELLNESS BALANCE

Name: _____ Date: _____

Instructor: _____ Section: _____

Purpose: To learn how to chart your current personal wellness balance and identify the wellness areas in which you would like to improve.

Materials: Results from Lab 1.1

Directions: Follow the instructions below.

SECTION I: YOUR PERSONAL WELLNESS BALANCE

1. Create a personal wellness balance chart with your scores from sections I–VI of Lab 1.1. Allocate a larger "piece of the pie" for dimensions of wellness where your scores are higher and a smaller slice for dimensions with lower scores. Another option: allocate a larger slice for areas where you spend most of your time during a week.

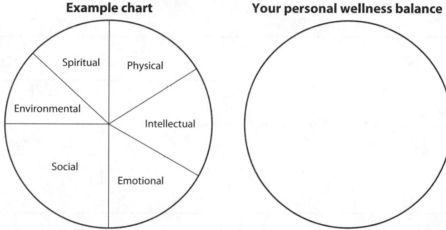

Example chart

Your personal wellness balance

2. Now create your **goal wellness balance chart.** Change your current balance chart to reflect your desired scores in each wellness dimension, or to reflect the optimal percentage of time you would like to allocate to each dimension.

Goal wellness balance chart

SECTION II: REFLECTION

Reflect on your answers, your wellness balance charts, and your wellness continuum (from the *Think! Act!* on page 5). What are your major areas of concern regarding your wellness? What two or three behaviors could you change easily to improve your wellness? Which one needs attention first?

_____

_____

_____

_____

_____

_____

_____

_____

_____

_____

_____

_____

_____

_____

_____

_____

LAB 1.3 • CREATE A BEHAVIOR CHANGE CONTRACT

Name: _____ Date: _____

Instructor: _____ Section: _____

Purpose: To introduce students to the process of writing a behavior change contract and planning for new life-style behaviors. This introduction will serve as a model for other behavior change plans in subsequent chapters.

Directions: Complete the following sections.

SECTION I: PERSONAL WELLNESS REVIEW

1. Review your answers from Lab 1.1 and Lab 1.2.

2. Consider the stages of change (precontemplation, contemplation, preparation, action, maintenance) and evaluate your readiness to make a behavior change.

3. Choose a target behavior to change. For this behavior, you should be in the contemplation or preparation stages. Write the behavior below.

My behavior to change is _____

SECTION II: SHORT- AND LONG-TERM GOALS

1. **Long-Term Goal:** Long-term goals are those set for six months to a year or more. These goals should be achievable and may take many steps and an extended time to reach. Be sure to use SMART (specific, measurable, action-oriented, realistic, time-oriented) goal-setting guidelines when creating your long-term goal. After writing out your long-term goal, choose an appropriate target date and a reward for completing your goal.

    a.   Long-Term Goal: _____

    b.   Target Date: _____

    c.   Reward: _____

2. **Short-Term Goals:** Short-term goals are those you want to achieve in less than six months. These goals will often help you reach your long-term goal. They may also be part of your long-term goal. Again, use SMART goal-setting guidelines when setting short-term goals. After writing out your short-term goals, choose appropriate target dates and rewards.

    a.   Short-Term Goal #1: _____

    b.   Target Date: _____

    c.   Reward: _____

    a.   Short-Term Goal #2: _____

    b.   Target Date: _____

    c.   Reward: _____

SECTION III: BEHAVIOR CHANGE OBSTACLES AND STRATEGIES

1. These are **three obstacles** to changing this behavior (things I am currently doing or situations that contribute to this behavior or make it harder to change):

a. _____

b. _____

c. _____

2. Here are **three strategies** I will use to overcome these obstacles:

a. _____

b. _____

c. _____

SECTION IV: GETTING SUPPORT

1. Resources I will use to help me change this behavior:

a. A friend/partner/relative: _____

b. A school-based resource: _____

c. A community-based resource: _____

d. A book or reputable website: _____

2. How will you use these supportive resources to help you with your goals?

_____

_____

SECTION V: CONTRACT, TRACKING, AND FOLLOW-UP

1. Contract: I intend to make the behavior change described above. I will use the strategies and rewards to achieve the goals that will contribute to a healthy behavior change.

Signed _____ Date _____

Witness _____ Date _____

2. Tracking: Tracking progress toward your goals is very important to ensure successful behavior change. As you move through this course, you will be asked to monitor your progress on several of your health, wellness, and fitness goals. Accurate and regular record-keeping is important.

3. Follow-up: When reaching your target date, it is important to follow up and reassess your program. During this course, you will be answering questions such as, Did you accomplish your goal? Do you need to set a new and more challenging goal? Do you need to alter your goals or program to make it more realistic? This section in your labs is important to modify your goals and your program and to set future goals.

2 Understanding Fitness Principles

Learning Outcomes

1. Describe the three primary levels of physical activity and their benefits.

2. Articulate the importance of each health-related component of fitness.

  Audio case study and audio Power-Point lecture

3. Identify the role that the skill-related components of fitness play in overall physical fitness.

4. Explain how following the fitness principles of overload, progression, specificity, reversibility, individuality, and recovery will increase your fitness program success.

5. Describe how much and the types of physical activity you should do for optimal health and wellness.

  Personal Fitness and Exercise

6. Incorporate general strategies for exercising safely.

7. Identify individual attributes that should be taken into account before beginning a fitness program.

 Lab 2.1 Assess Your Physical Activity Readiness

Lab 2.2 Identify Your Physical Activity Motivations and Obstacles

8. Individualize and implement strategies that will help you get started on your fitness and exercise goals.

  Lab 2.3 Changing Your Sedentary Time into Active Time

 Customizable 4-week starter walking programs

Pre- and post-quizzes and glossary flashcards

31

casestudy

LILY

"Hi, I'm Lily. I just started my junior year, and after a summer of lazing around, I want to get back into shape. I'm ready to put some serious time and energy into it, but the last time I started exercising, I tried to do too much and ended up injured. How do I keep from doing the same thing this time? How much exercise do I really need? And what does it actually mean to be fit, anyway—does it just mean being able to run a certain distance, or is there more to it than that?"

HEAR IT! ONLINE 🎧

. . . .

Fitness is a critical component of overall wellness. Being physically fit can improve your mood, give you more energy for daily activities, help you maintain a healthy weight, and reduce your risk of developing chronic diseases. All of these benefits can, in turn, help you live a longer, healthier life.

In this chapter, we cover the basic principles of fitness, address the question of how much exercise you need, introduce general guidelines for exercising safely, and discuss individual factors you should consider when designing your personal fitness program. Also, we go over strategies to help you get started exercising, including overcoming common obstacles to success.

> **physical fitness** A set of attributes that relate to one's ability to perform moderate to vigorous levels of physical activity without undue fatigue
>
> **physical activity** Any bodily movement produced by skeletal muscles that results in an expenditure of energy
>
> **exercise** Physical activity that is planned or structured, done to improve or maintain one or more of the components of fitness

What Are the Three Primary Levels of Physical Activity?

Physical fitness is the ability to perform moderate to vigorous levels of physical activity without undue fatigue. Note that *physical activity* and *exercise* are not the same thing: **physical activity** technically means any bodily movement produced by skeletal muscles that results in an expenditure of energy, whereas **exercise** specifically refers to planned or structured physical activity done to achieve and maintain fitness.

Physical activity is often measured in metabolic equivalents, or **MET** levels. A MET level of 1 is equivalent to the energy you use at rest or while sitting quietly. A MET level of 2 equals two times the energy used at a MET level of 1, while a MET level of 3 equals three times the energy used at a MET level of 1, and so forth. Levels of physical activity can be grouped into three primary categories: (1) *light/lifestyle/physical activities* (<3 METS), (2) *moderate physical activities* (3 to 6 METS), and (3) *vigorous physical activities* (>6 METS). Figure 2.1 illustrates examples of each of these levels of physical activity, and the benefits that are associated with them.

What Are the Health-Related Components of Physical Fitness?

The five **health-related components of physical fitness** are *cardiorespiratory endurance, muscular strength, muscular endurance, flexibility,* and *body composition*. Minimal competence in each of these areas is necessary for you to carry out daily activities, lower your risk of developing chronic diseases, and optimize your health and well-being.

Cardiorespiratory Endurance

Cardiorespiratory endurance (also called *cardiovascular fitness/endurance, aerobic fitness,* and *cardiorespiratory fitness*) is the ability of the cardiovascular and respiratory systems to provide oxygen to working muscles during sustained exercise. Achieving adequate cardiorespiratory endurance decreases your risk of diabetes, heart disease, obesity, and other chronic diseases.[1] Increased cardiorespiratory endurance also improves your ability to enjoy recreational activities, such as bicycling and hiking, and to participate in them for extended periods of time.

Muscular Strength

Muscular strength is the ability of your muscles to exert force. You may think of it as your ability to lift a

Light/Lifestyle Physical Activities (<3 METS)	Examples:	Benefits:
	Light yard work and housework, leisurely walking, self-care and bathing, light stretching, light occupational activity	A moderate increase in health and wellness in those who are completely sedentary; reduced risk of some chronic diseases

Moderate Physical Activities (3–6 METS)	Examples:	Benefits:
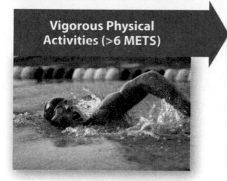	Walking 3–4.5 mph on a level surface, weight training, hiking, climbing stairs, bicycling 5–9 mph on a level surface, dancing, softball, recreational swimming, moderate yard work and housework	Increased cardiorespiratory endurance, lower body fat levels, improved blood cholesterol and pressure, better blood glucose management, decreased risk of disease, increased overall physical fitness

Vigorous Physical Activities (>6 METS)	Examples:	Benefits:
	Jogging, running, circuit training, backpacking, aerobic classes, competitive sports, swimming laps, heavy yard work or housework, hard physical labor/construction, bicycling over 10 mph up steep terrain	Increased overall physical fitness, decreased risk of disease, further improvements in overall strength and endurance

FIGURE **2.1** Examples and benefits of light/lifestyle physical activity, moderate physical activity, and vigorous physical activity.

heavy weight. Improved muscular strength decreases your risk of low bone density and musculoskeletal injuries.[2] In order to improve muscular strength, you need to tax your muscles in a controlled setting. This typically involves a weight room, as well as supervision to avoid injury.

Muscular Endurance

Muscular endurance is the ability of your muscles to contract repeatedly over time. Along with cardiorespiratory endurance, muscular endurance allows you to participate in recreational sports without undue fatigue. For example, in order to play a continuous game of basketball, you need to have good cardiorespiratory endurance to move up and down the court for the entire 90

minutes—and you need to have good muscular endurance to keep guarding, blocking, and shooting the ball effectively.

Flexibility

Flexibility is the ability to move your joints in a full range of motion. This component of fitness is often overlooked but maintaining a minimal level of flexibility is important for overall wellness. Flexibility in

MET The standard metabolic equivalent used to estimate the amount of energy (oxygen) used by the body during physical activity; 1 MET = resting or sitting quietly

health-related components of physical fitness Components of physical fitness that have a relationship with good health your joints increases your ability to do the activities you enjoy and work toward specific fitness goals. Although we don't know whether stretching reduces overall injury rates, it may reduce specific muscle and tendon injuries.[3] Having an adequate joint range of motion can be especially important to prevent neck and back pain when you are older[4] and help prevent the decreased physical function that often occurs with aging.[5]

Body Composition

Body composition refers to the relative amounts of fat and lean tissue in your body. Lean tissue consists of muscle, bone, organs, and fluids. A healthy body composition has adequate muscle tissue with moderate to low amounts of fat tissue. The recommendations for fat

percentages will vary based upon your gender and age. Increased levels of fat will put you at risk for diabetes, heart disease, and certain cancers.

What Are the Skill-Related Components of Physical Fitness?

In addition to the five health-related components of fitness, physical fitness also involves attributes that improve your ability to perform athletic and exercise tasks. These attributes are called the **skill-related components of fitness.** Often termed *sport skills,* these are qualities that athletes aim to improve in order to gain a competitive edge. Recreational athletes and general exercisers can also benefit from improving these skills. The six skill-related components of fitness are:

- *Agility*: The ability to rapidly change the position of your body with speed and accuracy

- *Balance*: The maintenance of equilibrium while you are stationary or moving

- *Coordination*: The ability to use both your senses and your body to perform motor tasks smoothly and accurately

- *Power*: The ability to perform work or contract muscles with high force quickly

- *Speed*: The ability to perform a movement in a short period of time

- *Reaction time*: The time between a stimulus and the initiation of your physical reaction to that stimulus

Although skill-related fitness is largely determined by heredity,[6] regular training can result in significant improvements. In order to improve skill-related components of fitness, athletes and exercisers first need to target the skills that will be important to their specific sport or exercise. For instance, a runner can benefit from increasing power for hill running and speed for winning races, whereas a tennis player can benefit from increased agility and reaction time.

Improving your fitness skills can be as easy as participating regularly in any sport or activity. Playing football will increase reaction time and power, while dancing will increase balance, agility, and coordination. Another way to increase these skills is to perform drills that mimic a sport-specific skill, or work specifically on any of the skill-related components of fitness. You can practice drills in group exercise classes, or you can work with a personal trainer. Specialized equipment is often used in such drills: for example, exercises utilizing obstacles such as hurdles or cones can help you improve your speed, agility, and coordination, while using balance boards or exercise balls can help you improve your balance.

What Are the Principles of Fitness?

In order to design an effective fitness program, you need to take into account the basic **principles of fitness** (also called *principles of exercise training*). These guiding principles explain how the body responds or adapts to exercise training.

Overload

The principle of **overload** states that in order to see improvements in your physical fitness, the amount or dose of training you undertake must be more than your body or specific body system is accustomed to. This applies to any of the components of physical fitness discussed earlier. For example, in order to increase your flexibility, you must stretch a little farther than you are used to.

Training Effects Consistent overloads or stresses on a body system will cause an *adaptation* to occur (Figure 2.2). An adaptation is a change in the body as a result of an overload. In exercise training this is called a *training effect*. For example, if you normally run two laps around a track each day but gradually increase this to four laps each day, the overload to your cardiorespiratory and muscular systems will cause adaptations in those systems. While you may feel tired and out of breath the first time you run four laps, after a few weeks of running those four laps the adaptations in your body will allow you to cover that distance with greater ease.

Dose-Response The amount of adaptation you can expect is directly related to the amount of overload or training dose that you complete. This is called the *dose-response relationship.* An increase in your "dose," or amount of training, will result in increased responses or adaptations to that training. How much response or adaptation you can expect is dependent upon the body system trained, the health or fitness outcome measured, and your individual physical and genetic characteristics.

Diminished Returns According to the concept of *diminished returns* (also called the *initial values principle*), the rate of fitness improvement diminishes over time

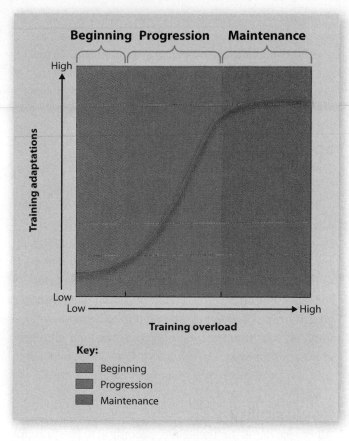

FIGURE **2.2** After adjusting to new training overloads at the beginning of your exercise program, you will see larger adaptations and improvements during the progression phase. As you approach your goal or genetic limits, your increases in overload will not result in further adaptations. This is a sign that you have reached a plateau and should maintain (if satisfied) or adjust your program for further improvement.

as fitness levels approach genetic limits. Initial fitness levels determine the amount of improvement that you can achieve from exercise training overloads. If you are sedentary and far from your genetic limits, you might experience large increases in fitness levels from moderate amounts of training. If you are active and closer to your genetic limits already, you may gain only small increases in fitness from larger amounts of training.

Progression

The principle of **progression** states that in order to effectively and safely increase fitness, you need to apply an optimal level of overload to the body within a certain time period. Simply stated, you need to increase your

principles of fitness General principles of exercise adaptation that guide fitness programming

overload Subjecting the body or body system to more physical activity than it is accustomed to

progression A gradual increase in a training program's intensity, frequency, and/or time workout levels enough to see results, but not so much that you increase your risk of injury. Your body will then progressively adapt to the overloads presented to it. To make sure that you are not progressing too quickly, follow the "10 percent rule": increase your program frequency, intensity, or duration by no more than 10 percent per week.

Specificity

The principle of **specificity** states that improvements in a body system will occur only if that specific body system is stressed or progressively overloaded by the physical activity. To follow this principle, make sure that you are training targeted muscle groups specific to your sport or that your program is specifically designed to meet your goals. For instance, if you are planning to walk a marathon, you should primarily *walk* during your training. If, instead, you decide to do lap swimming as your training, you may increase your cardiorespiratory fitness levels, but you will not be specifically training your lower body muscles to walk 26 miles.

Reversibility

All fitness gains are reversible, according to the principle of **reversibility**. This is the "use it or lose it" principle. If you do not maintain a minimal level of physical activity and exercise, your fitness levels will slip. Unfortunately, you cannot accumulate fitness or workout sessions in a "bank" for later. Doing a great deal of exercise in one week will not compensate for a subsequent month of doing no exercise. Whenever you stop exercising, it only takes one to two weeks to start losing fitness gains you may have made while training. Most of your improvements could be gone in a few months.[7] For example, if you spent four months running four miles three times a week, you could lose any fitness gains from those four months within two months of *no* training.

specificity The principle that only the body systems worked during training will show adaptations

reversibility The principle that training adaptations will revert toward initial levels when training is stopped

individuality Refers to the variable nature of physical activity dose-response or adaptations in different persons

rest and recovery Taking a short time off from physical activities to allow the body to recuperate and improve

overtraining Excessive volume and intensity of physical training leading to diminished health, fitness, and performance

Individuality

The principle of **individuality** states that adaptations to a training overload may vary greatly from person to person. Genetics influence all individual differences in training adaptations. Two people may participate in the same training program but have very different responses. While you cannot control your genetic makeup, understanding how you respond to exercise is important in designing your personal fitness plan. A person who responds well to a training program is considered a *responder*. One who does not respond well is considered a *nonresponder*. Of those individuals who show improvements, some may respond better to increases in total amount of physical activity, while others may show more improvement with increases in exercise intensity. Figuring out your individual responses to certain exercise programs is a trial-and-error process. Complete regular fitness assessments and training logs to track your progress and then adjust your program accordingly to meet your goals.

· ·

casestudy

LILY

"The last time I decided to start exercising, I started off slowly, jogging about half an hour twice a week. That went well. Then I got busy with school and stopped jogging for a whole month. To make up for it, I decided to run a 10k. It was a gorgeous day, and there were tons of other people running it. There were kids, and older people, and people who looked way more out of shape than I was—so even though I hadn't trained for it, I thought it'd be no problem. Well, three miles into it, my knees started to hurt. The pain came and went, and I managed to finish the six-mile race, but my knees hurt for two weeks afterward. That was the end of my big exercise plans."

THINK! What principles of fitness would you advise Lily to keep in mind before she attempts a new exercise routine? What mistakes did Lily make?

ACT! Tell a friend about or describe in your journal a past experience with exercise that was similar to Lily's. Tell your friend or write down what you intend to do differently this time around.

Rest and Recovery

The principle of **rest and recovery** (also called the *principle of recuperation*) is critical to ensuring continued progress toward your fitness goals. As you will recall, the overload principle states that you must subject your body to more exercise than it is accustomed to doing. However, your body also needs time to recover from the increased physiological and structural training stresses that you place on it. In *resistance training* (also called *weight training*) in particular, most of the training adaptations actually take place during the rest periods between workouts.

Constant training day after day with insufficient rest periods can result in reduced health benefits and can eventually lead to **overtraining**. If you are exercising consistently and start feeling more fatigue and muscle soreness than usual during and after exercise, you could be doing too much. Reduce the duration or intensity of your exercise and rest for a day or two. To prevent overtraining and to gain optimal benefits from your training program, schedule regular rest days (one to three per week) in any cardiorespiratory endurance program and every other day for any strength training program. Another important tip to avoid overtraining and injury is to alternate hard workout days with easier workout days during your weekly plan.

How Much Exercise Is Enough?

How much exercise or physical activity do you really need? The answers will vary, depending on which sources you turn to and on your individual fitness goals. Most agree that the first step is to avoid inactivity. *Any* amount of physical activity can confer basic health benefits. For increased health benefits, follow the minimal activity level recommendations below. For additional health benefits and fitness improvements, follow the guidelines outlined in the Physical Activity Pyramid and the FITT Principle.

Worksheet 26
How Much Do
I Move?

Minimal Physical Activity Level Guidelines

Personal
Fitness and
Exercise

Guidelines for physical activity and exercise are issued by various organizations that rely on credible scientific research in developing their recommendations. These organizations can be *government agencies* (such as the President's Council on Physical Fitness and Sports), *professional organizations* (such as the American College of Sports Medicine), or *private organizations* (such as the American Heart Association). In 2008, the U.S. Department of Health and Human Services issued the first ever national physical activity guidelines designed to "provide achievable steps for youth, adults, and seniors, as well as people with special conditions to live healthier and longer lives."[8] The recommendations are echoed by other leading organizations, such as the World Health Organization[9] and American College of Sports Medicine.[10]

As a nation we are doing better meeting these guidelines, but we can still improve. When the guidelines were released in 2008, 32 percent of adults reported participating in regular moderate physical activity and 24 percent of adults reported participating in regular vigorous physical activity.[11] Of these, 43 percent were meeting the recommended minimum physical activity levels (moderate or vigorous) and the goal is to increase that number to 48 percent by 2020.[12] Take a look at the guidelines in Table 2.1. How close are you to meeting these recommendations?

The Physical Activity Pyramid Guides Weekly Choices

The Physical Activity Pyramid (Figure 2.3) visually summarizes minimal physical activity and exercise guidelines for optimal health and wellness. The Physical Activity Pyramid's bottom layer represents light or lifestyle activities that you should strive to incorporate into your everyday life. Light physical activity every day, such as walking and gardening, is a great way to start and to ensure a strong "base" to your pyramid! The next layer of the pyramid represents moderate-to-vigorous aerobic and/or sports activities that you should try to do three to five times per week in order to build cardiorespiratory endurance and fitness. Aim to accumulate at least 150 minutes of moderate physical activity each week, such as quick walking or flat bicycling, or 75 minutes of vigorous activity each week, such as swimming or jogging. The third layer of the pyramid represents strength-training and flexibility-building exercises that you should try to incorporate at least two days per week. The top layer of the pyramid represents the activities that should ideally receive the least amount of your time—sedentary activities such as watching TV or surfing the Web—in favor of more active pursuits.

The box Six Easy Ways to Get More Active provides suggestions for how to incorporate more physical activity into your daily life.

TABLE 2.1 Physical Activity Guidelines for Americans			
	Key Guidelines for Health*	For Additional Fitness or Weight Loss Benefits*	PLUS
Adults	150 min/week moderate-intensity OR 75 min/week of vigorous-intensity OR Equivalent combination of moderate- and vigorous-intensity (i.e., 100 min moderate-intensity + 25 min vigorous-intensity)	300 min/week moderate-intensity OR 150 min/week of vigorous-intensity OR Equivalent combination of moderate- and vigorous-intensity (i.e., 200 min moderate-intensity + 50 min vigorous-intensity) OR More than the previously described amounts	Muscle strengthening activities for all the major muscle groups at least 2 days/week
Older Adults	If unable to follow above guidelines, then as much physical activity as your condition allows	If unable to follow above guidelines, then as much physical activity as your condition allows	In addition to muscle strengthening activities, those with limited mobility should add exercises to improve balance and reduce risk of falling
Children and Adolescents	60 min or more of moderate- or vigorous-intensity physical activity daily	Add vigorous-intensity physical activities within the 60 daily minutes at least 3 days/week	Include muscle and bone strengthening activities within the 60 daily minutes at least 3 days/week Activities should be age-appropriate, enjoyable, and varied

*Notes: Avoid inactivity, some activity is better than none; accumulate physical activity in sessions of 10 minutes or more at one time; and spread activity throughout the week.

Source: Office of Disease Prevention and Health Promotion, U.S. Department of Health and Human Services, *2008 Physical Activity Guidelines for Americans: Be Active, Healthy, and Happy!* ODPHP Publication no. U0036 (Washington, D.C.: U.S. Department of Health and Human Services, 2008), Available at www.health.gov .paguidelines.

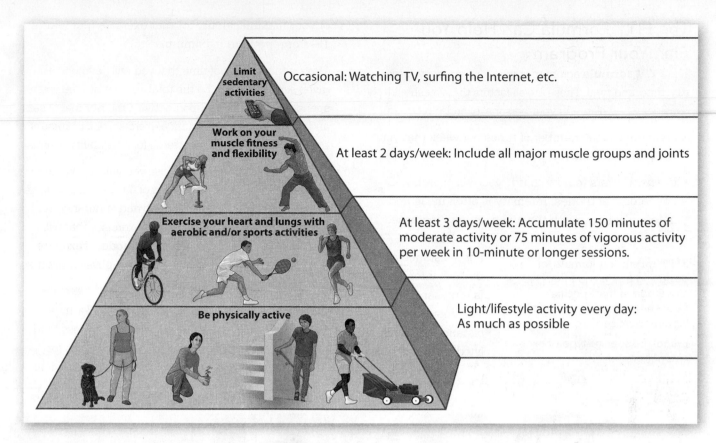

FIGURE **2.3** The Physical Activity Pyramid presents recommended levels of activity for optimal health and wellness.

TOOLS FOR **CHANGE** •

Six Easy Ways to Become More Active

You can improve your fitness level simply by adding more physical activity to your daily life. Below are a few ways you can incorporate more physical activity:

• Instead of driving your car to campus, ride your bike or walk.

• If you must drive to campus, park your car farther from your destination than usual.

• If you have a dog, walk it daily. If you already do that, add a second daily walk—your dog will love you for it!

• Carry a handbasket while grocery shopping instead of pushing a cart (assuming your grocery list is not very long).

• If you have children, play actively with them.

• If you have a desk job, get up, stretch, and walk around often.

THINK! Examine the Physical Activity Pyramid. How does your weekly physical activity match up to its recommendations? In which areas of the pyramid could you improve?

ACT! Draw your current physical activity pyramid. Now draw your physical activity pyramid incorporating the simple suggestions above. List the activities you could add to your week to become more active.

Source: U.S. Department of Health and Human Services, "Choices," Small Step Program, www.smallstep.gov/ga/choices.html (accessed September 2011).

The FITT Formula Can Help You Plan Your Program

The **FITT formula** acronym stands for *frequency, intensity, time,* and *type.* These are all factors that you should consider when planning your personal exercise program.

- *Frequency* is the number of times per week that you will perform an exercise.

- *Intensity* refers to how "hard" you will exercise. For aerobic activities, intensity is often measured in terms of how much the given activity increases your heart rate. For resistance activities, intensity is represented in the amount of resistance or weight lifted as a percentage of your maximal ability for that exercise (percent of 1RM or repetition maximum).

- *Time* is the amount of time that you will devote to a given exercise. It can be the total amount of time you spend on an aerobic or sport activity, the number of sets and repetitions for a resistance exercise, or the amount of time you spend holding a stretch for a flexibility exercise.

- *Type* refers to the kind of exercise you will do. Within each of the exercise components of fitness (cardiorespiratory endurance, muscular strength and endurance, and flexibility), there are many types of exercises that will increase fitness levels. Your type, or **mode**, of exercise will be determined by your preferences, physical abilities, environment, and personal goals.

See Figure 2.4 for a summary of the FITT guidelines for cardiorespiratory endurance, muscular fitness, and flexibility. If you are beginning a fitness program for the first time, you may want to start with the physical

> **FITT formula** A formula for designing a safe and effective program that specifies frequency, intensity, time, and type of exercise
>
> **mode** The specific type of exercise performed

	Cardiorespiratory Endurance	Muscular Fitness	Flexibility
Frequency	3–5 days per week	2–3 days per week	Minimally 2–3 days per week
Intensity	64%–95% of maximum heart rate	60%–80% of 1RM	To the point of mild tension
Time	20–60 minutes	8–10 exercises, 2–4 sets, 8–12 reps	10–30 seconds per stretch, 2–4 reps
Type	Any rhythmic, continuous, large muscle group activity	Resistance training (with body weight and/or external resistance) for all major muscle groups	Stretching, dance, or yoga exercises for all major muscle groups

FIGURE **2.4** The FITT principle applied to summary guidelines for cardiorespiratory endurance, muscular fitness, and flexibility.

Data from: C. E. Garner and others, "American College of Sports Medicine Position Stand: Quantity and Quality of Exercise for Developing and Maintaining Cardiorespiratory, Musculoskeletal, and Neuromotor Fitness in Apparently Healthy Adults: Guidance for Prescribing Exercise," *Medicine and Science in Sports and Exercise* 43, no. 7 (2011): 1334–59.

activity guidelines in Table 2.1. When you are ready, add appropriate levels of the Physical Activity Pyramid and then customize your program using the FITT formula to suit your personal goals.

What Does It Take to Exercise Safely?

Exercise-related injuries have risen in recent decades. More than seven million Americans receive medical attention for sports-related injuries each year, with the greatest numbers of injuries affecting 5- to 24-year-olds.[13] To reduce your risk of exercise injury, follow the guidelines below.

Warm Up Properly Before Your Workout

A proper warm-up consists of two phases: a general warm-up and a specific warm-up. In a *general warm-up*, your goal is to warm up the body by doing three to ten minutes of light physical activity similar to the activities you will be performing during exercise. During this period of time (called the *rest-to-exercise transition*), you are preparing your body to withstand the more vigorous exercise to come. Your core body temperature should rise a few degrees, and you should break a slight sweat. This movement and temperature rise will increase your overall blood flow, ready the joint fluid and structures, and improve muscle elasticity.

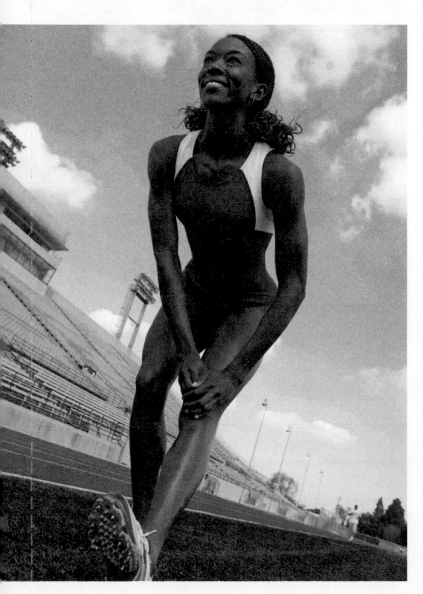

During a *specific warm-up,* your goal is to focus on the particular muscle groups and joints that you will be using during the activity set. This part of the warm-up should consist of three to five minutes of **range-of-motion** movements. You should move the joints involved in your exercise through the range of motion that they will experience during the activity. Move joints through a full range of motion in a relaxed and controlled manner. If you want to add light stretching to your warm-up, do so at the end of your specific warm-up.

> **range-of-motion** The movement limits that limbs have around a specific joint

Cool Down Properly After Your Workout

After you finish your workout, cool down in a manner that is appropriate to the activity that you performed. This *exercise-to-rest transition* should last anywhere from five to fifteen minutes. If your heart rate and temperature rose during your workout, you should perform a *general cool-down* in which your goal is to bring your heart rate, breathing rate, and temperature closer to resting levels. This cool-down is usually a less vigorous version of the activity you just performed. For example, if you jogged for 25 minutes, your general cool-down may consist of 10 minutes of walking.

If you have just finished a resistance-training program and your heart rate is not elevated, you should perform a *specific cool-down* for the joints and muscles you have exercised. A specific cool-down can be performed after a general cool-down for aerobic activities and right after exercise for resistance training activities. During a specific cool-down, you should stretch the muscle groups worked during the activity.

Take the Time to Properly Learn the Skills for Your Chosen Activity

There are hundreds of different activities that you can do to increase your health and fitness, each with a specific set of physical skills required for participation. You might choose simple activities such as walking or jogging, which require little skill and have short learning curves, or you might focus on activities that require more complex skills, such as fencing or hockey. Whatever you choose, properly learn the physical skills required for the activity to enhance your enjoyment and to avoid injury. If you are just beginning a sport for the first time—for example, skiing—do not immediately approach the sport the way a more experienced athlete would. Take lessons, start on the beginner slopes, and give yourself time to safely perform your chosen activity.

Consume Enough Energy and Water for Exercise

Deciding how much to eat and drink prior to exercise can be tricky. You need enough energy to work out, but you should not exercise on a full stomach. Eating a small meal 1 1/2 to 2 hours before exercise is a good way to make sure that you have energy (but not an upset stomach) during the workout. A light snack 30 to 60 minutes before your workout is acceptable as well.

Dehydration is more likely than food intake to affect your exercise performance. During the hours before your workout, be sure to drink enough water so that you do not feel thirsty as you go into your exercise session. Guidelines for drinking before, during, and after exercising should be tailored to the individual and the exercise session.[14] General guidelines are 17 to 20 oz. of fluid two to three hours before exercise and 7 to 10 oz. of fluid ten to twenty minutes prior to exercise.[15] During your workout, hydrate when you feel thirsty, and increase the amount of water you consume as you start to sweat more profusely.

Select Appropriate Footwear and Clothing

Consider this: Your feet will typically strike the ground 1,000 times during one mile of running. Over weeks of training, that translates to a great deal of wear and tear on your feet and lower body. Needless to say, proper footwear is critical to a safe and successful training program—regardless of the activity you choose.

While some sports require specialized footwear, most beginning exercisers just need one pair of good, all-around cross-trainers or running shoes. The most important aspect of footwear is proper fit and cushioning. Always try on shoes before purchasing them, and if possible, spend a few minutes mimicking the activity you will be doing in them. The best shoes are not always the most expensive ones, but you should aim to purchase the highest quality footwear you can afford. Ask for assistance from a knowledgeable salesperson—let him or her know what activities you are planning to pursue, and ask which shoes would be most appropriate for your plans.

Clothing for exercise can be very simple (e.g., shorts and a T-shirt) or very technical (e.g., clothing with wicking fibers or special treatments for protection against harsh weather). The most important thing is to dress appropriately for your chosen activity. Make sure that your clothing is comfortable and does not restrict your range of motion. Women may wish to wear supportive athletic bras, and men may want to consider wearing supportive compression shorts or undergarments. If you are planning to exercise outdoors, take temperature into consideration and dress accordingly. The longer you plan to exercise, the more carefully you should think about what to wear for a successful workout.

casestudy

LILY

"I've started jogging again! I'm back to jogging 30 minutes twice a week and thinking of bumping things up to three times a week. I'm hoping to eventually work my way up to jogging for 45 minutes straight, each time I go out. I'm not tempted to run a 10k again any time soon, but if I can keep this new routine going, maybe I will be ready for a 5k—without hurting my knees this time."

THINK! What kinds of things would you advise Lily to do, in order to reduce her chances of injury?

ACT! Describe Lily's exercise routine, using the FITT formula, and figure out what you might do the same or different from her.

What Individual Factors Should I Consider When Designing a Fitness Program?

There is no such thing as a "one-size-fits-all" physical fitness program. Different individuals have different needs, and general recommendations often need to be adapted to fit those individual needs. Your age, weight, current fitness level, and any disabilities and special health concerns are all factors that should be considered in order to design a safe and effective exercise routine.

Age

Older adults may require additional precautions in order to prevent injury while exercising. Men over age 45 and women over age 55 should obtain medical clearance before beginning an exercise program.[16] Moderate aerobic activity, muscle-strengthening exercises, and flexibility work are all recommended activities for older adults. In addition, balance exercises should be included to help prevent the risk of falls and injury.

Weight

Overweight individuals are at higher risk of musculo-skeletal injuries due to increased stress on their muscles and joints, and they should take precautions to ensure safe workouts. If you are overweight, consider a cross-training routine with a mix of moderate weight-bearing (e.g., walking, stair-climbing) and non-weight-bearing (e.g., bicycling, water exercise) activities. If you feel pain in your lower-body joints during exercise, shift to more non-weight-bearing activities during your workout.

Underweight individuals, on the other hand, should perform more strength-training and weight-bearing activities to ensure proper muscle and bone maintenance.

Current Fitness Level

Design a program that is appropriate to your current fitness level. If you already exercise regularly, consider gradually increasing the frequency or intensity of your workouts to realize more fitness gains.

If you are currently sedentary and are just beginning to think about starting an exercise routine, do not just suddenly attempt to participate in a triathlon! Pick an activity that you find enjoyable, start at a level that is comfortable for you, and proceed from there.

Disabilities

If you have mobility restrictions, poor balance, dizziness, or other conditions that are physically limiting, you can still incorporate activity into your daily life with alternative or adaptive exercises. Many colleges, community centers, parks and recreation facilities, and fitness centers offer adaptive courses, equipment, and instructors who are specially trained to help you meet your fitness goals. After obtaining medical clearance, seek out such facilities; your physician or a physical therapist may have good recommendations. The box Getting Active Despite Disability provides additional suggestions.

Special Health Concerns

Certain medical conditions may require you to exercise under medical supervision. Individuals with asthma, heart disease, hypertension, and diabetes all need medical clearance prior to beginning exercise and may need to be monitored by medical personnel

Getting Active Despite Disability

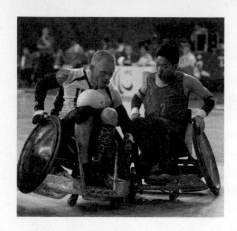

In the documentary film *Murderball*, muscular, aggressive rugby players compete in fierce, international competitions alongside other world-class athletes—all of them in wheelchairs. Their stories are an inspiration to disabled and nondisabled people alike, and demonstrate that while disability does pose undeniable obstacles, it does not have to hinder the achievement of even the highest levels of physical fitness.

With personal motivation, support from friends and family, and assistance from medical and fitness professionals, persons with disability can make exercise part of their daily routine and live physi-

cally active lives. In fact, the U.S. Department of Health and Human Services recommends that adults with disabilities follow the 2008 Physical Activity Guidelines for Americans, adjusting as necessary for varying abilities and physician recommendations.

There are various options available for modifying physical activities and helping all people achieve their health and fitness goals. For example, most strength-training machines are used from a seated position and can be operated by people in wheelchairs. Rubber exercise bands, meanwhile, can serve as alternative strength-building aids. Many companies offer modified sports equipment for people with disabilities: Handcycles allow people to ride bikes using arm power, and wakeboards and flotation devices enable waterskiing and swimming activities. Several kinds of seated skis make downhill skiing accessible to those with physical handicaps. And disabled people can play a long list of sports—with modified rules and equipment—including volleyball, tennis, golf, soccer, basketball, bowling, bocci, archery, tai chi, and karate.

---

during exercise. If you have special health concerns, seek out the advice of a qualified medical professional on how to exercise safely.

Individuals with significant bone or joint problems can benefit from selecting lower-impact activities such as swimming, water exercise, bicycling, walking, or low-impact aerobics. They can also benefit from resistance training exercises that can strengthen muscles and joint structures and contribute to bone-density maintenance and improvement (if their joint limitations will allow it).

If you are taking any prescription medications, ask your doctor whether there are side effects that you should consider before exercising. In addition, beware of over-the-counter medications and other products that may cause drowsiness (such as antihistamines, certain cough/cold medicines, and alcohol), as this will decrease your reaction time, coordination, and balance.

If you are pregnant, read the box Can I Exercise While I'm Pregnant? for advice on exercising safely while expecting.

How Can I Get Started Improving My Fitness Behaviors?

You know that exercise is good for you, but starting a fitness program and sticking with it over the long term can be a real challenge! According to a recent national survey, only 34 percent of adults in the United States participate in regular leisure-time physical activity.[17] College-aged adults (18 to 24 years) fared better, with 42 percent reporting regular physical activity patterns. The percentages drop as people age: Fewer than 27 percent of people 65 years and older reported regular leisure-time physical

Can I Exercise While I'm Pregnant?

Although pregnancy is not the time to start an intense fitness or weight-loss program, most pregnant women can maintain pre-pregnancy activities with just a few modifications. In fact, recent studies have shown that exercise during pregnancy benefits both the mother (improved cardiorespiratory function, decreased weight gain and discomfort, mood stability, and reduced gestational diabetes and high blood pressure risks) and fetus (improved stress tolerance and neurobehavioral maturation).[1] To exercise safely during pregnancy, follow the American College of Obstetricians and Gynecologists guidelines:[2]

• Get medical clearance for the activity you intend to do. Your physician may even have some specific recommendations for your fitness program.

• Seek out a pregnancy fitness exercise program where qualified instructors lead safe exercise sessions. These programs can also provide a good social support network for mothers-to-be.

• Choose fitness activities that do not increase risk of injury to you or the fetus. Avoid high-intensity sports, activities with the potential for falls or abdominal injury, and environmental extremes (such as temperature or barometric pressure—no scuba diving, in particular). Pay attention to your body temperature and avoid becoming too hot during exercise, especially during the first trimester. Choose low-impact activities such as swimming, water exercise, indoor cycling, yoga, and walking.

• In the absence of medical complications, perform at least 15 minutes of moderate exercise, gradually increasing to 30 minutes per day of accumulated moderate exercise. Aim for 150 minutes per week total.

• Monitor your exercise intensity levels by determining how you feel during exercise.

• In the third trimester, avoid supine exercises (i.e., exercises that require you to lie on your back), because these may restrict blood flow to the fetus.

• Do pelvic-floor exercises regularly. These exercises, called *kegels*, involve tightening the pelvic floor muscles for 5 to 15 seconds at a time; they will help with pregnancy-induced incontinence and delivery recovery. Add three to five sets of 10 to your daily routine.

Pregnancy can be both a wonder-filled and scary time. Maintaining a minimum level of fitness can help you cope with the stresses coming your way.

Sources:
1. K. Melzer and others, "Physical Activity and Pregnancy: Cardiovascular Adaptations, Recommendations and Pregnancy Outcomes," *Sports Medicine* 40, no. 6 (2010): 493–507.
2. American College of Obstetricians and Gynecologists, "ACOG Committee Opinion No. 267: Exercise during Pregnancy and the Postpartum Period," *Obstetrics & Gynecology* 99, no. 1 (2002): 171–173 (reaffirmed 2009).

activity. Despite the statistics, making fitness part of your daily life is within your reach—and can be tremendously fun and rewarding. However, preparing to exercise for the first time (or after a long sedentary period) can be daunting. If you are unsure how to start, what to do, or how much to exercise, you may have the impulse to just jump right in, do something your friends are doing, or try something you saw on TV or in a magazine. This haphazard approach often leads to disappointment and frustration—not to mention muscle soreness and even injury. A better approach is to think carefully about your exercise motivations, goals, and needs, select activities that will meet those needs (and that you enjoy!), apply the FITT formula to each of those activities, and then make a conscious long-term commitment to your exercise program.

As you plan your fitness program, ask yourself: what motivates you? What obstacles are in your way? What are reasonable fitness goals you can set for yourself? Are you prepared to commit to a fitness program? To begin, fill out **Lab 2.1** to assess your current readiness for a physical activity behavior change and to determine whether you need medical clearance to begin an exercise program.

Understand Your Motivations for Beginning a Fitness Program

If you understand your motivations for participating in a fitness program, you can plan activities in a way that makes you more likely to stick with the program. Below are some of the most common reasons people decide to exercise, along with tips for how to maximize your chances of long-term fitness success.

- *I want to gain health benefits.* If this is your main motivation, try to design a program centered on physical activities that you find enjoyable and easy to incorporate in your day-to-day life. If you don't like gyms, don't sign up for one! Instead, select an activity in which you genuinely take pleasure, such as walking with a friend or family member.

- *I want to have fun.* If your main motivation is fun, consider joining an intramural sports team on campus, or going on regular outdoor trips with friends. Seek out activities that, first and foremost, you know you will enjoy, and that have the beneficial "side effect" of fitness.

- *I want to meet new people or exercise with friends.* Participating in a fitness program can be a great way

to socialize. Even if you do not consider this one of your main reasons to start exercising, social motivations can often keep you coming back. Look for activity classes, clubs, or teams that you can join with friends or where you can meet new people with similar interests.

- *I like the challenge of setting goals and doing well in competition.* If this sounds like you, regardless of what activity you choose, be sure to set realistic, attainable goals. You may find a clearly defined target—such as an upcoming 5K race—to be just what you need to get started, so sign up!

- *I want to lose some weight.* If weight loss is your main motivation, you will need to consider your nutrition and diet plan along with your fitness plan. Choose fitness activities that burn plenty of calories and that you will enjoy doing often.

- *I would like to have a stronger, more toned body.* If this is your primary reason for exercise, select your favorite aerobic activity, begin strength training, or take a sport-specific class regularly.

Anticipate and Overcome Obstacles to Exercise

If you are not currently physically active, why not? Are you too busy? Do you simply dislike exercise? You can probably immediately identify several things that keep you from being as active as you want to be. Obstacles, or **barriers to physical activity**, can be categorized as either environmental or personal. *Environmental barriers* include both external/physical factors and social/interpersonal factors that may make it harder or easier for you to exercise. Do you feel safe exercising on the streets around your campus? Is the weather conducive to exercising? Are facilities open during the hours that you need them? Do you have friends who exercise and who might be interested in exercising with you? These external factors can greatly affect your exercise habits.

Likewise, *personal barriers* can play a role in whether you are successful in sticking to an exercise plan. Typical personal barriers include lack of self-motivation, injury, starting fitness levels and weight, disability, relationship difficulties, or psychological problems such as depression or anxiety. Older-than-average students, students with children, and those who work long hours while attending school often face unique challenges as they work to improve their fitness levels. The box Overcoming Common Obstacles to Exercise provides strategies for overcoming specific obstacles. **Lab 2.2** helps you assess your motivations for exercise and identify your obstacles to beginning a fitness program.

barriers to physical activity Personal or environmental issues that hinder your participation in regular physical activity

Make Time for Exercise

People often state that they don't exercise because they don't have enough time. That might be the case—or they may simply be assigning exercise a lesser priority in their life than other activities, such as watching TV or text-messaging friends. While socializing and scheduling downtime in a busy life *are* important, consider how much time you spend in your life on sedentary activities. Then consider the benefits to your health and sense of

TOOLS FOR **CHANGE** •

Overcoming Common Obstacles to Exercise

Below are lists of strategies for overcoming common obstacles to exercise.

Obstacle: Lack of Time

- Monitor your daily activities for one week. Identify at least three 30-minute time slots you could use for physical activity.

- Add physical activity to your daily routine. For example, walk or ride your bike to work or shopping, walk the dog, exercise while you watch TV, park farther away from your destination, and so on.

- Select activities requiring minimal time, such as walking, jogging, or stair-climbing.

Obstacle: Lack of Social Support

- Explain your interest in physical activity to friends and family. Ask them to support your efforts.

- Invite friends and family members to exercise with you. Plan social activities involving exercise.

- Develop new friendships with physically active people. Join a group, such as the YMCA or a hiking club.

Obstacle: Lack of Energy

- Schedule physical activity for times in the day or week when you feel energetic.

- Convince yourself that if you give it a chance, physical activity will increase your energy level; then try it.

Obstacle: Lack of Willpower

- Plan ahead. Make physical activity a regular part of your schedule and write it on your calendar.

- Invite a friend to exercise with you on a regular basis and write it on your calendar.

- Join an exercise group or class.

Obstacle: Fear of Injury

- Learn how to warm up and cool down to prevent injury.

- Learn how to exercise appropriately considering your age, fitness level, skill level, and health status.

- Choose activities involving minimum risk.

(Continued)

Obstacle: Lack of Skill

- Select activities requiring no new skills, such as walking, climbing stairs, or jogging.
- Exercise with friends who are at your skill level.
- Find a friend who is willing to teach you some new skills.
- Take a class to develop new skills.

Obstacle: Lack of Resources

- Select activities that require minimal facilities or equipment, such as walking, jogging, jumping rope, or calisthenics.
- Identify inexpensive, convenient resources available in your community (community education programs, park and recreation programs, worksite programs, etc.).

Obstacle: Weather Conditions

- Develop a set of regular activities that are always available regardless of weather (indoor cycling, aerobic dance, indoor swimming, stair-climbing, mall-walking, dancing, gymnasium games, etc.).

Obstacle: Travel

- Put a jump rope and resistance bands in your suitcase.
- Walk the halls and climb the stairs in hotels.
- Stay in places with swimming pools or exercise facilities.
- Join the YMCA or YWCA.
- Visit the local shopping mall and walk for half an hour or more.
- Pack your favorite aerobic exercise DVD.

Obstacle: Family Obligations

- Trade babysitting time with a friend, neighbor, or family member who also has small children.
- Exercise with the kids—go for a walk together, play tag or other running games, get an aerobic dance or exercise tape for kids and exercise together.
- Hire a babysitter and look at the cost as a worthwhile investment in your health.
- Jump rope, do calisthenics, ride a stationary bicycle, or use other home gymnasium equipment while the kids are busy playing or sleeping.
- Try to exercise when the kids are not around (e.g., during school hours or their nap time).

THINK! What are your main motivations to exercise? What are obstacles that you can anticipate?

ACT! For each obstacle, write down how you will get around it. Post reminders around your home and work to help you "stick" to your plan.

Source: Adapted from CDC, National Center for Chronic Disease Prevention and Health Promotion, Division of Nutrition, Physical Activity and Obesity, "Physical Activity for Everyone: Overcoming Barriers to Physical Activity," www.cdc.gov /physicalactivity/everyone/getactive/barriers.html (accessed January 2011).

well-being that would result if you replaced some of that sedentary time with physical activity.

To successfully stick with a fitness program, you need to prioritize exercise the same way that you prioritize your classes, homework, job, and social life. Schedule your exercise sessions into your calendar/appointment book. Prove to yourself that you are serious about getting fit by making the time for exercise. Get started by completing **Lab 2.3**, where you will make a plan to incorporate more physical activity into your daily life.

Select Fun and Convenient Activities

Even if you have committed to set aside time to exercise, you may not always *want* to. If you are accustomed to a sedentary lifestyle, it can be difficult to tear yourself away from the computer or to get off the couch. One way to counter a lack of motivation is to choose fun activities. If your workout is a form of play, you will look forward to it time and time again.

Choosing the best type of exercise is often also about convenience. Despite your good intentions and high level of motivation when starting a new activity, if it's not convenient for your existing lifestyle and commitments, you will have a hard time sticking with it. Look for activities, facilities, and workout times that make sense for your schedule.

Activities can be classified into three general categories or types: lifestyle physical activities, exercise training options, and sports and recreational activities.

Figure 2.5 illustrates sample moderate to vigorous lifestyle, exercise, and sports activities that you can choose from to meet activity guidelines and increase your fitness level.

Lifestyle Physical Activities Lifestyle physical activities are those that you perform during daily life. These include things such as walking the dog, bicycling to work, and so on. Lifestyle physical activities can be light, moderate, or vigorous, depending on what the task is and how long it takes you. For instance, watering your garden for 15 minutes may be a light activity, but raking leaves for four hours can be vigorous.

Exercise Training Options Most people think of typical exercise options when asked how they are going to increase their fitness. These include aerobics classes, jogging or running, weight training, indoor cardio workouts, yoga, tai chi, lap swimming, and water aerobics. These activities are great for specifically increasing your fitness. However, consider including a variety of activities to counter the boredom that may come from doing the same exercise week after week. Add a few sports and recreational activities every now and then to keep yourself motivated and your body challenged.

Sports and Recreational Activities Traditional team sports offer a great deal of fun, motivation, and fitness. Most cities have sports leagues for adult soccer, softball, basketball, ultimate Frisbee, and other team sports. If you like the camaraderie of working with a team and enjoy the challenge of team sports, strongly consider this option. You may be able to find team sports classes on campus, at community centers, and in sports clubs.

Individual sports activities can offer great fitness benefits as well. Court sports such as tennis, squash, and racquetball will increase your cardiorespiratory fitness and muscle endurance and will improve your agility, coordination, and reaction time. Many sports are recreational for some people but a competitive pastime for others.

If you are going to rely on a sport or recreational activity for your regular fitness routine, just make sure that it really is regular. For instance, skiing is great, but does not constitute a good fitness program if you only get to the mountain a few times a year. Golf, mountain biking, hiking, ice skating, and rock climbing are additional examples of recreational and competitive sports that can maintain or increase fitness if done regularly.

Choose Environments Conducive to Regular Exercise

A major obstacle to exercise for many people is having a suitable, convenient place to work out. The following are some factors to consider when deciding where to exercise.

Exercise Facility Options Exercise facilities are often located at colleges, community centers, health and fitness clubs, athletic and tennis clubs, parks and recreation facilities, YMCAs, corporate fitness centers, and

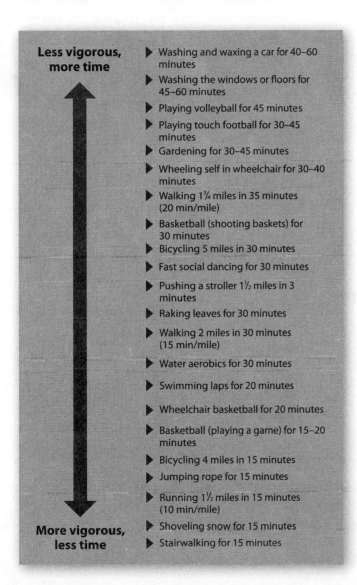

Less vigorous, more time

▶ Washing and waxing a car for 40–60 minutes
▶ Washing the windows or floors for 45–60 minutes
▶ Playing volleyball for 45 minutes
▶ Playing touch football for 30–45 minutes
▶ Gardening for 30–45 minutes
▶ Wheeling self in wheelchair for 30–40 minutes
▶ Walking 1¾ miles in 35 minutes (20 min/mile)
▶ Basketball (shooting baskets) for 30 minutes
▶ Bicycling 5 miles in 30 minutes
▶ Fast social dancing for 30 minutes
▶ Pushing a stroller 1½ miles in 3 minutes
▶ Raking leaves for 30 minutes
▶ Walking 2 miles in 30 minutes (15 min/mile)
▶ Water aerobics for 30 minutes
▶ Swimming laps for 20 minutes
▶ Wheelchair basketball for 20 minutes
▶ Basketball (playing a game) for 15–20 minutes
▶ Bicycling 4 miles in 15 minutes
▶ Jumping rope for 15 minutes
▶ Running 1½ miles in 15 minutes (10 min/mile)
▶ Shoveling snow for 15 minutes
▶ Stairwalking for 15 minutes

More vigorous, less time

FIGURE **2.5**   Sample moderate to vigorous physical activities.

Source: Centers for Disease Control and Prevention, "Physical Activity and Health: A Report of the Surgeon General," www.cdc.gov/nccdphp/sgr/ataglan.htm.

schools. Choosing a facility based upon its location is a good idea because the farther away a facility is from your home, the less likely you are to use it. Other things to consider when choosing a basic exercise facility are ease of parking (if you drive), variety of classes, quality of cardio and weight equipment, and hours that are compatible with your schedule. Additionally, you may be interested in facilities with a swimming pool, basketball and racquetball courts, locker rooms, showers, and spa.

Cost can be a big factor. Larger facilities with more offerings will likely be more expensive per month than a basic fitness center. Community centers and parks facilities often offer reasonable day use or multiday use fees. Almost all facilities offer day use passes for a fee, or even one-time free passes to check out the facility. Be sure to try the facility for several days to see whether you like the atmosphere, the equipment, and the instructors, and whether you feel safe and comfortable using the facility.

If you have not taken advantage of your college facilities yet, you may be missing out on a good deal. As a student, you can typically get access to classes, courts, leagues, equipment, and even personal trainers. College is the perfect time to try out new sports and activities.

Neighborhood When people live in safe neighborhoods where it is easy to exercise, they are more likely to be active.[18] This is becoming a bigger issue as growing cities and suburbs lead to a dramatic increase in urban sprawl. Some experts even suggest that urban sprawl is partially to blame for the rise in obesity in the United States in recent years. For example, researchers in New Jersey found that residents of sprawling counties were less likely to walk during leisure time, weighed more, and had high blood pressure more often than residents living in compact urban areas.[19] Living near streets that are conducive to physical activity (with sidewalks, bike lanes, street lights, slower traffic) and parks with bike and walking paths might make the difference between whether you stay regularly active or not.

Weather If you are an outside exerciser, the weather can create obstacles to regular physical activity. The impact of weather will, of course, depend on where you live and the time of year. If you are prepared, you can exercise in most weather conditions. Pay attention to your body. If you feel too hot when exercising outside, slow down, move into the shade, and consider suspending your workout for the day. Limit your exercise time in the rain if you become too wet and cold.

Safety Do you feel safe walking to the local gym to exercise? Do you feel comfortable jogging around your neighborhood? The box Adjusting to Your Environment presents tips for exercising safely in different environments.

TOOLS FOR **CHANGE** ●

Adjusting to Your Environment

In order to maintain a regular exercise routine, you need to feel safe and comfortable in your surroundings. Below are some suggestions for exercising safely in different environments:

- If your neighborhood is not safe, consider exercising with a friend or training group, or consider driving to a different nearby neighborhood to exercise.

- If you are exercising where there are many cars, wear bright clothing and face traffic when walking or running. Seek out areas that are less busy and where speed limits are lower.

- If you are heading into a wilderness area for a hike, trail run, or mountain-bike ride, plan your outing with a friend, or at least let someone know specifically where you are going and when you will return. Know your route and carry a map, a cell phone, and basic safety supplies, including food and water for at least a day, a flashlight or headlamp, first-aid supplies, a pocketknife, and a space or emergency blanket.

- Exercise facilities are typically safe places to work out. If you have any concerns for your safety in the locker room, workout areas, parking areas, or anywhere around the building, talk to the manager and get an escort to your car at night.

● ●

casestudy

LILY

"I've been following my new jogging routine for three weeks, but now the weather is cold and I cannot get motivated to run! I don't want to give up running but I don't live close to a gym and cannot afford a home treadmill. I just heard about a running group that uses the local track once a week and I know the school has a jogging and running class. Maybe I should try one of those to keep my motivation up and my running program on track? Perhaps I will meet someone I can run with that is just my speed."

THINK! What is Lily doing to increase her chances of sticking to her new exercise plans? What are three things you can do to make exercise a regular part of your life?

ACT! At the beginning of the chapter Lily asked ". . . *what does it actually mean to be fit?*" Given what you have explored in this chapter, write an answer to that question for yourself.

. . . .

Set Reasonable Goals for Increased Fitness

Setting appropriate, realistic goals can mean the difference between success and failure in fitness programming. People often start a fitness program and think they can train to run a 10k in three weeks—an unrealistic goal for a beginning exerciser. Make sure your goals are realistic; you may want to start with the sample plans in Activate, Motivate, & Advance Your Fitness: A Walking Program in this chapter (page 64). As you begin a fitness program, your progress may initially be slow, while your body adjusts to the new activity. Setting reasonable goals includes considering everything that you have assessed about yourself: your fitness level when you begin, your reasons for exercise, your motivations and attitudes about physical activity, and the constraints that other aspects of your life may impose.

Plan Your Rewards If you find yourself unmotivated to become active, try coming up with goal-related rewards to motivate yourself. Rewards can be highly individual; after all, different things motivate different people. The key is to come up with rewards that reinforce your new, more active lifestyle. A common reward for people trying to lose weight, for example, is to shop for new clothes. But rewards do not necessarily have to be material. If competition or personal challenge motivate you, for example, you may find the exhilaration of finishing a half-marathon or completing a race in the top 10 percent of contenders to be considerable reward of its own.

> **internal exercise rewards**
> Rewards for exercise that are based upon how one is feeling physically and mentally (sense of accomplishment, relaxation, increased self-esteem)
>
> **external exercise rewards**
> Rewards for exercise that come from outside of a person (trophy, compliment, day at the spa)

Rewards can be internal or external. **Internal exercise rewards** commonly involve feeling better about yourself, feeling healthier, and having better life satisfaction from exercising. Long-term exercisers often report that internal exercise rewards are their primary motivation. Studies have shown that exercise releases endorphins in your body that can fill you with a sense of well-being.[20] For many long-term exercisers, the physical activity itself is truly its own reward. New exercisers, however, often rely on **external exercise rewards**—at least initially. External exercise rewards can be anything from a new workout wardrobe to a celebratory dinner to the admiration and praise of your peers or fitness instructor.

As you incorporate regular physical activity and exercise into your lifestyle, you may find that just having fun and feeling good while exercising is reward enough. If this switch to an internal reward motivation does not happen right away, keep setting external rewards to keep yourself motivated until it does. Don't be surprised if the switch happens faster than you think.

Make a Personal Commitment to Regular Exercise

Deciding that you are going to lead a more physically active lifestyle is the first step to changing your exercise behaviors. The harder step is to commit to that decision. Examine what a more active lifestyle would mean to you and write out your personal commitment statement: a list of reasons to commit to fitness. Review this list regularly until your new behaviors become routine.

Remember that changing behavior takes perseverance. If you feel your commitment flagging, reread your personal commitment statement and remind yourself of the reasons you began your program in the first place.

chapterin**review**

videos

Log on to **www.pearsonhighered.com/hopson** or MyFitnessLab to view these chapter-related videos.
Personal Fitness and Exercise

onlineresources

Log on to **www.pearsonhighered.com/hopson** or MyFitnessLab for access to these book-related resources, and for links to other useful websites.

 Audio case study
Audio PowerPoint lecture

 Customizable 4-week walking programs
Take Charge of Your Health! Worksheets:
  Worksheet 26 How Much Do I Move?
Behavior Change Log Book and Wellness
Journal

 Lab 2.1 Assess Your Physical Activity
Readiness
Lab 2.2 Identify Your Physical Activity
Motivations and Obstacles
Lab 2.3 Changing Your Sedentary Time into
Active Time

 Pre- and post-quizzes
Glossary flashcards

reviewquestions

1. Moderate physical activity is best defined as activity that is
   a. less than 3 METS.
   b. 3–6 METS.
   c. 7–9 METS.
   d. over 10 METS.

2. Which health-related component of fitness involves moving your joints through a full range of motion?
   a. Cardiorespiratory fitness
   b. Muscular endurance
   c. Flexibility
   d. Body composition

3. Which skill-related component of fitness is most involved in braking quickly when a car in front of you stops suddenly?
   a. Agility
   b. Power
   c. Coordination
   d. Reaction time

4. The principle of individuality with respect to fitness states that
   a. adaptations to training overload may vary widely from person to person.
   b. all individuals respond the same way to exercise.
   c. genetic makeup has nothing to do with individual responses to exercise.
   d. nonresponders are individuals who do not benefit from exercise.

5. The 2008 Physical Activity Guidelines for Americans emphasize
   a. vigorous physical activity every day of the week.
   b. moderate physical activity for 150 minutes per week or vigorous physical activity for 75 minutes per week.
   c. resistance training for 300 minutes per week.
   d. limiting the amount of time you spend walking.

6. A proper warm-up consists of
   a. a few quick side bends.
   b. stretches that you hold for one minute or more.
   c. quick stair climbing.
   d. a gradual increase in body temperature and easy movements in the muscles and joints.

7. Experiencing knee pain can be categorized as having a(n) _____ barrier to physical activity.
   a. social
   b. scheduling
   c. environmental
   d. personal

8. Which of the following is an example of an internal exercise reward?
   a. Buying new workout clothing
   b. Having fun while exercising
   c. Placing third in your age group in the local 5K race
   d. Taking a celebratory trip after meeting an exercise goal

9. Which of the following is least likely to result in a successful long-term exercise routine?
   a. Making exercise a priority in your weekly schedule
   b. Setting up rewards for yourself
   c. Selecting fun and convenient activities
   d. Forcing yourself to go to a gym even though you don't enjoy it

10. Which fitness principle refers to subjecting the body or body system to more physical activity than it is accustomed to?
   a. Overload
   b. Adaptation
   c. Dose-response
   d. Specificity

critical**thinking**questions

 REVIEW IT! ONLINE

1. Give an example of how a training overload can lead to adaptations and training effects.
2. Describe the similarities and differences between the principle of diminished returns and the principle of progression.
3. Imagine you are about to begin a fitness program centered on bicycling. Apply the FITT formula to describe how you might set up your program.

4. If you are reluctant to increase your activity level due to fear of injury, what are five strategies that will help you overcome those fears and avoid injury?
5. Explain the difference between internal and external exercise rewards.

references

1. M. R. Carnethon, M. Gulati, and P. Greenland, "Prevalence and Cardiovascular Disease Correlates of Low Cardiorespiratory Fitness in Adolescents and Adults," *The Journal of the American Medical Association* 294, no. 23 (2005): 2981–88.
2. H. Suominen, "Muscle Training for Bone Strength," Aging *Clinical and Experimental Research* 18, no. 2 (2006): 85–93.
3. K. Small, L. McNaughton, and M. Matthews, "A Systematic Review Into the Efficacy of Static Stretching as Part of a Warm-Up for the Prevention of Exercise-Related Injury," *Research in Sports Medicine* 16, no. 3 (2008): 213–31.
4. L. O. Mikkelsson and others, "Adolescent Flexibility, Endurance Strength, and Physical Activity as Predictors of Adult Tension Neck, Low Back Pain, and Knee Injury: A 25 Year Follow Up Study," *British Journal of Sports Medicine* 40, no. 2 (2006): 107–13.
5. M. J. Spink and others, "Foot and Ankle Strength, Range of Motion, Posture, and Deformity Are Associated with Balance and Functional Ability in Older Adults," *Archives of Physical Medicine and Rehabilitation* 92, no. 1 (2011): 68–75.
6. T. D. Brutsaert and E. J. Parra. "What Makes a Champion? Explaining Variation in Human Athletic Performance." *Respiratory Physiology and Neurobiology* 151, no. 2–3 (2006): 109–23.
7. W. D. McArdle, F. I. Katch, and V. L. Katch, *Exercise Physiology: Energy, Nutrition, and Human Performance*, 7th Edition, (Baltimore: Lippincott Williams & Wilkins, 2010); K. Kubo and others, "Time Course of Changes in Muscle and Tendon Properties During Strength Training and Detraining," *Journal of Strength and Conditioning Research* 24, no. 2 (2010): 322–31.
8. Office of Disease Prevention and Health Promotion, U.S. Department of Health and Human Services, *2008 Physical Activity Guidelines for Americans: Be Active, Healthy, and Happy!* ODPHP Publication no. U0036 (Washington, DC: U.S. Department of Health and Human Services, 2008).
9. World Health Organization, "Global Recommendations on Physical Activity for Health," Global Strategy on Diet, Physical Activity and Health, www.who.int/dietphysicalactivity/factsheet_recommendations/en/index.html (accessed January 31, 2011).
10. C. E. Garner and others, "American College of Sports Medicine Position Stand: Quantity and Quality of Exercise for Developing and Maintaining Cardiorespiratory, Musculoskeletal, and Neuromotor Fitness in Apparently Healthy Adults: Guidance for Prescribing Exercise," *Medicine and Science in Sports and Exercise* 43, no. 7 (2011): 1334–59.
11. National Center for Health Statistics, Health Promotion Statistics Branch, CDC Wonder, *DATA2010 … the Healthy People 2010 Database* (Hyattsville, MD: Centers for Disease Control, 2009) http://wonder.cdc.gov/data2010/focus.htm (accessed January 2011).
12. Office of Disease Prevention and Health Promotion, U.S. Department of Health and Human Services, Healthy People 2020, "2020 Objectives and Goals: Physical Activity," http://healthypeople.gov/2020/topicsobjectives2020/objectiveslist.aspx?topicId=33 (2011).
13. J. M. Conn, J. L. Annest, and J. Gilchrist, "Sports and Recreation Related Injury Episodes in the U.S. Population, 1997–99," *Injury Prevention* 9, no. 2 (2003): 117–23.
14. M. N. Sawka and others, "American College of Sports Medicine Position Stand: Exercise and Fluid Replacement," *Medicine and Science in Sports and Exercise* 39, no. 2 (2007): 377–90.
15. H. H. Fink, A. E. Mikesky, and L. A. Burgoon, *Practical Applications in Sports Nutrition*. 2nd Edition (Sudbury, MA: Jones and Bartlett Publishers, 2009).
16. American College of Sports Medicine, *ACSM's Guidelines for Exercise Testing and Prescription*, 8th Edition (Baltimore: Lippincott Williams & Wilkins, 2010).
17. B. W. Ward and others, "Early Release of Selected Estimates Based on Data from the January–June 2010 National Health Interview Survey," National Center for Health Statistics, www.cdc.gov/nchs/nhis/released201012.htm (December 2010).

18. J. F. Sallis and K. Glanz, "The Role of Built Environments in Physical Activity, Eating, and Obesity in Childhood," *The Future of Children* 16, no. 1 (2006): 89–108; H. M. Grow and others, "Where Are Youth Active? Roles of Proximity, Active Transport, and Built Environment," *Medicine and Science in Sports and Exercise* 40, no. 12 (2008): 2071–9.

19. R. Ewing and others, "Relationship between Urban Sprawl and Physical Activity, Obesity, and Morbidity," *American Journal of Health Promotion* 18, no. 1 (2003): 47–57.

20. L. Carrasco, C. Villaverde, and C. M. Oltras, "Endorphin Responses to Stress Induced by Competitive Swimming Event," *The Journal of Sports Medicine and Physical Fitness* 47, no. 2 (2007): 239–45.

LAB 2.1 • ASSESS YOUR PHYSICAL ACTIVITY READINESS

Name: _____ Date: _____

Instructor: _____ Section: _____

SECTION I: THE PHYSICAL ACTIVITY READINESS QUESTIONNAIRE

Physical Activity Readiness
Questionnaire - PAR-Q
(revised 2002)

PAR-Q & YOU

(A Questionnaire for People Aged 15 to 69)

Regular physical activity is fun and healthy, and increasingly more people are starting to become more active every day. Being more active is very safe for most people. However, some people should check with their doctor before they start becoming much more physically active.

If you are planning to become much more physically active than you are now, start by answering the seven questions in the box below. If you are between the ages of 15 and 69, the PAR-Q will tell you if you should check with your doctor before you start. If you are over 69 years of age, and you are not used to being very active, check with your doctor.

Common sense is your best guide when you answer these questions. Please read the questions carefully and answer each one honestly: check YES or NO.

YES	NO		
☐	☐	1.	Has your doctor ever said that you have a heart condition <u>and</u> that you should only do physical activity recommended by a doctor?
☐	☐	2.	Do you feel pain in your chest when you do physical activity?
☐	☐	3.	In the past month, have you had chest pain when you were not doing physical activity?
☐	☐	4.	Do you lose your balance because of dizziness or do you ever lose consciousness?
☐	☐	5.	Do you have a bone or joint problem (for example, back, knee or hip) that could be made worse by a change in your physical activity?
☐	☐	6.	Is your doctor currently prescribing drugs (for example, water pills) for your blood pressure or heart condition?
☐	☐	7.	Do you know of <u>any other reason</u> why you should not do physical activity?

If

you

answered

YES to one or more questions

Talk with your doctor by phone or in person BEFORE you start becoming much more physically active or BEFORE you have a fitness appraisal. Tell your doctor about the PAR-Q and which questions you answered YES.

• You may be able to do any activity you want — as long as you start slowly and build up gradually. Or, you may need to restrict your activities to those which are safe for you. Talk with your doctor about the kinds of activities you wish to participate in and follow his/her advice.

• Find out which community programs are safe and helpful for you.

NO to all questions

If you answered NO honestly to <u>all</u> PAR-Q questions, you can be reasonably sure that you can:

• start becoming much more physically active – begin slowly and build up gradually. This is the safest and easiest way to go.

• take part in a fitness appraisal – this is an excellent way to determine your basic fitness so that you can plan the best way for you to live actively. It is also highly recommended that you have your blood pressure evaluated. If your reading is over 144/94, talk with your doctor before you start becoming much more physically active.

→

DELAY BECOMING MUCH MORE ACTIVE:

• if you are not feeling well because of a temporary illness such as a cold or a fever — wait until you feel better; or

• if you are or may be pregnant — talk to your doctor before you start becoming more active.

PLEASE NOTE: If your health changes so that you then answer YES to any of the above questions, tell your fitness or health professional. Ask whether you should change your physical activity plan.

<u>Informed Use of the PAR-Q</u>: The Canadian Society for Exercise Physiology, Health Canada, and their agents assume no liability for persons who undertake physical activity, and if in doubt after completing this questionnaire, consult your doctor prior to physical activity.

No changes permitted. You are encouraged to photocopy the PAR-Q but only if you use the entire form.

NOTE: If the PAR-Q is being given to a person before he or she participates in a physical activity program or a fitness appraisal, this section may be used for legal or administrative purposes.

"I have read, understood and completed this questionnaire. Any questions I had were answered to my full satisfaction."

NAME _____

SIGNATURE _____ DATE _____

SIGNATURE OF PARENT _____ WITNESS _____
or GUARDIAN (for participants under the age of majority)

Note: This physical activity clearance is valid for a maximum of 12 months from the date it is completed and becomes invalid if your condition changes so that you would answer YES to any of the seven questions.

CSEP
SCPE © Canadian Society for Exercise Physiology   Supported by: 🍁 Health   Santé
                                                                   Canada   Canada

Source: *Physical Activity Readiness Questionnaire (PAR-Q)* © 2002. Used with permission from the Canadian Society for Exercise Physiology. www.csep.ca.

SECTION II: HEALTH/FITNESS PRE-PARTICIPATION SCREENING QUESTIONNAIRE

Assess your health status by indicating all TRUE statements:

History—You have had:

_____ a heart attack

_____ heart surgery

_____ cardiac catheterization

_____ coronary angioplasty

_____ pacemaker/implantable cardiac defibrillator

_____ heart rhythm disturbance

_____ heart valve disease

_____ heart failure

_____ heart transplantation

_____ congenital heart disease

Symptoms:

_____ You experience chest discomfort with exertion.

_____ You experience unreasonable breathlessness.

_____ You experience dizziness, fainting, or blackouts.

_____ You take heart medications.

Other Health Issues:

_____ You have diabetes.

_____ You have asthma or other lung disease.

_____ You have burning or cramping sensations in your lower legs when walking short distances.

_____ You have musculoskeletal problems that limit your physical activity.

_____ You have concerns about the safety of exercise.

_____ You take prescription medication(s).

_____ You are pregnant.

If any of the above statements are true for you, consult your physician or other appropriate health care provider before engaging in exercise. You may need to use a facility with a medically qualified staff.

Cardiovascular Risk Factors:

_____ You are a man older than 45 years old.

_____ You are a woman older than 55 years, have had a hysterectomy, or are postmenopausal.

_____ You smoke, or quit smoking within the previous six months.

_____ Your blood pressure is higher than 140/90 mmHg.

_____ You do not know your blood pressure.

_____ You take blood pressure medication.

_____ Your blood cholesterol level is higher than 200 mg/dL.

_____ You do not know your cholesterol level.

_____ You have a close blood relative who had a heart attack or heart surgery before age 55 (father or brother) or age 65 (mother or sister).

_____ You are physically inactive (i.e., you get less than 30 minutes of physical activity on at least 3 days/week).

_____ You are more than 20 pounds overweight.

If you marked two or more of the statements in this section, you should consult your physician or other appropriate health care provider before engaging in exercise. You might benefit from using a facility with a professionally qualified exercise staff to guide your exercise program.

If you did not mark any of the above statements, you should not need medical clearance to exercise safely in a properly designed self-guided exercise program.

Source: American College of Sports Medicine, *ACSM's Guidelines for Exercise Testing and Prescription*, 8th ed. Lippincott Williams & Wilkins, Baltimore, MD, 2010.

SECTION III: PHYSICAL ACTIVITY STAGES OF CHANGE QUESTIONNAIRE

1. After carefully reading each of the following statements, please answer **YES** or **NO**.

(1) I am currently physically active.*	**NO**	**YES**
(2) I intend to become more physically active in the next six months.	**NO**	**YES**
(3) I currently engage in regular** physical activity.	**NO**	**YES**
(4) I have been regularly physically active for the past six months.	**NO**	**YES**

* Physical activity or exercise: Activities such as walking briskly, jogging, bicycling, swimming, or any other activity in which the exertion is at least as intense as these activities.

** Regular activity: Activity that adds up to a total of 30 minutes or more per day and is done at least five days per week.

2. Identify your physical activity stage of change (circle your stage):

→ If you answered NO to questions 1 and 2, you are in **PRECONTEMPLATION.**

(To move toward behavior change, it is important at this stage to start thinking about physical activity and its benefits.)

→ If you answered NO to question 1 and YES to question 2, you are in **CONTEMPLATION.**

(In order to move into preparation, you must gain information about how to get started moving toward your goal.)

→ If you answered YES to question 1 and NO to question 3, you are in **PREPARATION.**

(In this stage, it is important to remove barriers that are preventing regular physical activity.)

→ If you answered YES to questions 1 and 3, but NO to question 4, you are in **ACTION.**

(In order to maintain your new behavior, in this stage you need to track your progress, maintain your motivation, and head off potential relapses before they occur.)

→ If you answered YES to questions 1, 3, and 4, you are in **MAINTENANCE.**

(To keep your active lifestyle habits, try new activities and cross-training, make it fun, and strive to keep a consistent program despite life's obstacles.)

Source: B. H. Marcus and B. A. Lewis, "Physical Activity and the Stages of Motivational Readiness for Change Model," *President's Council on Physical Fitness and Sports Research Digest* 4, no.1 (2003): 1–8.

LAB 2.2 • IDENTIFY YOUR PHYSICAL ACTIVITY MOTIVATIONS AND OBSTACLES

Name: _____ **Date:** _____

Instructor: _____ **Section:** _____

Purpose: To identify your motivations for starting a physical activity, exercise, or sport (or maintaining your current fitness routine) and your obstacles to exercise, plus learn how to set up exercise-specific rewards to overcome those obstacles.

SECTION I: WHAT MOTIVATES YOU?

Assign a rating of 1–7 for each of the motivations listed below, using the following scale: 1 = not at all true, 7 = very true

I participate (or want to participate) in my physical activity or sport because:

_____ **1.** I want to be physically fit.

_____ **2.** It's fun.

_____ **3.** I like engaging in activities that physically challenge me.

_____ **4.** I want to obtain new skills.

_____ **5.** I want to maintain my weight and/or look better.

_____ **6.** I want to be with my friends.

_____ **7.** I like to do this activity.

_____ **8.** I want to improve existing skills.

_____ **9.** I like the challenge.

_____ **10.** I want to define my muscles so that I look better.

_____ **11.** It makes me happy.

_____ **12.** I want to keep up my current skill level.

_____ **13.** I want to have more energy.

_____ **14.** I like activities which are physically challenging.

_____ **15.** I like to be with others who are interested in this activity.

_____ **16.** I want to improve my cardiovascular fitness.

_____ **17.** I want to improve my appearance.

_____ **18.** I think it's interesting.

_____ **19.** I want to maintain my physical strength to live a healthy life.

_____ **20.** I want to be attractive to others.

_____ **21.** I want to meet new people.

_____ **22.** I enjoy this activity.

_____ **23.** I want to maintain my physical health and well-being.

_____ **24.** I want to improve my body shape.

_____ **25.** I want to get better at my activity.

_____ **26.** I find this activity stimulating.

_____ **27.** I will feel physically unattractive if I don't.

_____ **28.** My friends want me to.

_____ **29.** I like the excitement of participation.

_____ **30.** I enjoy spending time with others doing this activity.

SECTION II: SCORING MOTIVATIONS

Fill in your scores for the questions above in the appropriate boxes (for example, in the box for "Q 2," enter the numerical value you answered for question #2). Then add the totals for each type of motivation. Your total scores reflect which category motivates you the most.

Motivation Type	Interest/ Enjoyment	Competence	Appearance	Fitness	Social
	Q 2:	Q 3:	Q 5:	Q 1:	Q 6:
	Q 7:	Q 4:	Q 10:	Q 13:	Q 15:
	Q 11:	Q 8:	Q 17:	Q 16:	Q 21:
	Q 18:	Q 9:	Q 20:	Q 19:	Q 28:
	Q 22:	Q 12:	Q 24:	Q 23:	Q 30:
	Q 26:	Q 14:	Q 27:		
	Q 29:	Q 25:			
Totals:					

Source: R. M. Ryan, C. M. Frederick, D. Lepes, N. Rubio, and K. M. Sheldon, "Intrinsic Motivation and Exercise Adherence," *International Journal of Sport Psychology* 28 (1997): 335–354; C. M. Frederick and R. M. Ryan, "Differences in Motivation for Sport and Exercise and Their Relationships with Participation and Mental Health," *Journal of Sport Behavior* 16 (1993): 125–145.

SECTION III: WHAT KEEPS YOU FROM BEING ACTIVE?

Listed below are common reasons that people give to describe why they do not get as much physical activity as they would like. Read each statement and indicate how likely you are to state the same reason.

How likely are you to say?	Very likely	Somewhat likely	Somewhat unlikely	Very unlikely
1. My day is so busy now, I just don't think I can make the time to include physical activity in my regular schedule.	3	2	1	0
2. None of my family members or friends like to do anything active, so I don't have a chance to exercise.	3	2	1	0
3. I'm just too tired after work to get any exercise.	3	2	1	0
4. I've been thinking about getting more exercise, but I just can't seem to get started.	3	2	1	0
5. I'm getting older, so exercise can be risky.	3	2	1	0
6. I don't get enough exercise because I have never learned the skills for any sport.	3	2	1	0
7. I don't have access to jogging trails, swimming pools, bike paths, etc.	3	2	1	0
8. Physical activity takes too much time away from other commitments—work, family, etc.	3	2	1	0
9. I'm embarrassed about how I will look when I exercise with others.	3	2	1	0
10. I don't get enough sleep as it is. I just couldn't get up early or stay up late to get some exercise.	3	2	1	0
11. It's easier for me to find excuses not to exercise than to go out to do something.	3	2	1	0
12. I know of too many people who have hurt themselves by overdoing it with exercise.	3	2	1	0
13. I really can't see learning a new sport at my age.	3	2	1	0
14. It's just too expensive. You have to take a class or join a club or buy the right equipment.	3	2	1	0
15. My free periods during the day are too short to include exercise.	3	2	1	0
16. My usual social activities with family or friends do not include physical activity.	3	2	1	0
17. I'm too tired during the week, and I need the weekend to catch up on my rest.	3	2	1	0
18. I want to get more exercise, but I just can't seem to make myself stick to anything.	3	2	1	0
19. I'm afraid I might injure myself or have a heart attack.	3	2	1	0
20. I'm not good enough at any physical activity to make it fun.	3	2	1	0
21. If we had exercise facilities and showers at work, then I would be more likely to exercise.	3	2	1	0

Source: Centers for Disease Control and Prevention, "Barriers to Being Active Quiz," www.cdc.gov/nccdphp/dnpa/physical/life/barriers_quiz.pdf (accessed May 2, 2011).

SECTION IV: SCORING OBSTACLES

Follow these instructions to score your answers in Section III:

• Enter the circled number in the spaces provided, putting together the number for statement 1 on line 1, statement 2 on line 2, and so on.

• Add the three scores on each line. Your obstacles to physical activity fall into one or more of seven categories below. Circle any physical activity obstacles category with a score of 5 or above, because this is an important obstacle for you to overcome.

_____ +	_____ +	_____ =	_____
1	8	15	**Lack of time**
_____ +	_____ +	_____ =	_____
2	9	16	**Social influence**
_____ +	_____ +	_____ =.	_____
3	10	17	**Lack of energy**
_____ +	_____ +	_____ =	_____
4	11	18	**Lack of willpower**
_____ +	_____ +	_____ =	_____
5	12	19	**Fear of injury**
_____ +	_____ +	_____ =	_____
6	13	20	**Lack of skill**
_____ +	_____ +	_____ =	_____
7	14	21	**Lack of resources**

SECTION V: OVERCOME OBSTACLES TO EXERCISE

1. Do the results surprise you? Explain why or why not.

_____

_____

_____

2. How can you use these results to increase your likelihood of starting or sticking with an exercise program? What strategies can you think of to overcome your personal obstacles to exercise?

_____

_____

_____

LAB 2.3 • CHANGING YOUR SEDENTARY TIME INTO ACTIVE TIME

Name: _____ Date: _____

Instructor: _____ Section: _____

Purpose: To create a plan for reducing your sedentary time and replacing it with active time.

Directions:

1. On Worksheet A, list your typical activity for each hour of your day in the column labeled "Activity."

Worksheet A

Time of Day	Activity	Revised Activity
6:00 AM		
7:00 AM		
8:00 AM		
9:00 AM		
10:00 AM		
11:00 AM		
12:00 PM		
1:00 PM		
2:00 PM		
3:00 PM		
4:00 PM		
5:00 PM		
6:00 PM		
7:00 PM		
8:00 PM		
9:00 PM		
10:00 PM		
11:00 PM		

2. Now examine your list. What are your major sedentary activities? Highlight or circle them on Worksheet A.

3. List three physical activities that you would like to do but typically don't have time to do:

_____

_____

_____

4. Go back to Worksheet A and examine the sedentary activities you highlighted or circled in #2. Can you replace some of these sedentary activities with any of the physical activities you listed in #3? If so, write in the revised activity (in the "Revised Activity" column) next to the sedentary activity it is replacing.

5. If the physical activities you'd like to add to your schedule won't work in the time slots you have allotted for sedentary activity (for example, it may not be possible or safe to go out running at 11:30 PM), what are alternative physical activities you can safely pursue? Write them in.

activate, motivate,& ADVANCE YOUR FITNESS

A WALKING PROGRAM

ACTIVATE!

Walking is the most popular fitness activity in the United States and worldwide. If you are not currently active, walking is one of the best ways to start; you can participate at your own level, minimal equipment is required, and you can do the activity just about anywhere!

What Do I need for Walking?

SHOES: Obtain good-quality shoes. Visit a local running and walking store to get fitted for walking shoes or running shoes (which also work well for walking). A good fit is one of the most important determinants of the right shoe for you.

CLOTHING: Wear comfortable, non-restrictive clothing and cushioned socks that prevent blisters (avoid all-cotton socks). If you are walking outside, wear the right clothing for the weather, be it light clothing in the heat, waterproof clothing in the rain and snow, or warm clothing in the winter; dressing in layers is always a good idea. During the daytime wear sunscreen, sunglasses, and a hat; if you are walking outside at sunrise, dusk, or dark, wear reflective clothing and/or vest and lights.

How Do I Start a Walking Program?

HEALTH WALKING TECHNIQUE & SKILLS: Walking for *health* involves a basic walking stride with a focus on posture. Keep your head up and look straight ahead. Make sure that your shoulders are over your hips and you are not leaning too far forward or backward. Swing your arms easily at your sides, keeping your shoulders down and relaxed. Take natural strides and avoid overstriding (stepping out too far). Focus on being "light" on your feet; particularly avoid slapping your toes down. Instead, control your feet and roll your foot forward.

FITNESS WALKING TECHNIQUE & SKILLS: Increasing your walking pace for *fitness* involves a few adjustments to your walking stride. Follow the basic posture and foot recommendations above but add the following changes. Bend your elbows at ninety degrees and swing your arms in time with your stride. Avoid letting your elbows "chicken-wing" out to the side; instead, keep your elbows close to you. Your hands (in a loose fist) should swing from your lower chest back to your hips. Remember that the faster you swing your arms, the faster your legs will go to keep up! Shorten your stride and take faster steps instead of longer steps. Keep your light heel strike but exaggerate the roll through your foot even more.

Forcefully press off your toes with each stride to propel you forward.

Walking Tips

STREET AND TRAIL WALKING: Plan safe and interesting walking routes considering traffic and available walking paths. You can use an online mapping program to figure out your distance or to create a new route and calculate the distance. Carry a cell phone, ID, a few dollars, and a water bottle. Walk with a partner, if possible, and avoid wearing headphones or wear only one earpiece at a time. Always be aware of your surroundings and walk on the left facing traffic if possible. Follow traffic laws and do not assume that a car or bike operator has seen you.

TRACK WALKING: Walking on a track provides a nice flat, stable surface with a measured distance to walk. If you have a track near you, ensure that it is safe and that you have access to it. Most tracks are 400 meters around, with 4 laps being equal to a mile (on the innermost lane). When on the track, follow track etiquette by utilizing outside lanes for most of your training and leaving the inside lane (lane 1) for runners and sprinters or for timing yourself on a distance. If you are using the inside lane and a faster individual approaches behind you, move out to lane 2 or 3 to allow the person to pass on the inside.

TREADMILL WALKING: Walking inside on a treadmill can be a great option when the weather outside prohibits safe walking. When using the treadmill be sure to familiarize yourself with the controls before starting out. Learn to use the shut-off button (usually a large red button) and as a back-up wear the emergency shut-off clip on your clothing. Keep your body upright and avoid using the handrails or leaning forward too much. Keep your body in the center of the treadmill near the console. Most treadmills have pre-programmed workouts but you can also adjust the speed and incline manually. Start and stop by gradually increasing and decreasing the speed. When you finish, be careful exiting the treadmill; your legs may feel strange on the "non-moving" ground.

Walking Warm-Up and Cool-Down

A walking warm-up and cool-down include walking at a slower pace for three to ten minutes. After breaking a slight sweat in the warm-up, you can add range of motion exercises and 10- to 15-second light stretches. When you finish your walk, you can hold stretches longer for improved flexibility. In particular, focus on stretching the following muscle groups: quadriceps, hamstrings, gluteals, lower back, abductors, gastrocnemius, tibialis anterior, and the pectorals (see Chapter 5 for specific stretches to perform).

Four-Week Starter Walking Program

If you have been sedentary for a long time and need to start slowly, start with Program A below. If you are already able to walk 10–15 minutes continuously on three days a week, start with Program B below. Adjust time, intensity, and days of the walks to suit your personal fitness level and schedule; visit the companion website for customizable versions of these programs.

PROGRAM A **GOAL:** To walk 15–20 minutes continuously, 3–4 days a week

	Mon		Tue		Wed		Thurs		Fri		Sat		Sun	
	T*	I*	T	I	T	I	T	I	T	I	T	I	T	I
Week 1	5	L			5	L			8	M				
Week 2	5	L			8	M			10	M	8	M		
Week 3	10	M			12	M			10	M	12	M		
Week 4	15	M			15	M			20	M	15	M		

T*: Time. Total time is listed in minutes. Time does not include warm-up or cool-down time.
I*: Intensity. Intensity is listed as Light/Lifestyle (L), Moderate (M), or Vigorous (V) (see Figure 2.1).

PROGRAM B **GOAL:** To walk 25–30 minutes continuously, 4–5 days a week

	Mon		Tue		Wed		Thurs		Fri		Sat		Sun	
	T*	I*	T	I	T	I	T	I	T	I	T	I	T	I
Week 1	15	M			15	M			20	M				
Week 2	18	M			20	M			22	V	20	M		
Week 3	22	M	20	M	18	M			25	V	20	M		
Week 4	25	M	22	V	28	M			30	V	25	M		

T*: Time. Total time is listed in minutes. Time does not include warm-up or cool-down time.
I*: Intensity. Intensity is listed as Light/Lifestyle (L), Moderate (M), or Vigorous (V) (see Figure 2.1).

MOTIVATE!

Creating a plan and monitoring your progress are key motivators for any fitness program or behavior change project. Use an exercise log to track your walking program—make note of dates, times, distances, and intensity. Depending on your personal goals and the equipment available to you, you may also choose to keep track of heart rate, steps taken, or calories burned.

Sticking to a fitness plan can be tough, but there are plenty of things you can do to motivate yourself and overcome the obstacles that prevent you from achieving your goals. Here are a few; see the Tools for Change box: Overcoming Common Obstacles to Exercise on pages 47 and 48 for more ideas.

- **Is lack of time an obstacle for you?** If so, monitor your daily activities for 1 week to identify time slots of 15 minutes to half an hour that you could use for walking. Can you incorporate walking into any of your daily activities, such as walking between classes or when running errands? Figure out the timing in advance, and write your walking "appointments" into your schedule.

- **Do you need concrete numbers and immediate targets to keep you motivated?** If so, purchase a pedometer and start keeping track of the number of steps you take. Challenge yourself with mini-goals to increase your step count.

- **Is lack of willpower an obstacle for you?** If so, enlist a friend to join you on your walks, and schedule it into both of your calendars. Committing to another person can be a great motivator.

- **Is boredom an obstacle for you?** If so, look for ways to switch up your route or walk in places that offer sensory stimulation, such as a shopping mall or a wilderness trail. If you are walking on a treadmill, plan your walks to coincide with a favorite radio or television program (if your treadmill has a TV monitor) or download podcasts or audiobooks to listen to while you walk.

- **Is lack of energy or dislike of exertion an obstacle for you?** If so, create a special playlist of music to listen to while you walk, choosing up-tempo songs that will energize you, distract you from the minor discomforts of physical exertion, and help you keep pace.

- **Do you feel a need for more challenge or a long term goal?** If so, sign up for an upcoming charity walk and join a group that is training for it.

ADVANCE!

Ready for the next step? Once you have established your walking program, you may want to challenge yourself to try something new or take your activities to the next level. Below is a more advanced 4-week program you can follow; visit the companion website to personalize this or any of the programs in this book.

PROGRAM C **Goal:** To walk 40–45 minutes continuously, 5 days a week

	Mon		Tue		Wed		Thurs		Fri		Sat		Sun	
	T*	I*	T	I	T	I	T	I	T	I	T	I	T	I
Week 1	20	M			25	M			25	M				
Week 2	28	M			25	V			30	M	28	M		
Week 3	30	V	28	M	35	M			38	M	35	V		
Week 4	40	M	30	V	42	M			45	V	40	M		

T*: Time. Total time is listed in minutes. Time does not include warm-up or cool-down time.
I*: Intensity. Intensity is listed as Light/Lifestyle (L), Moderate (M), or Vigorous (V) (see Figure 2.1).

Disclaimer: These programs are designed for beginners and assume that all participants have been medically cleared for exercise via the procedures outlined in this chapter. Please also be sure that you have read and understand the basic fitness principles and procedures for starting a fitness program outlined in this chapter. This program is focused on the cardiorespiratory component of fitness, but remember that a well-rounded program will also include muscle strength, muscle endurance, flexibility, and back health components.

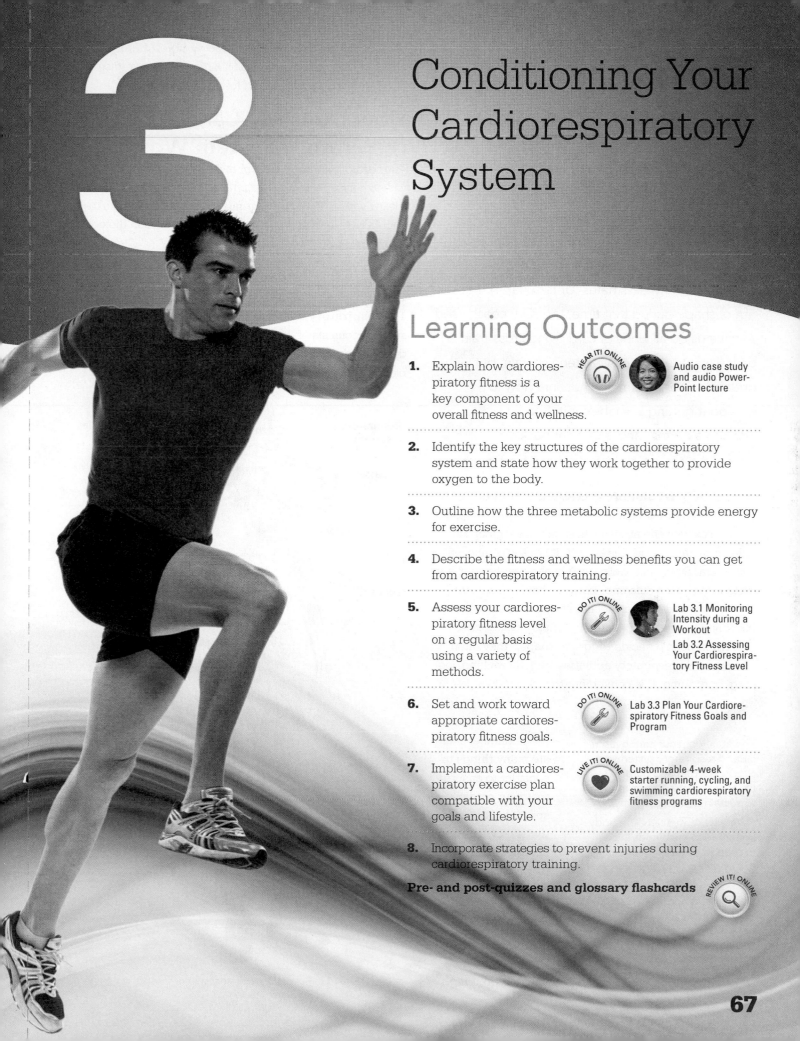

3

Conditioning Your Cardiorespiratory System

Learning Outcomes

1. Explain how cardiorespiratory fitness is a key component of your overall fitness and wellness.

   HEAR IT! ONLINE — Audio case study and audio PowerPoint lecture

2. Identify the key structures of the cardiorespiratory system and state how they work together to provide oxygen to the body.

3. Outline how the three metabolic systems provide energy for exercise.

4. Describe the fitness and wellness benefits you can get from cardiorespiratory training.

5. Assess your cardiorespiratory fitness level on a regular basis using a variety of methods.

   DO IT! ONLINE — Lab 3.1 Monitoring Intensity during a Workout
   Lab 3.2 Assessing Your Cardiorespiratory Fitness Level

6. Set and work toward appropriate cardiorespiratory fitness goals.

   DO IT! ONLINE — Lab 3.3 Plan Your Cardiorespiratory Fitness Goals and Program

7. Implement a cardiorespiratory exercise plan compatible with your goals and lifestyle.

   LIVE IT! ONLINE — Customizable 4-week starter running, cycling, and swimming cardiorespiratory fitness programs

8. Incorporate strategies to prevent injuries during cardiorespiratory training.

Pre- and post-quizzes and glossary flashcards

REVIEW IT! ONLINE

ANGELA

"Hi, I'm Angela. In high school, I was on the varsity tennis team; I played #2 singles and was pretty competitive! After high school, I spent a few years working and saving up money for college, so I'm a little older than most of my classmates. Unfortunately, I got out of shape during that time, too. Our coach used to have us do all kinds of cardio and cross-training drills. I want to start playing tennis again, but without a coach or a team, I'm not sure how to go about getting in shape for it. Should I just find a partner and dive right back in?"

HEAR IT! ONLINE

• •

Cardiorespiratory fitness is the ability of your cardiovascular and respiratory systems to supply oxygen and nutrients to large muscle groups in order to sustain continuous activity. It is a key component of your overall fitness and wellness. A healthy cardiorespiratory system can be the difference between having adequate energy to sustain daily, recreational, and sports activities and becoming tired out by performing simple physical tasks.

When people decide to "get in shape," they often choose cardiorespiratory activities such as walking, jogging, or running. It is convenient to just put on a pair of athletic shoes and head out the door, but remember there are many things to consider to ensure that your cardiorespiratory fitness activities are safe and effective. This chapter provides a brief overview of how the cardiorespiratory system works. We discuss the benefits of regular cardiorespiratory training.

cardiorespiratory fitness
The ability of your cardiovascular and respiratory systems to supply oxygen and nutrients to large muscle groups in order to sustain dynamic activity

respiratory system The body system responsible for the exchange of gases between the body and the air

cardiovascular system The body system responsible for the delivery of oxygen and nutrients to body tissues and the delivery of carbon dioxide and other wastes back to the heart and lungs

We then cover how to set goals for cardiorespiratory fitness and how to design a cardiorespiratory exercise program that is personalized for your needs.

How Does My Cardio-respiratory System Work?

The cardiorespiratory system is made up of the cardiovascular system and the respiratory system. Together, these systems deliver essential oxygen and nutrients to your body's cells and tissues and remove carbon dioxide and wastes.

An Overview of the Cardiorespiratory System

The **respiratory system** (also called the *pulmonary system*) consists of the air passageways and the lungs; the **cardiovascular system** consists of the heart and blood vessels (see Figure 3.1).

Respiratory system:
Air passages
Lungs

Cardiovascular system:
Heart
Veins
Arteries

FIGURE **3.1** The cardiorespiratory system consists of the cardiovascular and respiratory systems.

Air Passageways Air enters your body via your nose and mouth. It then continues through your throat (*pharynx*), voice box (*larynx*), and windpipe (*trachea*) (see Figure 3.2). These upper respiratory passageways warm, humidify, and filter the air, promoting optimal gas exchange. Mucus and small, hairlike projections called *cilia* filter out unwanted particles in the air; you expel these particles through your nose or mouth, or you swallow them. The inspired air travels down through the lower respiratory tract—the lower trachea, *bronchi,* and *bronchioles*—eventually reaching air sacs (*alveoli*) in the lungs, where gas exchange (i.e., the delivery of oxygen and the removal of carbon dioxide) occurs.

Lungs The air passageways in the lungs have extensive branching, similar to the branches on a large tree. At the very ends of the smallest branches (the bronchioles) are alveoli, which are surrounded by small blood vessels called *capillaries.* Because the walls of the alveoli and capillaries are very thin, oxygen moves easily from the alveolar sacs into the capillary blood. Vessels then transport oxygen to the heart and the rest of the body. Meanwhile, carbon dioxide moves from the capillaries into the alveoli and exits the body when you exhale. This exchange of oxygen and carbon dioxide is called **respiration**.

Heart The heart is a fist-sized pump consisting of four chambers: the *right atrium,* the *right ventricle,* the *left atrium,* and the *left ventricle* (Figure 3.3 on page 70). Small *valves* regulate the steady, rhythmic flow of blood between chambers and prevent the blood from flowing backward. The two **atria** are collecting chambers that receive blood from the rest of the body. The two **ventricles** pump blood out again. With each beat of the heart, the atria and ventricles fill and contract. The heart pumps blood through two different circulatory systems: in **pulmonary circulation**, blood circulates from the heart to the lungs and back; in **systemic circulation**, blood circulates from the heart to the rest of the body and back.

Blood returning to the heart from the body enters the heart through the right atrium. The right atrium pumps blood into the right ventricle. The right ventricle pumps blood through the **pulmonary artery** into the lungs. Blood returning from the lungs enters the heart through the left atrium. The left atrium pumps blood into the left ventricle. The left ventricle fills and contracts, pumping the blood out of the heart via the **aorta** and transporting it to the cells of the heart, brain, and body.

respiration The exchange of gases in the lungs or in the tissues

atria Upper chambers of the heart that collect blood from the rest of the body

ventricles Lower chambers of the heart that pump blood to the rest of the body

pulmonary circulation Blood circulation from the heart to the lungs and back

systemic circulation Blood circulation from the heart to the rest of the body and back

pulmonary artery The artery that carries blood from the right ventricle to the lungs

aorta The artery that carries blood from the left ventricle to the rest of the body

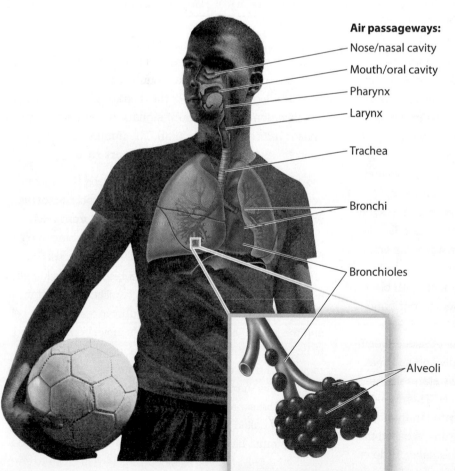

Air passageways:
Nose/nasal cavity
Mouth/oral cavity
Pharynx
Larynx
Trachea
Bronchi
Bronchioles
Alveoli

FIGURE **3.2** The respiratory system consists of the air passageways and the lungs.

1 Deoxygenated blood flows into the right atrium from the superior and inferior venae cavae.

3 Blood picks up oxygen and discards carbon dioxide in the lungs; it then goes through the pulmonary veins into the left atrium.

2 Blood moves from the right atrium into the right ventricle; from there it is pumped through the pulmonary artery into the lungs.

4 Oxygenated blood is forced from the left atrium into the left ventricle; from there it is pumped through the aorta into the rest of the body's blood vessels.

Aorta

Pulmonary artery

Superior vena cava

Pulmonary vein

Left atrium

Right atrium

Valves

Right ventricle

Inferior vena cava

Left ventricle

FIGURE **3.3** The heart is a four-chambered pump. The right atrium and left atrium collect blood from the rest of the body. The right and left ventricles pump blood back out. In pulmonary circulation, blood circulates from the heart to the lungs and back. In systemic circulation, blood circulates from the heart to the rest of the body and back.

Contraction of the ventricle chambers must be forceful enough to send blood out of the heart. In order to accomplish this task the ventricles are more muscular than the atria. The left ventricle is the most muscular chamber, because it must contract forcefully enough to send blood to the rest of the body.

The heart cycle consists of two phases: systole and diastole. During **systole**, the ventricles contract and blood is pumped out of the heart. During **diastole**, the ventricles relax and fill back up with blood from the right and left atria. Specialized heart tissue involuntarily and automatically starts the heart cycle. This tissue, located in the right atrium, is called the *pacemaker;* it determines how fast your heart beats. One "beat" of your heart consists of a full heart cycle. Through a stethoscope, you can hear your heartbeat as a "lub dub." The "lub" signals the end of the diastole phase (ventricular relaxation), and the "dub" signals the end of the systole phase (vertricular contraction). The number of times your heart beats in one minute is your **heart rate**.

Blood Vessels Blood vessels transport blood throughout your body. There are two types of blood vessels: **arteries**, which carry blood away from the heart, and **veins**, which carry blood back toward the heart. As arteries branch off from the heart, they divide into smaller blood vessels called *arterioles,* and then into even smaller blood vessels known as *capillaries*. As mentioned earlier, capillaries have thin walls that permit the exchange of substances between cells and the blood. Oxygen and nutrients move from the blood to body cells, while carbon dioxide and waste products move from body cells to the blood for transport to the lungs and kidneys through veins and *venules* (small veins).

The pressure that blood exerts on the walls of blood vessels is called **blood pressure**. The blood pressure in arteries must be high in order to drive the flow of blood to all your cells. (In veins, blood pressure is close to zero.) Due to the strength of the heart contraction, pressure in the arteries is higher during systole. The pressure

systole The contraction phase of the heart cycle

diastole The relaxation phase of the heart cycle

heart rate The number of beats of the heart in one minute

arteries High-pressure blood vessels that carry blood away from the heart to the lungs or cells

veins Low-pressure blood vessels that carry blood from the cells or lungs back to the heart

blood pressure The pressure that blood in the arteries exerts on the arterial walls measured in the arteries during this phase is called **systolic blood pressure**. When the heart is relaxed, pressure in the arteries drops; this pressure is called **diastolic blood pressure**. In addition to oxygen, working muscles need energy to keep contracting. The three primary energy systems are discussed next.

Three Metabolic Systems Deliver Essential Energy

All of the cells in your body need energy to function. The cellular form of energy is called *adenosine triphosphate,* or **ATP**. ATP must be constantly regenerated from energy stored in your body and from food. The energy stores in your body consist of fat in adipose tissues and muscles, glucose in the muscles and liver, and protein and **creatine phosphate** in muscles. The energy in food comes from fat, carbohydrates, and protein. Your body breaks down stored and consumed nutrients to ATP via three metabolic energy systems: the *immediate, nonoxidative* (anaerobic), and *oxidative* (aerobic) systems. To varying extents, your body draws upon all three systems while you are active, depending on the duration of the activity. Let's examine each of these systems in detail.

The Immediate Energy System When it needs quick, immediate access to energy, your body first draws upon the ATP stored in your muscles. "Explosive" activities such as a basketball jump shot, a 50-meter sprint, or a dive off a diving board are all examples of actions fueled by this immediate energy system. However, your body depletes energy stored in your muscles within a matter of seconds: ATP in muscle cells is typically used up in less than 10 seconds, and creatine phosphate (which is used to make more ATP) is typically gone within 30 seconds. As a result, your body must rely on other energy systems in order to sustain longer activities.

The Nonoxidative (Anaerobic) Energy System As soon as you start moving, the nonoxidative energy system begins breaking down glucose for energy. This system breaks down glucose quickly and *anaerobically* (without oxygen) in order to produce ATP. Although this system starts working immediately, it does not supply the majority of your needed ATP until about 30 seconds into an activity. Examples of nonoxidative, **anaerobic** activities include a sprint down a soccer field, running up a steep hill, and swimming a 100-meter sprint in the pool.

You may experience muscular fatigue with activities that use the nonoxidative energy system, because your body has a limited glucose supply and because the process

of breaking down glucose can produce high levels of **lactic acid**. Lactic acid accumulation in the muscles and blood can produce a burning sensation in the muscles during intense activity. The increase in lactic acid is temporary; contrary to popular belief, your body clears lactic acid from muscles within minutes or hours of exercise. Lactic acid does *not* cause the muscle soreness you may feel a day or two after an exercise session. In fact, during and after exercise, lactic acid cleared from the muscles and blood is reused for energy.

systolic blood pressure Blood pressure during the systole phase of the heart cycle

diastolic blood pressure Blood pressure during the diastole phase of the heart cycle

ATP Adenosine triphosphate; the cellular form of energy

creatine phosphate A molecule that is stored in muscle cells and used in the immediate energy system to donate a phosphate to make ATP

anaerobic Without oxygen (nonoxidative)

lactic acid An end-product of the nonoxidative breakdown of glucose that can increase acidity in muscles and the blood and cause muscular fatigue

casestudy

ANGELA

"I thought I would kick-start my plan to get back into shape by doing one of the workouts my tennis coach had us do in high school. I jogged for a mile, did some calisthenics on the court, and then played two sets of tennis with a friend. That was a mistake. My friend has a killer serve—it's like a bullet coming at you. She won every point she served because I couldn't move fast enough to return the ball. Also, I was surprised at how much that jog tired me out. I used to run a mile with no problem at all! By the end of the first set, I was completely exhausted. My friend won 6-1, 6-1."

THINK! Which energy system do you think Angela's friend relied on most while hitting her serves?

ACT! Write out activities you would do for a 10-minute cardiorespiratory warm-up. Now, try your 10-minute warm up and think about how the three energy systems are providing fuel to keep your muscles moving.

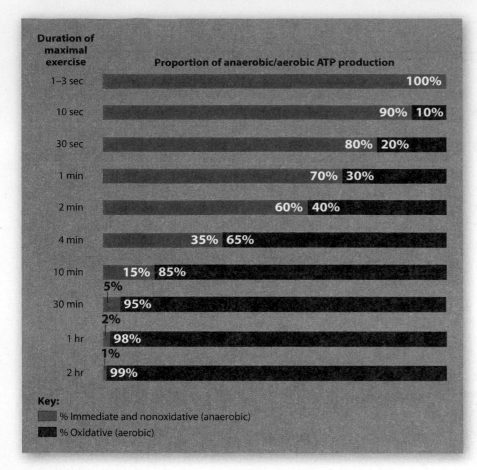

Duration of maximal exercise | **Proportion of anaerobic/aerobic ATP production**

1–3 sec	100%
10 sec	90% 10%
30 sec	80% 20%
1 min	70% 30%
2 min	60% 40%
4 min	35% 65%
10 min	15% 85%
30 min	5% 95%
1 hr	2% 98%
2 hr	1% 99%

Key:
- % Immediate and nonoxidative (anaerobic)
- % Oxidative (aerobic)

FIGURE **3.4** In the first two minutes of exercise, a body primarily uses ATP generated by the two nonoxidative (anaerobic) energy systems. After about three minutes into the exercise, a body begins to primarily use ATP generated by the oxidative (aerobic) energy system.

The nonoxidative energy system supplies your body with most of its needed ATP until about three minutes into an activity. At that point, the oxidative energy system becomes the primary provider of ATP.

The Oxidative (Aerobic) Energy System During the first three minutes of activity (when the immediate and nonoxidative systems are supplying most of the ATP you need), your body is also gradually increasing its *oxidative* production of ATP using oxygen in the **mitochondria** of your cells. The oxidative energy system is also called the **aerobic** energy system (*aerobic* means "with oxygen"). Mitochondria are often referred to as the "powerhouses of the cell," because most energy production occurs in these structures. The *complete* breakdown of fat, glucose, and protein occurs only in the mitochondria and the oxidative energy

mitochondria Cellular structures where oxidative energy production takes place

aerobic Dependent on oxygen (oxidative)

homeostasis A stable, constant internal environment

system yields more ATP from each energy source than any other system.

Aerobic activities are low- to moderate-intensity activities that are usually sustained for 20 minutes or longer. Examples of aerobic activities include cycling, treadmill walking, jogging, and water aerobics.

Figure 3.4 illustrates how the proportion of each energy system's contribution of ATP changes, depending on the duration of a given activity.

The Cardiorespiratory System at Rest and during Exercise

Your cardiorespiratory system must adapt in order to meet your body's needs during exercise.

Resting Conditions At rest, your body works to maintain **homeostasis**, a stable, constant internal environment. If you're healthy, your resting heart rate is between 50 to 90 beats per minute, your breathing rate is around 12 to 20 breaths per minute, and your resting blood pressure is below 120 systolic and below 80 diastolic. During homeostasis, your oxygen and nutrient delivery matches the needs of your cells. Your body breaks down fat via the oxidative energy system in order to supply ATP to the body. Although you "burn" fat for energy, your total energy expenditure is low.

Response to Exercise Physical activity disrupts your body's homeostasis. During exercise, your body must increase blood flow to working muscles in order to maintain adequate oxygen and nutrient delivery. Your heart rate increases, and stronger heart contractions result in an increase in **cardiac output**—the amount of blood exiting your heart in one minute. Your breathing rate also increases to ensure that adequate oxygen is transferred into the blood for working muscles.

The increased volume of blood moving from your heart into your blood vessels in exercise results in an increase in systolic blood pressure. The body directs this increased blood to contracting muscles and the vessels *dilate* (open up wider) to accommodate the increased blood flow. This arterial dilation allows diastolic blood pressure to stay the same or even decrease during aerobic exercise. In addition, capillaries that were not open at rest open up to allow for oxygen and nutrient exchange with muscles.

When you begin to exercise, it takes a few minutes for your body to increase blood flow and to fully engage the oxidative energy system. This is why your body must rely on the faster immediate and nonoxidative energy systems in the first few minutes of exercise. The slower ATP production of the oxidative system also means that during your exercise session, you may have to draw upon the nonoxidative energy system more than once. For example, if you are jogging and suddenly sprint to the end of the street, your oxidative energy system may not be able to supply ATP quickly enough. Your body will then draw upon the nonoxidative system (which breaks down glucose quickly) to supply the additional ATP you need.

How Does Aerobic Training Condition My Cardiorespiratory System?

Recall that aerobic activities are low- to moderate-intensity activities performed for an extended period of time (i.e., 20 minutes or longer). Regular aerobic training conditions your cardiorespiratory system by improving your body's ability to (1) deliver large amounts of oxygen

to working muscles, (2) transfer and use oxygen efficiently in the muscles, and (3) use energy sources for sustained muscular contractions. Figure 3.5 summarizes these and other adaptations that occur over time with aerobic training.

Aerobic Training Increases Oxygen Delivery to Your Muscles

With regular aerobic training, your body gets better at delivering oxygen to working muscles. Your respiratory muscles become more efficient and you experience less fatigue in an extended workout. You can carry more oxygen in your blood, due to an increase in **hemoglobin**, the oxygen-carrying protein. Since the fluid portion of your blood, the **plasma**, also increases with aerobic training, you will see an increase in your total blood volume. Your heart will adapt to this greater volume by increasing the blood-holding capacity of your left ventricle. The ventricle will not only hold more blood, but (with training) it will also have stronger contractions. All of this will allow you to pump more blood out of your heart with every heartbeat, thus increasing your heart's **stroke volume**.

cardiac output The volume of blood ejected from the heart in one minute; expressed in liters or milliliters per minute

hemoglobin A four-part globular, iron-containing protein that carries oxygen in red blood cells

plasma The yellow-colored fluid portion of blood that contains water, proteins, hormones, ions, energy sources, and blood gases

stroke volume The volume of blood ejected from the heart in one heartbeat; expressed in liters or milliliters per beat

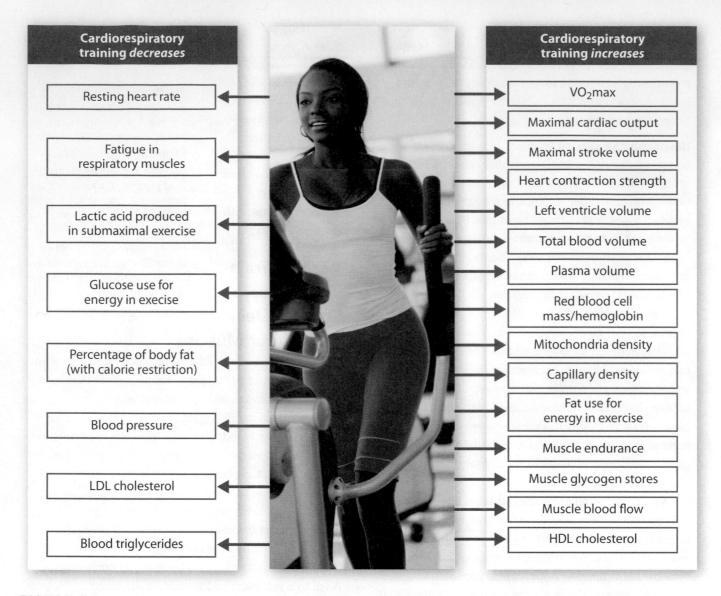

Cardiorespiratory training *decreases*

- Resting heart rate
- Fatigue in respiratory muscles
- Lactic acid produced in submaximal exercise
- Glucose use for energy in execise
- Percentage of body fat (with calorie restriction)
- Blood pressure
- LDL cholesterol
- Blood triglycerides

Cardiorespiratory training *increases*

- VO₂max
- Maximal cardiac output
- Maximal stroke volume
- Heart contraction strength
- Left ventricle volume
- Total blood volume
- Plasma volume
- Red blood cell mass/hemoglobin
- Mitochondria density
- Capillary density
- Fat use for energy in exercise
- Muscle endurance
- Muscle glycogen stores
- Muscle blood flow
- HDL cholesterol

FIGURE **3.5** Regular cardiorespiratory training results in numerous adaptations to the cardiovascular, respiratory, and muscle systems and an increase in overall health and wellness.

Aerobic Training Improves the Transfer and Use of Oxygen

Delivering oxygen to working muscles is only part of the picture. Your body also needs to transfer oxygen into the muscles and use it efficiently. With consistent aerobic training, your body increases the number of capillaries in the muscles that you train. This enables increased blood flow to these muscles and improves oxygen transfer from the blood into the muscles. Once inside the muscle cells, the oxygen is transported to mitochondria for use in the oxidative energy system. Mitochondria numbers increase within each muscle cell, improving oxygen use by muscles and subsequently improving oxidative production of ATP as well.

Aerobic Training Improves Your Body's Ability to Use Energy Efficiently

Regular aerobic training enhances your ability to store glycogen within muscles. When needed, glycogen can be broken down into glucose and used for energy during exercise. In fact, a minimal amount of glucose is needed during exercise to keep the oxidative energy system running efficiently.

Since fat breakdown for energy is accomplished within the mitochondria, an increase in the number of mitochondria will improve your body's ability to use fat for energy, sparing glucose and glycogen stores. Improving your body's ability to burn fat may allow you to have some glucose "left over" for that last-minute sprint to the finish! Less use of glucose and the nonoxidative energy system also means less lactic acid production during exercise and a delaying of fatigue.

What Are the Benefits of Improving My Cardiorespiratory Fitness?

There are many health-related reasons to improve your cardiorespiratory fitness.

Cardiorespiratory Fitness Decreases Your Risk of Disease

Having a low fitness level can put you at higher risk for disease and early death. The good news is that you don't need to increase your fitness to extremely high levels in order to see risk-reducing health benefits. Results of a multi-year federally funded trial indicate that just increasing your fitness to a moderate level can significantly reduce your risk of early mortality from several chronic diseases.[1] In particular, regular aerobic exercise helps protect you against the number-one killer in the world: cardiovascular disease. An increase in cardiorespiratory fitness can decrease your resting heart rate, decrease your blood levels of "bad" (LDL) cholesterol, and help prevent blood clots—all of which can lower your risk of heart attack and stroke. And it is never too early to start improving your fitness: in a study of children just nine to eleven years old, higher cardiorespiratory fitness levels were associated with healthier arteries.[2] If children learn to be active and sustain an active lifestyle, they can avoid the stiffer, less healthy arteries that tend to accompany a sedentary lifestyle in later years.[3]

Cardiorespiratory fitness can also help you manage your weight and blood pressure, thus reducing your chances of developing **metabolic syndrome** (a group of obesity-related risk factors associated with cardiovascular disease and type 2 diabetes).[4] It can also help lessen your risk of developing diabetes, since the regular rhythmic muscular contractions that occur in aerobic exercise improve your body's ability to use insulin and glucose.[5]

Regular physical activity stimulates hormones, anti-inflammatory agents, and immune responses that help protect against many forms of cancer. Studies have shown that regular physical activity and increased cardiorespiratory fitness can lower mortality rates in some of the most common cancers, including lung, colon, breast, and prostate.[6]

Cardiorespiratory Fitness Helps You Control Body Weight and Body Composition

Cardiorespiratory training burns calories. By increasing your calorie expenditure through exercise, you can more effectively manage your body weight and keep your level of body fat low. A high-intensity aerobic exercise session can elevate your metabolic rate for hours,[7] burning calories during the exercise session and long afterward. You can also burn many calories with light-to-moderate aerobic exercise by performing the activity for an extended period of time.

Cardiorespiratory Fitness Improves Self-Esteem, Mood, and Sense of Well-Being

Exercise makes you feel good! A single aerobic exercise session can improve mood and reduce tension and anxiety as a result of chemical changes in the brain and nervous system.[8] Since these benefits are primarily seen in regular exercisers,[9] don't be discouraged if you don't feel instantly "happy" after your first exercise session— stick with it! Long-term changes are even more dramatic. One study has shown that over the course of a 12-week aerobic fitness program, men and women reported improved self-concept, anxiety, mood, and depression scores, compared to a control group, and maintained their improved psychological health for

metabolic syndrome
A clustering of three or more heart disease and diabetes risk factors in one person (high blood pressure, impaired glucose tolerance, insulin resistance, decreased HDL cholesterol, elevated triglycerides, overweight with fat mostly around the waist)

resting heart rate The number of times your heart beats in a minute while the body is at rest; typically 50 to 90 beats per minute

pulse The pressure wave felt in the arteries due to blood ejection with each heartbeat

maximal oxygen consumption (VO$_2$max) The highest rate of oxygen consumption your body is capable of during maximal exercise; expressed in either liters per minute (L/min) or milliliters per minute per kilogram of body weight (ml/kg·min)

a year.[10] Numerous studies point to the importance of exercise in reducing symptoms of depression.[11,12]

Cardiorespiratory Fitness Improves Immune Function

Light to moderate exercise can boost your immune system.[13] Regular, moderate aerobic exercise can reduce stress and improve the quality of your sleep (stress and sleep are both tied to immune system health). Research has also shown that regularly participating in aerobic exercise can slow the reduction in immune system function that tends to occur as you get older.[14]

Cardiorespiratory Fitness Improves Long-Term Quality of Life

Cardiorespiratory fitness has a protective effect against age-related cognitive declines.[15] Research even suggests that aerobic exercise training can increase brain volume and thus *improve* cognitive function and memory as you age.[16,17]

Increased cardiorespiratory fitness can also improve the quality of life for individuals with chronic diseases or other medical conditions. Research has shown that after a six-month exercise program, men living with HIV improved their scores in cardiorespiratory fitness and in cognitive function and overall health.[18] Cardiorespiratory fitness has also been linked to better quality of life for survivors of breast cancer[19] and heart attacks.[20] Of course, the best time to incorporate a cardiorespiratory program into your life is *before* you show signs of disease.

How Can I Assess My Cardiorespiratory Fitness?

How fit is your cardiorespiratory system? Chances are, you already have a general idea. If you get easily winded after walking up a short flight of stairs or have trouble walking quickly for more than 10 minutes or so, you likely have a low cardiorespiratory fitness level.

Monitoring your **resting heart rate** is one way to keep track of general changes in your fitness level. Recall that your heart rate is the number of times your heart beats in one minute. Your resting heart rate decreases as your cardiorespiratory system becomes more conditioned. With an increase in stroke volume, your heart does not have to beat as many times per minute to deliver the same amount of blood to the body; at rest, your heart can slow down and still deliver adequate oxygen to all your cells.

When the heart contracts and pushes blood out, that wave of blood can be felt moving through the arteries. This is your **pulse**. To determine your heart rate, feel for your pulse at specific arteries around the body. The most common arteries to use for checking an exercise pulse are the *carotid* and the *radial* arteries (see Figure 3.6). Press your index and middle fingers gently against your skin and count the number of beats that you feel. Avoid using your thumb when taking your pulse, because the pulse in your thumb can interfere with your ability to count accurately. **Lab 3.1** walks you through how to take an accurate heart rate reading at rest and during exercise.

Understand Your Maximal Oxygen Consumption

Your body's maximal ability to utilize oxygen during exercise is called **maximal oxygen consumption** or **VO$_2$max**. Your VO$_2$max is the measure of your body's ability to deliver oxygen to the muscles and the muscles' ability to consume or use the oxygen. VO$_2$max numbers range from 20 to 94 ml/kg·min, with male athletes typically ranging from 50 to 70 ml/kg·min and female athletes ranging from 40 to 60 ml/kg·min. Your maximal oxygen consumption is largely determined by genetics and tends to decrease as

(a)   **(b)**

FIGURE **3.6** To determine your heart rate, feel for your pulse at either (a) the carotid artery, or (b) the radial artery.

you get older. That said, you can typically improve your VO_2max an average of 15 to 20 percent with training. The more deconditioned you are before beginning a training program, the more dramatic an improvement you can achieve with training.

The most accurate measurements of VO_2max are performed in a laboratory setting (see Figure 3.7). The test is usually completed on a treadmill or stationary bike and requires specialized equipment and technicians to ensure safety. The technicians measure the precise amount of oxygen that enters and exits the body during a maximal exercise session.

Test Your Submaximal Heart Rate Responses

An alternative to testing your true maximal oxygen consumption is to perform a *submaximal* test. Submaximal tests do not test your body's maximal oxygen

FIGURE **3.7** VO_2max can be most accurately measured in a laboratory setting, where direct gas analysis can determine the volume of oxygen a person's body is using while exercising at maximum capacity.

consumption but rather test for submaximal values that can be compared against norm charts or used to predict maximal values. Submaximal tests are safer, require less equipment and expertise, and are performed either in a laboratory or in a field/classroom setting.

Submaximal tests in the laboratory are usually performed on a stationary bike or treadmill. These tests predict your maximal effort level and oxygen consumption by assessing your heart rate response. A higher heart rate means higher oxygen consumption. By testing your heart rate response to different exercise intensities, an exercise technician can use your predicted **maximal heart rate (HRmax)** to estimate your maximal exercise intensity and oxygen consumption. Your maximal heart rate is the fastest your heart will beat in exhaustive exercise (a number that will decrease as you get older). One way to predict your HRmax is to subtract your age from the number 220. For example, if you are 18 years old, your predicted HRmax would be $220 - 18 = 202$ beats per minute. This formula is not as accurate as maximal laboratory tests, but it is used in many submaximal tests and heart rate training equations.

Test Your Cardiorespiratory Fitness in the Field/Classroom

Most classes in health and fitness enroll too many students to perform laboratory testing. More appropriate for these classes are classroom or field tests of cardiorespiratory fitness. Like laboratory tests, these tests either predict your maximal oxygen consumption from submaximal test results or allow you to compare your results with norm tables. In **Lab 3.2** you will perform three different assessments of cardiorespiratory fitness: the 3-minute step test, the 1-mile walking test, and the 1.5-mile running test.

DO IT! ONLINE

Three-Minute Step Test In this test, you will step up and down on a 12-inch-high step bench. At the end of three minutes, take your one-minute recovery heart rate and compare this to norm charts for your age and sex. The faster your heart recovers from exercise, the better conditioned you are.

One-Mile Walking Test In this test, you will walk as fast as you can for one mile. Record your finish time and your heart rate at the end of the one mile. Use your results to calculate an

> **maximal heart rate (HRmax)** The highest heart rate you can achieve during maximal exercise

estimated VO$_2$max and determine your fitness level for your age and sex. A faster time and lower heart rate indicate a higher level of fitness.

1.5-Mile Running Test In this test, you will run 1.5 miles as fast as you can. If you cannot run the entire course, you may take walking breaks. Use your finish time to calculate your estimated VO$_2$max and determine your fitness level for your age and sex. A faster time indicates a higher level of fitness.

How Can I Create My Own Cardiorespiratory Fitness Program?

Having a plan is one of the most important things you can do before beginning a personalized cardiorespiratory fitness program. Careful planning will help you reach your goals, prevent injuries, and ensure that you have fun while exercising!

Set Appropriate Cardiorespiratory Fitness Goals

Goal-setting for cardiorespiratory fitness should follow the SMART goal-setting guidelines (first introduced in Chapter 1). Recall that SMART goals are *s*pecific, *m*easurable, *a*ction-oriented, *r*ealistic, and *t*ime-oriented. Setting a vague goal such as "Build a stronger cardiorespiratory system" is not as useful as setting a specific goal that follows the SMART guidelines, such as "Improve my cardiorespiratory fitness from a 'fair' rating on my three-minute step test to a 'good' rating, by exercising on the elliptical machine three days a week for 30 minutes for the next two months."

In **Lab 3.3** you will set your own short- and long-term goals for cardiorespiratory fitness. Review the training adaptations and benefits of cardiorespiratory training discussed earlier to guide your goal-setting. Be realistic: If your goal is to run a marathon but you hate running, you will likely be setting yourself up for failure (unless your attitude toward running changes!). Choose goals that you can achieve, doing the types of activities that you enjoy most.

DO IT! ONLINE

Learn about Cardiorespiratory Training Options

There are a wide variety of cardiorespiratory training options available to you.

Classes If you enjoy the company of other people and like the motivating aspect of an instructor leading a workout, consider enrolling in a group exercise class. Classes that incorporate a continuous, rhythmic activity lasting more than 20 minutes will help you maintain or improve your cardiorespiratory fitness. Such classes can be found in colleges, recreational centers, and fitness centers in almost every community. Class formats and instructors can vary widely, so consider sampling a few different classes and instructors before deciding on a regular class. Choose classes where the instructors are not only motivating, but also experienced, certified, and knowledgeable about your current health/fitness levels.

Indoor Workouts If you are not sure about working out in a group or with an instructor, you can design your own cardiorespiratory workout using indoor cardio equipment. You can find cardio equipment at most gyms or fitness centers or purchase it for home use. Indoor cardio workout equipment includes stationary bicycles, treadmills, elliptical trainers, stair-climbing machines, recumbent bikes, arm cycle ergometers, rowing machines, and jump ropes. If you are using a machine in a fitness facility, get an introduction to the features, use, and safety from a facility employee. In addition, consider running on an indoor track, swimming in a pool, deep-water jogging, or participating in a racquet sport.

Outdoor Workouts If you like to be outside, explore outdoor options for a cardiorespiratory workout. It is not uncommon to pursue a combination of indoor and outdoor exercise routines, depending on the weather and the facility options available to you. Exercising outdoors can be very rewarding if you live in an area with interesting sights, safe routes, and beautiful trails. The options for outdoor cardio workouts are endless. Here are just a few ideas: walking, jogging, running, cycling, track workouts, trail running, hiking, tennis, cross-country skiing, open-water swimming, and inline skating.

Differing Workout Formats (Continuous, Interval, Circuit) Aerobic training is a type of *continuous* training—i.e., you perform a rhythmic activity and sustain it for a period of time (ideally 20 minutes or more). While aerobic training should be the cornerstone of your cardiorespiratory training program, other workout formats can add variety, intensity, and other fitness benefits.

An **interval workout** alternates periods of higher-intensity exercise with periods of lower-intensity exercise or rest. An interval workout method allows you to increase the intensity of your workout to a level that you might not otherwise be able to sustain for a long period of time. If done correctly, this type of workout can further develop your body's aerobic training adaptations. High intensity anaerobic intervals improve anaerobic conditioning but also have a greater injury potential.

A **circuit-training workout** involves moving from location to location in a circuit-training room and exercising for a certain amount of time (or number of repetitions) at each "station." You can enroll in a circuit-training class or circuit-train on your own. The circuit can contain alternating aerobic and weight-training activities, just weight stations, or just aerobic stations. The best circuit for cardiorespiratory conditioning is one with all aerobic exercise stations.

Apply FITT Principles to Cardiorespiratory Fitness

After setting goals and selecting the types of cardiorespiratory exercise that you want to do, you must decide how much, how hard, and how long to exercise. Recall the FITT principles (introduced in Chapter 2): *f*requency, *i*ntensity, *t*ime, and *t*ype. Let's look at how each of these principles applies to a cardiorespiratory fitness program.

Frequency According to the American College of Sports Medicine, you should spend three to five days per week on cardiorespiratory conditioning. If you are exercising at higher intensity levels, you can improve or maintain your VO_2max by working out only three days per week. If you are exercising at lower intensity levels, you may need more than three days per week (five is recommended) to improve cardiorespiratory fitness.

If your goals include weight loss or disease prevention, you will benefit from exercising more often but at a lower intensity in order to prevent injuries and overtraining.

Intensity Your workouts should be intense enough to tax your cardiorespiratory system, but not so difficult as to discourage you or increase your chances of injury. You can measure the intensity of your exercise by various methods, including determining your heart rate, assessing your **perceived exertion**, and self-administering a **talk test**.

Determining Your Heart Rate Your heart rate provides a good indication of how hard your cardiorespiratory system is working, since it is related to the amount of oxygen that your body is consuming. You can determine your heart rate by using a heart rate monitor or (as we discussed earlier) by counting your pulse.

Heart rate monitors can be found on cardio equipment and merely require you to place your hands on the receiving pads for a few seconds. Personal heart rate monitors, which consist of a chest strap transmitter and a wrist receiver, are also widely available.

Counting your pulse while you are exercising is an easy and low-cost way to measure your heart rate. Your heart rate decreases rapidly after stopping exercise, especially after 15 seconds; therefore, count your pulse for only 10 seconds, and try to keep moving as you count. Then multiply your 10-second count by six to convert to the number of beats per minute (bpm).

interval workout A workout that alternates periods of higher-intensity exercise with periods of lower-intensity exercise or rest

circuit-training workout A workout where exercisers move from one exercise station to another after a certain number of repetitions or amount of time

perceived exertion A subjective assessment of exercise intensity

talk test A method of measuring exercise intensity based on assessing your ability to speak during exercise

TABLE 3.1 ACSM's Training Guidelines for Cardiorespiratory Fitness	
Recommendations for the General Adult Population	
Frequency (days/week)	Moderate: 5 Vigorous: 3
Intensity (how hard)	Moderate: 64–76% of HRmax Vigorous: 77–95% of HRmax
Time (how long)	Moderate: 30–60 min (150 min/week) Vigorous: 20–60 min (75 min/week)
Type (exercises)	Large muscle group, dynamic activity

Data from: C. E. Garner and others, "American College of Sports Medicine Position Stand: Quantity and Quality of Exercise for Developing and Maintaining Cardiorespiratory, Musculoskeletal, and Neuromotor Fitness in Apparently Healthy Adults: Guidance for Prescribing Exercise," *Medicine & Science in Sports & Exercise* 43, no. 7 (2011): 1334–59.

What **target heart rate** should you aim for in a workout? The answer depends on your goals and fitness level. As you can see in Table 3.1, the American College of Sports Medicine's recommendations for exercise intensity level cites a wide range of target heart rates: 64 to 95 percent of HRmax. Use the following guidelines to determine where within this range you should aim:

- If your fitness level is low, you should follow the guidelines for moderate cardiorespiratory exercise or 64–76 percent of your HRmax. Start below or at the low end of this range if you are very deconditioned or brand new to exercise.

- If your fitness level is moderate, aim for the vigorous exercise guidelines or 77–95 percent of your HRmax or choose to do a mix of moderate and vigorous exercise.

Table 3.2 also provides target heart rate guidelines for exercise, using the HRmax method based on your age. Another method of determining your target heart rate is to measure your **heart rate reserve (HRR)**, the difference between your resting and maximum heart rates. **Lab 3.1** walks you through how to determine your HRR.

Perceived Exertion Another way to assess the intensity of your workout is by determining your perceived exertion; which is simply your perception of how hard you are working during exercise. One of the most well-known perceived exertion scales was developed by Gunnar Borg in 1970. His Rating of Perceived Exertion (RPE) scale is a subjective 15-point scale, from 6–20, that is related to heart rate responses to exercise.[21] The Borg RPE Scale can be a very valuable tool when it is not easy or appropriate to use heart rate monitoring to check your workout intensity. For example, if you participate in a water sport such as swimming, heart rate monitoring can be misleading; heart rates tend to slow down while exercising in water due to increased hydrostatic pressure and decreased temperature. For this reason, you may prefer to use RPE to determine your exercise intensity.

Another perceived exertion scale is the OMNI Scale of Perceived Exertion. Although originally developed for children, adult versions now exist and these provide a simple way to assess workout intensity on a 1-10 scale (see Figure 3.8). The OMNI Scale is correlated with the Borg RPE scale and heart rate responses.[22,23] As you become more experienced with a

target heart rate The heart rate you are aiming for during an exercise session; often a range with high and low heart rates called your *training zone*

heart rate reserve (HRR) The number of beats per minute available or in reserve for exercise heart rate increases; maximal heart rate minus resting heart rate

TABLE 3.2 Target Heart Rate Guidelines*		
Age	Target HR Range (bpm)	10-Sec Count
18–24	139–179	23–30
25–29	135–174	22–29
30–34	132–169	22–28
35–39	129–165	21–28
40–44	125–160	21–27
45–49	122–156	20–26
50–54	118–151	20–25
55–59	114–147	19–25
60–64	110–142	18–24
65+	108–140	18–23

*Based upon the *HRmax method,* where 220 − age = HRmax and the training zone is 70 to 90% of HRmax (moderate to vigorous). Individuals with low fitness levels should start below or at the low end of these ranges.

FIGURE **3.8** One method to determine your exercise intensity involves utilizing the OMNI Scale of Perceived Exertion for walking and running.

Source: A.C. Utter and others, "Validation of the Adult OMNI Scale of Perceived Exertion for Walking/Running Exercise," *Medicine & Science in Sports & Exercise* 36, no. 10 (2004): 1777. Used by permission of Wolters Kluwer/Lippincott, Williams & Wilkins.

particular cardiorespiratory activity and become more attuned to how your body feels during exercise, your ability to use the perceived exertion scales accurately will improve.

The Talk Test The talk test method of measuring exercise intensity is based on assessing how easily you can talk during exercise. While exercising at a *light* intensity, you should be able to talk easily and continuously. If you are exercising at a *moderate* intensity, you should be able to talk easily, but not continuously, during the activity. If you are too out of breath to carry on a conversation easily, you are working at a high or *vigorous* intensity. If you cannot talk at all, you are probably doing an anaerobic interval or sprinting.

To increase cardiorespiratory fitness, aim for at least a moderate intensity level for most of your workout or the highest level you can comfortably sustain for 20 to 30 minutes. You can incorporate short periods of light and vigorous activity for workout variety or interval training. Table 3.3 summarizes the most common intensity scales for cardiorespiratory endurance exercise. Use the one that works best for you and the type of exercise you have chosen.

Time For optimal cardiorespiratory conditioning, your exercise sessions should be 20 to 30 minutes long. If you are just starting out, exercise continuously for as long as you can, and then work your way up to the minimum guideline of 20 minutes. The box Can Shorter Workouts Benefit My Health? examines how workouts as short as 10 to 15 minutes can benefit health.

TABLE **3.3** Cardiorespiratory Intensity Scales*					
General	Talk Test	OMNI	Borg RPE	% HRR	% HRmax
Light	Easy conversation	0	6	30	57
		1	7	35	60
		2	8		
			9		
		3	10	40	
		4	11	44	64
Moderate	Brief sentences and words	5	12	45	65
			13		
		6	14	64	84
Vigorous	A few words	7	15	65	85
			16		
		8	17	84	94
Anaerobic	Barely or not able to talk	9	18	85	95
			19		
		10	20	100	100

*The various methods to quantify exercise intensity in this table may not be equivalent to one another.

Data are from: American College of Sports Medicine, *ACSM's Guidelines for Exercise Testing and Prescription*, 8th Edition (Baltimore, MD: Lippincott Williams & Wilkins, 2010); Office of Disease Prevention and Health Promotion, U.S. Department of Health and Human Services, *2008 Physical Activity Guidelines for Americans: Be Active, Healthy, and Happy!* ODPHP Publication no. U0036 (Washington, DC: U.S. Department of Health and Human Services, 2008), Available at: www.health.gov.paguidelines; R. J. Robertson and others, "Validation of the Adult OMNI Scale of Perceived Exertion for Cycle Ergometer Exercise," *Medicine & Science in Sports & Exercise* 36, no. 1 (2004): 102–108; A. C. Utter and others, "Validation of the Adult OMNI Scale of Perceived Exertion for Walking/Running Exercise," *Medicine & Science in Sports & Exercise* 36, no. 10 (2004): 1776–1780; G. Borg, *Borg's Perceived Exertion and Pain Scales* (Champaign, IL: Human Kinetics, 1998): 27–38.

Do Short Workouts Do Me Any Good?

The short answer is *yes*, they do! Experts once believed that long aerobic workouts, where the heart rate stays continuously in the target training zone, were more effective than short workouts for your health. Naturally, getting motivated for a long exercise session is not as easy as getting motivated for a short one. The good news? Recent research shows two important concepts: 1) you don't have to work out a long time to get benefits, and 2) a short *time* but a high *intensity* level of training can have a major impact on your health.

In one study, researchers instructed one group of obese women to walk briskly for 30 minutes three times per week and another group to walk intermittently for two 15-minute sessions five days per week.[1] The intermittent walkers gained nearly as much aerobic capacity as the continuous walkers—and in both groups, blood fats and insulin measurements improved significantly. The continuous walkers lost weight, however, while the intermittent walkers did not.

In another study, young (around 25 years old) but sedentary people were instructed to eat a high-fat meal and then exercise.[2] Half of the eaters then ran for 30 minutes on a treadmill, while the other half ran for three 10-minute stretches separated by rest periods. Intermittent exercise proved to be *better* at lowering fats in the bloodstream than continuous exercise. The experimenters speculate that this may happen because each exercise session independently speeds the metabolic rate, adding up to a greater overall effect than longer, single sessions.[3]

Newer research tells us that metabolic changes from 10 minutes of exercise persist for 60 minutes, providing a better blood glucose/insulin balance and catabolic (or calorie burning, lipolysis-fat breakdown) state as opposed to the anabolic state after eating.[4] The effects were more pronounced in individuals in the study who were more fit; if you get fit, you get even more metabolic benefits from intermittent exercise!

In addition to doing shorter bouts of exercise, you can also get a lot more out of your short exercise time by employing interval training as part of your exercise strategy. High intensity interval training means you exercise at almost maximum capacity for several shorts bursts and rest between bursts. Short amounts of interval training can be as effective as longer amounts of conventional training, so you can achieve your fitness goals in less time![5] Note that you shouldn't start doing intervals until after you have reached a minimal level of fitness. Your chance of injury increases with high intensity exercise and your body needs to be ready.

So squeeze in 10 minutes of aerobic exercise whenever you can, and remember the bottom line: Get moving, whether for short periods or long!

Sources:
1. J. E. Donnelly and others, "The Effects of 18 Months of Intermittent vs. Continuous Exercise on Aerobic Capacity, Body Weight and Composition, and Metabolic Fitness in Previously Sedentary, Moderately Obese Females," *International Journal of Obesity* 24, no. 5 (2000): 566–72.
2. T. S. Altena and others, "Single Sessions of Intermittent and Continuous Exercise and Postprandial Lipemia," *Medicine & Science in Sports & Exercise* 36, no. 8 (2004): 1364–71.
3. American College of Sports Medicine, "Short Bouts of Exercise Reduce Fat in the Bloodstream After Meals," News release, August 5, 2004, www.acsm.org.
4. J. P. Little and others, "A Practical Model of Low-Volume High-Intensity Interval Training Induces Mitochondrial Biogenesis in Human Skeletal Muscle: Potential Mechanisms," *The Journal of Physiology* 588, no. 6 (2010): 1011–22.

Type For optimal motivation, training adaptation, and injury prevention, choose activities that you enjoy. Alternate your participation in these activities by the day or week for a **cross-training** effect. Cross-training can help you maintain muscle balance by working different muscle groups.

Include a Warm-up and Cool-down Phase in Your Workout Session

A cardiorespiratory workout session should consist of three components: the **warm-up** phase, the main cardiorespiratory endurance conditioning set, and the **cool-down** phase. Figure 3.9 illustrates a sample workout for a moderately fit 20-year-old showing each of these components. Remember that your warm-up should ideally consist of light physical activity that mimics the movements of your main exercise set. For example, if your main exercise set is jogging, an ideal warm-up would be to walk briskly. Likewise, your cool-down should ideally be a less-vigorous version of your

main exercise set. (Review Chapter 2 for more guidelines on warming up and cooling down.) Keep in mind that when you are starting an exercise program, you should generally perform longer warm-up (15 to 20 minutes) and cool-down (10 minutes or more) segments.

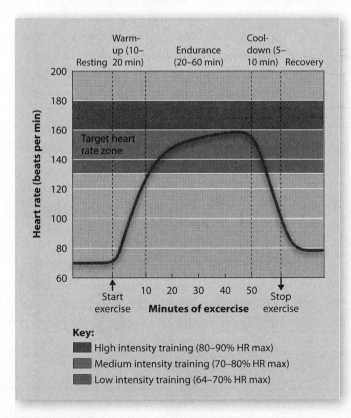

FIGURE 3.9 This graph charts the progression of a sample cardiorespiratory workout for a moderately fit 20-year-old. Note that it consists of a warm-up phase, an endurance phase, and a cool-down phase.

Adapted from *ACSM's Guidelines for Exercise Testing and Prescription*, 7th Edition (Baltimore, MD: Lippincott Williams & Wilkins, 2010).

> **cross-training** The practice of using different exercise modes or types in your cardiorespiratory training program
>
> **warm-up** The initial 5- to 20-minute preparation phase of a workout
>
> **cool-down** The ending phase of a workout where the body is brought gradually back to rest

Plan for Proper Progression of Your Program

When you are starting a new exercise program, it is easy to attempt to do too much too soon. A fitness program needs to be *progressive* in order for you to achieve results and avoid injury. As you begin a fitness program, your progress may initially be slow, while your body adjusts to the new activity. Eventually, consistent exercise will result in noticeable improvement.

In order to avoid injuring yourself, increase your workout by no more than 10 percent per week (the *10 percent rule*). That means that your weekly increases in frequency, intensity, and/or time should not total more than 10 percent. For example, if you are jogging for 30 minutes per exercise session, next week you could safely increase each session to 33 minutes (10 percent increase in time).

How Can I Maintain My Cardiorespiratory Program?

How many times have you started a fitness program only to quit after a few weeks? For many people, the biggest challenge to improving cardiorespiratory fitness is not beginning a program, but keeping it up. Next we discuss the stages of progression and the importance of tracking your progress and reassessing your needs.

Understand the Stages of Progression

Start-up In the *start-up* phase of a cardiorespiratory program, you will be adjusting to the new activity in your weekly routine. During this stage, it is important to pay attention to how you feel during exercise so that you can make adjustments if necessary. Do you prefer

casestudy

ANGELA

"After practically killing myself on the tennis court last week, I did some research into exactly what it means to 'get in shape.' I was really interested to learn about things like target heart rates and the different ways to measure cardiorespiratory fitness. I took the 1.5-mile run test and found out that my current fitness rating is only 'fair.' So my plan is to design a cardio workout that will get my rating up to 'good' or 'excellent' before challenging my friend to another match!"

THINK! Pretend you are Angela's fitness trainer and decide on an appropriate target goal for Angela. Does the goal you outlined for Angela follow the SMART guidelines?

ACT! Become your own personal fitness trainer and write yourself a target cardio-respiratory goal incorporating the SMART guidelines.

• •

exercising in the morning or in the evening? Is that aerobics class really right for you? In this first stage, your main concern should be fine-tuning your program until you settle on an activity and routine that is comfortable for you. Depending on your fitness level and exercise experience, this stage can last anywhere from two to four weeks.

Improvement Once you have the "kinks" worked out of your program, you are ready to move into the *improvement* phase. In this stage, your body starts adapting to the cardiorespiratory exercise. Some of these changes will be evident to you; some will not (refer to Figure 3.5). You should, however, start feeling better during exercise, have more energy when not exercising, and feel that you can exercise for longer periods of time without fatigue. As in the initial stage, listen to your body so that you can make changes as needed. The improvement stage can last anywhere from three to eight months, depending on your program and goals.

Maintenance After months of hard work you are at the fitness level you desire and you feel great! You

have reached the *maintenance* stage. The key to this stage is to keep your program consistent. If you stop exercising, you can lose your newly achieved fitness level in only half the time it took you to acquire it. In fact, athletes can start losing cardiorespiratory fitness within just two weeks of inactivity. If you need to cut back but don't want to lose your hard-earned improvements, cut back on exercise time but not intensity level. It is easier to maintain cardiorespiratory fitness with shorter but more intense workouts. The maintenance stage lasts for as long as you continue your program.

Record and Track Your Fitness Progress

Do you remember how you felt during that spinning workout three weeks ago? What was the speed and incline of your treadmill workout last week? One of the best ways to make sure that you stay on track with your fitness program is to record your activity and track your progress over time. Keeping a workout journal or log will encourage you to write down things such as the FITT components of your workout, how you felt during the workout, the time of day, and any other information that may be relevant. Record your successes as well as your setbacks—this will remind you of the progress you have made since beginning the program and help determine if your goals or workouts should be adjusted over time. The box Fitness Tracking Technology explains some of the technology and websites you can use to assess and log your fitness progress.

Troubleshoot Problems Right Away

Everyone will experience obstacles or problems when starting an exercise program. You may not have enough time in your day to work out, it may be difficult for you to physically get to your workout facility, you may be feeling pain in your knee, and so on. While these issues may set you back temporarily, they should not keep you from reaching your goals. Address the problems right away and brainstorm solutions; the sooner you acknowledge a problem and address it, the sooner you can get back on track.

Periodically Reassess Your Cardiorespiratory Fitness Level

Although you will certainly feel your progress by how your body responds to exercise, it is always nice to

Fitness Tracking Technology

There are countless electronic tools out there for tracking exercise, diet and nutrition, and weight management. Wearable monitors containing tiny motion sensors can track your baseline activity levels and workouts. The Fitbit tracker, for example, clips to your clothes and lets you count the number of steps you take in an exercise session or a day. It then calculates your mileage and total calories burned. With the DirectLife monitor, you assess your normal activity for a week or so, then dial up a 12-week activity plan and download it from a website. Before you buy a pedometer, heart rate monitor, or any other such device, ask your fitness instructor or you friends for recommendations, and consult equipment reviews in newspapers and on consumer websites.

If fussing with a gadget isn't for you, you can still take advantage of some useful online programs that help you log your physical activity online, track your progress, and access information about recommended guidelines for physical activity. For example, you can choose from thousands of smart phone applications to help you log miles run or laps swum, count calories taken in and burned, keep food diaries, calculate body fat and fat grams in foods, and track and share your weight via a social site. Many websites offer similar tools; below are just a few:

Lose It!: www.loseit.com/

LiveStrong.com: www.livestrong.com/

MyPyramid Tracker: www.mypyramidtracker.gov

Nike+: http://nikerunning.nike.com/nikeos /p/nikeplus/en_US/plus/#///runs/

President's Challenge: www.presidentschallenge.org

Runner's World Training Log: http://traininglog .runnersworld.com/landingpage.aspx

These high tech tools can't substitute for your own motivation and adherence. They can, however, offer portability and ease of tracking your personal data accurately. People often find these gadgets and programs fun to use and a way to give and receive support through social media connections.

• •

have quantitative measures of your progress as well. Complete the assessments in **Lab 3.2** at least twice—once after three months of your new program and again at six months. Keep in mind that you will see the most improvements in assessments that are similar to your chosen workout activity (e.g., if you are doing step aerobics, you will probably see more improvement in the step test than in the 1.5-mile run test). If you have not improved, look at your program again and figure out whether you need to redesign it.

Reassess Your Goals and Program as Needed

Once a target date arrives, review your goals for that date. Did you achieve what you set out to do? If not, list the reasons why. You may need to set more realistic goals with more realistic target dates, or select a different activity. If you need more motivation, consider finding a workout partner or working with a personal trainer. If you did reach your goal, set a new goal for maintenance or a more challenging goal to improve your fitness level even more. The sample running, cycling, and swimming programs in Activate, Motivate, & Advance Your Fitness at the end of this chapter (pages 105–114) can help you set new goals and develop new fitness plans.

How Can I Avoid Injury During Cardiorespiratory Exercise?

The fastest way to disrupt a training program is to get injured. Reduce your injury risk by understanding and following common exercise injury prevention methods.

Design a Personalized, Balanced Cardiorespiratory Program

The most common injuries from cardiorespiratory fitness programs are from overuse, such as strains and tendonitis, particularly in the lower body. If you attempt to do too much too soon, you put yourself at risk for such injuries. Make sure your exercise program considers your current level of fitness and make your FITT targets realistic and achievable. You may also want to consider incorporating cross-training into your program, since doing one activity exclusively can result in uneven muscle development, making you more vulnerable to injury.

Wear Appropriate Clothing and Footwear

Use common sense when you are dressing for your chosen cardiorespiratory activity. If you are cycling, a helmet and bright clothing are essential. If you are running, walking, taking a group fitness class, or participating in a racquet sport, pay particularly close attention to your footwear. You need shoes that will protect your feet and provide the right amount of support and cushioning. Here are some tips for finding the right shoes:[24]

- Shop for shoes after a workout or at the end of the day when your feet are their biggest.

- Wear the socks that you will use when you exercise.

- Be sure you can freely wiggle all of your toes.

- The shoes should feel comfortable as soon as you try them on.

- Try them out! Lace them up correctly and then walk or run around the store.

- Your heel should not slide up and down as you walk or run.

- If you participate in a sport three or more times a week or will be doing high-intensity workouts, choose a sport-specific shoe. Ask a knowledgeable salesperson for advice on purchasing sport-specific shoes.

What about those people you see running in bare feet, or with minimalist shoes? The box Barefoot Running: Is It Safe for Me? provides an overview of this style of running.

Pay Attention to Your Exercise Environment

Prevent Heat-Related Illness When exercising indoors, be sure the exercise room is well-ventilated and cool enough to prevent your body from overheating. When exercising outdoors in hot weather, take precautions to avoid heat-related illnesses such as **heat cramps**, **heat exhaustion**, or **heat stroke**. Your risk of heat-related illness increases if you (1) exercise too hard for your fitness level, (2) exercise in high heat, humidity, and sunshine, (3) have a low fitness level overall, (4) are lacking in adequate sleep, (5) are not

heat cramps Severe cramping in the large muscle groups and abdomen caused by high fluid and electrolyte loss in sustained exertion in the heat

heat exhaustion An elevated core body temperature, headache, fatigue, profuse sweating, nausea, and clammy skin brought on by sustained exertion in the heat with dehydration and electrolyte losses

heat stroke A core body temperature above 104°F, headache, nausea, vomiting, diarrhea, rapid pulse, cessation of sweating, and disorientation resulting from extreme exertion in very hot conditions

Is Barefoot Running Safe for Me?

Have you noticed people out on the street running without shoes or wearing "FiveFingers"—those funny-looking shoes with toes? What are these people up to? They are part of a new and growing trend: barefoot running. What's behind this trend? And should you be running barefoot?

Advocates of barefoot running point out that humans have been running without shoes or with minimal shoes since they stood up on two legs and indicate several perceived advantages to doing so. One claimed benefit is that the shorter stride in barefoot running reduces the number of running injuries.[1] Advocates say the less support you give to your arch, the stronger your arch becomes—barefoot activity builds up the muscles of the foot. And, they say, running barefoot makes you more aware of the terrain you are running through, encouraging a connection with the environment.[2] Researchers have shown that runners who run barefoot tend to strike the ground with their forefoot or midfoot rather than their heel;[3] there is anecdotal evidence that forefoot or midfoot striking can help avoid and/or mitigate repetitive stress injuries, especially stress fractures, plantar fasciitis, and runner's knee.[4]

Critics of the trend, though, point out that this is still a theory. As yet, there is no evidence that barefoot or minimalist running reduces injuries. Critics concede there is no evidence that running shoes reduce injuries either.[5] More research is needed before conclusions can be drawn about any of these opinions, pro or con. However, critics do point out that, unlike running in shoes, barefoot running can result in puncture wounds from sharp objects on the ground.

So, where does that leave you? Scientists do say that some barefoot running as a part of an overall training plan can be beneficial in strengthening the bones, ligaments, muscles, and tendons in the feet. And, using a barefoot *style* of running—striking the ground with the midfoot rather than the heel even when you're wearing running shoes—may also be beneficial.[6] The benefits of barefoot running in the sand or grass, for example, have been noted as a training tool, but not for every run. There is some validity to letting your foot move in a more natural way and steering away from shoes that don't allow your foot to move at all. Increasing the actual strength of your foot muscles is another benefit.

If you want to incorporate barefoot or "barefoot-like" running into your workout, some solid advice is to make the change slowly. Don't just throw out your running shoes and do a five-mile run! Start out by doing activities around the house barefoot, and walking barefoot to build up your foot and calf muscles slowly. Check with your doctor before adding barefoot running to your exercise program; people who have circulatory or nerve issues should not attempt to run barefoot, as they are at increased risk for injury. If your doctor clears you for incorporating barefoot running, you may want to try shoes with more flexibility and less cushioning and then gradually work your way to minimalist shoes for part of your weekly workout time. Then, do a portion of your running in bare feet to allow your feet to develop calluses for running on rough surfaces. As your muscles strengthen you can build on the time you spend running barefoot.[7]

Sources:
1. M. Warburton, "Barefoot Running," *Sportscience* 5, no. 3 (2001) www.sportsci.org/jour/0103/mw.htm.
2. R. Collier, "The Rise of Barefoot Running," *Canadian Medical Association Journal* 183, no. 1 (2011): E37–38.
3. D. E. Lieberman and others, "Foot Strike Patterns and Collision Forces in Habitually Barefoot Versus Shod Runners," *Nature* 463, no. 7280 (2010): 531–35.
4. D. E. Lieberman and others, "Running Barefoot, Forefoot Striking and Training Tips," www.barefootrunning.fas.harvard.edu/5BarefootRunning&TrainingTips.html (accessed February 2011).
5. R. Collier, "The Rise of Barefoot Running."
6. D. E. Lieberman and others, "Foot Strike Patterns and Collision Forces."
7. C. Pauls and L. Kravitz, "Barefoot Running," *IDEA Fitness Journal* 7, no. 5 (2010): 14–17.

accustomed to the environment, (6) have an underlying infection, or (7) are overweight.[25] You can decrease your risk by being more fit, wearing light, sweat-wicking clothing, picking cooler times of the day to exercise, avoiding hazardous conditions, letting your body gradually become accustomed to the environment, and increasing your workout slowly.

If you suspect you are developing a heat-related illness, act immediately. For heat cramps, cease activity, seek a cool environment, and restore your body's fluid and electrolyte balances by drinking water or a sports drink. For heat exhaustion, rest in a cool environment, apply cold packs to your head and neck, drink water or a sports drink, and seek medical attention. If you suspect heatstroke, you will need medical attention immediately; untreated heatstroke is very serious and can lead to death. In heatstroke illness the body can no longer cool itself and ice-water immersion and IV fluids may be necessary right away. Because exercise increases your core body temperature, your risk of heat illness is greater when you are active, even in lower temperatures. Take extra precautions during difficult workouts to take breaks and drink fluids.

Prevent Cold-Related Illness Exercising in extreme cold also presents risks. If you like to ski, hike in the mountains, swim in cold water, or just exercise in snowy, windy, rainy environments, you should take precautions to prevent **hypothermia**, a condition in which the body's internal temperature drops so low that it can no longer warm itself back up. If untreated, hypothermia leads to death. To avoid hypothermia, (1) minimize heat loss by wearing a warm hat and clothing, (2) keep yourself dry by wearing sweat-wicking clothing and changing out of wet clothes as quickly as possible, (3) exercise with a workout partner who can help recognize early warning signs of cold-related illness, (4) avoid exercising in poor weather conditions, (5) warm up thoroughly, (6) drink fluids to stay hydrated, and (7) get out of the cold and warm up if you start shivering.

The early warning signs of hypothermia include shivering, goose bumps, and fast, shallow breathing. The next stage involves violent shivering, muscle incoordination, mild confusion, pale skin, and potentially blue lips, ears, fingers, and toes. In the most dangerous and potentially fatal stage of hypothermia, shivering will

hypothermia A condition where the core temperature of the body drops below the level required for sustaining normal bodily functions

stop and the person will have trouble thinking, speaking, walking, and using his or her hands. If you suspect you are at risk of hypothermia, get dry and warm as soon as possible. If you are in an advanced stage of hypothermia, you will need medical attention immediately.

Be Aware of the Impact of Air Quality Air pollution can irritate your air passageways and lungs, particularly if you have asthma, allergies, bronchitis, or other pulmonary disorders. If you experience a disruption in your breathing pattern, irritated eyes, or a headache, stop exercising and go indoors. Avoid exercising outdoors when the air quality is poor, particularly if you have a smog or air-quality alert in your city that day. If you exercise outside on a regular basis, take measures to reduce your intake of air pollution. Exercise in wilderness areas, in parks, or on low-traffic streets. Try to exercise at times when the air quality is better, such as early in the morning and on weekends.

Watch for Hazards Watch for hazards in your exercise environment that may cause you to trip and fall. When exercising indoors, seek out a space with a well-maintained floor and where you can work out without obstructions. When exercising outdoors, seek out lower-impact surfaces such as a school track, running or bike path, or a dirt trail. Use your common sense: avoid slippery or muddy surfaces and areas with heavy vehicle traffic. If you exercise outdoors at night, wear reflective clothing and clip a light somewhere on your body so that drivers can easily see you.

• •

THINK! What hazards do you face in your exercise routine? Can cars really see you when you are running on the road at night? Do your shoes have decent soles, so you don't slip?

ACT! List three things about your workout routine, your clothing, or your environment that might put you at risk for injury or illness. For each thing, list what steps you need to take to reduce your risk.

• •

Drink Enough Water

If you sweat profusely and do not replace the lost fluid, you will become dehydrated. Your body needs a certain amount of water in order to function. Loss of body water will decrease your blood volume and will subsequently decrease the blood flow to muscles, lowering exercise performance. **Dehydration** will also slow your sweat

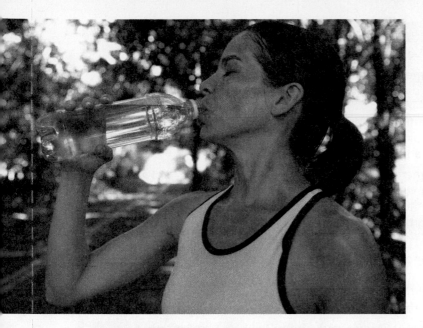

drinking additional fluid several hours before an exercise session and drink during exercise as

well. If you are exercising for more than an hour, you may benefit from drinking fluid with sugars and electrolytes (salts) in it, such as a sports drink.

Understand How to Prevent and Treat Common Injuries

Below are some of the most common exercise injuries, as well as guidelines for how to prevent and treat them. See also Table 3.4 for a summary of these and other common exercise injuries.

rate and significantly increase your susceptibility for heat-related illness.

According to the ACSM, you should lose no more than two percent of your body weight in fluid during an exercise session. A loss of fluid equivalent to one percent of your body weight will cause you to feel thirsty; losses over three percent may start to affect your exercise performance. Weigh yourself before and after exercise to determine how much water weight you have lost and adjust your fluid intake accordingly. Water loss is an individual issue. Everyone sweats at different rates in response to exercise. To decrease water loss, start

Delayed-Onset Muscle Soreness *Delayed-onset muscle soreness* (DOMS) is the muscle tightness and tenderness you may feel a day or two after a hard workout session. This soreness is due to microscopic tears in your muscle fibers and connective tissues; it occurs when the body sustains excessive overloads. Most people experience DOMS at one point or another and typically recover quickly. DOMS is a sign that you did too much too soon. If you experience DOMS (especially common when starting an exercise program), examine your program design. Find ways to decrease the time, intensity, resistance, or repetitions of the exercise.

TABLE 3.4 Common Exercise Injuries, Treatments, and Prevention		
Injury	Description	Treatment and Prevention
Delayed-Onset Muscle Soreness (DOMS)	Muscle tenderness and stiffness 24–48 hours after strenuous exercise	*Treatment:* Reduce exercise to light activity until the pain stops, gently stretch the area; for some, heat and anti-inflammatory medications help as well *Prevention:* Follow proper exercise programming guidelines
Back Pain	Sharp or dull pain and stiffness in the mid to lower back	*Treatment:* Reduce exercise until the acute pain stops; gently stretch the area; use ice, heat, anti-inflammatory medications *Prevention:* Strengthen abdominal and back muscles, stretch back and hip muscles, maintain a healthy body weight, have good posture and lifting techniques
Blisters	Red, fluid- or blood-filled pockets of skin, often on the feet after a long exercise session	*Treatment:* Change shoes that may have caused the blister, keep the area clean, and cover if needed; do not purposefully pop blisters *Prevention:* Use comfortable shoes that fit well and sweat-wicking socks (avoid all-cotton socks)
Muscle Cramps	Muscle pain, tightness, and uncontrollable spasms	*Treatment:* Stop activity; massage and stretch the affected area until the cramp releases *Prevention:* Follow warm-up, cool-down, and general exercise guidelines; stay fully hydrated for exercise

(Continued)

TABLE **3.4** (*Continued*)

Injury	Description	Treatment and Prevention
Muscle Strain	Damage to the muscle or tendon fibers due to injury or overtraining resulting in pain, swelling, and decreased function; varying levels of severity	*Treatment:* Reduce painful activity; apply ice or heat after a few days; use anti-inflammatory medications if desired; stretching *Prevention:* Follow warm-up, cool-down, and general exercise guidelines; reduce or stop activity if muscles feel overly weak and fatigued
Joint Sprain	Damage to ligaments or joint structures; the result of an acute injury resulting in pain, swelling, and loss of function; varying levels of severity	*Treatment:* Stop activity; use ice, compression, elevation; seek medical attention *Prevention:* Avoid high joint-stress activities, strengthen joint-supporting muscles, wear supportive bracing if necessary
Dislocation	Separation of bones in a joint causing structural alterations and potential ligament and nerve damage	*Treatment:* Stop activity; use ice, immobilization; seek medical treatment *Prevention:* Avoid high joint-stress activities, strengthen joint-supporting muscles, wear supportive bracing if necessary
Tendonitis	Chronic pain and swelling in tendons as a result of overuse	*Treatment:* Reduce exercise to light activity until the pain stops; apply ice, gently stretch the area; anti-inflammatory medications may help *Prevention:* Follow proper exercise programming guidelines, work for muscle balance in strength and flexibility
Plantar Fasciitis	Irritation, pain, and swelling of the fascia under the foot	*Treatment:* Reduce painful activities, gently stretch the area; for some people, ice, heat, and/or anti-inflammatory medications help *Prevention:* Wear good athletic shoes with adequate arch support and cushioning; warm up and stretch the plantar fascia prior to exercise
Runner's Knee	Patella-femoral pain syndrome where there is chronic pain behind or around the kneecap	*Treatment:* Reduce exercises that cause pain; use ice, anti-inflammatory medications if needed for pain and swelling *Prevention:* Work for balance in strength and flexibility in all of the knee-supporting muscles; wear good athletic shoes with support and foot control; exercise on softer surfaces; control weight
Shin Splints	Chronic pain in the front of the lower leg (the shins); can also occur as pain on the sides of the lower leg	*Treatment:* Reduce painful exercise; apply ice, gently stretch the area, switch to less weight-bearing activities *Prevention:* Work for balance in strength and flexibility in the lower-leg muscles, wear good athletic shoes with support and cushioning, exercise on softer surfaces
Stress Fracture	Small crack or breaks in the bone in overused areas of the body causing chronic pain; must be medically diagnosed via X-ray	*Treatment:* Perform non-weight-bearing exercise until the acute pain stops, seek medical attention, rest *Prevention:* Follow proper exercise programming guidelines to avoid overtraining, wear good athletic shoes with support and cushioning, exercise on softer surfaces

Muscle and Tendon Strains A muscle or tendon strain is a soft-tissue injury that can be acute or chronic. An acute, sudden strain occurs due to a trauma or sudden movement/force that you are not accustomed to. A chronic, perpetual strain occurs from overstressed muscles that are worked in the same way over and over. Muscle strains involve damage to the muscle fibers; tendon strains involve damage to the tissue that connects muscles to bones. The primary symptoms of a strain are muscle pain, spasms, and weakness. In addition, there may be swelling of the area, cramping, and difficulty moving the muscle involved. Commonly strained areas of the body are the lower back and the back of the thighs (hamstrings).

Ligament and Joint Sprains A sudden movement or trauma can cause a sprain (damage to joint structures.) A *mild* or *first-degree sprain* involves overstretching or slight tearing of the ligament(s), resulting in some pain and swelling but little or no decrease in joint stability. In a *moderate* or *second-degree sprain,* ligaments are partially torn, and the area is painful, swollen, and bruised. In this level of sprain, mobility is limited and medical attention should be sought to determine the true severity of the injury. A *severe* or *third-degree sprain* involves a complete tearing or rupturing of the ligament or joint structures. Excessive pain, swelling, bruising, and an inability to move or put any weight on the joint are symptoms of a third-degree sprain. Immediate medical attention is necessary to determine whether bones were broken during the injury process. The most common sprains occur in the ankle while landing from a jump, in the knee from a fall or a blow to the side, and in the wrist during a fall.

Overuse Injuries Overuse injuries are due to repetitive use. You are at an increased risk of an overuse injury if you are new to sports and exercise, if you dramatically change your exercise routine, or if you do the same type of activity day in and day out.

Tendonitis is a typical overuse injury that can result from overusing the lower- or upper-body muscles. The repetitive contractions of skeletal muscles can cause pain and swelling in the tendons near joints. Common tendonitis locations are the elbow, ankle, and shoulder; these often result from tennis ("tennis elbow"), running, and weight-lifting, respectively.

A frequent overuse injury in runners and walkers is *plantar fasciitis,* or inflammation in the fascia on the underside of the foot. Pain in the arch and the heel of the foot, particularly when you are not warmed up (stepping out of bed in the morning), is the hallmark of this overuse injury.

Another injury common in runners is "runner's knee," or *patella-femoral pain syndrome.* Pain behind the kneecap (patella), inflammation, and tenderness can result from an imbalance in knee-stabilizing muscles that will cause the patella to get "off track" with your other knee joint structures. Women tend to have more problems with this syndrome than men due to the greater dynamic flexibility of their hips and knees.

Shin splints is the general term used to describe any pain that occurs in the front or sides of the lower legs. It may be tendonitis, a muscle strain, connective tissue inflammation, or a stress fracture. In response to repetitive stresses on hard surfaces, the muscles, tendons, and connective tissues of your lower leg muscles become inflamed and painful. Shin splints are common in runners and high-mileage walkers. Over time, repeated stress to the lower leg can lead to a *stress fracture,* a small crack or break in a bone. If you think you have shin splints but the pain won't go away with rest, ice, and therapy, you should get medical attention to rule out a stress fracture.

Treating Injuries with RICE The **RICE** treatment for injuries involves *rest, ice, compression,* and *elevation.* After an injury, you should *rest* or stop using that body part and allow for treatment and recovery. Most injuries will require *ice* immediately to reduce blood flow, acute inflammation, and pain. Apply ice or an ice pack for 10 to 30 minutes at a time, three to five times a day until symptoms lessen. *Compression* or applying pressure to the injury can be helpful for injuries that are bleeding or swelling. Using an elastic bandage around the injury will reduce swelling but still allow for adequate blood flow to the area. Tingling or discolored skin can be a sign that your wrapping is too tight. In order to promote blood flow back to the heart and lower the amount of swelling, *elevate* the injury above heart level. Following the RICE treatment is a good start for most exercise and sports-related injuries. Seek further medical attention if you are unsure how injured you are or if symptoms do not cease within a few hours.

> **RICE** Acronym for rest, *ice,* compression, and elevation; a method of treating common exercise injuries

chapterin**review**

videos

Log on to **www.pearsonhighered.com/hopson** or MyFitnessLab to view these chapter-related videos.

Personal Fitness and Exercise   3-Minute Step Test Assessment   Heart Rate: Carotid Pulse

Heart Rate: Radial Pulse

onlineresources

Log on to **www.pearsonhighered.com/hopson** or MyFitnessLab for access to these book-related resources and for links to other useful websites.

Audio case study
Audio PowerPoint lecture

Lab 3.1 Monitoring Intensity during a Workout
Lab 3.2 Assessing Your Cardiorespiratory
Fitness Level
Lab 3.3 Plan Your Cardiorespiratory Fitness
Goals and Program
Alternate Aerobic Fitness Assessment:
2-Minute Marching Test
Alternate Aerobic Fitness Assessment:
Adapted for Swimming
Alternate Aerobic Fitness Assessment:
Adapted for Wheelchair Users

Customizable four-week running programs
Customizable four-week biking programs
Customizable four-week swimming programs
Take Charge of Your Health! Worksheets
Behavior Change Log Book and Wellness
Journal

Pre- and post-quizzes
Glossary flashcards

reviewquestions

1. Cardiorespiratory fitness would be most improved by which of the following?
   a. Stretching your leg muscles every day
   b. A 90-minute yoga class, three times per week
   c. Vigorously riding your bicycle every day for 30 minutes
   d. Walking to and from classes across campus

2. Regular cardiorespiratory fitness activities reduce your chance of developing
   a. metabolic syndrome.
   b. HIV.
   c. athlete's foot.
   d. dehydration.

3. Which circulation delivers blood to the lungs?
   a. Pulmonary
   b. Systemic
   c. Hepatic
   d. Cardiac

4. Which energy system will provide most of the ATP during an hour-long bicycle ride?
   a. The immediate energy system
   b. The nonoxidative energy system
   c. The creatine phosphate energy system
   d. The oxidative energy system

5. Which of the following will decrease with regular aerobic training?
   a. Muscle cell size
   b. Blood volume
   c. Resting heart rate
   d. Maximal cardiac output

6. Which of the following is an example of vigorous exercise?
   a. Gardening
   b. Running a fast mile
   c. A one-mile leisurely walk
   d. Bowling

7. The bulk of your cardiorespiratory training program should include
   a. interval training.
   b. circuit training.
   c. hill run training.
   d. continuous target heart rate training.

8. Which OMNI Scale of Perceived Exertion value is associated with training in your target heart rate range?
   a. 1
   b. 3
   c. 7
   d. 9

9. Which of the following is the *best* way to plan for cardiorespiratory program progression?
   a. Follow the 10 percent rule
   b. Increase your exercise duration each time you work out
   c. Schedule re-assessments of your cardiorespiratory fitness every four weeks
   d. Increase your exercise intensity with every work-out session

10. What is the most common type of injury or illness in cardiorespiratory exercisers?
    a. Heat illness
    b. Hypothermia
    c. Overuse injuries
    d. Head injuries

critical**thinking**questions

1. Name three benefits of having a high level of cardiorespiratory fitness and explain how each impacts your overall health and wellness.

2. What are the pros and cons of each method of intensity monitoring: target heart rate, perceived exertion, and the talk test?

references

1. J. L. Johnson and others, "Exercise Training Amount and Intensity Effects on Metabolic Syndrome," *American Journal of Cardiology* 100, no. 12 (2007): 1759–66.
2. K. E. Reed and others, "Arterial Compliance in Young Children: The Role of Aerobic Fitness," *European Journal of Cardiovascular Prevention and Rehabilitation* 12, no. 5 (2005): 492–97.
3. J. M. McGavock, T. J. Anderson, and R. Z. Lewanczuk, "Sedentary Lifestyle and Antecedents of Cardiovascular Disease in Young Adults," *American Journal of Hypertension* 19, no. 7 (2006): 701–07.
4. C. E. Finley and others, "Cardiorespiratory Fitness, Macronutrient Intake, and the Metabolic Syndrome: The Aerobics Center Longitudinal Study," *Journal of the American Dietetic Association* 106, no. 5 (2006): 673–79.
5. C. R. Bruce and others, "Endurance Training in Obese Humans Improves Glucose Tolerance and Mitochondrial Fatty Acid Oxidation and Alters Muscle Lipid Content," *American Journal of Physiology: Endocrinology and Metabolism* 291, no. 1 (2006): E99–E107.
6. X. Sui and others, "Influence of Cardiorespiratory Fitness on Lung Cancer Mortality," *Medicine and Science in Sports and Exercise* 42, no. 5 (2010): 872-8; S. W. Farrell and others, "Cardiorespiratory Fitness, Different Measures of Adiposity, and Total Cancer Mortality in Women," *Obesity (Silver Spring)* (Feb 2011). [Epub ahead of print].

7. G. R. Hunter and others, "Increased Resting Energy Expenditure after 40 Minutes of Aerobic but Not Resistance Exercise," *Obesity (Silver Spring)* 14, no. 11 (2006): 2018–25.
8. S. M. Markowitz and S. M. Arent, "The Exercise and Affect Relationship: Evidence for the Dual-Mode Model and a Modified Opponent Process Theory," *Journal of Sport & Exercise Psychology* 32, no. 5 (2010): 711–30.
9. M. D. Hoffman and D. R. Hoffman, "Exercisers Achieve Greater Acute Exercise-Induced Mood Enhancement than Nonexercisers," *Archives of Physical Medicine and Rehabilitation* 89, no. 2 (2008): 358–63.
10. T. M. DiLorenzo and others, "Long-Term Effects of Aerobic Exercise on Psychological Outcomes," *Preventative Medicine* 28, no. 1 (1999): 75–85.
11. P. J. Carek, S. E. Laibstain, and S. M. Carek, "Exercise for the Treatment of Depression and Anxiety," *International Journal of Psychiatry in Medicine* 41, no. 1 (2011): 15–28.
12. V. S. Conn, "Depressive Symptom Outcomes of Physical Activity Interventions: Meta-Analysis Findings," *Annals of Behavioral Medicine* 39, no. 2 (2010): 128–38.
13. J. Romeo and others, "Physical Activity, Immunity and Infection," *The Proceedings of the Nutrition Society* 69, no. 3 (2010): 390–99.
14. M. H. Arai, A. J. Duarte, and V. M. Natale, "The Effects of Long-Term Endurance

Training on the Immune and Endocrine Systems of Elderly Men: The Role of Cytokines and Anabolic Steroid Hormones," *Immunity and Aging* 3 (2006): 9.
15. R. S. Newson and E. B. Kemps, "Cardiorespiratory Fitness as a Predictor of Successful Cognitive Ageing," *Journal of Clinical and Experimental Neuropsychology* 28, no. 6 (2006): 949–67.
16. S. J. Colcome and others, "Aerobic Exercise Training Increases Brain Volume in Aging Humans," *Journal of Gerontology Series A: Biological Sciences and Medical Sciences* 61, no. 11 (2006): 1166–70.
17. K. I. Erickson and others, "Exercise Training Increases Size of Hippocampus and Improves Memory," *Proceedings of the National Academy of Sciences U.S.A.,* 108, no. 7 (2011): 3017–22.
18. S. Fillipas and others, "A Six-Month, Supervised, Aerobic and Resistance Exercise Program Improves Self-Efficacy in People with Human Immunodeficiency Virus: A Randomized Controlled Trial," *Australian Journal of Physiotherapy* 52, no. 3 (2006): 185–90.
19. M. McNeely and others, "Effects of Exercise on Breast Cancer Patients and Survivors," *Canadian Medical Association Journal* 175, no. 1 (2006): 34–41.
20. M. Benetti, C. L. Araujo, and R. Z. Santos, "Cardiorespiratory Fitness and Quality of Life at Different Exercise Intensities after Myocardial Infarction," *Arquivos Brasileiros de Cardiologia* 95, no. 3 (2010): 399–404.

21. G. Borg, *Borg's Perceived Exertion and Pain Scales.* (Champaign: Human Kinetics, 1998) 27–38.
22. R. J. Robertson and others, "Validation of the Adult OMNI Scale of Perceived Exertion for Cycle Ergometer Exercise," *Medicine & Science in Sports & Exercise* 36, no. 1 (2004): 102–108.
23. A. C. Utter and others, "Validation of the Adult OMNI Scale of Perceived Exertion for Walking/Running Exercise," *Medicine & Science in Sports & Exercise* 36, no. 10 (2004): 1776–1780.
24. American Academy of Orthopaedic Surgeons, "Your Orthopaedic Connection: Athletic Shoes," http://orthoinfo.aaos.org/topic.cfm?topic=A00318 (accessed September 2011).
25. M. Rav-Acha and others, "Fatal Exertional Heat Stroke: A Case Series," *American Journal of the Medical Sciences* 328, no. 2 (2004): 84–87.

LAB 3.1 • MONITORING INTENSITY DURING A WORKOUT

Name: _____ Date: _____

Instructor: _____ Section: _____

Materials: Calculator and a stopwatch

Purpose: (1) To measure your resting heart rate (RHR); (2) to calculate your personal target heart rate range for exercise; (3) to assess the intensity of your workout

SECTION I: DETERMINING YOUR RESTING HEART RATE

1. **Practice Taking Your Pulse** Press your middle and index fingers gently on the side of your throat to take your *carotid pulse.* You can also take a *radial pulse* by placing your middle and index fingers at the thumb side of your wrist. Measure your resting heart rate (RHR) by counting your pulse for 60 seconds, then 30 seconds, then 10 seconds. Record your counts and complete the calculations below.

Pulse Rate #1 (60 sec) _____ × 1 = _____ 1 full minute RHR

Pulse Rate #2 (30 sec) _____ × 2 = _____ 1 calculated minute RHR

Pulse Rate #3 (10 sec) _____ × 6 = _____ 1 calculated minute RHR

2. **Determine Your True Resting Heart Rate**
Take your pulse first thing in the morning on four different days. Record and average the results below. For an accurate resting heart rate, always count your pulse for a full minute. Ideally, you should take your pulse after waking up *without an alarm* and after a good night's rest.

	Resting Heart Rate (RHR)	Time of Day
Day 1		
Day 2		
Day 3		
Day 4		

Average RHR = _____

SECTION II: CALCULATE YOUR TARGET HEART RATE RANGE FOR EXERCISE

Calculate your personal target heart rate range for exercise using two methods: the maximum heart rate (HRmax) method and the heart rate reserve (HRR) method. Your target heart rate will provide a guideline for how many beats per minute (bpm) your heart should be beating during exercise, in order to achieve improvements in cardiorespiratory fitness. Note that you must count your pulse within 15 seconds of stopping exercise in order for your heart rate to reflect the exercise rate. Thus, if you take five seconds to find your pulse and start counting, that leaves you 10 seconds to take an exercise heart rate.

Method #1: Maximum Heart Rate (HRmax)

1. Find your predicted HRmax = 220 − _____ = _____
                                              (age)   (predicted HRmax)

2. Find your low HR target = _____ × .70 = _____ bpm ÷ 6 = _____
                                  (predicted HRmax)   *Low HR target*   *Low 10 sec target*

3. Find your high HR target = _____ × .90 = _____ bpm ÷ 6 = _____
                                   (predicted HRmax)   *High HR target*   *High 10 sec target*

Method #2: Heart Rate Reserve (HRR)

1. Find your HRR = _____ – _____ = _____

      (predicted HRmax)   RHR   HRR

              (from Section I)

2. Find 50% of HRR = (_____ × .50) = _____ – _____ bpm ÷ 6 = _____

        HRR   RHR   *Low HR target*   *Low 10 sec target*

3. Find 80% of HRR = (_____ × .80) = _____ – _____ bpm ÷ 6 = _____

        HRR   RHR *High HR target*   *High 10 sec target*

SECTION III: MONITOR YOUR WORKOUT INTENSITY LEVEL

Practice monitoring your workout intensity during a 30-minute exercise session. You can choose any form of individual exercise that allows you to easily monitor your heart rate via a pulse check.

1. Calculate your estimated heart rate goal as a 10-second count for each time interval in the chart below.

2. Conduct your exercise session. Take your pulse and record your actual exercise heart rates.

3. In the last column of the chart, write your perceived exertion scores (1–10 OMNI Scale) scores 30 seconds before the end of the time period indicated on the workout schedule.

Time	Planned Intensity	Calculated HR 10 sec Count	Actual 10 sec HR	Perceived Exertion (1–10)
5 min warm-up	Slowly up to 55% HRmax	Predicted HRmax × .55 = _____ ÷ 6 = _____		
5 min	65% HRmax	Predicted HRmax × .65 = _____ ÷ 6 = _____		
4 min	75% HRmax	Predicted HRmax × .75 = _____ ÷ 6 = _____		
3 min	85% HRmax	Predicted HRmax × .85 = _____ ÷ 6 = _____		
4 min	75% HRmax	Predicted HRmax × .75 = _____ ÷ 6 = _____		
5 min	65% HRmax	Predicted HRmax × .65 = _____ ÷ 6 = _____		
4 min cool-down	55% HRmax	Predicted HRmax × .55 = _____ ÷ 6 = _____.		

SECTION IV: REFLECTION

1. How close were your calculated and actual heart rates during your 30-minute exercise session?

2. Did the intensity levels feel higher or lower than you thought they would at each percentage of HRmax?

LAB 3.2 • ASSESSING YOUR CARDIORESPIRATORY FITNESS LEVEL

Name: _____   **Date:** _____

Instructor: _____   **Section:** _____

Materials: Calculator, 12-inch step, stopwatch, metronome

Purpose: To measure (1) recovery from physical activity, (2) walking speed, and (3) current level of cardiorespiratory fitness.

SECTION I: THE THREE-MINUTE STEP TEST

For this test, you will be stepping on a 12-inch high step bench for three minutes and then measuring your recovery pulse for one full minute.

1. Setup and preparation. Set up a 12-inch-high step bench in a place that will be safe to perform the test. Set the metronome to a pace of 96 beats per minute, which means you will be doing 24 steps up and down in a minute. Listen to the metronome and do a couple of practice steps to ensure that you can step with the right cadence ("up, up, down, down"). One foot will be stepping up or down with each beat of the metronome. Have a stopwatch available to time your three minutes on the step and your one minute HR afterward.

2. Step up and down for three minutes. Start the metronome and march in place to the beat. Start stepping up on the bench and down to the floor after starting the stopwatch. Maintain this exact pace for the entire three minutes.

3. Stop and count your pulse for one full minute. At the end of three minutes, stop stepping, turn off the metronome, sit down on your bench, and find your carotid or radial pulse immediately. Within five seconds of stopping the exercise, start counting your recovery pulse and count for one full minute.

4. Record your results and your fitness rating. Record your recovery heart rate below in beats per minute (bpm). Locate your fitness rating on the chart below and record that as well.

The 3-Minute Step Test RESULTS

1-Minute Recovery HR: _____ **(bpm)**   **Fitness Rating:** _____

YMCA 3-Minute Step Test Ratings (bpm)							
Men	Excellent	Good	Above Average	Average	Below Average	Poor	Very Poor
18–25 yrs	50–76	79–84	88–93	95–100	102–107	111–119	124–157
26–35 yrs	51–76	79–85	88–94	96–102	104–110	114–121	126–161
36–45 yrs	49–76	80–88	92–98	100–105	108–113	116–124	130–163
46–55 yrs	56–82	87–93	95–101	103–111	113–119	121–126	131–159
56–65 yrs	60–77	86–94	97–100	103–109	111–117	119–128	131–154
66+ yrs	59–81	87–92	94–102	104–110	114–118	121–126	130–151

YMCA 3-Minute Step Test Ratings (bpm)							
Women	Excellent	Good	Above Average	Average	Below Average	Poor	Very Poor
18–25 yrs	52–81	85–93	96–102	104–110	113–120	122–131	135–169
26–35 yrs	58–80	85–92	95–101	104–110	113–119	122–129	134–171
36–45 yrs	51–84	89–96	100–104	107–112	115–120	124–132	137–169
46–55 yrs	63–91	95–101	104–110	113–118	120–124	126–132	137–171
56–65 yrs	60–92	97–103	106–111	113–118	119–127	129–135	141–174
66+ yrs	70–92	96–101	104–111	116–121	123–126	128–133	135–155

SECTION II: THE ONE-MILE WALK TEST

You will walk one mile and determine your heart rate response to the exercise immediately after. IMPORTANT REMINDERS: The accuracy of this test depends on three things: (1) Walk during this test. Do not run. (2) Walk the mile as fast as you can. (3) Keep a steady pace throughout the mile. Do not "sprint" at the end.

1. **Preparation and warm-up.** Make sure that you have an accurate one-mile course to complete (four laps around a standard track) and a stopwatch. Warm up with three to five minutes of light walking and range-of-motion activities.

2. **Walk one full mile as fast as you can.** After completing the one mile, record your finish time (from your watch, stopwatch, or someone calling out the time) below. Convert the time from minutes and seconds to minutes with a decimal fraction.

3. **Immediately take an exercise heart rate and cool-down.** Within five seconds of finishing the walk, find your carotid or radial pulse and count your pulse for 10 seconds. Multiply the number by 6 and record your HR below. After recording your finish time and your HR, cool down by walking slowly for another five minutes and doing some light stretching.

4. **Calculate your estimated maximal oxygen consumption (VO$_2$max).** Use the formula below to calculate your estimated VO$_2$max. This number will more accurately reflect your fitness level if you followed the test instructions carefully.

5. **Find the cardiorespiratory fitness level that corresponds to your predicted VO$_2$max.** Use the chart at the end of Section III to determine your cardiorespiratory fitness level, as determined by this one-mile walking test.

The One-Mile Walk Test RESULTS

One-Mile Walk Time: _____ (min:sec); divide sec by 60 = _____ (min w/decimal)

Exercise HR: _____ (beats) × 6 = _____ (bpm)
                    (10 sec count)

Estimated VO$_2$max: Use the following equation to estimate VO$_2$max, where gender = 0 for female and 1 for male; time = walk time to the nearest hundredth of a minute; and HR = heart rate (bpm) at the end of the walking test. Plug in your weight and numbers from above and calculate the numbers in parentheses first. Complete the calculation to find your estimated VO$_2$max.

- VO$_2$max = 132.853 − [0.0769 × body weight (lb)] − [0.3877 × age (yr)] + [6.3150 × gender] − [3.2649 × time (min)] − [0.1565 × HR (bpm)]

- $VO_2max = 132.853 - [0.0769 \times \underline{\hspace{1.5cm}} \text{ (lb)}] - [0.3877 \times \underline{\hspace{1.5cm}} \text{ (yr)}] + [6.3150 \times \underline{\hspace{1.5cm}} \text{(gender)}] - [3.2649 \times \underline{\hspace{1.5cm}} \text{ (min)}] - [0.1565 \times \underline{\hspace{1.5cm}} \text{ (bpm)}]$

- $VO_2max = 132.853 - \underline{\hspace{1.5cm}} - \underline{\hspace{1.5cm}} = \underline{\hspace{1.5cm}} - \underline{\hspace{1.5cm}} - \underline{\hspace{1.5cm}}$

- $VO_2max = \underline{\hspace{1.5cm}} \text{ (ml/kg·min)}$

Walk Test VO₂max Fitness Rating: _____

SECTION III: 1.5-MILE RUN TEST

1. **Preparation and warm-up.** Make sure that you have an accurate 1.5-mile course to complete (six laps around a standard track) and a stopwatch. Warm up with 5 to 10 minutes of walking/jogging and range-of-motion activities.

2. **Run (with walk breaks if needed) 1.5 miles as fast as you can.** After reaching 1.5 miles, mark your finish time (from your watch, stopwatch, or someone calling out the time) below. Convert the time from minutes and seconds to minutes with a decimal fraction.

3. **Cool-down.** After recording your finish time, cool down by walking for five minutes and doing some light stretching.

4. **Calculate your estimated maximal oxygen consumption (VO₂max).** Use the formula below to calculate your estimated VO₂max.

5. **Find your cardiorespiratory fitness level that corresponds to your predicted VO₂max.** Use the chart at the end of this section to determine your cardiorespiratory fitness level, as determined by this 1.5-mile running test.

The 1.5-Mile Run Test RESULTS

1.5-Mile Run Time: _____ (min:sec); divide sec by 60 = _____ (min w/decimal)

Estimated VO₂max: You will use the following equation to estimate VO₂max, where time = run time to the nearest hundredth of a minute. Plug in your time from above, compute the number in parentheses first, and complete the calculation to find your estimated VO₂max.

- $VO_2max = [483 \div \text{time (min)}] + 3.5$

- $VO_2max = [483 \div \underline{\hspace{3cm}} \text{ (min)}] + 3.5$

- $VO_2max = \underline{\hspace{3cm}} + 3.5$

- $VO_2max = \underline{\hspace{3cm}} \text{ (ml/kg·min)}$

Run Test VO₂max Fitness Rating: _____

Estimated VO₂max Fitness Ratings (ml/kg·min)						
Men	Superior	Excellent	Good	Fair	Poor	Very Poor
18–29 yrs	>56.1	51.1–56.1	45.7–51.0	42.2–45.6	38.1–42.1	<38.1
30–39 yrs	>54.2	48.9–54.2	44.4–48.8	41.0–44.3	36.7–40.9	<36.7
40–49 yrs	>52.8	46.8–52.8	42.4–46.7	38.4–42.3	34.6–38.3	<34.6
50–59 yrs	>49.6	43.3–49.6	38.3–43.2	35.2–38.2	31.1–35.1	<31.1
60–69 yrs	>46.0	39.5–46.0	35.0–39.4	31.4–34.9	27.4–31.3	<27.4

Estimated VO$_2$max Fitness Ratings (ml/kg·min)						
Women	Superior	Excellent	Good	Fair	Poor	Very Poor
18–29 yrs	>50.1	44.0–50.1	39.5–43.9	35.5–39.4	31.6–35.4	<31.6
30–39 yrs	>46.8	41.0–46.8	36.8–40.9	33.8–36.7	29.9–33.7	<29.9
40–49 yrs	>45.1	38.9–45.1	35.1–38.8	31.6–35.0	28.0–31.5	<28.0
50–59 yrs	>39.8	35.2–39.8	31.4–35.1	28.7–31.3	25.5–28.6	<25.5
60–69 yrs	>36.8	32.3–36.8	29.1–32.2	26.6–29.0	23.7–26.5	<23.7

Reprinted with permission from The Cooper Institute, Dallas, Texas, from Physical Fitness Assessments and Norms for Adults and Law Enforcement, available online at www.CooperInstitute.org.

You may also use the chart below to estimate your fitness level using only your run time.

Estimated Run Time Ratings				
Men	Excellent	Good	Fair	Poor
Ages 20–29	<10:10	10:10–11:29	11:30–12:38	>12:38
Ages 30–39	<10:47	10:47–11:54	11:55–12:58	>12:58
Ages 40–49	<11:16	11:16–12:24	12:25–13:50	>13:50
Ages 50–59	<12:09	12:09–13:35	13:36–15:06	>15:06
Ages 60–69	<13:24	13:24–15:04	15:05–16:46	>16:46
Women	Excellent	Good	Fair	Poor
Ages 20–29	<11:59	11:59–13:24	13:25–14:50	>14:50
Ages 30–39	<12:25	12:25–14:08	14:09–15:43	>15:43
Ages 40–49	<13:24	13:24–14:53	14:54–16:31	>16:31
Ages 50–59	<14:35	14:35–16:35	16:36–18:18	>18:18
Ages 60–69	<16:34	16:34–18:27	18:28–20:16	>20:16

Reprinted with permission from The Cooper Institute, Dallas, Texas, from *Physical Fitness Assessments and Norms for Adults and Law Enforcement*, available online at www.CooperInstitute.org.

LAB 3.3 • PLAN YOUR CARDIORESPIRATORY FITNESS GOALS AND PROGRAM

Name: _____ Date: _____

Instructor: _____ Section: _____

Materials: Results from cardiorespiratory fitness assessments, calculator, lab pages.

Purpose: To learn how to set appropriate cardiorespiratory fitness goals and create a personal cardiorespiratory fitness program designed to meet those goals.

SECTION I: SHORT- AND LONG-TERM GOALS

Create short- and long-term goals for cardiorespiratory fitness. Be sure to use SMART goal-setting guidelines (specific, measurable, action-oriented, realistic, time-oriented). Select appropriate target dates and rewards for completing your goals.

Short-Term Goal (3–6 Months)

_____

_____

Target Date: _____

Reward: _____

Long-Term Goal (12+ Months)

_____

_____

Target Date: _____

Reward: _____

SECTION II: CARDIORESPIRATORY FITNESS OBSTACLES AND STRATEGIES

1. What **barriers or obstacles** might hinder your plan to improve your cardiorespiratory fitness? Indicate your top three obstacles below:

    a. _____

    b. _____

    c. _____

2. Overcoming these barriers/obstacles to change will be an important step in reaching your goals. Write down three **strategies** for overcoming the obstacles listed above:

    a. _____

    b. _____

    c. _____

SECTION III: GETTING SUPPORT

1. List resources you will use to help you change your cardiorespiratory fitness:

Friend/partner/relative: _____

School-based resource: _____

Community-based resource: _____

Other: _____

2. How will you use these supportive resources to help you meet your cardiorespiratory fitness goals?

_____

_____

_____

_____

_____

_____

_____

_____

SECTION IV: CARDIORESPIRATORY FITNESS PROGRAM REFLECTIONS

1. How realistic are the short- and long-term target dates you have set for achieving your cardiorespiratory fitness goals?

_____

_____

_____

2. How many days per week are you planning to work on your cardiorespiratory fitness program? _____

3. What types of workouts are you planning to try?

_____

_____

_____

4. Do you have a workout partner? Do you plan to work with a workout partner, personal trainer, or instructor to help get you started?

_____

_____

_____

SECTION V: CARDIORESPIRATORY TRAINING PROGRAM DESIGN

Plan a four-week cardiorespiratory training program, using resources available to you (facility, instructor, text) and completing the following training calendar (A = activity, I = intensity, T = time).

Four-Week Cardiorespiratory Training Program						
Sun	Mon	Tues	Wed	Thurs	Fri	Sat
Date: _____	Date: _____	Date: _____	Date: _____	Date: _____	Date: _____	Date: _____
A:	A:	A:	A:	A:	A:	A:
I:	I:	I:	I:	I:	I:	I:
T:	T:	T:	T:	T:	T:	T:
Date: _____	Date: _____	Date: _____	Date: _____	Date: _____	Date: _____	Date: _____
A:	A:	A:	A:	A:	A:	A:
I:	I:	I:	I:	I:	I:	I:
T:	T:	T:	T:	T:	T:	T:
Date: _____	Date: _____	Date: _____	Date: _____	Date: _____	Date: _____	Date: _____
A:	A:	A:	A:	A:	A:	A:
I:	I:	I:	I:	I:	I:	I:
T:	T:	T:	T:	T:	T:	T:
Date: _____	Date: _____	Date: _____	Date: _____	Date: _____	Date: _____	Date: _____
A:	A:	A:	A:	A:	A:	A:
I:	I:	I:	I:	I:	I:	I:
T:	T:	T:	T:	T:	T:	T:

SECTION VI: TRACKING YOUR PROGRAM AND FOLLOWING THROUGH

1. **Goal and Program Tracking:** Use the following chart to monitor your progress. Change the activity, intensity, or time of your workout plan to reflect your progress as needed.

2. **Goal and Program Follow-up:** At the end of the course or at your short-term goal target date, reevaluate your cardiorespiratory fitness and ask yourself the following questions:

   a.   Did you meet your short-term goal or your goal for the course? If so, what positive behavioral changes contributed to your success? If not, which obstacles blocked your success?

   b.   Was your short-term goal realistic? What would you change about your goals or training plan?

	Five-Week Cardiorespiratory Training Log					
	Dates	Activity	Time	Av. HR	RPE	Comments
Week 1						
Week 2						
Week 3						
Week 4						
Week 5						

activate, motivate, & ADVANCE YOUR FITNESS

A RUNNING PROGRAM

ACTIVATE!

Whether this is your first attempt at running or you want to take your current run workouts to the next level, there is a program built just for you.

Running Program Preparation & Safety

Going too far or too fast right away is the number-one cause of injury among new runners. Focus on the minutes instead of miles, and use these programs to gradually increase your run time.

What Do I need for Running?

SHOES: Visit your local running store to find your most important running tool, your shoes! The employees are generally experienced runners who can assist you in finding a good fit for your foot, running style, gait, running surface and, of course, your goals.

CLOTHING: Wear comfortable and supportive clothing. Choose materials that wick moisture away from your skin. In cold weather, wear layers. In the sun, wear sunscreen, sunglasses, and a hat or visor. At sunrise, dusk, or night, wear reflective clothing and/or a vest and lights.

How Do I Start a Running Program?

TECHNIQUE: Relax your shoulders and gently swing your arms (90-degree elbow) up to your chest and down to your hips. Keep hands loose and relaxed. Look forward, rather than down at the ground. Stay light on your feet and use shorter, quicker steps. Land on the mid-foot or balls of your feet and push off. Aim for a stride rate (your turnover) of 180 steps per minute. Count the number of times your right foot strikes the ground in a minute and multiply that by two.

ETIQUETTE: Follow a few basic guidelines whether you are running alone or with a group, especially if you run in a high-traffic area. On a sidewalk or a multi-use path or trail, run on the right and pass on the left, after alerting others you are passing. Say, "On your left" as you approach. No matter where you run, remember to never run more than two abreast. If you need to stop, step off to the right to allow others to get by.

Running Tips

ROAD RUNNING: Plan safe and interesting routes that consider both traffic and available running paths. Check with your local running store or club for routes and running partners. Let someone know where you are going and when you will return. Carry a cell phone, ID, a few dollars, and a water bottle. Stay aware of your surroundings by wearing only one piece of your earphones. Run facing traffic and pay attention to traffic signals and signs.

TRACK RUNNING: A track will give you a stable and soft running surface. Other benefits? Tracks are usually well lit and you won't have to plan a route. Plus, you may have access to a rest room and a place to keep your water bottle and phone nearby. On a track, you can test pacing, adjust your run/walk ratios, and re-test your cardiorespiratory fitness level regularly. Most tracks are 400 meters; four laps on the inner lane equal a mile. Follow track etiquette by utilizing outside lanes for most of your training and leave the inside lane (lane 1) for faster runners and sprinters and for timing yourself on a specific distance. If you are using the inside lane and a faster individual approaches behind you, move out to lane 2 or 3 to allow the person to pass. Finally, try to change your running direction every few runs to vary the stresses on your body of going around turns.

TREADMILL RUNNING: Treadmills offer convenience, efficiency, and a safe environment when the weather is less than ideal. Be sure to familiarize yourself with the controls before starting out. Remember to maintain good form and avoid both the handrails and the back of the treadmill belt.

TRAIL RUNNING: Take a break from the asphalt jungle to run in nature. Ease into trail running by starting with flat, soft, easy-to-navigate trails (dirt, bark dust, pine needles, wood chips) and work your way up to more challenging ones. Take smaller steps, slow down, and constantly scan the trail to find the best footing. If possible, trail run with a buddy. If not, be sure that you know your route, take water, and tell someone of your location, start time, and anticipated end time.

Running Warm-Up and Cool-Down

Walk or jog at a slower pace for 5–10 minutes to warm-up or cool-down. After breaking a light sweat in your warm-up, you may want to add dynamic range-of-motion exercises. After you finish your cool-down, you can hold static stretches longer for improved flexibility.

Four-Week Running Programs

If you are new to running, if you want to transition from walking to running, or if you have taken a break from running for six months or more, then build your run program gradually and start with Program A. If you are already running 15 minutes continuously on two days a week, start with Program B below. Adjust time, intensity, and training days to suit your personal fitness level and schedule; visit the companion website for more options.

PROGRAM A

GOAL: Transition from walking to running. Increase run minutes while maintaining a moderate intensity level three to four days a week.

	Mon		Tue		Wed		Thurs		Fri		Sat		Sun	
	T*	I*	T	I	T	I	T	I	T	I	T	I	T	I
Week 1	20 1/4	L			20 1/4	L			20 1/4	L–M				
Week 2	24 1/5	M			24 1/5	M			24 1/5	M				
Week 3	32 1/7	M			32 1/7	M			32 1/7	M				
Week 4	24 2/10	M			24 2/10	M			24 2/10	M	24 2/10	M		

T*: Time. Total time is listed in minutes with the Walk/Run minute ratio below.
I*: Intensity. Intensity is listed as Light/Lifestyle (L), Moderate (M), or Vigorous (V). (See Table 3.3.)
** Workouts do not include warm-up or cool-down time.

INTENSITY LEVEL | L | M | V |
Light Moderate Vigorous

PROGRAM B

GOAL: Run at a moderate to vigorous intensity level three to five days a week, complete a 30-minute continuous run, and incorporate vigorous interval training sessions.

	Mon T*	Mon I*	Tue T	Tue I	Wed T	Wed I	Thurs T	Thurs I	Fri T	Fri I	Sat T	Sat I	Sun T	Sun I
Week 1	20	L–M 3–5	20	M 5–6	20	M 5–6			20	L–M 3–5				
Week 2	20	M 5–6			25	M 5–6			20	M 5–6	25	L–M 3–5		
Week 3	25	M 5–6			20	M 5–6	Interval	L–M–V			30	M 5–6		
Week 4	25	M 5–6	Interval	L–M–V	20	L–M 3–5	Interval	L–M–V			30	L–M 3–5		

T*: Time. Total time is listed in minutes.
I*: Intensity. Intensity is listed as Light/Lifestyle (L), Moderate (M), or Vigorous (V) and the OMNI scale of 0–10. (See Figure 3.8 and Table 3.3.)
** Workouts do not include warm-up or cool-down time.

INTENSITY LEVEL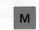
Light   Moderate   Vigorous

Program B Interval Workout—3 Miles

800m (.5 mile) at 7–8 on the OMNI scale (V)
800m (.5 mile) recovery (easy jog or walk/jog) at 2–5 on the OMNI scale (L–M)
**REPEAT this 1:1 ratio two more times for a total of 4800m or 3 miles.

MOTIVATE!

Create your own exercise log to track your running program—make note of dates, times, distances, intensity level—or use the one on the companion website. Here are a few tips to keep you running:

MORNING WORKOUTS: Try running first thing in the morning. That way, you can check it off your to-do list, and nothing can push your run off your day's schedule. Tip for success: organize your running clothes, shoes, gear, water bottle, and breakfast the night before.

DON'T PUT AWAY YOUR GEAR: Place your workout log, shoes, workout clothes, water bottle, and stretching mat in plain sight, in your work bag, or your car. Visual cues can help you remember your goals and prioritize your run.

DO IT FOR CHARITY: Need a reason or just more support? Name your cause and chances are there is a local run or race to raise awareness and funds for it. Committing to run for worthy causes reminds you that you are fortunate to be healthy and able to run. Fuel your motivation by knowing you're doing good for more than just yourself.

ADVANCE!

Now that you have established your running program, challenge yourself to try something new or take your running to the next level. How about participating in your first 5k? If you've been there, done that, how about actually racing (picking up your pace to set a new personal record)? On the next page is a more advanced four-week program you can follow; visit the companion website to find more options or simply to personalize this or any of the programs in this book.

PROGRAM C GOAL: Run 5k/3.1miles!

	Mon		Tue		Wed		Thurs		Fri		Sat		Sun	
	T/D*	I*	T/D	I	T/D	I	T/D	I	T/D	I	T/D	I	T/D	I
Week 1	25	L–M 3–5 62–70	25	L–M 3–5 62–70			25	M 5–6 65–85	25	M 5–6 65–85				
Week 2	25	M 5–6 65–85			Interval	L–M–V			2 miles	M 5–6 65–85	30	M 5–6 65–85		
Week 3	25	M 5–6 65–85	Interval	L–M–V	2.5 miles	L–M 3–5 62–70	Interval	L–M–V	3 miles	M 5–6 65–85				
Week 4	30	M 5–6 65–85			35	L–M 3–5 62–70					Goal 5k Run!			

T/D*: Time/Distance. Total time/distance is listed in minutes or miles.
I*: Intensity. Intensity is listed as Light/Lifestyle (L), Moderate (M), or Vigorous (V), the OMNI scale of 0–10, and % of HRmax. (See Figure 3.8 and Table 3.3.)
** Workouts do not include warm-up or cool-down time

INTENSITY LEVEL

Light Moderate Vigorous

Program C Interval Workout

Alternate two minutes hard and two minutes easy for one mile:

2 minutes at 85% HRmax or 7–8 on the OMNI scale (V)
2 minutes at <60% HRmax or 2–3 on the OMNI scale (L)
5 minutes at 65–84% HRmax or 5–6 on the OMNI scale (M)
**REPEAT twice more (total of three sets)

activate, motivate, & ADVANCE YOUR FITNESS

A CYCLING PROGRAM

LIVE IT! ONLINE

ACTIVATE!
Whether you cycle indoors or take your bike out on the road or trail, you can get a fun and amazing workout.

Cycling Program Preparation & Safety
Sure, cycling can be an intense, calorie-burning workout, but it can also be a simple way to take care of errands, commute, meet up with friends, or just enjoy the great outdoors. Follow the programs below to get started. As you get stronger, you can increase your mileage and speed.

What Do I Need for Cycling?
GEAR: Safe cycling requires quite a bit of equipment (helmet, padded cycling shorts, gloves, shoes, reflective gear, racks) and, of course, the bike. You can start on almost any style of bicycle, but most importantly, you need a bike that fits. Visit your local bike shop to get the right bike for you. When indoor cycling, adjust both seat and handlebar height to create a comfortable and safe fit. If you are new to indoor cycling or unfamiliar with the stationary bikes at your facility, be sure to ask a trained instructor to assist you with proper bike setup.

How Do I Start a Cycling Program?
TECHNIQUE: Work on developing a smooth and efficient pedaling technique. Lighten up, pedal in a smooth circle, and pull through the back of the stroke. *Cadence* is pedaling speed in revolutions per minute (RPM). A cadence of 60 RPM means that one pedal makes a complete revolution 60 times in one minute. Monitor your cadence with periodic cadence checks. Count the revolution of one leg for 15 seconds and then multiply by four. The cadence range is 80–110 RPM for cycling on a flat road and 60–80 RPM for climbing hills.

ETIQUETTE: Participating in group rides will teach you the etiquette for road cycling and mountain biking. Inquire about weekly rides or a beginners' cycling group at your local bike shop.

Cycling Tips
INDOOR CYCLING: Weather, traffic, flat tires ... with indoor cycling you won't have these excuses for missing your workout. Indoor cycling also allows you to precisely control your workout and mix periods of higher-intensity cycling with resting pedal strokes.

OUTDOOR CYCLING: Whether you choose streets, bike paths, or trails, plan safe routes that take into consideration both traffic and terrain. Try using a mapping program or stop by your local bike shop to learn more about the routes and popular riding areas in your neighborhood. Safety tips: brush up on your cycling skills, have proper reflective equipment, learn how to use a bike repair kit (fixing flat tires), and know local traffic laws and trail usage rules.

Cycling Warm-Up and Cool-Down

Cycle at a slow cadence for 5 to 15 minutes to warm-up or cool-down. After the cool-down portion of your ride, perform a few light stretches that focus on your low back muscles, hamstrings, quadriceps, and calves.

Four-Week Cycling Programs

If you are new to cycling or are coming back after time off, start with Program A to build your cardiorespiratory fitness base. If you are already riding for 15 or more continuous minutes at least twice a week, then start with Program B. Adjust time, intensity, and training days to suit your personal fitness level and schedule; visit the companion website for more options.

PROGRAM A

GOAL: Increase cycling minutes while maintaining a moderate intensity level three to four days a week, building to 100 total minutes by week four.

	Mon		Tue		Wed		Thurs		Fri		Sat		Sun	
	T*	I*	T	I	T	I	T	I	T	I	T	I	T	I
Week 1	20	L			20	L			20	L–M				
Week 2	25	M			25	M			25	M				
Week 3	20	M			25	M			15	M	30	L–M		
Week 4	25	M			25	M			25	M	25	L–M		

T*: Time. Total time is listed in minutes.
I*: Intensity. Intensity is listed as Light/Lifestyle (L), Moderate (M), or Vigorous (V). (See Table 3.3.)
** Workouts do not include warm-up or cool-down time.

INTENSITY LEVEL

Light Moderate Vigorous

PROGRAM B

GOAL: Cycle at a moderate intensity level three to five days a week, build to a 40-minute ride, and incorporate vigorous interval training sessions each week.

	Mon		Tue		Wed		Thurs		Fri		Sat		Sun	
	T*	I*	T	I	T	I	T	I	T	I	T	I	T	I
Week 1	25	L–M 3–5			25	L–M 3–5			25	M 5–6	25	M 5–6		
Week 2	25	M 5–6			30	M 5–6			25	L–M 3–5	35	M 5–6		
Week 3	30	M 5–6	Interval	L–M–V	20	L–M 3–5	Interval	L–M–V	30	M 5–6				
Week 4	30	M 5–6	Interval	L–M–V	25	M 5–6	30	M 5–6			40	L–M 3–5		

T*: Time. Total time is listed in minutes.
I*: Intensity. Intensity is listed as Light/Lifestyle (L), Moderate (M), or Vigorous (V) and the OMNI scale of 0–10. (See Figure 3.8, and Table 3.3.)
** Workouts do not include warm-up or cool-down time.

INTENSITY LEVEL

Light Moderate Vigorous

Program B Interval Workout—25 Minutes

2 minutes of flat cycling (cadence 80–110 RPM) at 7–8 on the OMNI scale (V)
1 minute of recovery (pedal easy, below 80 RPM) at 3 on the OMNI scale (L)
**REPEAT this 2:1 ratio four more times for a total of 15 minutes
30 seconds of hill work (increase tension and drop cadence to 60–80 RPM) at 7–8 on the OMNI scale (V)
90 seconds of recovery (pedal easy, below 80 RPM with little or no resistance) at 3 on the OMNI scale (L)
**REPEAT this 1:3 ratio four more times for a total of 10 minutes

MOTIVATE!

Create your own exercise log to track your cycling program—note dates, times, distances, cadence, intensity level—or use the one on the companion website. Here are a few tips to keep you cycling:

RIDE FOR 10: If you lack energy or motivation for a spin, give yourself 10 minutes. Tell yourself that you can quit after 10 minutes if you still don't feel like riding. Chances are that once you have made the effort to start, you'll complete your workout. If not, at least you managed a solid 10 minutes and you can feel good about listening to your body and taking a rest day.

REWARD YOURSELF: Promise yourself a healthy treat or fun experience at week's end if you stick to your cycling program. Maybe a pedicure or a massage or a scoop of frozen yogurt; hard work makes a reward that much more satisfying.

INDOOR GROUP RIDE: Sometimes just knowing that others are expecting you is enough to help you show up for your workout. Try an indoor cycling class at your gym. You'll develop new friendships with other physically active people and increase your cardiorespiratory fitness. Win-Win!

ADVANCE!

Ready to be challenged in your cycling program or try a new approach? Below is a more advanced four-week program you can follow. Visit the companion website to find more options or to personalize this or any of the programs in this book.

PROGRAM C

GOAL: Ride 20k/12.4mi in ≤ 60 minutes (indoors or out)!

	Mon		Tue		Wed		Thurs		Fri		Sat		Sun	
	T/D*	I*	T/D	I	T/D	I	T/D	I	T/D	I	T/D	I	T/D	I
Week 1	25	L–M 3–5 62–70	25	M 5–6 65–85	25	L–M 3–5 62–70	25	M 5–6 65–85			35	M 5–6 65–85		
Week 2	30	M 5–6 65–85	20	V 7–8 85–94	6 miles	L–M 3–5 62–70	30	M 5–6 65–85			40	M 5–6 65–85		
Week 3	35	M 5–6 65–85	Interval	L–M–V			Interval	L–M–V	35	L–M 3–5 62–70	45	M 5–6 65–85		
Week 4	40	M 5–6 65–85	20	L–M 3–5 62–70	40	M 5–6 65–85	Interval	L–M–V			Goal 20k Ride!	M 5–6 65–85		

T/D*: Time/Distance. Total time/distance is listed in minutes or miles.
I*: Intensity. Intensity is listed as Light/Lifestyle (L), Moderate (M), or Vigorous (V), the OMNI scale of 0–10, and % of HRmax. (See Figure 3.8 and Table 3.3.)
** Workouts do not include warm-up or cool-down time

INTENSITY LEVEL

Light   Moderate   Vigorous

Program C Interval Workout—30 Minutes

3 minutes of flat cycling (cadence 80–110 RPM) at 85% HRmax or 7–8 on the OMNI scale (V)
1 minute of recovery (pedal easy, below 80 RPM) at 3 on the OMNI scale (L)
**REPEAT this 3:1 ratio four more times for a total of 20 minutes
1 minute of hill work (increase tension and drop cadence to 60–80 RPM) at 85% HRmax or 7–8 on the OMNI scale (V)
1 minute of recovery (pedal easy, below 80 RPM with little or no resistance) at 3 on the OMNI scale (L)
**REPEAT this 1:1 ratio four more times for a total of 10 minutes

activate, motivate, & ADVANCE YOUR FITNESS

A SWIMMING PROGRAM

ACTIVATE

Low-impact and fun, swimming is an excellent way to improve your overall fitness!

Swimming Program Preparation & Safety:

If you have access to a pool, all you really need are two key items—swimsuit and goggles—and you're set to hit the water. Start and build slowly, focusing on minutes, not laps, and, as you gain strength, you will swim further and faster.

What Do I Need for Swimming?

GEAR: Look for a swimsuit that stays in place and moves with you, and be sure to try on goggles to ensure a good fit. You may want a swim cap to keep your hair out of your face. In addition, various pieces of equipment are commonly used to help swimmers improve technique and performance: kickboards, pull buoys, fins, and a stopwatch or the pool's pace clock. Lastly, don't forget your shatter-proof water bottle.

How Do I Start a Swimming Program?

TECHNIQUE: Taking a lesson is the best way to become more comfortable in the water and develop a more efficient technique. Inquire at your local college or American Red Cross chapter about adult swim classes or private swim coaches in your area.

ETIQUETTE: Pools are busy at open swim times and you will rarely get a lane to yourself. Aim to share a lane with other swimmers close to your same speed. You will most likely encounter *circle swimming* (swimming in a counter clockwise direction in the pool lane). Allow faster swimmers to take the lead, make sure there is a five second gap between you and the person in front of you, and avoid swimming in the middle of the lane. If you need to take a break at the wall, keep to the side of the lane so that others can turn or rest as well.

Swimming Tips

OPEN WATER: Although it takes strong skills, open-water swimming can be exciting and invigorating! Check with your local swim store or a swim or triathlon club to find swim partners and learn more about safe open water swim areas. Remember, the water temperature is generally much cooler than a pool; many open-water swimmers wear neoprene wetsuits to stay warm. Practice "sighting" (looking up to see where you are in relation to land, buoys, docks) and swimming in a straight line before heading out.

Swimming Warm-Up and Cool-Down

A swimming warm-up and cool-down consists of slow water walking, water jogging, or swimming at a slower pace for 5–10 minutes. You can also warm-up on deck with light, dynamic full range movements. After your cool-down, you can hold basic stretches for 10–30 seconds to improve flexibility.

Four-Week Swimming Programs

As you start a new swimming program, rest often, use resting swim strokes (elementary backstroke, sidestroke) as needed, and monitor your intensity periodically. Heart rates are typically 10–13 beats per minute lower when swimming than when performing exercise on land, so evaluate intensity using perceived exertion level. If even one length of the pool is tiring for you, start with Program A and focus on swim time, not distance or number of laps. If you are already able to swim comfortably at a moderate intensity level for close to 15 minutes (continuously or with minimum rest) and you are swimming at least twice a week, then start with Program B. Adjust time, intensity, and days of the swims to suit your personal fitness level and schedule; visit the companion website for more options.

PROGRAM **A**   **GOAL:** Increase continuous swim minutes at a light-to-moderate intensity level three to four days a week, building to 100 total minutes by week four.

	Mon		Tue		Wed		Thurs		Fri		Sat		Sun	
	T*	I*	T	I	T	I	T	I	T	I	T	I	T	I
Week 1	15	L			20	L			20	M				
Week 2	20	M			25	M			25	M				
Week 3	25	M			20	M			15	M	25	M		
Week 4	25	M			25	M			25	M	25	M		

T*: Time. Total time is listed in minutes.
I*: Intensity. Intensity is listed as Light/Lifestyle (L), Moderate (M), or Vigorous (V). (See Table 3.3.)
** Workouts do not include warm-up or cool-down time.

INTENSITY LEVEL
Light   Moderate Vigorous

PROGRAM **B**   **GOAL:** Increase continuous swim minutes at a moderate intensity level three to five days a week, build to a 30-minute swim, and incorporate vigorous interval training sessions each week.

	Mon		Tue		Wed		Thurs		Fri		Sat		Sun	
	T*	I*	T	I	T	I	T	I	T	I	T	I	T	I
Week 1	25	L–M 3–5			25	M 5–6			25	M 5–6	25	M 5–6		
Week 2	25	M 5–6			Intervals	L–M–V			25	M 5–6				
Week 3	20	M 5–6			25	M 5–6			20	M 5–6	30	L–M 3–5		
Week 4	25	M 5–6	Intervals	L–M–V	30	M 5–6	Intervals	L–M–V	25	M 5–6				

T*: Time. Total time is listed in minutes.
I*: Intensity. Intensity is listed as Light/Lifestyle (L), Moderate (M), or Vigorous (V) and the OMNI scale of 0–10. (See Figure 3.8 and Table 3.3.)
** Workouts do not include warm-up or cool-down time.

INTENSITY LEVEL
Light   Moderate Vigorous

Program B Interval Workout—700 m/yds

3 × 100 m/yds with 60 seconds of rest between [100s at 7–8 on the OMNI scale (V) and rest at 0–2 (L)]
2 × 75 m/yds with 45 seconds of rest between [75s at 7–8 on the OMNI scale (V) and rest at 0–2 (L)]
3 × 50 m/yds with 30 seconds of rest between [50s at 7–8 on the OMNI scale (V) and rest at 0–2 (L)]
4 × 25 m/yds with 15 seconds of rest between [25s at 7–8 on the OMNI scale (V) and rest at 0–2 (L)]

MOTIVATE!

Create your own exercise log to track your swimming program—note dates, times, laps, intensity level—or use the one on the companion website. Here are a few tips to keep you swimming:

LEARN SOMETHING NEW: Taking a lesson can help you develop confidence, which leads to more efficient swimming and increased enjoyment. The more you enjoy your workout, the better the results will be and the more likely you are to stick with it.

JOIN A TEAM: Lacking the support you need to swim regularly? Masters Swimming is a national program where adults 18 and older can swim in a team setting. You can swim at your own pace and be competitive or non-competitive—your choice! There are teams and clubs in communities across the country and all of them offer multiple practice options, workouts, and coaching; you will gain a new group of friends who will be expecting you at the pool.

TRY A WATER EXERCISE CLASS: Getting bored? Mix things up, make new friends, and take a break from swimming laps while still getting a great workout in the water. Most pools have different types of group water exercise classes; chances are one will be right for you.

ADVANCE!

Congratulations! You have established your swim fitness program. Are you ready to challenge yourself with a new goal and take your swimming to the next level? Below is a more advanced four-week program that you can follow; visit the companion website to find more options or to personalize this or any of the programs in this book.

PROGRAM C

GOAL: Swim a mile, continuous (or with minimum rest)! (1650 yards/1508 meters)

	Mon		Tue		Wed		Thurs		Fri		Sat		Sun	
	T/D*	I*	T/D	I	T/D	I	T/D	I	T/D	I	T/D	I	T/D	I
Week 1	25	L–M 3–5 62–70	700	M 5–6 65–85	25	L–M 3–5 62–70	700	M 5–6 65–85	25	M 5–6 65–85				
Week 2	30	M 5–6 65–85	1000	M 5–6 65–85	Interval	L–M–V	1000	M 5–6 65-85	30	L–M 3–5 62–70				
Week 3	25	M 5–6 65–85	Interval	L–M–V	30	L–M 3–5 62–70	Interval	L–M–V			35	M 5–6 65–85		
Week 4	30	M 5–6 65–85	1500	M 5–6 65–85	Interval	L–M–V	20	L–M 3–5 62–70			Goal Mile Swim!			

T/D*: Time/Distance. Total time/distance is listed in minutes or yards/meters.
I*: Intensity. Intensity is listed as Light/Lifestyle (L), Moderate (M), or Vigorous (V), the OMNI scale of 0–10, and % of HRmax. (See Figure 2.1, Figure 3.8, and Table 3.3.)

INTENSITY LEVEL

L — Light   M — Moderate   V — Vigorous

** Workouts do not include warm-up or cool-down time
*** Heart rates are typically 10–13 beats per minute lower when swimming, than when performing exercise on land, adjust heart rate targets accordingly.

Program C Interval Workout—1200 m/yds

3 × 100 m/yds with 60 seconds of rest between [100s at 65–84% HRmax, 5–6 on the OMNI scale (M), and rest at 0–2 (L)]
2 × 200 m/yds with 2 minutes of rest between [200s at 85% HRmax, 7–8 on the OMNI scale (V), and rest at 0–2 (L)]
1 × 500 m/yds [at 65–84% HRmax, 5–6 on the OMNI scale (M)]

4

Building Muscular Strength & Endurance

Learning Outcomes

1. Explain how muscular strength and muscular endurance relate to life-long fitness and wellness.

 HEAR IT! ONLINE Audio case study and audio Power-Point lecture

2. Identify key skeletal muscle structures and explain how they work together to allow for basic muscle function.

3. Articulate the fitness and wellness improvements you can make with regular resistance training.

4. Evaluate your changes in muscle fitness over time by assessing your muscular strength and muscular endurance at regular intervals.

 DO IT! ONLINE Lab 4.1 Assessing Your Muscular Strength
Lab 4.2 Assessing Your Muscular Endurance

5. Set and work toward appropriate muscular fitness goals.

 DO IT! ONLINE Lab 4.3 Setting Muscular Fitness Goals
Lab 4.4 Your Resistance-Training Workout Plan

6. Implement a safe and effective resistance-training exercise program compatible with your goals and lifestyle.

 LIVE IT! ONLINE Customizable 4-week starter and intermediate resistance-training programs

7. Observe safety precautions when resistance training.

 SEE IT! ONLINE More than 100 videos demonstrating proper technique and resistance-training safety

8. Incorporate strategies to avoid the risks associated with supplement use.

 SEE IT! ONLINE The Mitchell Report on Steroids in Baseball

Pre- and post-quizzes and glossary flashcards REVIEW IT! ONLINE

casestudy

GINA

"Hi, I'm Gina. I'm from San Francisco and I'm a sophomore majoring in economics. I'm taking a fitness and wellness class this semester, and this week we're starting the section on muscular fitness. I'm curious about it because I've never lifted weights before! I like to go hiking and I take yoga classes from time to time, but I wouldn't call myself an athlete. Does it really make sense for someone like me to start a strength-training program?"

HEAR IT! ONLINE

• •

Whether you're a beginner like Gina or an athlete interested in conditioning, this chapter answers common questions about muscular fitness, explains the benefits of resistance training, and gives you the tools for designing a program that is custom-made for you.

Muscular fitness is the ability of your musculoskeletal system to perform daily and recreational activities without undue fatigue and injury. Muscular fitness involves having adequate muscular strength and endurance. **Muscular strength** is the ability of a muscle or group of muscles to contract with maximal force. It describes how strong a muscle is or how much force it can exert. Exercise professionals often measure muscular strength by determining the maximum weight

muscular fitness The ability of your musculoskeletal system to perform daily and recreational activities without undue fatigue and injury

muscular strength The ability of a muscle to contract with maximal force

muscular endurance The ability of a muscle to contract repeatedly over an extended period of time

resistance training Controlled and progressive stressing of the body's musculoskeletal system using resistance (i.e., weights, resistance bands, body weight) exercises to build and maintain muscular fitness

a person can lift at one time. **Muscular endurance** is the ability of a muscle to contract repeatedly over an extended period of time. It describes how long you can sustain a given type of muscular exertion. One way that fitness professionals measure muscular endurance is by determining the maximum weight a person can lift 20 times consecutively.

You can build better muscular strength and endurance through resistance training. **Resistance training** is also referred to as *weight training* or *strength training* and can be done with measured weights, body weight, or other resistive equipment (i.e., exercise bands or exercise balls). Resistance exercises stress the body's musculoskeletal system, which enlarges muscle fibers and improves neural control of muscle function, resulting in greater muscular strength and endurance.

Are you already participating in a resistance-training program? If so, you are not alone. In 2008, 22–27 percent of adults over the age of 18 reported regular participation in muscular strength and endurance activities.[1] The numbers are up from 1998, when 18 percent of adults reported participating in muscle fitness activities and 2004, when 17.5 percent of women and 21.5 percent of men reported regular resistance training.[2] However, participation numbers are still much lower than the *Healthy People 2020* target: 30 percent of adults participating in muscle strengthening exercises two or more times per week.[3] If you are not participating, now may be the perfect time to start because facilities and classes are readily available at most colleges and universities and you may have a group of peers who want to support each other in getting fit and healthy.

Resistance training offers such varied benefits that exercise professionals recommend it in nearly all health-related fitness programs. Regular resistance training can make daily activities easier: carrying around a backpack full of heavy textbooks won't tire you as much; bringing in a bag of groceries will be less taxing; and taking the stairs will seem natural and feel better than riding in an elevator. No matter what your age or goals, resistance training is an important part of staying healthy and functional throughout your life.

How Do My Muscles Work?

The human body contains hundreds of muscles, each of which belongs to one of three basic types: (1) voluntary *skeletal muscle,* which allows movement of the skeleton and generates body heat; (2) involuntary *cardiac muscle,* which exists only in the heart and facilitates the pumping of blood through the body; and (3) involuntary *smooth muscle,* which lines some internal organs and moves food through the stomach and intestines. Resistance training and cardiorespiratory exercises benefit your skeletal and cardiac muscles. Here we focus on skeletal muscles and the signals from the nervous system that coordinate and control their contraction.

An Overview of Skeletal Muscle

Each skeletal muscle is surrounded by a sheet of connective tissue that draws together at the ends of the muscle, forming the **tendons** (see Figure 4.1). Muscular contractions allow for skeletal movement because muscles are attached to bones via tendons. These attached muscles pull the bones, which pivot at joints, creating a specific body movement.

Within each skeletal muscle are individual muscle cells called **muscle fibers**. Bundles of muscle fibers are called *fascicles.* Each muscle fiber extends the full length of the muscle. Within each muscle fiber are many **myofibrils**, each containing contractile protein filaments. These filaments are made up of two kinds of protein—*actin* and *myosin*—which partially overlap at rest and give the whole cell a striped appearance. The microscopic structure and function of actin and myosin

allow them to slide across each other and shorten the muscle. You can picture this sliding and shortening as similar to the way your forearms can slide past each other inside the front pocket of a hooded sweatshirt, pulling your elbows closer together. Simultaneous shortening of the many fibers within a whole muscle causes the pattern of muscular tension we call *contraction.* It is this whole-muscle contraction that moves bones and surrounding body parts.

Every muscle fiber can be categorized as either *slow* or *fast,* depending on how quickly it can contract. **Slow-twitch muscle fibers** (Type I) depend on oxygen and contract relatively slowly, but can contract for longer periods of time without fatigue. In slow-twitch fibers, the energy for contraction primarily comes from the breakdown of fat from the blood, muscle cells, and adipose

tendons The connective tissues attaching muscle to bone

muscle fibers The cells of the muscular system

myofibrils Thin strands within a single muscle fiber that bundle the skeletal muscle protein filaments and span the length of the fiber

slow-twitch muscle fibers Muscle fiber type that is oxygen dependent and can contract over long periods of time

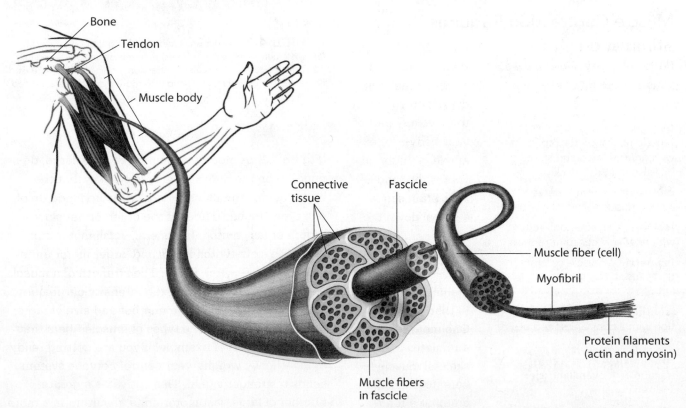

FIGURE **4.1** Muscle is attached to bones via tendons. Tendons are a continuation of the connective tissue that surrounds the entire muscle as well as each muscle bundle (fascicle). A fascicle is made up of many muscle cells (muscle fibers). Within each muscle fiber, myofibril strands contain actin and myosin proteins.

tissue. For efficient fat breakdown, oxygen and minimal levels of glucose breakdown are required. **Fast-twitch muscle fibers** (Type II) are not oxygen-dependent and contract more rapidly than slow-twitch fibers, but tire relatively quickly (they also produce greater muscle power). In fast-twitch fibers, the energy for contraction primarily comes from phosphocreatine and glycogen reserves within the muscles, glycogen stored within the liver, and glucose in the blood.

All fiber types exist in skeletal muscles, but some muscles within the body (such as postural trunk muscles) have more slow-twitch fibers, while other muscles (such as those in the calves) have more fast-twitch fibers. The proportion of muscle fiber types varies from person to person based on both genetics and training. Elite athletes have muscle fiber compositions that complement their sport. Marathoners, for instance, have higher levels of slow-twitch fibers that supply them with optimal muscular endurance. Power weight lifters, on the other hand, have more fast-twitch fibers that allow feats of enormous muscular strength over short periods of time. Sedentary individuals and people who do general resistance training typically have 50 percent slow-twitch and 50 percent fast-twitch fiber composition.

Muscle Contraction Requires Stimulation

For a voluntary skeletal muscle to contract, the nervous system must send a signal directly to the muscle. When you want to move any part of your body—for example, a finger on your right hand—your brain sends a signal down the spinal cord and through motor nerves to the skeletal muscle fibers in that finger. One motor nerve stimulates many skeletal muscle fibers, together creating a functional unit called a **motor unit**

fast-twitch muscle fibers Muscle fiber type that contracts with greater force and speed but also fatigues quickly

motor unit A motor nerve and all the muscle fibers it controls

isotonic A muscle contraction with relatively constant tension

isometric A muscle contraction with no change in muscle length

isokinetic A muscle contraction with a constant speed of contraction

concentric A muscle contraction with overall muscle shortening

eccentric A muscle contraction with overall muscle lengthening

FIGURE **4.2** Motor units and muscle contraction strength. (a) Motor unit X is smaller (5 fibers) than motor unit Y (15 fibers). (b) The strength of a muscular contraction increases with increased fibers per motor unit (X vs. Y) and with more motor units activated (X + Y).

(Figure 4.2). A motor unit can be small or large, depending on the number of muscle fibers that the motor nerve stimulates. Motor units are made up of one type of muscle fiber or the other, either slow-twitch or fast-twitch. In general, small motor units comprise slow-twitch fibers and larger motor units comprise fast-twitch fibers. The strength of a muscle contraction depends upon the intensity of the nervous system stimulus, the number and size of motor units activated, and the types of muscle fibers that are stimulated. For example, if you are getting ready to lift a heavy weight, your central nervous system sends a stronger signal. This activates a greater number of large, fast motor units, resulting in a more forceful muscle contraction than if you were merely picking up an apple.

(a)

(b)

FIGURE 4.3 (a) Isotonic contractions include concentric (shortening) and eccentric (lengthening) contractions. (b) Isometric contractions produce force in the muscle with no movement.

Three Primary Types of Muscle Contractions

Muscle contractions all result in an increase in tension or force within the muscle, but some contractions move body parts while others do not. There are three primary types of contractions: isotonic, isometric, and isokinetic. **Isotonic** contractions are characterized by a consistent muscle tension as the contraction proceeds and a resulting movement of body parts (Figure 4.3a). An arm curl with a 10-pound hand weight involves isotonic contractions throughout your arm. **Isometric** contractions are characterized by a consistent muscle length throughout the contraction with no visible movement of body parts. An example of an isometric contraction occurs when you hold a hand weight at arm's length in front of you; your arm is not moving, but you feel tension in your arm muscles (Figure 4.3b). **Isokinetic** contractions are characterized by a consistent muscle contraction speed within a moving body part. In order to perform isokinetic contractions, you need specialized equipment that holds the speed of movement constant as your arm, leg, or other muscles contract with varying forces.

Isotonic contractions are the most common in exercise programs. Lifting free weights, working on machines, and doing push-ups are all examples of isotonic contractions. Isotonic contractions can be either concentric or eccentric. **Concentric** contractions occur when force is developed in the muscle as the muscle is shortening—for example, when you curl a free weight up toward your shoulder. In **eccentric** muscle contractions, force remains in the muscle while the muscle is lengthening. This occurs as you lower a free weight back to its original position. Figure 4.3a illustrates these muscular contractions, using a bicep-curl exercise as an example.

• •

casestudy

GINA

"I love to go on short hikes. There are some gorgeous trails in the San Francisco Bay Area. Some of them are hilly but I don't mind—the views from the top are always worth it. My calves definitely get a workout! I'd like to be able to do longer hikes, but the truth is that I usually get tired after about three miles. I know there are some longer hikes with spectacular views, but I don't feel ready for them yet."

THINK! Given what you've learned so far, what would you tell Gina about how resistance training can benefit her? Which type of muscle fibers would you guess that Gina has more of: slow-twitch fibers or fast-twitch fibers?

ACT! Go outside and enjoy a favorite activity. During the activity, name the muscle contractions that occur: are they isotonic or isometric contractions?

How Can Regular Resistance Training Improve My Fitness and Wellness?

People used to think that weight lifting was solely a means of improving body shape and producing bigger muscles. We now know that, in addition to improving physical appearance, resistance training can also result in specific physiological changes that have significant fitness and wellness benefits. Figure 4.4 summarizes these changes. We discuss the benefits of resistance training in detail in the section that follows.

Regular Resistance Training Increases Your Strength

Regular resistance training with an adequate load, or amount of weight lifted, will result in an increase in muscle strength. Although men tend to realize greater gains in muscle size due to higher testosterone levels, women often have a larger capacity to improve relative strength over time.[4] Stronger lower- and upper-body muscles benefit both men and women.

hypertrophy An increase in muscle cross-sectional area

Neural Improvements When you start a resistance-training program, you will gain muscular strength before noticing any increase in muscle size. This is because internal physiological adaptations to training take place before muscle enlargement. The strength of a muscular contraction depends, in large part, on effective recruitment of the motor units needed for that contraction. The better your body is at recruiting the necessary motor units through voluntary neural signaling, the stronger your muscles will be. In the first few weeks or months of a resistance-training program, most of the adaptation involves an increased ability to recruit motor units, which causes more muscle fibers to contract.

Increased Muscle Size With consistent resistance training, the amount of actin and myosin within your muscle fibers increases. This results in **hypertrophy**, an increase in the size or cross-sectional area of the protein filaments. With more contractile proteins, a muscle can contract more forcefully; in other words, larger muscles are stronger muscles. While both slow- and fast-twitch muscles will increase in size with resistance training, greater increases in strength will result from hypertrophy of fast-twitch muscle fibers.

Muscle hypertrophy in response to resistance training takes longer than neural improvements, but

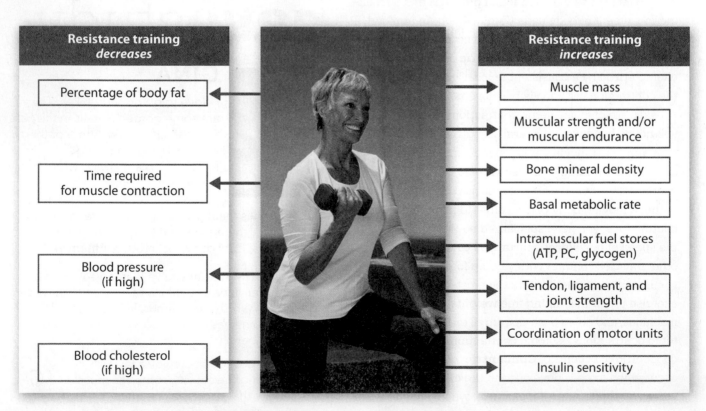

Resistance training *decreases*	Resistance training *increases*
Percentage of body fat	Muscle mass
Time required for muscle contraction	Muscular strength and/or muscular endurance
Blood pressure (if high)	Bone mineral density
Blood cholesterol (if high)	Basal metabolic rate
	Intramuscular fuel stores (ATP, PC, glycogen)
	Tendon, ligament, and joint strength
	Coordination of motor units
	Insulin sensitivity

FIGURE **4.4** Physiological changes from resistance training.

is the most important contributor to strength gains over time. The degree of hypertrophy or enlargement you can expect with weight training depends upon your gender, age, genetics, and how you design your training program. Some individuals will develop larger muscles more quickly than others; some will experience only limited hypertrophy. In particular, women and men with smaller builds will realize less muscle development than those with larger builds, even with identical training programs (see the box What Are the Benefits of Strength Training for Women?). Older individuals will also have slower progress and overall less muscle development, though they can still see significant improvements.

A program with heavier weights, longer durations, or more frequent training can produce greater gains than a more standard fitness-training program. People who stop resistance training will experience some degree of **atrophy**, a shrinking of the muscle to its pretraining size and strength. To avoid atrophy, you need to make a long-term commitment to resistance training.

Regular Resistance Training Increases Your Muscular Endurance

Muscular endurance helps you perform both cardio-respiratory activities, such as hiking and running, and muscular fitness activities, such as circuit or sports training. In fact, just doing these activities will improve your muscular endurance. Muscular endurance exercises trigger physiological adaptations that improve your ability to regenerate ATP efficiently and thus sustain muscular contractions for a longer period of time. The end result will be the ability to snowboard a long run instead of having to rest halfway down; to walk up three flights of stairs with ease; or to rake leaves vigorously for an hour without difficulty.

Regular Resistance Training Improves Your Body Composition, Weight Management, and Body Image

Improved body composition is an important outcome of resistance training: the amount of lean muscle tissue increases, the amount of fat tissue decreases, and thus the ratio of lean to fat improves. Research has

demonstrated that such higher lean-to-fat ratios improve your overall health profile and reduce your risk of heart attack, diabetes, and death from cardiovascular diseases.[5] Fat does not turn into muscle or vice versa; the number of fat and muscle cells remains the same, with cells merely enlarging or shrinking depending on food intake and activity levels.

atrophy A decrease in muscle cross-sectional area

More muscle means a faster metabolic rate; pound for pound, muscle tissue expends more energy than fat tissue.[6] With more total calories being expended during the day, weight control becomes easier and more effective.[7] Resistance training should be combined with aerobic exercise for overall weight loss,[8] but resistance training during weight loss helps ensure that you will lose fat and not precious muscle tissue;[9] your body can be lighter, stronger, and leaner (i.e., more toned) instead of just lighter (and potentially still flabby), as often happens with traditional diet-only weight-loss methods.

When you begin a resistance-training program, you may experience a slight initial weight gain as muscle tissue grows. If you focus only on the scale, this can be discouraging. It is better to focus on how much stronger and more toned your muscles feel. With a consistent fitness and nutrition program, fat loss will eventually "catch up" to muscle gain and will be reflected in weight loss as well. Since muscle tissue is more compact than fat tissue, your body size will gradually decrease over time as muscles become toned and fat tissues shrink. This, in turn, can improve your body image. In one study, college students realized measurable increases in overall body image after circuit weight training (a form of resistance training) for six weeks.[10]

Regular Resistance Training Strengthens Your Bones and Protects Your Body from Injuries

Bone health is an important issue for everyone, from children to older adults. Osteoporosis-related fractures are common among older women and men and can cause dramatic decreases in a person's mobility, independence, and quality of life. By putting stress and controlled-weight loads on the muscles, joint structures, and supporting bones, resistance training

What Are the Benefits of Strength Training for Women?

College-age men are much more likely to participate in strength training than college-age women (47% for men and 28% for women, ages 18–24).[1] Although fewer women in the United States engage in strength-training than men overall, the gap narrows as people age; 16 percent of men and 11 percent of women over 75 years of age report strength training activities. Despite this gender gap, the benefits of strength training for women are just as great as men. Many of these benefits are especially appealing to women for reasons that may differ from men. For example, strength training promotes stronger bones and this helps prevent osteoporosis in the long-term, something women are at a greater risk for than men.[2, 3] In addition, the maintenance of lean tissue helps you keep your functional independence as you age; this is another long-term risk for women.[4, 5] Immediate benefits of weight training include reduced body fat and greater ability to control body weight; improved stamina and decreased fatigue; better sleep and less insomnia; and increased self-confidence, body image, and sense of well-being. Plus, there is a bonus for your weekend and vacation plans! People who strength train also find that their ability to enjoy recreational activities and sports—playing ultimate Frisbee, for example—improves.

Now let's address common myths about strength training for women.

Myth 1: Women don't benefit much from resistance exercise. It's true that on average, men's muscles are larger and more powerful than women's; men produce 5 to 10 times more testosterone, which promotes muscle development. Men's nervous systems also signal muscle contraction more rapidly, producing greater power. Because they have more total muscle tissue, men's absolute strength is greater than women's. However, when muscle mass is compared pound for pound, women are equally strong. Women will increase strength and muscle endurance through strength training, just as men do.

Myth 2: Strength training will cause women to "bulk up." In truth, women who do regular resistance training rarely look heavily muscled. Very few women build large, bulky muscles without major effort (or the use of dangerous steroid drugs) because they have different natural hormone levels than men. Strength training will make your muscles leaner and, with additional strategies for fat loss, you can even "slim down" if that is your goal!

Myth 3: The weight room is a place primarily for men. Some women find it intimidating to go to a weight room. It is true that weight rooms can be dominated by men who seem to know exactly what they are doing. Although men typically lift greater amounts of weight and seem to have different training strategies than most women, many will welcome new weight training participants of both genders. Once you are comfortable, ask to join in on a set of exercises with a group. Many women also find it helpful to go to the gym with a friend (man or woman) who has similar resistance-training goals. This is a great motivation tip for everyone. You can also go to the gym when it's less busy, find an instructor for guidance, do strength training at home, or try a gym exclusively for women. Whatever it takes, begin strength training to experience the amazing benefits throughout your life, it's worth it!

THINK! What's keeping you from strength training? What obstacles are preventing you from going to the weight room?

ACT! Write down your obstacles to strength training (in a weight room or at home). Now figure out and write down a way you can tackle each one!

Sources:
1. Centers for Disease Control (CDC), "QuickStats: Percentage of Adults Aged ≥18 Years Who Engaged in Leisure-Time Strengthening Activities, by Age Group and Sex—National Health Interview Survey, United States, 2008," *Morbidity and Mortality Weekly Report* 58, no. 34 (2009): 955.
2. A. Guadalupe-Grau and others, "Exercise and Bone Mass in Adults," *Sports Medicine* 39, no. 6 (2009): 439–68.
3. J. E. Layne and M. E. Nelson, "The Effects of Progressive Resistance Training on Bone Density: A Review," *Medicine and Science in Sports and Exercise* 31, no. 1 (1999): 25–30.
4. K. Ogawa and others, "Resistance Exercise Training-Induced Muscle Hypertrophy Was Associated with Reduction of Inflammatory Markers in Elderly Women" *Mediators of Inflammation* 2010 (2010).
5. M. D. Phillips and others, "Resistance Training at Eight-Repetition Maximum Reduces the Inflammatory Milieu in Elderly Women," *Medicine and Science in Sports and Exercise* 42, no. 2 (2010): 314–25.

stimulates muscle tissue growth and the generation of harder, stronger bones, thereby reducing the risk of fracture.

Building strong bones is especially important in the period starting with childhood skeletal growth and development and ending at about age 30. The "reservoir" of bone tissue you lay down in those years and then maintain throughout life will help prevent weak, brittle bones as you age. Even the bones of older individuals can benefit from strength training; in one study, eight months of resistance training positively affected hip bone density in older women, whereas no change occurred with moderate-impact aerobic exercise over the same time period.[11]

Getting hurt will put you on the sidelines. Whether you exercise for fun, fitness, or competition, preventing injuries is a key to continued participation. Injury prevention tips are often specific to your chosen activity; however, strong muscles, bones, and connective tissues are the common denominator for preventing injury in any activity. Regular resistance training improves not only muscular strength and endurance, but also the strength of tendons, ligaments, and other supporting structures around each joint. As they grow stronger, the joints themselves are better protected from injury. A stronger body can handle the physical stresses of everyday life (carrying heavy books or groceries, lifting laundry baskets, moving furniture, etc.)

with less chance of injury. A strong, pain-free back and proper posture are crucial to daily functioning without injury. Individuals who participate in regular resistance-training exercise have stronger postural muscles and report less low back pain.

Imbalanced muscles around a joint may result in a change in joint alignment with subsequent pain or injury. Muscular balance will reduce this risk. A well-designed muscle fitness program will work toward improving strength and muscle endurance in opposing muscular groups, promoting overall muscle balance.

> **sarcopenia** The degenerative loss of muscle mass and strength in aging

Regular Resistance Training Helps Maintain Your Physical Function with Aging

Starting between the ages of 25 and 30, men and women begin to lose muscle mass. As they age, they lose up to one-third of their muscle mass due to changes in hormones, activity levels, and nutrition. Injury and chronic diseases can cause people to exercise less and accelerate typical muscle loss. **Sarcopenia**, literally "poverty of flesh," is the term applied to this age-related loss in skeletal muscle (see Figure 4.5).

CT scan of healthy young adult shows normal amount of muscle area

CT scan of sedentary older adult shows greatly reduced muscle area, indicating sarcopenia

Muscle
Bone

FIGURE **4.5** CT scans showing the difference in muscle mass in a healthy young adult vs. an older adult with sarcopenia. Age-related muscle loss can be slowed with resistance training.

muscle power The ability of a muscle to quickly contract with high force

Sarcopenia reduces overall physical functioning by decreasing muscular strength and endurance and causing losses in **muscle power**, or the capacity to exert force rapidly. While no one is immune from the aging process, resistance training throughout one's life can significantly slow natural muscle loss. In fact, older individuals who do resistance training can show a rate of improvement equal to that of younger people. The increase in muscular fitness and the improvements it brings to everyday physical functioning help individuals live independently for a longer portion of their lives.

Regular Resistance Training Helps Reduce Your Cardiovascular Disease Risk

Regular resistance training can lower your risk of cardiovascular disease by increasing blood flow to working muscles and vital tissues throughout your body. In fact, people who perform regular resistance-training exercise have lower blood pressure and blood cholesterol readings than sedentary people. Since being overfat (having a higher than recommended percentage of body fat) increases your risk of cardiovascular disease and adult-onset diabetes, an improved body composition achieved through resistance training can help you lower your risk of both of these diseases.

Regular Resistance Training Enhances Your Performance in Sports and Activities

Achieving muscular fitness through resistance training has yet another benefit: A stronger body is more resistant to fatigue, moves more quickly, and recovers more quickly from illness or injury. All of these traits contribute to better performance in sports, recreational activities, and other fitness pursuits. Resistance training is often the common denominator among training programs for different sports and activities. Because of these benefits, physically active adults often incorporate some form of resistance training that builds strength and endurance in the muscle groups most crucial to their sport.

casestudy

GINA

"I've always wanted to hike to the top of Nevada Falls in Yosemite National Park. I'm told that it can be done as a day hike, but it is about seven miles round trip. There is also a steep section of rocks near another waterfall along the way—apparently you get completely soaked while hiking that part of the trail! Even on dry trails, I'm always extra careful hiking downhill, because I once sprained my ankle on a hike, which was not fun.

If resistance training can help me take on Nevada Falls, I'm interested. I've also always wished I had better muscle tone, but to be honest, I don't want to 'bulk up' . . . "

THINK! Name at least two ways that resistance training can help Gina realize her goal of safely hiking to the top of Nevada Falls. How would you respond to Gina's concerns about "bulking up"?

ACT! What's your "Nevada Falls"? That is, what is something you have always wanted to do, if only you were in better physical shape? Write down your ideas and post the note somewhere you can see it each day for motivation. Start an action plan to reach your goal!

HEAR IT! ONLINE

How Can I Assess My Muscular Strength and Endurance?

Before you can plan an appropriate resistance-training program, it is important to assess your current muscular strength and endurance. You can then compare the results to norm charts for your age and gender, or simply use them as a starting point for designing your program. After you've followed your program for a while, follow-up assessments will help you evaluate your progress and make adjustments to stay on track.

Test Your Muscular Strength

Tests of muscular strength gauge the maximum amount of force you can generate in a muscle. People usually carry out these tests in a weight room where measured weights of all sizes are readily available.

1 RM Tests One repetition maximum (1 RM) tests are the most common tool fitness instructors and personal trainers use to assess their clients' muscular strength. To participate in the tests safely, you must be medically cleared to lift heavier weights than you have in the past, have detailed instructions for the test procedure, know general weight-training guidelines, have a few weeks of weight-training experience, and have qualified **spotters** standing nearby to watch and assist if necessary. If you are weight training on campus or at a gym, an instructor will be able to help you through these preliminary steps.

These 1 RM tests are performed by discovering the maximum amount of weight you can lift one time on a particular exercise. You must accurately determine your 1 RM within three to five trials so that muscle fatigue from repetitions does not change your result. In general health and fitness classes or beginning weight-training programs, instructors often tell students to predict their 1 RM instead of actually attempting a maximum lift. This is particularly true when students are new to resistance training and unfamiliar with weight-training guidelines. To predict your 1 RM, you will lift, press, or pull a weight that will fully fatigue your upper- or lower-body muscles in 2 to 10 repetitions. You can then use a formula that

converts actual weight lifted and real number of repetitions to a prediction of your 1 RM capacity for that exercise. In **Lab 4.1** (at the back of this chapter), you will use chest-press and leg-press exercises to determine your predicted 1 RM. You can perform these tests for any weight-training exercise and then convert to the predicted 1 RM value. Many weight-training programs use a percentage of your 1 RM or predicted 1 RM to determine a safe starting level for weight lifting.

Grip Strength Test Another common test of muscle strength is the hand grip strength test using a piece of equipment called a *grip strength dynamometer*. As you squeeze the dynamometer (with one hand at a time), it measures the static or isometric strength of your grip-squeezing muscles in pounds or kilograms (kg).

Test Your Muscular Endurance

Muscular endurance tests evaluate a muscle's ability to contract for an extended period of time. Some of these tests must be performed in a weight room, whereas others require only your body weight for resistance and can be performed anywhere.

20 RM Tests You can use any weight-training exercise to find your **20 repetition maximum (20 RM).** This test determines the maximal amount of weight you can lift exactly 20 times in a row before the muscle becomes too fatigued to continue. Twenty repetition maximum tests are particularly useful for setting muscular endurance goals and then tracking your progress. Try to discover your 20 RM within one to three tries to avoid fatiguing your muscles and altering your results. **Lab 4.2** walks you through the steps of finding your 20 RM for the chest-press and leg-press exercises.

Calisthenic Tests Calisthenics are conditioning exercises that use your body weight for resistance. Calisthenic tests use sit-ups, curl-ups, pull-ups, push-ups, and flexed arm support/hang exercises to assess muscular endurance. The procedures for these tests vary. You will learn how to perform curl-up and push-up assessments in Lab 4.2. Calisthenic tests allow you to test yourself outside of a weight-training facility and to compare your results to well-established physical fitness norms.

> **one repetition maximum (1 RM)** The maximum amount of weight you can lift one time
>
> **spotter** A person who watches, encourages, and, if needed, assists a person who is performing a weight-training lift
>
> **20 repetition maximum (20 RM)** The maximum amount of weight you can lift 20 times in a row
>
> **calisthenics** A type of muscle endurance and/or flexibility exercise that employs simple movements without the use of resistance other than one's own body weight

How Can I Design My Own Resistance-Training Program?

Designing an effective resistance-training program takes some knowledge, and many people enlist the help of a personal trainer or fitness professional. You can become your own personal trainer, however, by using the guidelines in this section to plan a safe and effective muscular fitness program.

Set Appropriate Muscular Fitness Goals

Remember to use SMART goal-setting guidelines: Goals should be *s*pecific, *m*easurable, *a*ction-oriented, and *r*ealistic and should have a *t*imeline. Your goals may be appearance-based, function-based, or a combination of the two.

Appearance-Based Goals Many people have appearance-based goals for muscular fitness: they want larger muscles, or muscles that are more toned and less flabby. "Spot reduction" (i.e., trimming down just one area of the body) is another often-voiced goal. Researchers have proven spot-reduction to be a myth. Several carefully controlled studies show that fat doesn't disappear through repeated exercise to one area.[12]

In order to judge your progress toward appearance-based goals, be sure to include some sort of measure of progress in your resistance-training plan. For muscle size, measure the circumference of your biceps or calves, for example, and then set a goal to increase or decrease this number. For overall body size, your goal may be to increase lean tissue weight but decrease fat tissue and percentage of body fat. If your goal is to become more "toned," quantify this in some way. Look in the mirror and make notes about the way your body looks and moves. After you reach the target date for your plan, reread your notes, look in the mirror, and then reevaluate whether your muscle tone has improved.

Function-Based Goals Include some specific goals for improving muscle function in your fitness plan. Function-based goals focus on your muscular capabilities and include gaining better muscular strength, greater muscular endurance, or both. **Lab 4.3** will guide you in setting goals for realistic changes in muscle function, and then help you to assess your improvements.

Explore Your Equipment Options

Should you use weight machines in your resistance-training program? Free weights? Other equipment? No equipment at all? These are important decisions, and they will be determined by your fitness goals, the type of equipment available to you, your experience with weight-training exercises, and your preferences.

dumbbells Weights intended for use by one hand; typically one uses a dumbbell in each hand

barbells Long bars with weight plates on each end

many others allow you to isolate and strengthen specific muscle groups as well as to train without a spotting partner.

Machines If you are new to resistance training, weight machines can be very useful. Systems such as Cybex®, Nautilus®, Life Fitness®, and

Free Weights Personal trainers and exercise physiologists consider free-weight exercises to be a more advanced approach to weight training than machine-weight exercises. Free-weight exercises use **dumbbells**; **barbells**; incline, flat, or decline benches; squat racks; and related equipment. Free-weight exercises allow your body to move through its natural range of motion instead of the path predetermined by a weight machine. This both requires and promotes development of more muscle control. Some athletes prefer free-weight exercises because the balance and movement patterns needed to successfully lift free weights are closer to their sport movement patterns, whether that be tossing a football, putting a shot, or doing the breaststroke. Since workout facilities often have both free weights and weight machines, many people start their resistance-training program exclusively with machine-weight exercises and then progress to free weights within the first few months. Table 4.1 compares machine-weight training and free-weight training.

Alternate Equipment You can increase resistance on your body with equipment other than machines or free weights. Resistance bands made of tubing or flat strips of rubber allow you to simultaneously increase resistance throughout a range of motion and to improve muscular endurance. You can perform many different exercises with these bands. They fold up and pack perfectly in a suitcase or gym bag for a portable workout. Stability balls (also called Swiss, fitness, or exercise balls) are 18-inch to 30-inch diameter vinyl balls that have various uses for muscular fitness, endurance, and balance. Ball routines involve performing exercises while sitting, lying, and/or balancing on the ball. The ball exerciser must use core trunk muscles to counteract the natural instability of the ball, which enhances overall body function. People sometimes use heavily weighted balls called medicine balls to increase resistance, either individually, with a partner, or in a group. You can hold a medicine ball while doing calisthenic or free-weight exercises or pass a ball from partner to partner for a functional increase in muscle endurance.

No-Equipment Training Calisthenics such as push-ups, pull-ups, lunges, squats, leg lifts, and curl-ups do not involve equipment. Instead, they use your body weight to provide the resistance. Like resistance bands, these exercises are perfect for maintaining muscular strength and endurance while traveling.

TABLE 4.1 Machine-Weight vs. Free-Weight Training

Machine Weights	Free Weights
PROS	**PROS**
Safe and less intimidating for beginners	Can be tailored for individual workouts
Quicker to set up and use	Range of motion set by lifter, not machine
Spotters not typically needed	Some exercises can be done anywhere
Support of standing posture not needed	Standing and sitting postural muscles worked
Adaptable for those with limitations	Movements can transfer to daily activities
Variable resistance is possible	Good for strength and power building
Good isolation of specific muscle groups	Additional stabilizer muscles worked
Only good option for some muscle groups	Lower cost and more available for home use
CONS	**CONS**
Machine sets range of motion	More difficult to learn
May not fit every body size and type	A spotter may be needed
Some people lack access to weight machines	Incorrect form may lead to injuries
Posture supporting muscles used less	More time may be needed to change weights
Limited number of exercises/machines	More training needed to create program

Understand the Different Types of Resistance-Training Programs

You can plan a resistance-training program with various types of equipment and numerous exercise routines. The right program for you will be determined by your goals, experience, and personal preference.

Traditional Weight Training Traditional weight training takes place in a weight room and usually includes a combination of machine-weight, free-weight, and calisthenic exercises. Individuals may work alone or with a partner and will usually perform multiple **sets** and **repetitions** of a particular exercise before moving on to the next exercise. Guidelines for setting up your traditional weight training program are outlined in the next section and sample traditional weight training programs are available at the end of the chapter.

Circuit Weight Training Circuit weight training is done in a specialized circuit-training room, a general workout room, or a weight room. Exercisers move from one station to another in a set pattern (the "circuit") after a certain amount of time at a station or after performing a certain number of repetitions of an exercise such as a biceps curl, leg press, or chest press. Some circuits include only resistance-training exercises and have the single goal of improving muscular fitness. Some circuits involve cardiorespiratory or aerobic training equipment, such as stair-steppers or stationary bicycles, mixed in with the resistance exercises to improve both cardiorespiratory and muscular fitness.

sets Single attempts at an exercise that include a fixed number of repetitions

repetitions The number of times an exercise is performed within one set

In circuit training, it is important to remember the specificity training principle: In order to get optimal muscle fitness benefits, you must focus on the resistance exercises; in order to realize added cardiorespiratory benefits, you must spend a minimal amount of time on the cardio machines (20 to 30 minutes total per exercise session).

Circuit exercises should be organized properly in order to ensure a safe and effective exercise session. For example, multi-joint exercises (bench press, leg press) are often performed before single-joint exercises (bicep curl, leg extension) and muscle groups worked are spread out to allow recovery between sets. Exercises that stress the core postural muscles are reserved for the end of the workout because these muscles provide important trunk support during seated and standing exercises.

Plyometrics and Sports Training Resistance-training programs designed to support specific sports can be quite different from general resistance training. Athletes may use many of the general weight-training exercises illustrated in this chapter, but they usually also perform exercises or exercise methods that specifically benefit their sports performance. Plyometrics, power lifts, and speed and agility drills are examples.

A **plyometric exercise** program incorporates explosive exercises that mimic the quick transition movements needed in many sports (e.g., basketball, wrestling, and gymnastics). These exercises are characterized by a landing and slowing down of the body mass followed immediately by a rapid movement in the opposite direction (for instance, jumping down off of a box and then immediately jumping back up as high as you can). Plyometrics is a highly specialized training method that should be performed under proper direction and only by

individuals who have achieved a high level of muscular fitness.

Power lifting is a type of resistance training that incorporates fast and forceful actions to improve strength and speed. Lifting for **power** stresses the nervous system to act quickly and the tendons, ligaments, and joint structures to become more stable. Sports that require high levels of explosive movement and power (football, wrestling, gymnastics, and track-and-field events) may require power-lifting training to build strength with speed. Power lifting is a competitive sport in itself. Competitive power lifts include the bench press, the squat, the dead lift, and the Olympic lifts (the clean and jerk and the snatch). Like plyometrics, power lifting should be practiced only by experienced athletes or those with comparable weight-training experience.

The training regimens for certain athletes may include **speed** and **agility** drills. These drills are making their way into mainstream sports training and boot-camp-style group exercise classes. Speed and agility drills improve muscle responsiveness, speed, footwork, and coordination. Typical speed and agility drills include line sprints, high-knee runs, fast-foot-turnover running, and hopping quickly through

plyometric exercise An exercise that is characterized by a rapid deceleration of the body followed by a rapid acceleration of the body in the opposite direction

power The ability to produce force quickly

speed The ability to rapidly accelerate; exercises for speed will increase stride length and frequency

agility The ability to rapidly change body position or body direction without losing speed, balance, or body control

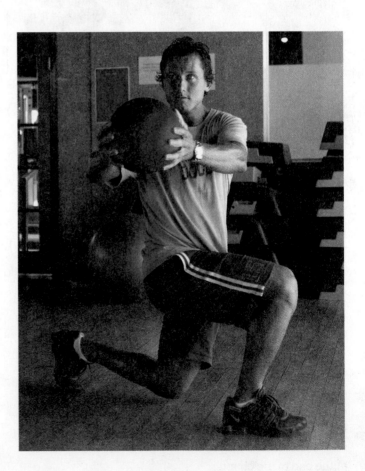

varying foot patterns (using agility dots or other markers). Speed and agility drills can be performed by anyone who is physically fit enough to learn and perform the skills. Proper instruction and modification of the drills for differing ability levels is essential to prevent injuries.

Whole-Body Exercise Programs The increasing popularity of "functional" training, training that carries over to life activities, has given rise to exercise programs that focus on whole-body exercises. These programs, such as CrossFit and kettlebell, focus on exercises that integrate various muscle groups into one exercise rather than isolate a muscle group, as do some traditional weight-room exercises. The exercises aim to address three planes of movement (forward and back, side to side, and rotational) for increased crossover into daily activities and enhanced sports and recreation performance. There has been initial evidence that this type of training can reduce neck and back pain.[13] It's not necessary to join a special gym or exercise class (although those are available) to take advantage of this type of training. Take the concepts presented in the previous section on plyometrics and sports training, think about your current resistance-training program, and integrate the concepts to add more whole-body and functional exercises. For instance, instead of limiting yourself to stationary lunges, add a walking forward movement with a twist to the opposite side to every lunge step.

Learn and Apply FITT Principles

FITT stands for *frequency*, *intensity*, *time*, and *type*. The acronym represents a checklist for determining how often, how hard, and how long to exercise, and what types of exercise to choose at your current level of muscular fitness.

Frequency of Training Your goals and your schedule determine how often you will train each week. At a minimum, you should work each muscle group twice per week. A full-body muscle workout means two sessions in the weight room each week. If you split your muscle workouts (for example, into upper body and lower body), then you would go to the weight room four times per week. Table 4.2 presents American College of Sports Medicine (ACSM) guidelines for muscular fitness programs.

It is important to let each muscle group rest for 48 hours before taxing it again with resistance training. Especially when you are just beginning, schedule your workouts so that they are at least two days apart.

When you perform an intense weight-training session, micro-damage occurs within the muscle cells

TABLE 4.2 ACSM's Guidelines for Resistance Training in Healthy Adults

Goal	Level	Intensity (% 1 RM)	Repetitions	Sets	Rest (min between sets)[b]	Frequency (days/week)[c]	Number and Types of Exercises
Improve Muscular Fitness[a]	Beginner/novice	40–70	8–12	1–3	2–3	2–3	8–10+ emphasizing multiple-joint exercises for opposing muscle groups in the lower body, upper body, and trunk; add single-joint exercises as needed for muscle balance
	Intermediate/advanced	60–80	8–12	2–4	2–3	2–3	
Increase Muscular Endurance	All levels	<50	15–25	1–2	2–3	2–3	
Further Increase Muscular Strength	Intermediate	70–80	1–12	2–4	2–3	2–5	
	Advanced	>80	1–6	2–4	2–3	2–5	

[a]Muscular strength, mass, and to some extent, muscular endurance.
[b]Rest a particular muscle group 48 hours between workout sessions
[c]2–3 days/week = total body workouts, 4–5 days/week = split routine to train each major muscle group twice per week

Data from: American College of Sports Medicine. *ACSM's Guidelines for Exercise Testing and Prescription.* 8th Edition. Baltimore, MD: Lippincott Williams & Wilkins, 2010; and Ratamess N. A., Alvar B. A., Evetovich T. K., et al. "ACSM Position Stand: Progression Models in Resistance Training for Healthy Adults," *Medicine and Science in Sports and Exercise* 341, no. 3 (2009): 687–708; C. E. Garner and others, "American College of Sports Medicine Position Stand: Quantity and Quality of Exercise for Developing and Maintaining Cardiorespiratory, Musculoskeletal, and Neuromotor Fitness in Apparently Healthy Adults: Guidance for Prescribing Exercise," *Medicine and Science in Sports and Exercise* 43, no. 7 (2011): 1334–59.

and rest time is needed for muscle repair and adaptation. Your muscles will adapt by constructing new actin and myosin contractile proteins and other supporting structures. Over time, this adaptation results in stronger, leaner, larger muscles. Intense workouts of the same muscle group on subsequent days will disrupt the repair and adaptation process. Rather than faster muscle development, this overtraining is more likely to cause injuries, muscle fatigue, and weakening. An exception can be made for lower intensity muscular fitness classes or calisthenics, which can be done daily as long as they are not overly fatiguing.

Muscle soreness that sets in within a day or two is called delayed-onset muscle soreness (DOMS); it is a sign that your body was not ready for the amount of overload you applied. Contrary to popular belief, it is not lactic acid that causes DOMS; accumulated lactic acid is cleared from the muscle cells within hours of exercise. If you choose weight amounts correctly, your muscles will sustain small amounts of micro-damage that does not result in soreness and that your body can repair within 48 hours after the workout.

Intensity of Training The intensity of a weight-training program refers to the amount of **resistance** you apply through any given exercise. For each exercise, the intensity you choose will depend on your fitness goals for that particular muscle group or your body as a whole. The ACSM guidelines in Table 4.2 for muscular fitness can help you choose weight-training

intensities (shown as a percentage of your 1 RM or percentage of predicted 1 RM).

The intensity or weight chosen for each exercise should be enough to overload the muscle group you are working; that means you should feel slight discomfort or muscle fatigue near the end of your exercise set. If you feel no fatigue during the entire set of repetitions and feel you could lift the weight another 3 to 10 times, then the intensity is too low. Aim for muscle fatigue but not complete exhaustion.

Resting between sets will affect your weight-training intensity and performance on subsequent exercises. The greater the weight you lift for strength building, the longer the rest period you may want between sets. Resting periods can be shorter for muscular endurance-building exercises. In fact, shorter rests may help build better muscular endurance.

Time: Sets and Repetitions Choosing the appropriate number of repetitions or lifts within each set is yet another important part of setting up your resistance-training program. Once again, your fitness goals help determine the number of sets you will execute for each exercise and the number of repetitions within each set. Your weight-training experience and the time you have available to work out will affect your planning as well. ACSM recommends that you perform two to four sets of each exercise during a given workout session (see Table 4.2). However, if you are new to resistance training, you will see progress with just one set per muscle group. As you progress in your resistance-training program, you can increase your sets from one to two, and eventually to three or more. You can execute two, three, or four sets for all your exercises, or perform two sets of certain exercises, three of

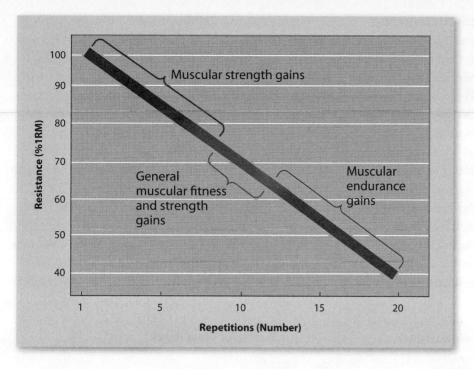

Muscular strength gains

General muscular fitness and strength gains

Muscular endurance gains

Resistance (%1RM)

Repetitions (Number)

FIGURE **4.6** Fewer repetitions with higher resistance will produce gains in muscular strength. More repetitions with lower resistance will produce gains in muscular endurance.

others, and so on. Keep in mind, however, that overtraining one particular muscle group can lead to muscle imbalance and injury.

Intensity and repetitions have an inverse relationship relative to muscular strength and endurance (see Figure 4.6): For muscular strength development, you will lift heavier weights and do fewer repetitions; for muscular endurance, you will lift lighter weights with more repetitions.

Type: Choosing Appropriate Exercises Which exercises should you do during each workout session? The final part of designing a muscular fitness program is choosing exercises that will help you achieve your goals and muscle balance. Create your own muscular fitness goals in Lab 4.3 and use Figure 4.7 to start planning your resistance-training program. Next, decide which specific exercises will help you attain your muscular fitness goals: Complete **Lab 4.4** to plan a muscular fitness program using Figures 4.8 and 4.9 to assist you in exercise selection.

Muscle balance requires a selection of upper-body exercises, trunk exercises, and lower-body exercises. Choose exercises from Figure 4.9 that work *opposing muscle groups,* muscles on both the front and back of your

Determine muscular fitness goal

Increase muscular strength	Improve general muscular fitness and strength	Increase muscular endurance
Choose 5–10 key weight training exercises to do in a gym	Choose 8–10 basic resistance training exercises (full body) to do in a gym or at home	Choose 8–10 basic resistance training exercises (full body) to do in a gym or at home
Write out your plan per exercise: 60–80% 1RM 2–4 sets 8–10 reps 2–3 min rests	Write out your plan per exercise: 50–70% 1RM 1–3 sets 10–12 reps 2–3 min rests	Write out your plan per exercise: 40–50% 1RM 1–2 sets 15–20 reps 2–3 min rests

FIGURE **4.7** Use this flowchart as you design your muscular fitness program. Just starting? Begin at the lower end of all recommended ranges (for rest periods, begin at the upper end).

body. Emphasize exercises that are **multiple-joint exercises**—exercises that affect more than one muscle group—since these exercises tend to be more functional and time-efficient. Examples of multiple-joint exercises include chest press, overhead press, leg press, and lunges. **Single-joint exercises** can be added as needed to target major muscle groups further. Examples of single-joint exercises include biceps curl, lateral raise, leg curl, and heel raise.

For a starting program, choose between 8 and 10 exercises, remembering that each additional exercise will add time to your exercise session; with too many exercises, you may need to split your workout into alternating selections of exercises on different days. In choosing exercises, you may select weight machines, free weights, calisthenics, or a combination of all three. Most weight-training programs will include all three and will be determined by the equipment available to you. As mentioned earlier, focus on weight-training machines if you are new to resistance training. See Activate, Motivate, & Advance Your Fitness: A Resistance-Training Program at the end of the chapter (page 169) for sample resistance-training programs to help you get started.

multiple-joint exercises
Exercises that involve multiple joints and muscle groups to achieve an overall movement

single-joint exercises
Exercises that involve a single joint and typically focus on one muscle group

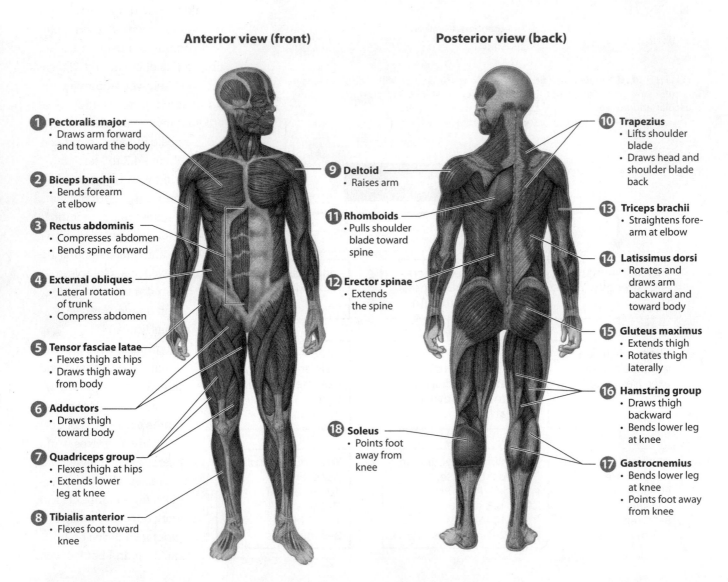

Anterior view (front)

1 Pectoralis major
- Draws arm forward and toward the body

2 Biceps brachii
- Bends forearm at elbow

3 Rectus abdominis
- Compresses abdomen
- Bends spine forward

4 External obliques
- Lateral rotation of trunk
- Compress abdomen

5 Tensor fasciae latae
- Flexes thigh at hips
- Draws thigh away from body

6 Adductors
- Draws thigh toward body

7 Quadriceps group
- Flexes thigh at hips
- Extends lower leg at knee

8 Tibialis anterior
- Flexes foot toward knee

9 Deltoid
- Raises arm

11 Rhomboids
- Pulls shoulder blade toward spine

12 Erector spinae
- Extends the spine

18 Soleus
- Points foot away from knee

Posterior view (back)

10 Trapezius
- Lifts shoulder blade
- Draws head and shoulder blade back

13 Triceps brachii
- Straightens forearm at elbow

14 Latissimus dorsi
- Rotates and draws arm backward and toward body

15 Gluteus maximus
- Extends thigh
- Rotates thigh laterally

16 Hamstring group
- Draws thigh backward
- Bends lower leg at knee

17 Gastrocnemius
- Bends lower leg at knee
- Points foot away from knee

FIGURE **4.8** These muscles or muscle groups are commonly used in resistance-training exercises. Figure 4.9 illustrates exercises you can use to work the muscle groups shown.

FIGURE **4.9**

RESISTANCE-TRAINING EXERCISES

Videos for these exercises and more are available online at www.pearsonhighered.com/hopson and on MyFitnessLab.

Lower-Body Exercises

1. Squat

(a) Free weight squat and

(b) Machine squat: Place the barbell or pad on your upper back and shoulders. Stand with feet shoulder-width apart, toes pointing forward, hips and shoulders lined up, abdominals pulled in. Looking forward and keeping your chest open, bend your knees and press your hips back. Lower until the angle created between your thigh and calf is between 45 degrees and 90 degrees. Keep your knees behind the front of your toes. To return to the start position, contract your abdominals, press hips forward, and extend your legs until they are straight.

(c) Ball squat: Place the ball between your mid-back and a smooth wall. Your feet should be six to twelve inches in front of your hips, shoulder-width apart, and toes pointing forward. Contract your abdominals, look forward, and keep your shoulders and hips lined up as you lower your torso. Lower until the angle created between your thigh and calf is about 90 degrees. Your knees should be just above your toes (but not in front of them) or directly above your ankles depending upon your starting position, strength, and ankle flexibility. If not, reposition your feet before the next repetition. Return to the starting position by contracting your legs and pushing the ball into and back up the wall.

(a)

(b)

(c)

Muscles targeted:

7 Quadriceps

15 Gluteus maximus
16 Hamstrings

2. Leg Press

SEE IT! ONLINE

Sit with your back straight or firmly against the backrest. Place your feet on the foot pads so that your knees create a 60- to 90-degree angle. Stabilize your torso by contracting your abdominals and holding the hand grips or seat pad. Press the weight by extending your legs slowly outward to a straight position without locking your knees. Return the weight slowly back to the starting position. If your buttocks rise up off of the seat pad, you may be lifting too much weight.

Muscles targeted:

7 Quadriceps

15 Gluteus maximus
16 Hamstrings

3. Lunge

SEE IT! ONLINE

Stand with feet shoulder-width apart. Step forward and transfer weight to the forward leg. Lower your body straight down with your weight evenly distributed between the front and back legs. Keep your front knee in line with your ankle by striding out far enough. Make sure the front knee does not extend over your toes. Repeat with the other leg.

Muscles targeted:

7 Quadriceps

15 Gluteus maximus
16 Hamstrings

4. Leg Extension

SEE IT! ONLINE

Sit with your back straight or firmly against the backrest and place your legs under the foot pad. Stabilize your torso by contracting your abdominals and holding the handgrips or seat pad. Lift the weight by extending your legs slowly upward to a straight position without locking your knees. Return the weight slowly to the starting position. If your buttocks rise up off the seat pad, you may be lifting too much weight.

Muscles targeted:

7 Quadriceps

5. Leg Curl

(a) Machine: Lie on your stomach so that your knees are placed at the machine's axis of rotation and the roller pad is just above your heel. Keep your head on the machine pad. Grasping the hand grips for support, lift the weight by contracting your hamstrings and pulling your heels toward your buttocks. Slowly lower the weight back to the start position.

(b) Calisthenics with ball: Lie on your stomach with knees bent and place the ball between your feet. Keep your head on the mat. Lower the ball to the ground and lift it back up by contracting your hamstrings and pulling your heels toward your buttocks.

(a)

(b)

Muscles targeted:

🔟⑯ Hamstrings

6. Hip Abduction

(a) Machine: Sit with your back straight or firmly against the back-rest and place your legs against the pads. Grasping the hand grips or seat pad for support, press your legs outward slowly by contracting your outer thighs or hip abductors. Be careful not to extend the legs further than your normal range of motion. Slowly lower the machine weight by bringing your legs back together.

(b) Calisthenics with resistance band: Connect the resistance band to a low point on a machine and attach the free end to your outside leg. Stand with good posture and hold onto a wall or machine for support. Contract your hip abductors and extend your leg out to the side of your body. Slowly release the outside leg back to the starting position beside or crossed slightly in front of the standing leg.

(a)

(b)

Muscles targeted:

⑤ Tensor fasciae latae

7. Hip Extension

(a) Machine: Stand tall with your working leg extended in front of you and connected to the cable machine. Support yourself by contracting your abdominals and holding on to the machine or handrails. Press the working leg behind you, contracting the gluteals and hamstrings. Hold the end position for 1 to 3 seconds before slowly returning to the starting position.

(b) Calisthenics with resistance band: Connect the resistance band to a low point on a machine and attach the free end to your lower leg. Stand with good posture and hold on to a wall or machine for support. Contract your gluteals and hamstrings and extend the working leg behind your body. Slowly release the leg back to the starting position slightly in front of the standing leg.

(a)

(b)

Muscles targeted:

15 Gluteus maximus
16 Hamstrings

8. Heel Raise

(a) **Straight-leg:** Stand tall with good posture and place your heels lower than the toes (you should feel just a slight stretch in the calf muscle). Looking forward and contracting your trunk muscles for balance and support, lift your heels up by contracting your gastrocnemius muscle. Be sure to do a full range of motion and slow, controlled repetitions.

(b) **Bent-leg:** Place your body in the machine with your heels lower than the toes and the weight pad placed comfortably on your thighs. Lift your heels up slightly and release the weight support bar with your hand. Slowly lower and lift the weight by contracting your soleus calf muscle through its full range of motion.

(a)

(b)

Muscles targeted:

17 Gastrocnemius

18 Soleus

9. Hip Adduction

(a) Machine: Sit with your back straight or firmly against the backrest and place your legs against the pads set at a comfortable range of motion. Grasping the hand grips or seat pad for support, press your legs together slowly by contracting your inner thighs or hip adductors. Slowly return your legs to the starting position.

(b) Calisthenics with resistance band: Connect the resistance band to a low point on a machine and attach the free end to your inside leg. Stand with good posture and hold onto a wall or machine for support. Contract your hip adductors and cross your leg in front of your body to the opposite side of your body. Slowly release the leg back to the starting position beside or slightly to the side of the standing leg.

(c) Calisthenics with ball: Lie on your back with a ball pressed between your knees. Press your knees firmly together, squeezing the ball. Hold the squeeze for 3 to 10 seconds and release.

Muscles targeted:

6 Adductors

(a)

(b)

(c)

Upper-Body Exercises

10. Push-Up

(a) Full push-ups and

(b) Modified push-ups: Support yourself in push-up position (from the knees or feet) by contracting your trunk muscles so that your neck, back, and hips are completely straight. Place hands slightly wider than shoulder-width apart. Slowly lower your body toward the floor, being careful to keep a straight body position. Your elbows will press out and back as you lower to a 90-degree elbow joint angle. Press yourself back up to the start position. Be careful not to let your trunk sag in the middle or your hips lift up during the exercise. Continually contract the abdominals to keep a strong, straight body position.

(a)

(b)

Muscles targeted:

1 Pectoralis major

13 Triceps brachii

11. Chest Press

(a) Free-weight: Lie down on the bench and position yourself with the weight bar directly above your chest. Stabilize your legs and back by placing your feet firmly on the ground and keeping your lower back flat. Grasp the bar with your hands slightly wider than shoulder-width apart and lift the bar off the rack. Slowly lower the bar to just above your chest. Press the weight up to a straight arm position and return the bar to the rack when your set of repetitions is complete. Use a spotter when lifting heavier free weights.

(b) Machine: Place yourself on the chest press machine and adjust the seat height so that the hand grips are at chest height. Stabilize your torso by firmly pressing your upper back against the seat back and planting your feet on the ground or foot supports. Press the hand grips away from the body until the arms are straight. Slowly return your hands to the starting position.

(a)

(b)

Muscles targeted:

1 Pectoralis major

13 Triceps brachii

12. Chest Fly

(a) Machine: Sit with your back straight or firmly against the back-rest, plant your feet on the ground or place on the foot pads, and grab the handles or place your arms behind the machine pads. Your arms should be directly to the side but not behind your body. Press your arms together slowly by contracting your chest and shoulder muscles. Slowly return your arms to the starting position.

(b) Bench chest flys: Lie down on the bench and position yourself with the dumbbells directly above your chest. Stabilize your legs and back by placing your feet firmly on the ground and keeping your lower back flat against the bench. Holding the dumbbells with a slight bend in the elbow joint, slowly lower them out to the side until your upper arms are parallel with the floor. Don't extend the arms beyond this position. Return your arms to the starting position by contracting your chest and shoulder muscles.

(a)

(b)

Muscles targeted:

1 Pectoralis major

13. Lat Pull-Down

(a) Machine: Position the seat and leg pad on the lat pull-down machine so that your thighs are snug under the pad while your feet are flat on the ground. Grab the pull-down bar with a wide overhand grip on your way down to a seated position. Sitting directly under the cable, pull the bar down to your upper chest. Focus on contracting the mid-back first and then the arms by pulling the shoulder blades and elbows back and down. Slowly straighten your arms back to the starting position.

(b) Calisthenics with resistance band: Hold the resistance band above your head with your arms straight up and your hands shoulder-width apart. Pull down and outward with your hands. Focus on contracting the mid-back first and then the arms by pulling the shoulder blades and elbows back and down. End with the band at the top of your chest, hold for 1 to 3 seconds, then slowly straighten your arms back to the starting position.

(a)

(b)

Muscles targeted:

1 Pectoralis major
2 Biceps brachii

14 Latissimus dorsi

14. Assisted Pull-Up

Grab the pull-up bar with a wide overhead grip. Contract the back and arms in order to pull your body up until the bar is at chin height. Slowly straighten your arms back to the starting position.

Muscles targeted:

1 Pectoralis major
2 Biceps brachii

14 Latissimus dorsi

15. Row

(a) Machine compound row: Position the seat height until the handles are at the level of your shoulders. Sit upright and place your feet on the ground or foot pads. Grab the handgrips and pull your elbows back. Hold this position for 1 to 3 seconds, then slowly return to the starting position.

(b) Row on cable machine: Grab the cable machine handles, ropes, or bar. Make sure that you are seated so that your arms and shoulders are fully extended forward. Position your feet on foot pedals or firmly on the ground with your heels. Make sure there is a slight bend in your knees. Pull your shoulder blades and elbows back until your hands are just in front of your chest. Hold this position for 1 to 3 seconds, then slowly return to the starting position.

(c) Free-weight dumbbell: Position right hand and right knee on bench as shown. Keep your back flat and head in a straight line. Pull dumbbell up to the side of your chest with your left hand, contracting your mid-back and leading with your elbow. Return to starting position and repeat on other side.

(d) Calisthenics with resistance band: Wrap the resistance band low around a weight machine or around your feet in the seated position. Hold the resistance band with your arms straight out and initial tension on the band. Pull back with your hands, focusing on contracting the mid-back first. Pull the shoulder blades and elbows back until your hands are at the lower chest, hold for 1 to 3 seconds, then slowly straighten your arms back to the starting position.

(a)

(b)

(c)

(d)

Muscles targeted:

2 Biceps brachii

11 Rhomboids
14 Latissimus dorsi

9 Deltoids (posterior)
10 Trapezius

16. Upright Row

Stand with your feet in a shoulder-width position. Keep your hips and shoulders aligned and your abdominals pulled in. Hold a barbell down in front of the body with straight arms and your hands positioned shoulder-width apart. Lift the weight to chest height keeping your elbows out, wrists straight, shoulders down. Return slowly to the starting position and repeat.

Muscles targeted:

9 Deltoids (posterior)
10 Trapezius

17. Overhead Press

SEE IT! ONLINE

(a) **Machine** and

(b) **Free-weight dumbbell:** Sit with your back straight or firmly against the backrest, plant your feet firmly on the ground, and pull in your abdominals. Position your hands just wider than shoulder-width width and just above the shoulders. Carefully press the weight over your head until your arms are straight but your elbows are not locked out. Slowly return the weight to the starting position and repeat.

(a)

(b)

Muscles targeted:

9 Deltoids (anterior and medial)

13 Triceps brachii

18. Lateral Raise

SEE IT! ONLINE

(a) **Machine:** Position yourself in the machine and sit with a tall, straight back. Contract your shoulders and lift your arms out to the side until they are parallel with the ground. Slowly lower your arms back down to your sides.

(b) **Free-weight dumbbell:** Stand with your feet shoulder-width apart. Hold the dumbbells to your sides or slightly in front of you. Lift your arms out to the side until they are parallel with the ground. While lifting, your elbows should have a slight bent to avoid over-extension of the elbow joint. Keep the weights at the same height as your elbows and keep your shoulders down. Slowly return the dumbbells back down to the starting position.

(a)

(b)

Muscles targeted:

9 Deltoids (anterior and medial)

19. Biceps Curl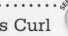

(a) Machine: Position yourself in the machine so that your feet are on the ground and your elbows are placed at the axis of rotation for the exercise. Grab the hand grips with an underhand grip and start with your arms straight but not over-extended. Lift your hands toward your head until your biceps are fully contracted. Slowly lower the weight back down to the starting position.

(b) Free-weight barbell: Stand with your feet either in a stride or a shoulder-width position and your knees slightly bent. Keep your hips and shoulders aligned and your abdominals pulled in. Hold a barbell down in front of the body with an underhand grip, straight arms, and your hands at shoulder-width. Lift the weight up to your shoulders while keeping your back straight and abdominal muscles tight. If you are leaning back to perform the lift, you may be lifting too much weight. Return the weight to the starting position slowly and repeat.

(c) Free-weight dumbbell: For one-arm concentration curls, sit on a bench and hold a dumbbell in one hand. Start with the working arm extended toward the ground and your elbow pressed into your inner thigh. Lift the dumbbell up to the shoulder and then return slowly to the starting position.

(d) Alternating free-weight dumbbell: Sit on a bench or chair with a dumbbell in each hand. Sit with good posture (ears and shoulders over hips and abdominals contracted) and your feet planted on the ground for balance. Lift one dumbbell up to your shoulder turning your palm toward your shoulder as you lift. Slowly lower the dumbbell to the starting position as you lift the dumbbell in your other hand.

(e) Calisthenics with resistance band: Place the center of a resistance band under one foot and grab the free ends of the band with a straight arm on the same side. Stand tall with your feet either in a stride or a side-to-side position and your knees soft. Keep your hips and shoulders aligned and your abdominals pulled in. Lift the resisted hand toward your shoulder until the biceps are fully contracted. Slowly lower the hand back to the starting position and repeat.

Muscles targeted:

2 Biceps brachii

(a)

(b)

(c)

(d)

(e)

20. Pullover

SEE IT! ONLINE

(a) Free-weight barbell: Lie on your back on a flat bench with your feet on the floor. Move the bar to the starting position with your upper arms just above your ears and your elbows slightly bent. Pull the weight back up and over the body without changing your elbow angle. Stop when the weight bar is directly over the chest.

(b) Machine: Adjust seat so that the machine pivots at your shoulder joints. Sit with your elbows against the pads and grasp the bar behind your head. Press forward and down with your arms until the bar is in front of your chest or abdomen. Slowly return to the starting position.

(a)

(b)

Muscles targeted:

1 Pectoralis major

13 Triceps brachii

14 Latissimus dorsi

21. Triceps Extension

SEE IT! ONLINE

(a) Machine: Grab the hand grips and start with your arms bent to at least 90 degrees. Press your hands away and down until your elbows are straight but not locked out. Slowly release the weight back to the starting position.

(b) Free-weight dumbbell: Start with the weight behind your head and your elbows lifted to the ceiling. Contract the triceps muscles to lift the weight over the head until the arms are straight. Slowly return to the starting position and repeat.

(c) Calisthenics with resistance band: Grasp the middle of a resistance band with one hand and the free ends with the other hand. Place one hand behind you and "anchor" the band at your hips or low back. Press the hand near your head upward by contracting the triceps muscle and extend the arm until straight. Slowly return the working arm to the starting position and repeat.

(a)

(b)

(c)

Muscles targeted:

13 Triceps brachii

Trunk Exercises

22. Back Extension

(a) Machine: Position yourself in the machine so that your hips are pressed all the way back, the back pad is on your mid to upper back, and your back is rounded over. Stabilize with your legs but try to refrain from pushing with the legs and hips during the exercise. Contract your back extensors and straighten out your back until you are in an upright position.

(b) Calisthenics on a mat: Start in a prone position with arms and legs extended and your forehead on the mat. Lift and further extend your arms and legs using your back and hip muscles. If you are free of low-back problems, you can lift a little further up for increased intensity. Hold the position for 3 to 5 seconds and then slowly lower to the mat.

(c) Calisthenics on a ball: Lie with your stomach over the ball, anchoring your feet and knees on the ground. Place your hands behind your head or extend the arms out straight for increased exercise intensity. Lift the head, shoulders, arms, and upper back until you have a slight curve in the back. Hold this position for 3 to 5 seconds and then lower to the ball.

(a)

(b)

(c)

Muscles targeted:

12 Erector spinae

23. Abdominal Curl

(a) Machine: Place yourself in the sitting or lying abdominal machine according to the machine instructions. Place your feet on the ground or foot pads and grab the hand grips and/or place your arms or chest behind the machine pads. Contract your abdominals while flexing your upper torso forward. Slowly return to the starting position and repeat.

(b) Calisthenics on a ball: Lie back with the ball placed at your low- to mid-back region. Place your feet shoulder-width apart on the ground so that your knees are bent at about 90 degrees. Cross your hands at your chest or place them lightly behind your head. Contract your abdominals while flexing your upper torso forward. Slowly return to the starting position and repeat.

(a)

(b)

Muscles targeted:

3 Rectus abdominis

24. Reverse Curl

SEE IT! ONLINE

Lie on your back and place your hands near your hips. Lift your legs up so that your body creates a 90-degree angle to the floor. Your knees may be bent or straight for this exercise. Contract your abdominals while lifting your hips up off the mat. Slowly return to the starting position and repeat. Be careful not to rock the hips and legs back and forth when doing this exercise; instead, perform a controlled lifting of the hips upward.

Muscles targeted:

3 Rectus abdominis

25. Oblique Curl

SEE IT! ONLINE

Lie on your back with one foot on the mat and knee bent to 90 degrees. Rest the opposite ankle on the bent knee. With one arm providing support on the ground and the other hand behind the head, contract your oblique abdominals and lift your opposite shoulder toward the lifted knee (elbow stays out). Keep the supporting arm and elbow on the floor and refrain from pulling on the head and neck with your hand. Return to the starting position slowly and repeat on the other side.

Muscles targeted:

4 External obliques

26. Side Bridge

SEE IT! ONLINE

(a) Modified side bridge and

(b) Forearm side bridge and

(c) Intermediate side bridge:
Lie on your side with your legs together and straight or bent behind you at 90 degrees. Support your body weight with your forearm or a straight arm. Lift your torso to a straight body position by contracting your abdominal and back muscles. Hold this position for a number of seconds or slowly drop the hip to the mat and lift back up for repeated repetitions.

(a)   (b)

(c)

Muscles targeted:

4 External obliques

27. Plank

SEE IT! ONLINE

(a) Modified plank and

(b) Forearm plank and

(c) Push-up position plank: Lie on your stomach and support yourself in plank position (from the forearms or hands) by contracting your trunk muscles so that your neck, back, and hips are completely straight. Your forearms or hands should be under your chest and placed slightly wider than shoulder-width apart. Hold this position for 5 to 60 seconds, increasing duration as you gain muscular endurance.

(a)

(b)

(c)

Muscles targeted:

3 Rectus abdominis   **4** External obliques

What If I Don't Reach My Goals?

Once you've applied FITT principles, chosen training levels, designed a program, and set target dates, you may find that your muscular development is not keeping up with your ambitions or that you cannot follow through consistently with training sessions. What other steps can you take to ensure success in your muscular fitness program?

Track Your Progress Use a weight-training log or a notebook to track your progress. Lab 4.4 provides you with a log that allows you to (1) see your week-to-week progress, (2) stay motivated, (3) detect problems with your program design or goals, and (4) know where to redesign your program if needed.

Evaluate and Redesign Your Program as Needed Periodically reevaluate your muscular fitness program. Common times to reassess are at your target completion date, when you feel you aren't making progress, when your improvement rate is faster than anticipated, and when you feel overtraining fatigue or injury. First, retake the initial tests for muscular strength and endurance. Second, reassess your goals: accomplished

or not? Third, evaluate your overall program and write out what you like and don't like about it. If you have met your goals and enjoy your program, continue but set more challenging goals based on FITT parameters. If you have not met your goals or don't like your program, rewrite the goals and target dates, redesigning to solve your issues. Get help from an exercise professional if needed. Evaluating and redesigning should allow you, once again, to move toward your muscular fitness goals successfully. Lab 4.4 provides practice at evaluation and redesign.

THINK! Many people find group exercise classes to be motivating. Do you?

ACT! Find classes that will help you meet your muscular fitness goals (such as Pilates, fitness "boot camp," or muscle pump). Some classes are designed solely for muscular fitness, while others address both muscular fitness and cardiovascular training. Be sure to use enough resistance or weight to elicit a muscle training response.

casestudy

GINA

"My main goals in resistance training are to improve my muscle endurance so that I can go on longer hikes and to strengthen my muscles and joints so that I can reduce the chance I'll be injured on the trail. I live close to campus and there is a gym with weight equipment available, but how do I decide what equipment to use and what exercises to focus on?"

THINK! What would you say to Gina about the benefits of using free weights versus machines? What would you tell her about the differences between traditional weight training, circuit weight training, and plyometrics programs? Which would you advise her to begin with?

ACT! Verbalize your own resistance-training goals. Are they appearance based or function based? Write out your initial ideas for applying the FITT principles to your goals.

What Precautions Should I Take to Avoid Resistance-Training Injuries?

Greater muscular fitness achieved through resistance training helps prevent general injury during sports or daily activity. However, weight training itself can cause injuries such as muscle or tendon strains, ligament sprains, fractures, dislocations, and other joint problems. This is especially true if the lifter pushes for an unrealistic overload. Injuries tend to occur while using free weights, but you can prevent them by getting proper instruction and guidance and by heeding a few basic suggestions.

Follow Basic Weight-Training Guidelines

When starting your resistance-training program, be conservative. Resist the temptation to begin with too many exercises or sets or with too much weight! Before increasing your resistance-training intensity or duration, observe how your body responds to the training over a few weeks. After that, you can safely increase the number of repetitions and/or the amount of weight. The safest approach is to follow the "10 percent rule." Limit increases in exercise frequency, intensity, or time to no more than 10 percent per week. Gentle increases will help prevent injury, overtraining, or soreness. Break this rule only if the initial intensity you selected was very low or a certified fitness professional instructs you to do otherwise.

Be Sure to Warm Up and Cool Down Properly

Weight-training guidelines include a warm-up and a cool-down before and after training sessions. A proper weight-training warm-up includes a general warm-up and a specific warm-up. The general warm-up consists of 3 to 10 minutes of cardiorespiratory exercises—walking, jogging (on or off a treadmill), biking, stationary biking, elliptical trainer use, or any activity that increases body temperature (breaking a light sweat) and blood flow to muscles. The specific warm-up should include range-of-motion exercises that mimic (without weight added) the resistance exercises you'll be performing. Move your limbs through a full range of motion before using a given weight machine or lifting free weights. Then, do a warm-up set with very light resistance. Now you are ready to perform your serious sets.

Some people also like to stretch before weight training. If you want to add stretching to your warm-up, do so only after a general warm-up to be sure your body has been adequately warmed up in preparation for stretching. Pre-exercise stretching should be light, and you should hold each stretch no more than 10 to 15 seconds. A proper cool-down for resistance training includes general range-of-motion exercises and stretches for the muscle groups applied during the weight-training session.

Know How to Train with Weights Safely

Get a proper introduction to weight training before you begin. Learn the proper grips and postures; the right way to isolate some muscle groups and stabilize others; the correct way to adjust machines for your height; and the safe way to sit, stand, and move during weight lifting to prevent injury. Learn the proper use of weights and weight machines. Use safety collars at the ends of weight bars to secure the weights on the bar.

When lifting free weights, use a spotter to watch, guide, and assist you. Perform all exercises in a slow and controlled manner. Some personal trainers recommend using a count of two up and four down to control the weight-lowering phase. Ask the spotter to watch your control and to make sure you are lifting safely and can return the bar safely after the lift. The object is to avoid fast, jerky, or bouncy motions that can injure your muscles or allow the weight to get away from you and cause injury.

Spotters typically assist when a weight lifter is attempting to lift a weight near his or her maximal fatigue level and the lift requires full-body balance. Exercises such as squats and the bench press require the weight to be lifted over the head or in a position that could present a danger to the lifter. When performing these exercises, always work out with a spotter.

Perform all exercises through a full range of motion. With free weights, you must determine the range yourself. Be sure to request extra training and attention if you need help.

Stay balanced: Set up in a relaxed, balanced position and maintain that position after a lift or set of lifts. Lifting while off balance is an easy way to create strain on one side and to pull or tear a muscle. Balance your exercise to build equal strength on both sides and from front to back.

Breathe in deeply in preparation for a lift and breathe out continuously as you lift. Some weight lifters use a **Valsalva maneuver** (that is, they exhale forcibly with a closed throat so no air exits) as a way to stabilize the trunk during a lift. However, holding your breath this way can cause an unhealthy blood pressure increase and slow blood flow to the heart, lungs, and brain. Breathe out during the push or pull part of a lift, particularly while lifting heavy weights, to avoid a Valsalva maneuver.

Use lighter weights when attempting new lifts or after taking time off from your routine. You can build up by three to five percent per session or 10 percent per week. Don't assume

Valsalva maneuver The process of holding one's breath while lifting heavy weight; this practice can increase chest cavity pressure and result in light-headedness during the lift; excessively increased blood pressure can result after the lift and breath are released you can pick up where you left off before a break in your training; that's asking for muscle strain or injury.

Do not continue resistance training if you are in pain. Learn to differentiate the effort of lifting from the pain of an injury, particularly to a joint.

Muscle strains are common among people who use improper lifting techniques and machine setups. Eccentric contractions, in particular, tend to cause microtears in the muscle fibers and connective tissue within and surrounding the muscles. Eccentric contractions typically take place during the lowering of a weight, so it is important not to "drop" a weight to its starting position, whether lifting free weights or using a machine.[14] Wear gym shoes to protect your feet and wear gloves to improve your grip and protect your hands.

Get Advice from a Qualified Exercise Professional

A qualified trainer can help you learn the proper head and body position for lifting each type of weight (with or without the help of a spotter) and for using weight machines of each type. Learning to adjust the machines properly is part of this training. Seek out people qualified to provide accurate resistance-training information, especially if you are just getting started or before significantly changing aspects of your routine, such as amount of weight, number of repetitions, speed of movement, or body posture.

How can you recognize a qualified exercise professional? Ask any potential personal trainer or instructor questions such as the following:

- Are you certified as a personal trainer or fitness instructor by a reputable, nationally recognized organization such as ACSM, National Strength and Conditioning Association (NSCA), and the American Council on Exercise (ACE)?

- Do you have a certificate or degree in exercise science from an accredited two- or four-year college?

- What types of experience have you had as an instructor or personal trainer?

- How long have you been working in the field of fitness and wellness?

- What are your references from employers and past/present clients?

ergogenic aids Any nutritional, physical, mechanical, psychological, or pharmacological procedure or aid used to improve athletic performance

- How current are you with the changing guidelines and emerging trends in exercise and fitness, and how can you demonstrate this currency?

You'll want to look at practical details such as how much the personal trainer charges, whether he or she has liability insurance, and how well his or her schedule will accommodate yours. Intangibles are equally important: How well do you get along with this potential trainer, and how motivated does he or she help you feel?

Consider enrolling in a specific weight-training class at your college or university. Instructors in such courses are already screened for the qualifications listed here, and the cost will be significantly lower than hiring your own personal trainer.

Persons with Disabilities May Have Different Weight-Training Guidelines

Weight-training programs benefit virtually everyone, including people with some limitations or disabilities. Resistance training can decrease pain and increase mobility in people with joint and muscle disabilities and orthopedic conditions such as arthritis, multiple sclerosis, or osteoarthritis.

Safety guidelines and appropriate exercises will vary and will be determined by the disability or limitation of each person. Everyone will need medical clearance before beginning a resistance-training program, and those with certain chronic conditions and muscle disorders may need specific exercise recommendations and directions from a physician. If your gym lacks specialized equipment, look for a trainer who can help you perform modified exercises on the available machines. Wheelchair exercisers can perform many seated resistance-training exercises in the gym or at home. Visit this book's website to view demonstrations of easily adaptable resistance-training exercises for people of all abilities.

Is It Risky to Use Supplements for Muscular Fitness?

Dietary supplements marketed as promoters of muscle conditioning are called performance aids or dietary **ergogenic aids**. Some supplements are safe but ineffective; some are both unsafe and ineffective. Few, if any, are worth the risk and expense. Manufacturers of nutritional supplements need not prove their products are safe or effective before offering them for sale on the open market. The FDA may remove unsafe products, but this occurs after the product is "tested" on the buying public. To avoid being an inadvertent subject in an uncontrolled experiment, look into the risks of a supplement very carefully before considering its use. Some ergogenic aids, such as anabolic steroids, are controlled substances. This means they require a prescription for legal use and should not be used for nonprescription purposes. Their use can get you banned from athletic competitions.

Anabolic Steroids

The Mitchell Report on Steroids in Baseball

Anabolic steroids are synthetic drugs that are chemically related to the hormone testosterone. Physicians sometimes prescribe small doses within a medical setting for people with muscle diseases, burns, some cancers, and pituitary disorders. Some athletes and recreational weight trainers take anabolic steroids—illegally, outside of a medical setting, and without a prescription—to increase muscle mass, strength, and power. Anabolic steroids can produce some of these results in some users, but with overwhelmingly negative side effects that far outweigh the benefits. Besides being illegal, steroids increase the risk of liver and heart disease, cancer, acne, breast development in men, and masculinization in women. Because dramatically stronger muscles may exert more force than the body can handle, anabolic steroid use can also promote connective tissue and bone injuries. Steroid use can also be habit forming, lead to other drug addictions, and even cause death, as explained in the box Why Are Steroids Dangerous?

Creatine

Creatine is a legal nutritional supplement containing amino acids. It is most often sold as creatine monohydrate in powder, tablet, capsule, or liquid form. The body's natural form of creatine (phosphocreatine) is generated by the kidneys and stored in muscle cells. You can also consume creatine in the diet by eating meat products.

Creatine taken at recommended levels can improve performance by temporarily increasing the body's normal muscle stores of phosphocreatine. Since this natural energy substance powers bursts of activity lasting less than 60 seconds, creatine users sometimes find they can train more effectively in power activities and may be able to maintain higher forces during lifting. This can result in increased training adaptations such as strength and muscle size. Creatine intake also causes a temporary retention of water in muscle tissue that produces a small temporary increase in size, strength, and ability to generate power. Creatine has no effect on performance of aerobic endurance exercise.

So far, there have been few serious side effects reported in studies of people using creatine for up to four years. Since the long-term effects of creatine use are unknown, however, potential users should proceed with caution.

Adrenal Androgens (DHEA, Androstenedione)

Dehydroepiandrosterone (DHEA) is the body's most common hormone; it occurs naturally in the body and acts as a weak steroid chemical messenger (a conveyor of internal control signals and information).

• •

casestudy

GINA

"I'm a big baseball fan. While growing up in San Francisco, I went to Giants and A's games all the time. So I was shocked to hear about the allegations of steroid and drug use among professional baseball players. I'm confused about the health risks of steroids and supplements. Are they all dangerous? What about the products you can buy in a health store, like creatine?"

THINK! How would you answer Gina's questions about steroids and creatine? Give two other examples of ergogenic supplements. How safe are they?

ACT! Talk with a friend or your instructor about ergogenic supplements. Outline the pros and cons of taking certain supplements.

Why Are Steroids Dangerous?

Why are government drug regulators—not to mention parents, educators, and coaches—so worried about steroid use in young people? Steroid use in teens and young adults is a problem for several major reasons:

1. Steroid use can lead to the abuse of other drugs. Some of the side effects of steroid use are so disruptive that people turn to opiate drugs such as cocaine and heroin to relieve their distress.
2. Anabolic steroids can permanently disrupt normal development. A person's body and brain are still developing during adolescence and into their early twenties. Steroids interfere with the normal effects of sex hormones. Most of these changes are irreversible.
3. Steroid use can lead to behavioral changes, including irritability, hostility, aggression, and depression. These changes can continue even after the user stops using steroids.[1,2]
4. Steroids promote heart disease, heart attacks, and strokes, even in athletes younger than thirty. The drugs also cause blood-filled cysts in the liver that can burst and cause serious internal bleeding.
5. Injecting steroids and sharing needles with other users can lead to the transmission of dangerous infections. The disease risks include hepatitis, HIV, and endocarditis, a bacterial infection of the heart.

Problems in men	Problems in both	Problems in women
• Baldness	• Strokes and blood clots	• Increase in facial and body hair
• Headaches	• Aggressive behavior	• Deepened voice
• Development of breasts	• Mood swings	• Reduced breast size
• Shrinkage of testicles	• Severe acne on face and back	• Menstrual problems
• Enlarged prostate	• High blood pressure and heart disease	• Enlarged clitoris
• Reduced sperm count	• Liver damage	
	• Nausea	
	• Bloating	
	• Urinary and bowel problems	
	• Impotence	
	• Increased risk of tendon injuries	
	• Aching joints	

Sources:
1. American Psychological Association (APA), Press Release, "Animal Models Show that Anabolic Steroids Flip the Adolescent Brain's Switch for Aggressive Behavior," www.apa.org/news/press/releases/2006/02/steroids.aspx (February 26, 2006).
2. J. M. Grimes and others, "Plasticity in Anterior Hypothalamic Vasopressin Correlates with Aggression during Anabolic–Androgenic Steroid Withdrawal in Hamsters," *Behavioral Neuroscience* 120, no. 1 (2006): 115–24.

Manufacturers produce and sell it as a supplement in a synthetic concentrated form despite the lack of definitive proof of its safety or effectiveness. DHEA proponents claim that it increases muscle mass and strength, lowers body fat, alters natural hormone levels, slows aging, and boosts immune functions. However, research studies have produced conflicting results on DHEA and overall do not provide strong evidence of a large positive effect on muscle mass and strength or on body fat levels.

Androstenedione (nickname "andro") is another naturally occurring steroid hormone with a structure related to both DHEA and testosterone. It is found naturally in meats and some plants. Even though manufacturers claim "andro" will increase testosterone levels, one pivotal study found that it actually lowered the body's natural production of testosterone, did not increase the body's adaptations to resistance training, and increased heart disease risk in men.[15] Androstenedione was ordered off the market by the FDA in 2004, and its use is dwindling. Both DHEA and androstenedione appear to decrease HDL or "good" cholesterol, which helps explain why these substances increase heart attack risks and other cardiovascular problems.[16] Both also increase the risk of developing certain cancers and accelerating the growth of existing cancers. These serious side effects strongly argue against the use of DHEA or "andro."

Growth Hormone (GH)

Your body's pituitary gland produces human growth hormone (GH), which promotes bone growth and muscle growth and decreases fat stores. Drug manufacturers produce GH synthetically for medical use in children and young adults with abnormally slow or reduced growth and related disorders. Although the FDA regulates growth hormone, athletes wanting to gain an edge over their competitors sometimes obtain and use it illegally. Marketers claim that growth hormone supplementation will counteract the muscle mass lost with disuse and aging, among other alleged benefits. However, GH side effects include irreversible bone growth (acromegaly/gigantism), increased risk of cardiovascular disease and diabetes, and decreased sexual desire, among others.

Marketers of oral GH supplements claim the same positive benefits to lean muscle mass and fat mass, but this is not borne out in tests or actual use. Oral GH, in fact, cannot even be absorbed from your digestive tract into your bloodstream! A far better way to increase natural levels of growth hormone is to perform regular exercise. In a study of women who ran for exercise, baseline resting GH levels increased by 50 percent in those training at higher compared to lower intensities.[17]

Amino Acid and Protein Supplements

Many bodybuilders and weight lifters take amino acid supplements because they believe that consuming protein or its building blocks (amino acids) will lead to enhanced muscle development. However, evidence is mixed that high intake of protein or taking protein-based supplements will improve training or exercise performance or build muscle mass beyond the levels achieved through normal dietary protein. When combined with resistance training, moderate increases in protein intake may lead to small increases in lean muscle mass and strength beyond resistance training alone.[18] In contrast, supplementation with the amino acid glutamine produces no beneficial effect above and beyond resistance training itself.[19] Taking moderate doses of these supplements has no dramatic side effects, but large doses of either the supplements or protein itself can create amino acid imbalances, alter protein and bone metabolism, and be dangerous to individuals with liver or kidney disease.[20] See the box Should I Increase My Protein Intake Immediately after Resistance Training? for more on protein supplementation.

Should I Increase My Protein Intake Immediately after Resistance Training?

If you are looking to increase muscle strength and size, then definitely YES! Even if your goals are health and muscle maintenance, a balanced recovery meal or drink is beneficial. After resistance training, the muscles worked are depleted of nutrients and are in a state of muscle breakdown from the exercise. Providing muscles with nutrients and correcting protein imbalances helps repair breakdown damage and promotes recovery.[1] Eating protein after exercise, particularly essential amino acids, promotes protein synthesis.[2] Protein synthesis is even more pronounced when protein consumption is accompanied by easily digestible carbohydrates.[3] Carbohydrates will increase the release of insulin into the blood, which will in turn enhance protein storage in cells.[4]

Timing is important. Immediately after resistance training the muscles are receptive to bringing protein into cells. That increased protein helps with repair and recovery and promotes increases in the strength and size of the muscle. Increasing your intake a little bit right *before* exercise can also help.[5] In one study, subjects who took protein supplements immediately before and after resistance training had 86 percent greater increase in lean tissue mass and 30 percent greater overall strength after 10 weeks of resistance training than those who had the same supplements in the morning and night (not close to the exercise session).[6]

Tips for post–resistance-training nutrition:

- Consume 100–500 calories—depending upon your body size, workout length and intensity, and goals.

- Consume something that is digested rapidly—a liquid source is great!

- Drink or eat something with essential amino acids for your protein source—whey protein is a great source and you can get this in milk and chocolate milk.

- Make sure your snack is easily digested and has high-glycemic load carbohydrates—again, chocolate milk fills the bill!

- Consume about two parts carbohydrate to one part protein. Healthy fats can also be included.

- For the greatest effect, consume your post-exercise drink or snack within an hour, preferably within 30 minutes, of stopping your exercise session.

- After an hour or later in the day, eat a full recovery meal with a balance of protein, carbohydrates, and healthy fats.

Sources:
1. S. M. Phillips, J. W. Hartman, and S. B. Wilkinson, "Dietary Protein to Support Anabolism with Resistance Exercise in Young Men," *Journal of the American College of Nutrition* 24, no. 2 (2005): 134S–9S.
2. S. L. Miller and others, "Independent and Combined Effects of Amino Acids and Glucose after Resistance Exercise," *Medicine and Science in Sports and Exercise* 35, no. 3 (2003): 449–55.
3. K. Pritchett and others, "Acute Effects of Chocolate Milk and a Commercial Recovery Beverage on Postexercise Recovery Indices and Endurance Cycling Performance," *Applied Physiology, Nutrition, and Metabolism* 34, no. 6 (2009): 1017–22.
4. S. M. Phillips, "Physiologic and Molecular Bases of Muscle Hypertrophy and Atrophy: Impact of Resistance Exercise on Human Skeletal Muscle (Protein and Exercise Dose Effects)," *Applied Physiology, Nutrition, and Metabolism* 34, no. 3 (2009): 403–10.
5. K. D. Tipton and others, "Stimulation of Net Muscle Protein Synthesis by Whey Protein Ingestion before and after Exercise," *American Journal of Physiology: Endocrinology and Metabolism* 292, no. 1 (2006): E71–6.
6. P. J. Cribb and A. Hayes, "Effects of Supplement Timing and Resistance Exercise on Skeletal Muscle Hypertrophy," *Medicine and Science in Sports and Exercise* 38, no. 11 (2006): 1918–25.

chapterin**review**

videos

Log on to **www.pearsonhighered.com/hopson** or MyFitnessLab to view these chapter-related videos.

Free-Weight Exercises
Safety Tips: Dumbbells
Bench/Chest Press
Biceps Curl
Dumbbell Flys
Dumbbell Row
Front Raise
Lateral Raise
Lunges
Pullover
Shoulder Press
Shoulder Shrugs
Squats
Straight-Leg Heel Raise
Triceps Extension
Triceps Kickback
Upright Rows
Walking Lunges
Resistance Band Exercises
Safety Tips: Resistance Bands
Bench/Chest Press
Biceps Curl
Flys
Front Raise
Lat Pull-Down
Lateral Raise
Leg Abduction
Leg Adduction
Leg Curl
Leg Press
Seated Row

Shoulder Press
Shoulder Shrug
Squats
Triceps Extension
Triceps Kickback
Upright Row
Stability Ball Exercises
Safety Tips: Stability Balls
Abdominal Curl
Abdominal Tuck
Back Extension
Bridge Leg Curl
Bridge Up
Dumbbell Fly/Press
Hip Adduction
Lat Roll-Out
Leg Curl
Oblique Side Crunch
Pike-Up
Plank
Reverse Dumbbell Fly
Wall Squat
Strength Exercises
Requiring No Equipment
Arm/Leg Extensions
Back Bridge
Bench Dips
Modified Push-Ups
Oblique Curl
Pelvic Tilt
Plank (Forearm Position)

Plank (Push-Up Position)
Push-Ups
Reverse Curl
Side Bridge (Beginner)
Side Bridge (Intermediate)
Side Bridge (Advanced)
Machine Exercises
Abdominal Curl
Assisted Pull-Up
Biceps Curl
Chest Flys
Chest Press
Hip Extension
Lat Pull-Down
Lateral Raise
Leg Curl
Leg Extension
Leg Press
Machine Row
Overhead Press
Smith Machine Squat
Triceps Extension
Assessments
Curl-Up Assessment
Grip Strength Assessment
One Repetition Maximum (1RM)
    Prediction Assessment
Push-Up Assessment

The Mitchell Report on
Steroids in Baseball

onlineresources

Log on to **www.pearsonhighered.com/hopson** or MyFitnessLab for access to these book-related resources and for links to other useful websites.

Audio case study
Audio PowerPoint lecture

Customizable 4-week resistance-training programs
Behavior Change Log Book and
Wellness Journal

Lab 4.1 Assessing Your Muscular Strength
Lab 4.2 Assessing Your Muscular
Endurance
Lab 4.3 Setting Muscular Fitness Goals
Lab 4.4 Your Resistance-Training
Workout Plan
Alternate Lab: Assessing Grip Strength

Pre- and post-quizzes
Glossary flashcards

reviewquestions

1. Muscular strength is the ability to
   a. contract your muscles repeatedly over time.
   b. run a six-minute mile.
   c. look "toned" in a swimsuit.
   d. contract your muscle with maximal force.

2. Which of the following benefits of resistance training will reduce your risk of cardiovascular diseases?
   a. Increased bone density
   b. Increased muscle power
   c. Reduced body fat levels
   d. Better sports recovery

3. What is a single muscle cell called?
   a. Muscle fiber
   b. Muscle fascia
   c. Fascicle
   d. Contractile bundle

4. Which of the following will result in a stronger muscle contraction?
   a. Eating more protein before your workout
   b. Activating slow, smaller motor units
   c. Taking DHEA before your workout
   d. Activating more motor units overall

5. Sitting down in a chair and standing up again is an example of which type of exercise?
   a. Isotonic
   b. Isokinetic
   c. Isometric
   d. Isostatic

6. Muscle strength improvements in the first few weeks of a program are due to
   a. increased size of muscle fibers.
   b. increased activation and coordination of motor units
   c. increased ability of muscles to move through a full range of motion.
   d. increased blood flow to working muscles.

7. A test of muscular endurance includes
   a. a 1 RM test.
   b. a grip-strength test.
   c. a 20 RM test.
   d. a pull-up test.

8. One disadvantage of using machines for resistance-training exercises is
   a. it takes time to adjust the machine for your height and desired resistance level.
   b. the machine does not promote the use of postural and stabilizing muscles during the exercise.
   c. spotters are needed.
   d. it can be hard to isolate specific muscle groups.

9. Which of the following is part of the criteria you should use when selecting a personal trainer?
   a. Certified by ACSM, NSCA, or ACE
   b. Looks like someone who works out a lot
   c. Recommended by a friend who was sore after a workout with the trainer
   d. Able to provide dietary supplements at a reduced cost

10. Which of the following supplements/drugs promotes irreversible bone growth, cardiovascular disease, diabetes, and decreased sexual desire?
    a. Anabolic steroids
    b. Creatine
    c. Growth hormone
    d. Androstenedione

critical**thinking**questions

1. Why is weight training a popular activity among college students and adults of all ages?

2. Define sarcopenia and discuss how it can be reversed through exercise. How are sarcopenia and atrophy different?

3. What is the predominant fiber type in the postural trunk muscles and why does this make sense?

4. Discuss the role of resistance training in preventing injuries.

5. How does circuit weight training differ from regular weight training? What are the specific benefits of doing circuit weight training?

references

1. Centers for Disease Control and Prevention (CDC), "QuickStats: Percentage of Adults Aged ≥ 18 Years Who Engaged in Leisure-Time Strengthening Activities, by Age Group and Sex—National Health Interview Survey, United States, 2008," *Morbidity and Mortality Weekly Report* 58, no. 34 (2009): 955; National Center for Health Statistics, Health Promotion Statistics Branch, CDC Wonder, *DATA2010...the Healthy People 2010 Database* (Hyattsville, MD; Centers for Disease Control, 2010), http://wonder.cdc.gov/data2010/focus.htm (accessed May 2011).

2. National Center for Health Statistics, CDC Wonder, *DATA2010...the Healthy People 2010 Database*, 2010; CDC, "Trends in Strength Training: United States, 1998–2004," *Morbidity and Mortality Weekly Report* 55, no. 28 (2006): 769–72.

3. Office of Disease Prevention and Health Promotion, U.S. Department of Health and Human Services, "Healthy People 2020 Topics and Objectives: Physical Activity," http://healthypeople.gov/2020/topicsobjectives2020/objectiveslist.aspx?topicid=33 (accessed April 2011).

4. M. J. Hubal and others, "Variability in Muscle Size and Strength Gain after Unilateral Resistance Training," *Medicine and Science in Sports and Exercise* 37, no. 6 (2005): 964–72.

5. K. Davison and others, "Relationships between Obesity, Cardiorespiratory Fitness, and Cardiovascular Function," *Journal of Obesity* 2010 (2010); M. Fogelholm, "Physical Activity, Fitness and Fatness: Relations to Mortality, Morbidity and Disease Risk Factors. A Systematic Review," *Obesity Reviews* 11 no. 3 (2010): 202–21; J.G. Stegger and others, "Body Composition and Body Fat Distribution in Relation to Later Risk of Acute Myocardial Infarction: A Danish Follow-up Study," *International Journal of Obesity* (February 2011) [Epub ahead of print].

6. Z. Wang and others, "Specific Metabolic Rates of Major Organs and Tissues across Adulthood: Evaluation by Mechanistic Model of Resting Energy Expenditure," *American Journal of Clinical Nutrition* 92, no. 6 (2010): 1369–77.

7. S. M. Fernando and others, "Myocyte Androgen Receptors Increase Metabolic Rate and Improve Body Composition by Reducing Fat Mass," *Endocrinology* 151 no. 7 (2010): 3125–32; R. R. Wolfe, "The Underappreciated Role of Muscle in Health and Disease," *American Journal of Clinical Nutrition* 84, no. 3 (2006): 475–82.

8. J. E. Donnelly and others, "American College of Sports Medicine Position Stand: Appropriate Physical Activity Intervention Strategies for Weight Loss and Prevention of Weight Regain for Adults," *Medicine and Science in Sports and Exercise* 41 no. 2 (2009): 459–71; B. L. Marks and others, "Fat-free Mass Is Maintained in Women Following a Moderate Diet and Exercise Program," *Medicine and Science in Sports and Exercise* 27, no. 9 (1995): 1243–51.

9. W. W. Campbell and others, "Resistance Training Preserves Fat-free Mass without Impacting Changes in Protein Metabolism after Weight Loss in Older Women," *Obesity* 17, no. 7 (2009): 1332–9.

10. P. A. Williams and T. F. Cash, "Effects of a Circuit Weight Training Program on the Body Images of College Students," *International Journal of Eating Disorders* 30, no. 1 (2001): 75–80.

11. E. A. Marques and others, "Effects of Resistance and Aerobic Exercise on Physical Function, Bone Mineral Density, OPG, and RANKL in Older Women," *Experimental Gerontology* 46, no. 7 (2011): 524–32.

12. American Council on Exercise (ACE), ACE FitnessMatters, "Why Is the Concept of Spot Reduction Considered a Myth?" www.acefitness.org/fitnessqanda /fitnessqanda_display.aspx?itemid=341 (2004).

13. K. Jay and others, "Kettlebell Training for Musculoskeletal and Cardiovascular Health: A Randomized Controlled Trial," *Scandinavian Journal of Work, Environment, and Health* 37, no. 3 (2010): 196–203.

14. M. Bird, American College of Sports Medicine, "Building Strength Safely" *Fit Society Page* (Fall 2002): 3.

15. C. E. Brodeur and others, "The Andro Project: Physiological and Hormonal Influences of Androstenedione Supplementation in Men 35–65 Years Old Participating in a High-Intensity Resistance Training Program," *Archives of Internal Medicine* 160, no. 20, (2000): 3093–104.

16. M. L. Kohut and others, "Ingestion of a Dietary Supplement Containing Dehydroepiandrosterone (DHEA) and Androstenedione Has Minimal Effect on Immune Function in Middle-Aged Men," *Journal of the American College of Nutrition* 22, no. 5 (2003): 363–71.

17. A. Weltman and others, "Endurance Training Amplifies the Pulsatile Release of Growth Hormone: Effects of Training Intensity," *Journal of Applied Physiology* 72, no. 6 (1992): 2188–96.

18. D. G. Candow and others, "Effect of Whey and Soy Protein Supplementation Combined with Resistance Training in Young Adults," *International Journal of Sport Nutrition and Exercise Metabolism* 16, no. 3 (2006): 233–44.

19. D. G. Candow and others, "Effect of Glutamine Supplementation Combined with Resistance Training in Young Adults," *European Journal of Applied Physiology* 86, no. 2 (2001): 142–9.

20. E. L. Knight and others, "The Impact of Protein Intake on Renal Function Decline in Women with Normal Renal Function or Mild Renal Insufficiency," *Annals of Internal Medicine* 138, no. 6 (2003): 460–7.

LAB 4.1 • ASSESSING YOUR MUSCULAR STRENGTH

Name: _____ **Date:** _____

Instructor: _____ **Section:** _____

Materials: Calculator, leg press machine, chest press machine

Purpose: To assess your current level of muscular strength

Note: This lab should be performed in the presence of an instructor to ensure proper form and safety.

MUSCULAR STRENGTH ASSESSMENT

One Repetition Maximum (1 RM) Prediction Assessment

ACSM recommends measuring muscular strength by performing one repetition maximum (1 RM) or multiple RM assessments. This lab estimates 1 RM for the chest press and leg press by finding the amount of weight you can maximally lift 2 to 10 times.

1. **Warm up.** Complete 3 to 10 minutes of light cardiorespiratory activity to warm the muscles. Perform range-of-motion exercises and light stretches for the joints and muscles that you will be using.

2. **Use proper form while executing the chest press and leg press exercises.** For the chest press, position yourself so the bar or handles are across the middle of your chest. Spread your hands slightly wider than shoulder width. Bring the handles/bar to just above your chest and then press upward/outward until your arms are straight. For the leg press, position yourself so that your knees are at a 90-degree angle. Press the weight away from your body until your legs are straight.

3. **Perform one light warm-up set.** Set the machine at a very light weight and lift this weight about 10 times as a warm-up for your assessment.

4. **Find the appropriate strength-assessment weight and number of repetitions.** Set a weight that you think you can lift at least 2 times but no more than 10 times. Perform the lift as many times as you can (to complete fatigue) up to 10 repetitions. If you can lift more than 10 repetitions, try again using heavier weight. Repeat until you find a weight you cannot lift more than 2 to 10 times. In order to prevent muscle fatigue from affecting your results, attempt this assessment no more than three times to find the proper weight and number of repetitions. If you experience muscle fatigue, rest and perform the test again on another day. Record your results in the Muscular Strength Results section (see step 7).

5. **Find your predicted 1 RM.** Predict your 1 RM based upon the number of repetitions you performed. If the weight you lifted was between 20 and 250 pounds, use the 1 RM Prediction Table to find your predicted 1 RM. If you lifted over 250 pounds, use the Multiplication Factor Table to find your predicted 1 RM. You can find these tables at the end of this lab.

6. **Find your strength-to-body weight ratio.** Divide your predicted 1 RM by your body weight for your strength-to-body-weight ratio (S/BW). Since heavier people often have more muscle, this is a better indicator of muscular strength than just the weight lifted alone. Record your results in the Muscular Strength Results section.

7. **Find your muscle strength rating by using the Strength-to-Body Weight Ratio chart provided on the last page of this lab.** Finding your rating tells you how you compare to others who have completed this test in the past. Record your results on the next page.

Muscular Strength Results

Chest Press: Weight lifted _____ Repetitions _____

$$\underline{\hspace{6cm}} \times \underline{\hspace{6cm}} = \underline{\hspace{5cm}}$$

Weight lifted (lb)   Multiplication factor*   Predicted 1 RM (lb)

$$\underline{\hspace{6cm}} \div \underline{\hspace{6cm}} = \underline{\hspace{5cm}}$$

Predicted 1 RM (lb)   Body weight (lb)   S/BW ratio

Rating _____

Leg Press: Weight lifted _____ Repetitions _____

$$\underline{\hspace{6cm}} \times \underline{\hspace{6cm}} = \underline{\hspace{5cm}}$$

Weight lifted (lb)   Multiplication factor*   Predicted 1 RM (lb)

$$\underline{\hspace{6cm}} \div \underline{\hspace{6cm}} = \underline{\hspace{5cm}}$$

Predicted 1 RM (lb)   Body weight (lb)   S/BW ratio

Rating _____

*Multiplication factor from the Multiplication Factor Table on the last page of this lab.

1 RM Prediction Table

Wt (lb)	Repetitions									
	1	2	3	4	5	6	7	8	9	10
20	20	21	21	22	23	23	24	25	26	27
25	25	26	26	27	28	29	30	31	32	33
30	30	31	32	33	34	35	36	37	39	40
35	35	36	37	38	39	41	42	43	45	47
40	40	41	42	44	45	46	48	50	51	53
45	45	46	48	49	51	52	54	56	58	60
50	50	51	53	55	56	58	60	62	64	67
55	55	57	58	60	62	64	66	68	71	73
60	60	62	64	65	68	70	72	74	77	80
65	65	67	69	71	73	75	78	81	84	87
70	70	72	74	76	79	81	84	87	90	93
75	75	77	79	82	84	87	90	93	96	100
80	80	82	85	87	90	93	96	99	103	107
85	85	87	90	93	96	99	102	106	109	113
90	90	93	95	98	101	105	108	112	116	120
95	95	98	101	104	107	110	114	118	122	127
100	100	103	106	109	113	116	120	124	129	133
105	105	108	111	115	118	122	126	130	135	140
110	110	113	116	120	124	128	132	137	141	147
115	115	118	122	125	129	134	138	143	148	153

(Continued)

1 RM Prediction Table (Continued)

					Repetitions					
Wt (lb)	1	2	3	4	5	6	7	8	9	10
120	120	123	127	131	135	139	144	149	154	160
125	125	129	132	136	141	145	150	155	161	167
130	130	134	138	142	146	151	156	161	167	173
135	135	139	143	147	152	157	162	168	174	180
140	140	144	148	153	158	163	168	174	180	187
145	145	149	154	158	163	168	174	180	186	193
150	150	154	159	164	169	174	180	186	193	200
155	155	159	164	169	174	180	186	192	199	207
160	160	165	169	175	180	186	192	199	206	213
165	165	170	175	180	186	192	198	205	212	220
170	170	175	180	185	191	197	204	211	219	227
175	175	180	185	191	197	203	210	217	225	233
180	180	185	191	196	203	209	216	223	231	240
185	185	190	196	202	208	215	222	230	238	247
190	190	195	201	207	214	221	228	236	244	253
195	195	201	206	213	219	226	234	242	251	260
200	200	206	212	218	225	232	240	248	257	267
205	205	211	217	224	231	238	246	255	264	273
210	210	216	222	229	236	244	252	261	270	280
215	215	221	228	235	242	250	258	267	276	287
220	220	226	233	240	248	256	264	273	283	293
225	225	231	238	245	253	261	270	279	289	300
230	230	237	244	251	259	267	276	286	296	307
235	235	242	249	256	264	273	282	292	302	313
240	240	247	254	262	270	279	288	298	309	320
245	245	252	259	267	276	285	294	304	315	327
250	250	257	265	273	281	290	300	310	322	333

Multiplication Factor Table for Predicting 1 RM

Repetitions	1	2	3	4	5	6	7	8	9	10
Multiplication Factor	1.0	1.07	1.11	1.13	1.16	1.20	1.23	1.27	1.32	1.36

Table and multiplication factors generated using the Bryzcki equation:
1 RM = weight (kg) /[1.0278−(0.0278 × repetitions)].

Source: Adapted from M. Brzycki, "Strength Testing: Predicting a One-Rep Max from a Reps-to-Fatigue," *Journal of Physical Education, Recreation, and Dance* 64, no. 1 (1993): 88–90.

Strength-to-Body Weight Ratio Ratings

Chest Press						
Men	**Superior**	**Excellent**	**Good**	**Fair**	**Poor**	**Very Poor**
<20 yrs	1.75	1.34–1.75	1.19–1.33	1.06–1.18	0.89–1.05	0.89
20–29 yrs	1.62	1.32–1.62	1.14–1.31	0.99–1.13	0.88–0.98	0.88
30–39 yrs	1.34	1.12–1.34	0.98–1.11	0.88–0.97	0.78–0.87	0.78
40–49 yrs	1.19	1.00–1.19	0.88–0.99	0.80–0.87	0.72–0.79	0.72
50–59 yrs	1.04	0.90–1.04	0.79–0.89	0.71–0.78	0.63–0.70	0.63
>60 yrs	0.93	0.82–0.93	0.72–0.81	0.66–0.71	0.57–0.65	0.57
Women	**Superior**	**Excellent**	**Good**	**Fair**	**Poor**	**Very Poor**
<20 yrs	0.87	0.77–0.87	0.65–0.76	0.58–0.64	0.53–0.57	0.53
20–29 yrs	1.00	0.80–1.00	0.70–0.79	0.59–0.69	0.51–0.58	0.51
30–39 yrs	0.81	0.70–0.81	0.60–0.69	0.53–0.59	0.47–0.52	0.47
40–49 yrs	0.76	0.62–0.76	0.54–0.61	0.50–0.53	0.43–0.49	0.43
50–59 yrs	0.67	0.55–0.67	0.48–0.54	0.44–0.47	0.39–0.43	0.39
>60 yrs	0.71	0.54–0.71	0.47–0.53	0.43–0.46	0.38–0.42	0.38
Leg Press						
Men	**Superior**	**Excellent**	**Good**	**Fair**	**Poor**	**Very Poor**
<20 yrs	2.81	2.28–2.81	2.04–2.27	1.90–2.03	1.70–1.89	1.70
20–29 yrs	2.39	2.13–2.39	1.97–2.12	1.83–1.96	1.63–1.82	1.63
30–39 yrs	2.19	1.93–2.19	1.77–1.92	1.65–1.76	1.52–1.64	1.52
40–49 yrs	2.01	1.82–2.01	1.68–1.81	1.57–1.67	1.44–1.56	1.44
50–59 yrs	1.89	1.71–1.89	1.58–1.70	1.46–1.57	1.32–1.45	1.32
>60 yrs	1.79	1.62–1.79	1.49–1.61	1.38–1.48	1.25–1.37	1.25
Women	**Superior**	**Excellent**	**Good**	**Fair**	**Poor**	**Very Poor**
<20 yrs	1.87	1.71–1.87	1.59–1.70	1.38–1.58	1.22–1.37	1.22
20–29 yrs	1.97	1.68–1.97	1.50–1.67	1.37–1.49	1.22–1.36	1.22
30–39 yrs	1.67	1.47–1.67	1.33–1.46	1.21–1.32	1.09–1.20	1.09
40–49 yrs	1.56	1.37–1.56	1.23–1.36	1.13–1.22	1.02–1.12	1.02
50–59 yrs	1.42	1.25–1.42	1.10–1.24	0.99–1.09	0.88–0.98	0.88
>60 yrs	1.42	1.18–1.42	1.04–1.17	0.93–1.03	0.85–0.92	0.85

Source: Reprinted with permission from The Cooper Institute, Dallas, Texas from PHYSICAL FITNESS ASSESSMENTS AND NORMS FOR ADULTS AND LAW ENFORCE-MENT, available online at www.CooperInstitute.org.

LAB 4.2 • ASSESSING YOUR MUSCULAR ENDURANCE

Name: _____   **Date:** _____

Instructor: _____   **Section:** _____

Materials: Leg press machine, bench press machine, exercise mat, yardstick or ruler, tape

Purpose: To assess your current level of muscular endurance

Note: This lab should be performed in the presence of an instructor to ensure proper form and safety.

SECTION I: MUSCULAR ENDURANCE WEIGHT-LIFTING ASSESSMENT

Twenty Repetition Maximum (20 RM) Assessment

The 20 RM assessment is a weight-lifting assessment of your muscular endurance. By performing the assessments before and after completing 8 to 12 weeks of muscular fitness exercises, you can measure your improvement.

1. Prepare for the muscle endurance assessments. If you have just completed the muscular strength assessments in Lab 4.1, you will already be warmed up. If not, follow the position, form, and warm-up instructions for bench press and leg press in Lab 4.1.

2. Find your 20 RM for chest press and leg press. Set a weight that you think you can lift a maximum of 20 times. Perform the lift to see whether you were correct. If not, increase or decrease the weight and try again until you find your 20 RM. In order to be sure that muscle fatigue does not affect your results, try to find your 20 RM within three tries. If it takes longer, rest and perform the test again on another day. Record your results below.

Muscular Endurance Weight Lifting Results

Chest Press: 20 RM weight lifted _____

Leg Press: 20 RM weight lifted _____

SECTION II: MUSCULAR ENDURANCE CALISTHENIC ASSESSMENT

Push-Up Assessment

In this muscular endurance assessment, you will perform as many push-ups as you can. This test will assess the muscular endurance of your pectoralis major, anterior deltoid, and triceps brachii muscles. If you work with a partner, your partner can check your positioning and form and count your repetitions.

1. Get into the correct push-up position on an exercise mat. Support the body in a push-up position from the knees (women) or from the toes (men). The hands should be just outside the shoulders and the back and legs straight.

2. Start in the "down" position with your elbow joint at a 90-degree angle, your chest just above the floor, and your chin barely touching the mat. Push your body up until your arms are straight and then lower back to the starting position (count one repetition). Complete the push-ups in a slow and controlled manner.

3. Complete as many correct technique push-ups as you can without stopping and record your results in the Muscular Endurance Calisthenic Results section below.

4. Find your muscle endurance rating for push-ups in the chart at the end of this lab and record your results.

Curl-Up Assessment

In this muscular endurance assessment, you will perform as many curl-ups as you can (up to 25). This test will assess the muscular endurance of your abdominal muscles.

1. Lie on a mat with your arms by your sides, palms flat on the mat, elbows straight, and fingers extended. Bend your knees at a 90-degree angle. Mark the start and end positions with tape. Your instructor or partner will mark your starting finger position with a piece of tape under each hand. He or she will then mark the ending position 10 cm (or close to 4 inches) away from the first piece of tape, one ending position tape for each hand. Your goal is to rise far enough on the curl-up to achieve a 30-degree trunk elevation.

2. Your instructor or partner will set a metronome to 50 beats/min and you will complete the curl-ups at this slow, controlled pace: one curl-up every three seconds (25 curl-ups per minute).

3. To start the test, curl your head and upper back upward, reaching your arms forward along the mat to touch the ending tape. Then curl back down so that your upper back and shoulders touch the floor. During the entire curl-up, your fingers, feet, and buttocks should stay on the mat. Your partner will count the number of correct repetitions you complete. Any curl-ups performed without touching the ending position tape will not be counted in the final results.

4. Perform as many curl-ups as you can without pausing, to a maximum of 25. Record your score below. Determine your muscular endurance rating for curl-ups using the chart below and record your results.

**Alternative: One-minute timed curl-ups. Your instructor may choose to have you complete as many curl-ups as you can within one minute (without the metronome pacing). Using the same start and end positions, perform controlled repetitions of curl-ups for one minute and record your results below.

Muscular Endurance Calisthenic Results

Push-Ups: Repetitions_____   Rating_____

Curl-Ups: Repetitions_____   Rating_____

**Alternative: One-minute timed curl-ups: Repetitions _____

SECTION III: REFLECTION

1. What was surprising about your muscular fitness results, if anything?

_____

_____

2. Based upon your assessment results, which aspect of muscular fitness will your program focus on, muscular strength or muscular endurance?

_____

_____

Muscluar Endurance Rating

Push-ups						
Men	**Superior**	**Excellent**	**Good**	**Fair**	**Poor**	**Very Poor**
20–29 yrs	>36	31–36	24–30	21–23	16–20	<16
30–39 yrs	>30	24–30	19–23	16–18	11–15	<11
40–49 yrs	>25	19–25	15–18	12–14	9–11	<9
50–59 yrs	>21	15–21	12–14	9–11	6–8	<6
60–69 yrs	>18	13–18	10–12	7–9	4–6	<4
Women	**Superior**	**Excellent**	**Good**	**Fair**	**Poor**	**Very Poor**
20–29 yrs	>30	22–30	16–21	14–15	9–13	<9
30–39 yrs	>27	21–27	14–20	12–14	7–11	<7
40–49 yrs	>24	16–24	12–15	10–11	4–9	<4
50–59 yrs	>21	12–21	8–11	6–8	1–5	<1
60–69 yrs	>17	13–17	6–12	4–6	1–3	<1
Curl-ups						
Men	**Superior**	**Excellent**	**Good**	**Fair**	**Poor**	**Very Poor**
20–29 yrs	>25	22–25	16–21	13–15	10–12	<10
30–39 yrs	>25	19–25	15–18	13–14	10–12	<10
40–49 yrs	>25	19–25	13–18	8–12	5–7	<5
50–59 yrs	>25	18–25	11–17	9–10	7–8	<7
60–69 yrs	>25	17–25	11–16	8–10	5–7	<5
Women	**Superior**	**Excellent**	**Good**	**Fair**	**Poor**	**Very Poor**
20–29 yrs	>25	19–25	14–18	7–13	4–6	<4
30–39 yrs	>25	20–25	10–19	8–9	5–7	<5
40–49 yrs	>25	20–25	11–19	6–10	3–5	<3
50–59 yrs	>25	20–25	10–19	8–9	5–7	<5
60–69 yrs	>25	18–25	8–17	5–7	2–4	<2

Source: Adapted from Canadian Society for Exercise Physiology. *The Canadian Physical Activity, Fitness & Lifestyle Approach: CSEP-Health & Fitness Program's Health-Related Appraisal & Counseling Strategy*, 3rd ed. Canadian Society for Exercise Physiology: 2003.

Name: _____ Date: _____

Instructor: _____ Section: _____

Purpose: To learn how to set appropriate muscular fitness goals (short- and long-term).

SECTION I: SHORT- AND LONG-TERM GOALS

Create short- and long-term goals for muscular strength and muscular endurance. Be sure to use SMART (*Specific*, *Measurable*, *Action-Oriented*, *Realistic*, *Timed*) goal-setting guidelines. Apply information from the Chapter 4 text and use your results from Labs 4.1 and 4.2. Remember that aiming to improve your assessment scores is a measurable way to set goals. Select appropriate target dates and rewards for completing your goals.

Short-Term Goals (3–6 months)

1. Muscular Strength Goal:

_____

   Target Date: _____

   Reward: _____

2. Muscular Endurance Goal:

_____

   Target Date: _____

   Reward: _____

Long-Term Goals (12+ months)

1. Muscular Strength Goal:

_____

   Target Date: _____

   Reward: _____

2. Muscular Endurance Goal:

_____

   Target Date: _____

   Reward: _____

SECTION II: MUSCULAR FITNESS OBSTACLES AND STRATEGIES

What barriers or obstacles might hinder your plan to improve your muscular fitness? Indicate your top three obstacles below and list strategies for overcoming each obstacle.

a. _____

b. _____

c. _____

SECTION III: GETTING SUPPORT

1. List resources you will use to help change your muscular fitness:

Friend/partner/relative: _____   School-based resource: _____

Community-based resource: _____   Other: _____

SECTION IV: REFLECTION

1. How realistic are the short- and long-term target dates you have set for achieving your muscular fitness goals?

_____

_____

_____

_____

2. Are there any other strategies not listed above that could assist you in reaching your goals?

_____

_____

_____

_____

3. Think about all of the opportunities that present themselves in your daily life to work toward muscular fitness. List as many of these as you can think of:

_____

_____

_____

_____

LAB 4.4 • YOUR RESISTANCE-TRAINING WORKOUT PLAN

Name: _____ **Date:** _____

Instructor: _____ **Section:** _____

Purpose: To create a basic, personal resistance-training workout plan. Forms for following up and tracking your muscular fitness and your resistance-training program are included.

Directions: Complete the following sections.

SECTION I: MUSCULAR FITNESS PROGRAM QUESTIONS AND MOTIVATIONS

1. How many days per week are you planning to work on your muscular fitness program? _____

2. How experienced are you at resistance training? (select one below)

Novice **Intermediate (training 1 to 2 years)** **Advanced (training 3+ yrs)**

3. Which will you focus on first? (select one) **Muscular strength** **Muscular endurance**

4. The best muscular fitness programs are well rounded and work the entire body. However, some people want to focus more heavily on one area than another. Which muscle groups do you want to focus on?

_____

5. Which type of equipment do you plan to use and why? (check all that apply)

☐ **Weight machines**

☐ **Free weights**

☐ **No equipment (calisthenic exercises)**

6. How much time do you plan for your resistance-training program on each workout day? _____

7. Do you have a workout partner? Do you plan to work with a partner, trainer, or instructor to help you get started?

_____

*See **Activate, Motivate, Advance Your Fitness: A Resistance-Training Program** on page 169 for a sample resistance-training program that will match your preferences and goals outlined above.

SECTION II: RESISTANCE-TRAINING PROGRAM DESIGN

In the table on the following page, plan your resistance-training program using resources available to you (facility, instructor, text). Complete one line for each exercise you have chosen to do in your program.

Exercise	Muscle(s) Worked	Frequency (days/week)	Intensity (weight in lb)	Sets (number)	Reps (number per set)	Rest (time between sets)
LOWER BODY						
1.						
2.						
3.						
4.						
5.						
6.						
7.						
8.						
UPPER BODY						
1.						
2.						
3.						
4.						
5.						
6.						
7.						
8.						
9.						
10.						
11.						
12.						
TRUNK						
1.						
2.						
3.						
4.						
5.						

SECTION III: TRACKING YOUR PROGRAM AND FOLLOWING THROUGH

1. Goal and program tracking: Use a resistance-training chart (see next page) to monitor your progress. Change the amount of resistance, sets, or repetitions frequently to ensure continuing progress toward your goals.

2. Goal and program follow-up: At the end of the course or at your short-term goal target date, reevaluate your muscular fitness and answer the following questions:

    a. Did you meet your short-term goal or your goal for the course?

    b. If so, what positive behavioral changes contributed to your success? If not, which obstacles blocked your success?

    c. Was your short-term goal realistic? After evaluating your progress during the course, what would you change about your goals or resistance-training plan?

DATE																							
EXERCISE	Wt.	Sets	Reps	Wt.	Sets	Reps	Wt.	Sets	Reps	Wt.	Sets	Reps	Wt.	Sets	Reps	Wt.	Sets	Reps	Wt.	Sets	Reps
1.																					
2.																					
3.																					
4.																					
5.																					
6.																					
7.																					
8.																					
9.																					
10.																					
11.																					
12.																					
13.																					
14.																					

activate, motivate, & ADVANCE YOUR FITNESS

A RESISTANCE-TRAINING PROGRAM

ACTIVATE!

With the long list of health, wellness, and fitness benefits associated with resistance training, there is no doubt you want to get started now and give it all you've got! Just as with your cardiorespiratory program, don't make the mistake of trying to do too much, too soon. Doing too much too soon in a new resistance-training program is a leading cause of injury! Follow these programs to gradually increase the number of times you train each week, the number of exercises you incorporate into your weekly routine and, of course, the load (weight) and the volume (sets/repetitions).

What Do I Need for Resistance Training?

SHOES: For most resistance-training programs, you will want a pair of shoes with good traction and a non-slip sole. This gives you a stable base and prevents slipping when you lift.

CLOTHING: Wear comfortable, supportive clothing that allows for full range-of-motion movements. Choose materials that wick moisture away from your skin to help you regulate your body temperature and stay dry. In addition, you might find a pair of weight lifting gloves helpful for increasing your grip strength and preventing blisters and calluses.

How Do I Start a Resistance-Training Program?

TECHNIQUE: Safe and effective resistance training really depends on proper technique. Please be sure to read through each exercise description carefully and learn the proper technique for each exercise to ensure good form. If you need assistance with how to properly use or set up a weight machine or if you need an exercise demonstration, ask your instructor or the fitness specialist at your facility. In addition to maintaining good form, it is important to perform each exercise in a slow and controlled manner through the full range of motion, taking care to avoid "locking out" your joints. If you are unable to maintain good form, decrease the weight or even the number of repetitions. Keep the weight balanced and use collars on weight bars to keep weights stable and secure. When it comes to proper breathing technique, keep it simple.

In general, you will want to exhale during the exertion phase (when the exercise is hardest). Finally, when lifting free weights it is always advisable to have a spotter. This is especially important for heavier weight loads, for maximal efforts, and for exercises that require the weight to pass over your head, face, or chest and even when a weight actually rests on your shoulders.

ETIQUETTE: Most facilities will have posted regulations for all patrons, and there are a few basic guidelines to keep in mind when you are resistance training.

Remember, safety first. Place weights, collars, and other equipment back when you finish using them. The next user may not be as strong as you are and may not be able to move the weight plates. The last thing anyone in the gym needs is to be tripping over free weights, so put your weights back on the rack when you finish with them. Be sure to wipe down machines, equipment, and benches after use. Most gyms supply wipes or have spray bottles and rags spread out throughout the weight room, so you shouldn't use your personal sweat towel.

Another common courtesy is to let others use the machines or weights during your rest intervals between sets.

Resistance-Training Tips

AT THE GYM: One of the advantages of resistance training at a gym is access to the wide variety of equipment and the amount of actual weight: weight machines, barbells (long bars with weights attached or slots to add weight plates), dumbbells (smaller, hand-held weights), benches (flat, incline, decline), cable stations, the latest the industry has to offer. Utilizing essentials (machines and free weights) and the extras (balls, bands, etc.) provides exercise variety, which reduces boredom and increases exercise adherence. Another advantage to having a wide array of equipment and exercise options available relates to your specific muscular fitness goal and your progression. The exercise options included in the programs below and at the end of the chapter show options and modifications based on the equipment you have available. Feel free to mix up the mode you use for a basic exercise to challenge your body and increase your resistance or effort. Sometimes it is the little changes you make to an exercise that lead to the biggest progress.

AT HOME: You really have everything you need to get started. There are dozens of exercises that use your own bodyweight against gravity to increase your muscular endurance and strength. That being said, you can always add a few pieces of equipment to your home gym as you progress. Items you might consider include bands or tubing, a stability ball, medicine balls, suspension training systems, kettlebells, etc. These all store easily and most travel well. Each of these is simply one of many tools available to help you create a resistance to overcome. Training with different exercises and different exercise equipment allows you the opportunity to challenge your body with dynamic or functional exercises that mimic your movements in your activities of daily living (ADL) or your sport by introducing a fresh stimulus for physiological adaptation. For example, training with a medicine ball helps to develop total body power, muscular endurance, and flexibility. Bands can provide exercise options for beginning to advanced exercisers and athletes, an effective yet inexpensive way for your entire family to incorporate resistance training into their weekly routine. Stability balls can be used for everything from improving core stability, static and dynamic balance, strength, and flexibility and can enhance functional and sport performance. You can do an entire workout with a stability ball or use one as part of a well-rounded exercise program for greater variety and effective progression in your resistance-training program.

Resistance-Training Warm-Up and Cool-Down

A resistance-training warm-up and cool-down should include light cardiorespiratory exercises for 5 to10 minutes. After breaking a light sweat in your warm-up, you will want to add dynamic exercises for increasing your range of motion and maybe a bit of foam rolling. Before you begin your lifts with full weight, you should complete a few repetitions with little or no weight to ensure proper form, posture, and body alignment. After you finish your cool-down, you can hold static stretches longer for improved flexibility.

Resistance-Training Programs

If you are new to resistance training or if you have taken a lay-off of more than three months, start slowly and build gradually. Start with Program A. This will help you increase overall muscular fitness (both muscular endurance and strength) and help to keep you injury free! If you are already resistance training two days a week (full body routine), then start with Program B. Adjust intensity, volume and training days to suit your personal fitness level and schedule; visit the companion website for more options.

PROGRAM A

GOAL: Improve overall muscular fitness by performing 8 exercises twice a week.

| Frequency | Intensity | Time | | | Number & Type of Exercises |
		Reps	Sets	Rest	
2 non-consecutive days a week	60% 1RM	12	2	2 minutes between sets	8 multiple-joint exercises

Order of Exercises:

Leg Press
Heel Raises (can be performed through ankle plantar flexion while completing Leg Press)
Chest Press

Compound Row
Overhead Press
Lat Pull-Down
Abdominal Curl
Back Extension

PROGRAM B

GOAL: Continue to improve muscular fitness by performing a split resistance-training program (upper/lower) four days of the week.

| Frequency | Intensity | Time | | | Number & Type of Exercises |
		Reps	Sets	Rest	
4 days a week: Upper body M/W Lower body T/Th	70% 1RM	10	3	2.5 minutes between sets	Upper body: 7 multiple-joint exercises 1 single-joint exercise Lower body: 4 multiple-joint exercises 3 single-joint exercises

M/W Upper Body Order of Exercises:

Chest Press
Row
Chest Fly
Overhead Press
Lat Pull-Down
Upright Row
Biceps Curl
Triceps Extension

T/Th Lower Body Order of Exercises:

Squat
Lunge
Leg Extension
Leg Curl
Heel Raise
Abdominal Curl
Oblique Curl
Back Extension

MOTIVATE!

Create your own exercise log to track your resistance-training program—make note of days, actual exercises, sets, reps, load amounts, and rest intervals—or use the log available through the companion website. Here are a few other tips to keep you training strong.

ADJUST YOUR TRAINING ROUTINE: Boredom is a motivation killer. Regular changes to your training exercises, incorporating different equipment, and changing your training location from time to time are all ways to keep you engaged and ready for a new challenge.

MOTIVATION THROUGH MEDIA: Listen to music or podcasts during your rest intervals. In your downtime, try reading articles, blogs, or books about fitness, resistance training, healthy lifestyles, or your favorite sport. This helps to keep you interested and engaged to reach your goals.

STAY POSITIVE: Turn around your negative thoughts and self-talk and low energy days by surrounding yourself with positive affirmations and training partners. Stay focused and remember your goals. Take a moment to acknowledge how much you have already accomplished.

JOIN A FITNESS MESSAGE BOARD: Check out the message boards of fitness websites for inspiration from others who have accomplished their goals or who are working toward exercise goals similar to yours. Most message boards are designed to foster encouragement, discipline, and accountability.

MAKE A HEALTH CONTRACT WITH YOUR FAMILY MEMBERS: Everyone gets one private hour every day to exercise guilt-free. This will help establish your family's goal of a happy, healthy, and active lifestyle.

ADVANCE!

Now that you have established your resistance-training program, challenge yourself. Maybe it is time to try a few new exercises or new equipment. You may want to retake the estimated 1 RM and 20 RM tests and set new goals to take your training to the next level. Remember to follow the "10 percent rule" to safely progress to a new goal: do not increase frequency, intensity, or time more than 10 percent per week. Below are two more advanced resistance-training programs. You can follow these or log onto the companion website to find more options or to personalize this program or any of the programs in this book.

PROGRAM C

GOAL: Increase muscular endurance by performing 12 exercises three days a week.

Frequency	Intensity	Time			Number & Type of Exercises
		Reps	Sets	Rest	
3 non-consecutive days a week	50% 1RM	15	3	45–60 seconds between sets	10 multiple joint and 2 single joint

Order of Exercises:

Push-Up
Assisted Pull-Up
Squat
Lunge
Chest Fly
Row

Upright Row
Overhead Press
Biceps Curl
Pullover
Plank
Side Bridge (each side)

PROGRAM D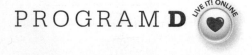

GOAL: Build muscular strength and mass by performing a high-intensity split resistance-training program (upper/lower) four days of the week.

Frequency	Intensity	Time			Number & Type of Exercises
		Reps	Sets	Rest	
4 days a week: Upper body M/W Lower body T/Th	80% 1RM	8	4	3 minutes between sets	Upper body: 7 multiple-joint exercises 1 single-joint exercise Lower body: 4 multiple-joint exercises 3 single-joint exercises

M/W Upper Body
Order of Exercises:

Chest Press
Row
Overhead Press
Lat Pull-Down
Lateral Raise
Biceps Curl
Tricep Extension
Back Extension

T/Th Lower Body
Order of Exercises:

Leg Press
Leg Extension
Leg Curl
Hip Abduction
Hip Adduction
Heel Raise
Abdominal Curl
Reverse Curl
Oblique Curl

5

Maintaining Flexibility & Back Health

Learning Outcomes

1. Articulate how regular stretching and being flexible can benefit your lifelong fitness and wellness.

 HEAR IT! ONLINE
Audio case study and audio PowerPoint lecture

2. Identify the body structures, body systems, and individual factors that will determine your joint flexibility and back health over time.

  DO IT! ONLINE
Lab 5.1 Assess Your Flexibility

3. Use safe and effective stretching exercises and techniques, reducing stretching-related injuries.

  SEE IT! ONLINE
Demonstration videos of stretching exercises

 Twist to Get Fit

4. Implement a safe and effective stretching program that will maintain or improve your flexibility.

 DO IT! ONLINE
Lab 5.3 Planning a Flexibility Program

 LIVE IT! ONLINE
Customizable 4-week starter and intermediate flexibility training programs

5. Evaluate your personal risk for the primary causes of lower-back pain.

 DO IT! ONLINE
Lab 5.2 Assess Your Posture

6. Incorporate strategies to reduce your risk for (or manage existing) lower-back pain.

 LIVE IT! ONLINE
Customizable 4-week back health exercise programs

Pre- and post-quizzes and glossary flashcards REVIEW IT! ONLINE

casestudy

MARK

"Hi, I'm Mark. I live in Colorado Springs, at the foothills of the Rocky Mountains. I love the outdoors. I've been a backpacker, fisherman, and skier my whole life. My girlfriend is a fitness instructor and has been telling me that I should really stretch more, but I'm skeptical. What's so important about stretching? Will it help me be a better hiker or skier? How do I figure out what kind of stretches I should do? And when and how often should I stretch?"

Flexibility is the ability of joints to move through a full **range of motion**. Flexibility tends to decrease as we get older,[1] so a good time to start a stretching program—if you don't stretch already—is when you are younger. Starting to stretch now will help you feel good and will increase your chances of staying flexible as you get older. A complete fitness program should include **stretching** and range-of-motion exercises to help you maintain flexibility and prevent joint problems.

Flexibility can be classified as static or dynamic. **Static (passive) flexibility** is a measure of the limits of a joint's overall range of motion. **Dynamic (active) flexibility** is a measure of overall joint stiffness during movement (i.e., with muscular contraction). Active movement such as swinging a tennis racket or leaping over a hurdle on a track requires good dynamic flexibility.

flexibility The ability of a joint (or joints) to move through a full range of motion

range of motion The movement limits of a specific joint or group of joints

stretching Exercises designed to improve or maintain flexibility

static (passive) flexibility A joint's range-of-motion limits with an external force applied

dynamic (active) flexibility A joint's range-of-motion limits with muscular contraction applied

In this chapter, we will cover how maintaining your flexibility can improve your mobility, keep your joints healthy, and help you relax. We will discuss the factors that determine how flexible a person is, present strategies for stretching safely and effectively, and provide guidelines for developing a personalized stretching program. We will also discuss the common problem of lower-back pain and offer strategies for incorporating a back-health component into your regular fitness plan.

What Are the Benefits of Stretching and Flexibility?

Like Mark, many people are not in the habit of stretching and are not sure why stretching is important. There are many benefits to stretching, but the most compelling is simple: Being flexible will help you move freely and complete activities you want to do with greater ease.

Improved Mobility, Posture, and Balance

A regular stretching program helps you maintain joint mobility throughout your body. Your joints allow you to *move*—whether you are bending your knees to tie a shoelace, riding a bicycle around campus, or reaching for a bowl on the top shelf of a cupboard. A reduction in your flexibility can result in a reduction in your ability to move about freely as you perform daily activities. Likewise, an improvement in your flexibility can result in greater freedom of movement. Keeping your body flexible and strong also helps you maintain your balance. Individals who have better ankle strength and range of motion not only have better balance, but also a greater functional ability—which means fewer falls and injuries.[2]

Regular stretching can also help you maintain a balance of muscle strength and muscle flexibility, which is important for proper joint alignment and posture. For example, if the muscles on the front of your hips get too tight, your pelvis can get pulled forward and cause a larger sway in your lower back. This will alter your posture and could even affect your balance. Good flexibility, developed through stretching, helps you keep your joints and spine aligned and promotes overall body stability.

Healthy Joints and Pain Management

As many as 28 percent of all adults report pain or stiffness in joints. That number increases dramatically with age, and women are more likely to have those joint symptoms. Many adults also have or will develop **arthritis** at some point in their lives; 54 percent of people 75 years and older have been diagnosed with arthritis.[3] Regular exercise, including range-of-motion and flexibility exercises, is essential for people with arthritis to maintain function and manage joint pain.[4] Even in people without arthritis, stretching will increase joint flexibility, improve joint function, and decrease periodic joint pain.[5]

Possible Reduction of Future Lower-Back Pain

Having an adequate level of flexibility may reduce your risk of lower-back pain in the future; however, research on the subject is inconclusive. While poor flexibility has been linked to lower-back pain in adolescents, these relationships are less clear in adults.[6,7,8,9] Despite the mixed evidence, most experts agree that having a minimal level of joint mobility and flexibility through the hips and back is one of the strategies for reducing the risk of developing chronic lower-back pain.[10] We will discuss lower-back pain in more detail later in this chapter.

Muscle Relaxation and Stress Relief

After sitting at a computer for hours working on a term paper, doesn't it feel great to stand up and stretch? Staying in one position for too long, repetitive movement, and other stressors can result in stiff and "knotted" muscles. Gentle stretching and relaxation increases blood flow to tight muscles, stimulates the nervous system to decrease stress hormones, and ultimately helps relax areas of tension in your body.

What Determines My Flexibility?

What makes one person a human pretzel, while others can barely touch their toes? Is flexibility genetic, or can it be attributed entirely to the amount of stretching that you do? Many factors can affect your individual level of flexibility. Your joints, muscles, **tendons**, and nervous system—along with other characteristics such as age, gender, genetics, and activity level—can all influence your flexibility.

arthritis An umbrella-term for more than 100 conditions characterized by inflammation of a joint

tendons Connective tissues that attach muscle to bone

joint The articulation or point of contact between two or more bones

Joint Structures, Muscles and Tendons, and the Nervous System

The range of motion possible in a particular **joint** is limited by the structures that comprise that joint, the muscles and tendons that cross over the joint, and the nervous system.

Joint Structures The individual components of a joint all affect the joint's mobility and stability (Figure 5.1). *Cartilage* is a strong, smooth tissue that cushions the ends of the bones, preventing them from rubbing directly against one another and providing impact protection. *Ligaments* are fibrous connective tissues that connect bone to bone. Some ligaments form the outer layer of the *joint capsule* to provide a reinforcing structure to the overall joint. Other ligaments, not part of the joint capsule, provide further stability to the joint. The *synovial membrane* forms the inner layer of the joint capsule and secretes *synovial fluid* into the *joint cavity*. Synovial fluid

FIGURE **5.1** Joints are surrounded by a supportive joint capsule made of ligaments and synovial membranes. The joint cavity is filled with synovial fluid that (along with cartilage and bursa sacs) cushions and protects bones during movement. The stability of a joint is strengthened by muscle-tendon insertions surrounding the joint.

lubricates and protects the joint. *Bursae (singular, bursa)* are small fluid-filled sacs that lubricate the movement of muscles over one another or muscles over bone.

Muscles and Tendons Overall joint structure accounts for 47 percent of the resistance to movement around a joint (dynamic flexibility), while individual *soft tissues* (muscles, connective tissue, ligaments, tendons, and skin) account for 53 percent of the resistance to movement.[11] With regular activity and stretching, connective tissues within muscles remain supple and able to easily lengthen. With disuse and age, connective tissues become stiffer, limiting flexibility. Temperature can also affect the flexibility of soft tissues. When muscle temperature rises, connective tissues become softer and allow muscles to more easily lengthen.

The Nervous System Your nervous system is responsible for stimulating muscle contractions, and it also triggers muscle relaxation. Muscles and tendons contain nervous-system receptors that interpret information about the tension and length of muscles at any given moment. These receptors protect the muscle from damage caused by excessive amounts of tension or by stretching too far. If there is too much tension or force within a muscle, receptors in the tendon (called **golgi tendon organs**) will trigger your muscle to relax.

If your muscle is stretching too far, receptors in the muscle fibers (called **stretch receptors** or **muscle spindles**) will trigger your muscle to contract. This reflexive contraction is called the **stretch reflex**. Have you ever had a doctor tap your knee and watch your leg kick out in response? The doctor was striking your *patellar tendon*. This rapidly stretches your quadriceps muscle, which triggers stretch receptors in the quadriceps to signal your nervous system. Your leg then kicks out because of a reflex contraction of your quadriceps muscle stimulated by the nervous system.

Reducing the stretch reflex

golgi tendon organs Muscle tension receptors located in tendons that are responsible for triggering muscle relaxation to relieve excessive muscle tension

stretch receptors (muscle spindles) Muscle length receptors located within muscle fibers that trigger muscle contractions in response to rapid, excessive muscle lengthening

stretch reflex The reflex contraction of a muscle triggered by stretch receptors (muscle spindles) in response to a rapid overextension of that muscle

and activating the golgi tendon organs allows your muscles to relax, elongate, and gain improvements in flexibility.

Individual Factors

Beyond the anatomical structures and physiological mechanisms that we all share, individual factors such as genetics, gender, age, body type, and activity level also affect flexibility.

Genetics Most people have a moderate level of flexibility. They have flexible and less-flexible areas of their bodies and need to work to maintain their present level of flexibility. However, some people are extremely flexible by nature, while others are exceptionally inflexible. Genetic differences in body structure and the elasticity of soft tissues help account for the wide variety of flexibility levels.

Gender Although it is widely assumed that females are more flexible than males, this may only be true for specific joints, as discussed in the box Men, Women, and Flexibility.

Age Flexibility changes throughout the lifespan. Flexible preschool children experience a decrease in joint range of motion until the preteen years, when flexibility increases again to its peak by 18 years of age.[12] In adulthood, flexibility decreases with age due to physical changes in muscles, joints, and connective tissues. These changes are joint specific and are primarily related to inactivity and disuse.

The good news is that with regular exercise, people of all ages can improve their current level of flexibility. In a study of men over 65 years of age, researchers observed flexibility improvements when the men participated in a regular resistance-training program.[13] These improvements disappeared when the men stopped training, reinforcing the notion that regular and sustained exercise is the key to maintaining and improving flexibility.

Body Type Body type can affect flexibility but typically only at the extremes of body shape and size. For example, body type may affect range of motion if an excessive amount of muscle or fat physically interferes with full joint movement. That said, genetics and training are far more influential factors in determining flexibility than is body type. There are people with long, lean bodies whom you might expect to be flexible but who actually are not due to genetics or inactivity.

DIVERSITY

Men, Women, and Flexibility

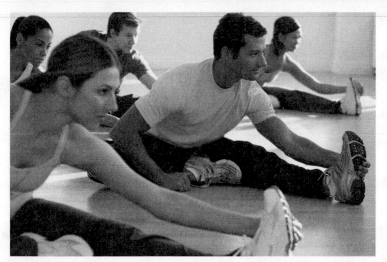

Women are more flexible than men, right? Not necessarily! This commonly held belief is not always true and may lull men into thinking that being inflexible is normal and okay. Women generally *are* more flexible in the hip joint and hamstrings, which are the most common sites for flexibility testing.[1] Women may have greater flexibility in these areas than males due to their wider hips, hormonal influences, and

tendency to participate in activities that develop greater flexibility. In other joints and areas of the body, however, there is not a large difference between males and females. In fact, males may have greater flexibility in other areas. For example, males may have greater trunk rotation capabilities.[2]

Interestingly, greater joint range of motion and flexibility may increase the chances of injury. Because women tend to have greater hip flexibility and internal rotation of the hip joint, they are more likely to have knee problems.[3] The bottom line is that adequate range of motion should be a goal for everyone, men and women. Being able to move your body without restriction opens up activity options and makes life easier!

Sources:
1. J. T. Manire and others, "Diurnal Variation of Hamstring and Lumbar Flexibility," *Journal of Strength and Conditioning Research* 24, no. 6 (2010): 1464–71.
2. J. T. Blackburn and others, "Sex Comparison of Hamstring Structural and Material Properties," *Clinical Biomechanics* 24, no. 1 (2009): 65–70.
3. R. H. Brophy and others, "The Core and Hip in Soccer Athletes Compared by Gender," *International Journal of Sports Medicine* 30, no. 9 (2009): 663–7.

Meanwhile, there are people with stocky, muscular builds who are exceptionally flexible, including many gymnasts.

Activity Level Inactivity can result in low levels of flexibility as muscles and connective tissues tighten and shorten with disuse. Overly repetitive physical activity can also result in muscle "stiffness." However, when done properly, stretching and regular physical activity can improve flexibility. We will introduce effective stretches and exercises later in this chapter.

Health Status Certain medical conditions can affect your joint health and range of motion. Diseases that affect your **collagen** and connective tissues can produce overly mobile or exceptionally inflexible joints. For example, arthritis speeds up the destruction of collagen and cartilage, leading to joint inflexibilty. In some genetic syndromes, reduced or ineffective collagen causes hypermobility. During pregnancy, many women will experience more flexible joints. Injuries or scar tissue can also affect your ability to move your

joints through their full range of motion.

collagen The primary protein of connective tissues throughout the body

casestudy

MARK

"I've heard that physical activity is supposed to improve your flexibility. If that's true, why do my muscles feel really stiff after a long day of skiing or hiking? I've noticed that this happens especially when I've gone for my first ski or hike of the season. Are my muscles just out of shape?"

THINK! What might explain Mark's muscle stiffness?

ACT! Make a list of at least five different factors that might play a role in Mark's flexibility.

How Can I Assess My Flexibility?

Flexibility levels vary from joint to joint. As a result, most flexibility tests are designed to measure the flexibility of specific muscles and joints, not to measure your body's overall level of flexibility. However, if you take a variety of flexibility tests, you can get a sense of how your body's overall level of mobility is measuring up to recommended target ranges.

Perform the "Sit-and-Reach" Test

One of the most common measures of flexibility is the "sit-and-reach" test. This test measures the flexibility of your lower back, hip, and hamstring muscles. These areas are often tight in individuals who are inactive. This muscular imbalance can negatively influence posture, balance, and risk of back pain. **Lab 5.1** provides instructions for the sit-and-reach test.

Perform Range-of-Motion Tests

Having an adequate range of motion in your joints and maintaining that range over time should be the primary goal of a flexibility fitness program. Lab 5.1 provides instructions for performing range-of-motion tests on joints located in your neck, shoulders, trunk, hips, and ankles. By performing these tests, you can evaluate how the range of motion of your joints compares to those of the general population and determine whether your joints are more flexible or less flexible than average. This information will help you design a personalized program for developing flexibility. You can measure your progress over time by retaking the tests after months of training.

How Can I Plan a Good Stretching Program?

Regardless of whether you already stretch regularly, keep in mind the following guidelines to ensure a safe and effective program.

Set Appropriate Flexibility Goals

Decide up front what your goal is. Do you want to *maintain* your current level of flexibility (which is all that many people want to do), or do you want to *improve* your flexibility? Complete the sit-and-reach test and the range-of-motion tests described in Lab 5.1 before making this decision.

Once you've decided on your overall goal, follow the SMART guidelines for setting more specific goals. Recall that SMART stands for *specific*, *measurable*, *action-oriented*, *realistic*, and *time-oriented*. An example of a SMART goal designed to *maintain* your flexibility is, "My goal for the next year is to maintain the joint flexibility and range-of-motion levels recorded on my flexibility assessments by incorporating stretching into my workouts at least four times per week." An example of a SMART goal designed to *improve* your flexibility is, "My goal is to regularly stretch so that I can increase my lower-back, hip, and hamstring flexibility from 'poor' to 'good' on the sit-and-reach test by the end of the school semester." For most people, the primary goal should be the ability to move their joints through a normal range of motion. Achieving exceptionally high levels of flexibility may be desirable for some sports and activities but is not necessary for the average person.

Apply the FITT Program Design Principles

Recall that FITT stands for frequency, intensity, time, and type. Use the FITT principles to design your own personalized stretching program. Table 5.1 provides general guidelines from the American College of Sports Medicine. Refer to this table as a starting point for designing your own program.

Frequency Notice that the ACSM guidelines in Table 5.1 recommend stretching at least 2 to 3 days per week. If you've determined that your current level of flexibility is already within "normal" ranges and you

TABLE **5.1** ACSM's Flexibility Training Guidelines for Healthy Adults	
Frequency	2–3 days/week minimum
Intensity	Stretch to the point of feeling tightness or slight discomfort
Time	10–30 seconds per static stretch repetition 2–4 repetitions of each stretching exercise
Type	Static, dynamic, or PNF stretching of all major muscle groups*

*Ballistic stretching may be appropriate for some individuals in certain sports and recreational activities.

Source: C. E. Garner and others, "American College of Sports Medicine Position Stand: Quantity and Quality of Exercise for Developing and Maintaining Cardiorespiratory, Musculoskeletal, and Neuromotor Fitness in Apparently Healthy Adults: Guidance for Prescribing Exercise," *Medicine and Science in Sports and Exercise* 43, no. 7 (2011): 1334–59.

When Should I Stretch?

Many people incorrectly think that they have to stretch before a workout. In general, it is actually better to perform most of your static stretching *after* a workout, when your muscles are warm and your joint structures are more receptive to stretching.

For *most* individuals, light pre-exercise static stretches will not negatively affect exercise or recreational performance. If you are an athlete, though, you may want to avoid too much static stretching before a competition or high-intensity workout. Some studies have shown that extensive static stretching can result in a reduction in muscle strength and power that lasts 30 minutes or more.[1] The implications of this research are still unknown: A more recent study showed that stretching did not alter the 1 repetition maximum bench press performance in collegiate male athletes.[2]

It is also now generally accepted that pre-exercise stretching does not reduce over-use injuries.[3] This is a surprise to many people, but it doesn't mean that you have to give up your warm-up stretches. If you warm up properly first, you can stretch at any time of day and improve your flexibility.[4] More research must be done, but the recommendations now include stretching for maintaining joint mobility, but not as a primary means to reduce injury or enhance performance.

Key points:

- If you perform static stretches, stick to *light* static stretching (10 to 15 seconds)

- If you want to stretch before a workout, be sure to warm up beforehand. Stretching cold muscles can result in injury.

- Emphasize dynamic stretches in your warm-up and make sure the movements are similar to your exercise, sport, or recreational activity.

Sources:
1. T. Yamaguchi and K. Ishii, "Effects of Static Stretching for 30 Seconds and Dynamic Stretching on Leg Extension Power," *Journal of Strength and Conditioning Research* 19, no. 3 (2005): 677–83.
2. Z.D. Molacek, D. S. Conley, T. K. Evetovich, and K. R. Hinnerichs, "Effects of Low- and High-Volume Stretching on Bench Press Performance in Collegiate Football Players," *Journal of Strength and Conditioning Research* 24, no. 3 (2010): 711–16.
3. M. P. McHugh and C. H. Cosgrave, "To Stretch or Not to Stretch: the Role of Stretching in Injury Prevention and Performance," *Scandinavian Journal of Medicine & Science in Sports* 20, no. 2 (2010): 169–81.
4. G. G. Haff (ed.), "Round Table Discussion: Flexibility Training," *Strength and Conditioning Journal* 28, no. 2 (2006): 64–85.

merely want to maintain that level, you should stretch two days per week. If you've determined that your current level of flexibility needs improvement to reach a "normal" range, you should stretch three or more days per week. Should you stretch before a workout, after a workout, or both? The box When Should I Stretch? explores these questions and others.

Intensity The ACSM guidelines (see Table 5.1) state that you should stretch "to the point of feeling tightness or slight discomfort." If you are feeling pain, you are stretching too far and risking injury. Pay close attention to your body whenever you stretch; your flexibility level may vary slightly from day to day.

Time The ACSM guidelines state that you should perform your stretching program for at least 10 minutes at a time. In that time, stretch all major muscle groups, hold stretches for 10 to 30 seconds each, and repeat stretches two to four times. As soon as you start to stretch, your stretch reflex will activate: You can feel this as a slight increase in muscle tension when you move into a stretch position. By holding your stretches for at least 10 seconds, you are giving the stretch reflex time to lessen. You are also giving your golgi tendon organs time to activate and, thus, allow your muscles to lengthen farther.

By repeating stretches multiple times, you enable your muscles to relax and lengthen a little bit more each time. If you are beginning a stretching program for the first time and feel uncomfortable with multiple repetitions, you can perform one repetition of each stretch and still obtain benefits. After a few weeks of stretching consistently, gradually increase the number of repetitions to the recommended two to four times per session. Aim to have your total stretching time for each exercise add up to sixty seconds.

Type There are numerous kinds of stretching techniques. The most common are highlighted below.

- **Static stretching** involves moving slowly into a stretch and holding it for a prescribed amount of time. This is the simplest and safest method for individuals who are just starting a stretching program. Static stretching is effective, because the activity of slow stretching and holding reduces the activation of stretch receptors. After a workout, static stretching can help muscles recover and help you to maintain or improve your flexibility.

- **Dynamic stretching** involves stretching through movement. During dynamic stretching, you mimic the motions of your workout or

sports activity with slow, fluid movements. Dynamic stretching increases dynamic flexibility and can enhance muscle action during sports and recreational activities.[14] The warm-up phase of an exercise session is a good time to implement dynamic stretching, because it helps prepare the body for the more intense physical activity to come.

- **Ballistic stretching** is a stretching method characterized by bouncing, sometimes jerky, movements and high momentum. Ballistic stretching increases dynamic flexibility and can benefit trained athletes in sports requiring fast, explosive movements such as wrestling, gymnastics, tennis, and basketball. However, the bouncing movements in ballistic stretching rapidly activate the stretch receptors, making this method less effective at increasing static flexibility.

- **Proprioceptive neuromuscular facilitation (PNF)** uses the voluntary contraction of muscle

static stretching Stretching characterized by slow and sustained muscle lengthening

dynamic stretching Stretching characterized by controlled, full-range-of-motion movements that mimic exercise session movements

ballistic stretching Stretching characterized by bouncing, jerky movements and momentum to increase range of motion

proprioceptive neuromuscular facilitation (PNF) Stretching that is facilitated or enhanced by the voluntary contraction of the targeted muscle group or contraction of opposing muscles

casestudy

MARK

"The ski season just started. Out of curiosity, I asked a ski instructor for his opinions on stretching. He was surprised that I have been skiing my whole life but wasn't in the habit of stretching! He explained how stretching can help reduce muscle tension, improve my ability to make quick turns, and help prevent strains and stiffness. He recommended quadriceps and hamstrings stretches, for starters. He also suggested some stretching exercises that mimic the motion of skiing, in case I ever wanted to try skiing at a more advanced level."

THINK! Look at the quadriceps and hamstrings stretches in Figure 5.3. Are these static or dynamic stretches? What is the difference?

ACT! Assume that Mark wants to begin a general stretching program in the "off" season when he is not skiing, with the goal of improving his flexibility. Given the ACSM guidelines you have learned, write out a basic flexibility program for him.

HEAR IT! ONLINE

groups to help facilitate relaxation and stretching in target muscles. The most common method of PNF stretching is called *contract-relax PNF.* In contract-relax PNF, the exerciser experiences an isotonic or isometric contraction of the target muscle just prior to slow, passive stretching of that muscle. An example of contract-relax PNF in action is shown in Figure 5.2.

Table 5.2 lists some of the pros and cons of each stretching method. For most people starting a flexibility program on their own, static stretches are the safest option. Figure 5.3 illustrates some common stretching exercises you can select from, and Activate, Motivate, & Advance Your Fitness: A Flexibility Training Program located at the end of the chapter (page 210) offers options for sequencing and combining stretches. **Lab 5.3** walks you through the process of designing your own program.

(a) Lie on your back with one leg bent and the other extended toward the ceiling. Have a partner hold your lifted leg as you try to press your leg to the ground for 6 seconds. Your partner can resist enough to allow no movement at all (isometric contraction) or just enough to allow gradual movement toward the ground (isotonic contraction). The contraction stimulates the golgi tendon organs to activate and promote muscle relaxation.

(b) Immediately following the 6-second contraction, relax your muscles and have your partner move your leg up and toward your chest into a passive stretch for the hips, hamstrings, and low back. Hold this stretch for 10–30 seconds and release.

FIGURE **5.2** An example of a contract-relax proprioceptive neuromuscular facilitation (PNF) partner exercise.

TABLE 5.2 Pros and Cons of Common Stretching Methods		
Stretching Method	Pro	Con
Static	Safe, simple to use, effective at increasing static flexibility	Can reduce muscle strength and power immediately after stretching, can be time consuming
Dynamic	Increases dynamic flexibility, functional movements	Takes time to learn correct movement patterns
Ballistic	Can be beneficial for ballistic sports, increases dynamic flexibility	Not as effective at increasing overall flexibility
PNF	Effective at increasing flexibility levels	Need a partner or equipment to perform, complicated method

FIGURE **5.3**

STRETCHES TO MAINTAIN OR INCREASE FLEXIBILITY

All standing stretches should be started or performed from a good posture position (abs pulled in, feet facing forward, knees slightly bent). All one-arm or one-leg stretches should be performed on both sides.

Hold stretches for 10 to 30 seconds. (Refer to Figure 4.8 on page 132 for the full-body muscle diagram.)

Videos for these exercises and more are available online at www.pearsonhighered.com/hopson and on MyFitnessLab.

Upper-Body Stretches

1. Neck Stretches

(a) Head turn: Gently turn your head to look over one shoulder, keeping both of your shoulders down.

(b) Head tilt: Keeping your chin level and your shoulders down, tilt your head to one side.

(a)   (b)

Muscles targeted:

10 Trapezius

2. Pectoral and Biceps Stretch

Stand arm's length away from a wall. Reach your arm out to the side and place your palm flat on the wall. Turn your body away from the wall until you feel a comfortable stretch.

Muscles targeted:

1 Pectoralis major
2 Biceps brachii

3. Upper-Back Stretch

Reach your arms out in front of you and clasp your hands while rounding out your back and lowering your head.

Muscles targeted:

10 Trapezius   **11** Rhomboids
14 Latissimus dorsi

4. Side Stretch

SEE IT! ONLINE

Reach one straight arm over your head and bend sideways at the waist. Focus on reaching up and over with your arm. The opposite hand can reach for the floor or be placed at your hip.

Muscles targeted:

14 Latissimus dorsi   **4** External obliques

5. Shoulder Stretch

SEE IT! ONLINE

Reach one arm across the chest and hold it above or below the elbow with the other hand. Keep both shoulders pressed down.

Muscles targeted:

9 Deltoids

6. Triceps Stretch

SEE IT! ONLINE

Lift your arm overhead, reaching the elbow toward the ceiling and the hand down the back. Assist the stretch by using your other hand to either **(a)** press the arm back from the front or **(b)** reach over your head, grasp your arm just below the elbow, and pull back and toward your head.

(a)   **(b)**

Muscles targeted:

13 Triceps brachii

Lower-Body Stretches

7. Low-Back Knee-to-Chest Stretch

Lie on your back on a mat and lift either **(a)** one knee or **(b)** two knees toward the chest, grasping the leg(s) from behind for support.

(a)

(b)

Muscles targeted:

12 Erector spinae

8. Torso Twist and Hip Stretch

(a) Seated twist: Sit on a mat with your legs straight out in front of you. Bend one knee and cross that leg over your other leg. Turn your body toward the bent knee and twist your body to look behind you. Place the opposite arm on the bent leg to gently press into the stretch further.

(b) Lying cross-leg twist: While lying on your back, bend the knee and hip of one leg to 90 degrees. Keep the other leg straight and slowly move the bent leg across your body toward the floor. Keep your arms wide for balance and both shoulders down.

(a)

(b)

Muscles targeted:

12 Erector spinae

4 External obliques

5 Tensor fasciae latae

15 Gluteus maximus

9. Gluteal Stretch

Lie on your back with one leg bent and the foot on the floor. Place the ankle of the other leg on your thigh just below the knee. Lift both legs toward the chest and support them with your hands clasped behind your thigh.

Muscles targeted:

15 Gluteus maximus

10. Hip Flexor Stretch

SEE IT! ONLINE

(a) Standing stretch: Stand tall with one foot forward and one foot back in a lunge position. Lift up the heel of the back leg and press your hips forward.

(b) Low-lunge stretch: Lunge forward and gently place your back knee on a mat and release your foot to point back. Lean forward into the hip and thigh stretch but make sure that your front ankle is directly under your front knee.

(a)　　　　　　(b)

Muscles targeted:

7 Quadriceps

---

11. Inner-Thigh Stretch

SEE IT! ONLINE

(a) Side lunge stretch: With a wide stance, shift your weight over onto one leg, bending that knee. Press your hips back to ensure that your bent knee does not extend beyond your ankle. Place your hands on your thigh, and keep your chest lifted and back straight.

(b) Butterfly stretch: Sitting on a mat, bring the bottoms of your feet together and pull your feet gently toward you. Actively contract your hip muscles to lower your knees closer to the ground. A slight lean forward will stretch the gluteal and low-back muscles as well.

(a)　　　　　　(b)

Muscles targeted:

6 Adductors

---

12. Outer-Thigh Stretch

SEE IT! ONLINE

Stand arm's length next to a wall. Place your outside foot on the floor closer to the wall, crossing over the inside leg. Lean your hip closer to the wall while you lean your upper body away from the wall for balance.

Muscles targeted:

5 Tensor fasciae latae

13. Quadriceps Stretch

SEE IT! ONLINE

Grab your foot from behind and pull it back toward your rear until you feel a stretch in the front of your thighs. Maintain straight body alignment and keep your thighs parallel to one another. When **(a)** standing, assist your balance by holding a wall, a chair, or another form of support. The stretch can also be done from a **(b)** lying down position.

(a)

(b)

Muscles targeted:

7 Quadriceps

14. Hamstrings Stretch

SEE IT! ONLINE

(a) Modified hurdler stretch: Sit with one leg extended and the other leg bent. The bent leg should have the knee facing sideways and the foot placed next to the extended leg near the calf, knee, or thigh. Keeping your back as straight as possible, lean your body forward, moving your chest closer to your extended leg. Your hands can be placed on the floor next to your knee, calf, or ankle for support.

(b) Supine lying: Lying on your back, bend one knee and extend the other toward the ceiling. Support the stretch by placing your hands or a towel above or below the knee. As you become more flexible, work at bringing your leg closer to your chest.

(a)

(b)

Muscles targeted:

16 Hamstrings

15. Calf Stretches

(a) Gastrocnemius lunge: Lean into a wall in a lunge position, extending one leg straight behind you. Press the heel of your straight leg into the floor as you lean your body and hips into the wall.

(b) Gastrocnemius heel drop: Stand tall and place your toes on a raised surface (mat or step) that will not tip over. Balance by holding on to a wall for support as you lower your heels toward the floor.

(c) Soleus stretch: Starting in a lunge position (a), bend the back knee until you feel a stretch in the soleus muscle.

Muscles targeted:

17 Gastrocnemius   **18** Soleus

(a) (b) (c)

16. Shin Stretch

Reach one leg behind you and place the tips of your toes on the ground. Bend both knees and lower the body slightly as you press the top of your back foot toward the ground. You can use a wall for support if needed.

Muscles targeted:

8 Tibialis anterior

Can I Become Flexible without Stretching?

If a regular stretching routine doesn't appeal to you, try one of these classes to help you reach your flexibility goals:

Yoga originated in India about 5,000 years ago and has become a popular activity in the United States. The forms of yoga most commonly practiced in the United States today require a combination of mental focus and physical effort while performing a variety of postures, or *asanas*. The physical aspect of yoga results in improvements in flexibility, posture, agility, balance, stamina, muscle endurance, and coordination. The mental aspect of yoga promotes attention, controlled breathing, relaxation, a union of mind and body, and an overall psychological sense of well-being.

Tai chi is a martial art that was developed in ancient China by monks wanting to defend themselves. Tai chi practice involves a slow-moving, smooth, and continuous series of positions or forms. These exercises increase balance, muscle endurance, flexibility, and coordination; they also reduce anxiety and stress.[1] Tai chi has become popular with many people, but older individuals in particular are drawn to this safe and effective way to exercise. There are other forms of martial arts that will develop flexibility, as well. You may want to look into classes for one of these popular martial arts: capoeira, karate, jujitsu, or tae kwon do.

Pilates was developed by Joseph Pilates in New York City in the 1920s. Pilates involves performing a sequence of exercises on a mat or specialized equipment designed to stretch and strengthen muscles. Specific breathing patterns are combined with stretching and resistance exercises to increase flexibility and muscle endurance, particularly in the core trunk-supporting muscles.

Dance is a fantastic and fun way to improve your flexibility and your overall fitness level. A group exercise class, such as aerobic dance, will usually give you a chance to work on your flexibility during the cool-down phase.

All of the activities described above require instruction by a trained professional, especially since some exercises can be risky for the untrained or novice participant.

Source:
1. C. Lan, S. Y. Chen, and J. S. Lai, "Changes of Aerobic Capacity, Fat Ratio, and Flexibility in Older TCC Practitioners: A Five-year Follow-up," *American Journal of Chinese Medicine* 36, no. 6 (2008): 1041–50; H. Liu and A. Frank, "Tai Chi as a Balance Improvement Exercise for Older Adults: a Systematic Review," *Journal of Geriatric Physical Therapy* 33, no. 3 (2010): 103–9.

Consider Taking a Class

LIVE IT! ONLINE

Twist to Get Fit

If you would like more structure and instruction in your stretching program, consider enrolling in a class. Yoga, tai chi, Pilates, dance, and martial arts classes can be fun, effective ways to maintain or improve your flexibility. For more information on these types of classes, see the box Can I Become Flexible without Stretching?. You may have heard of whole-body vibration or seen one of these machines in your college's gym. The box What Is Whole Body Vibration? gives more information about these machines.

What Is Whole Body Vibration?

In the 1960s, scientists who were looking for a way to help astronauts maintain or increase muscle and bone mass while in space started using whole body vibration (WBV) platforms as a solution. A motor under the whole body vibration platform transmits vibrations to the person using the platform. The vibrations occur quickly in one or more directions and stimulate muscle fiber contractions. The platforms are becoming more common in workout centers, and it makes sense: there is quite a bit of evidence to support the use of these vibration platforms for increased flexibility and muscle action. The evidence seems to be consistent for flexibility gains,[1] even over some of the other benefits such as bone density and muscle strength. Stretching during vibration on a WBV platform appears to be a good adjunct to static stretching and may help you retain the flexibility you gain.[2]

The down side with these machines is that they are expensive and they take up space. Given their cost, they probably aren't worth the investment for most people. If your gym has a WBV platform, talk with a fitness instructor or personal trainer about designing a program for you. Standing or lying muscle fitness exercises can be performed on the platform. Time on the platform should amount to 20 to 30 minutes a day, but work your way up to this. Use the platform a few times per week or every day to increase range of motion, muscle fitness, and bone density. If your gym doesn't have one, don't worry: just focus on incorporating well-balanced flexibility and muscle fitness routines into your schedule.

Sources:

1. D. G. Dolny and G. F. Reyes, "Whole Body Vibration Exercise: Training and Benefits," Current Sports Medicine Reports 7, no. 3 (2008): 152–7; R. Di Giminiani and others, "Effects of Individualized Whole-Body Vibration on Muscle Flexibility and Mechanical Power," Journal of Sports Medicine Physical Fitness 50, no. 2 (2010): 139–51; F. Fagnani and others, "The Effects of a Whole-Body Vibration Program on Muscle Performance and Flexibility in Female Athletes," American Journal of Physical Medicine and Rehabilitation 85, no. 12 (2006): 956–62.
2. J. B. Feland and others, "Whole Body Vibration as an Adjunct to Static Stretching," International Journal of Sports Medicine 31, no. 8 (2010): 584–9.

How Can I Avoid Stretching-Related Injuries?

We used to think of stretching as a way to avoid injury, but we now know that stretching can actually *cause* injury if done improperly. To avoid a stretching-related injury, adhere to the following guidelines.

Stretch Only Warm Muscles

An increase in body temperature prepares the joint fluid and structures for stretching and improves muscle elasticity. These changes allow you a greater range of motion while stretching. Static stretches, in particular, should be performed *after* a workout, when the muscles have been sufficiently warmed up.

Perform Stretches Safely

One of the keys to safe and effective stretching is to avoid activating stretch receptors when you want a muscle to relax. Stretch receptors are activated when muscles are lengthened rapidly. Muscle injury can occur from quick, bouncing movements, because the muscle is lengthening too far too quickly and the stretch reflex is creating tension at the same time. Avoid the stretch reflex by stretching carefully and slowly. Holding your stretches for at least 15 seconds will allow the stretch receptors and golgi tendon organs to make nervous system adjustments. These adjustments will allow further relaxation and lengthening of the muscles involved.

Know Which Exercises Can Cause Injury

Figure 5.4 shows common high-risk or **contraindicated** stretches with safer alternatives. Note that this figure

contraindicated Not recommended

Higher risk exercises:

Full neck circles

Yoga plough/plow

Unsupported forward flexion

Double leg lifts

Hurdler's stretch

Deep knee bends

Alternative exercises:

Head tilt and head turn (Figure 5.3 Exercise 1)

Low-back knee-to-chest stretch (Figure 5.3 Exercise 7)

Hamstring stretch (Figure 5.3 Exercise 14)

Reverse curl (Figure 4.9 Exercise 24)

Quadriceps stretch (Figure 5.3 Exercise 13)

Squat (Figure 4.9 Exercise 1)

Cervical neck

Problem: Hyperextension or extreme flexion of the neck that puts pressure on the cervical vertebrae, discs, and other supporting structures.

Avoid: Tipping your head too far back, making full circles with your head, and bending your head forward under tension.

Lumbar spine

Problem: Hyperextension or flexion of the low back that puts pressure on the lumbar vertebrae, discs, and other hip and back supporting structures.

Avoid: Back positions where your muscle strength and endurance is questionable and any positions where you feel pain.

Knee joint

Problem: Extreme flexion of the knee that puts pressure on the joint and other supporting structures.

Avoid: Bending the knees too far under weight or pressure.

FIGURE **5.4** Choose safer alternatives to these common higher-risk exercises and stretches. Take into account your personal goals, experience, and limitations.

is *not* an all-inclusive list. Choosing safe exercises is a highly individual process. Consider your personal limitations and health issues when deciding which exercises are best for your body.

Be Especially Cautious If You Are a Hyperflexible or Inflexible Person

If you are really flexible, you may need to be more careful while stretching than the average exerciser. Excessive hypermobility increases joint laxity or looseness, decreases joint stability, and can lead to permanent changes in connective tissue. Take precautions to avoid overstretching, which may lead to injury or decreases in exercise performance. For example, if you are taking a yoga class, let your instructor know that you are hyperflexible and ask if there are any modified poses that would reduce your risk of overstretching.

Inflexibility is common in many people. If you have limited range of motion in one or more joints, avoid stretching beyond your abilities. Work gradually to improve your range of motion and overall flexibility. People with a very limited range of motion may be more susceptible to sudden acute injuries during sports, to activity-related injuries during daily-living tasks, and to lower-back injuries.

How Can I Prevent or Manage Back Pain?

While you are young, back pain is probably the furthest thing from your mind. However, lower-back pain affects at least 70 percent of the general U.S. population at some point in life, and about 28 percent of Americans at any given moment.[15] Some 31 percent of all Americans report limitations due to chronic back conditions.[16] In fact, back and spine problems are the self-reported cause of disability for 7.6 million Americans (16.8 percent), with women affected more often.[17] While Americans spend more than $86 billion each year treating back pain symptoms, the number and symptoms of sufferers continue to rise.[18]

Research has shown that college students are not immune to back-health issues. In recent studies, 29 to 43 percent of students reported regular lower-back pain, with higher numbers in students who were feeling sad, exhausted, or overwhelmed and those carrying heavy backpacks.[19,20] According to a recent American College Health Association survey of nearly 96,000 students, 12.5 percent reported having seen a physician in the last year for low back pain.[21]

Factors that increase your risk of lower-back pain include obesity, smoking, pregnancy, stress, inactivity, weak and inflexible muscles, and poor posture. In addition, a number of events can trigger back pain or cause a back injury, including accidents, sports injuries, repetitive movements, work trauma, and excessive sitting—especially if you already have other risk factors.

In the next sections, we will cover the causes of back pain, explain how the spine is structured and supported, and present strategies to reduce your risk of back pain. For those who already experience regular episodes of back pain, the next sections will also discuss ways to effectively manage, resolve, and prevent future recurrences of back pain.

Understand the Primary Causes of Back Pain

You experience back pain when your movement causes a sprain, strain, or spasm in one of the muscles, tendons, or ligaments in the back. You may also feel pain when your spine structures become misaligned or injured and the spinal nerves become compressed or irritated. Back pain can also result from age- or disease-related degeneration of the bones and joints of the spine. Ultimately, most back pain is caused by a *sedentary lifestyle*, which results in muscle weakness, inflexibility, and imbalance—all conditions that can lead to poor posture and body mechanics and to a higher risk of back pain and injury.

Muscular Weakness, Inflexibility, and Imbalance The supporting musculature of the spine is important for maintaining healthy posture, mobility, and spine structures. Weakness and inflexibility in key muscles can lead to muscular imbalances that affect the alignment of your spine. Weak abdominals, for instance, can cause your pelvis to rock forward and create a greater curvature in your lower back. This puts more pressure on spine structures and other spine-supporting muscles, potentially leading to back pain. Inflexible, tight hip flexor muscles can also cause a forward tilt of the pelvis and an increased curvature of the lower back.

Muscles become weak when they are not used on a regular basis. Repetitive movements or long hours of sitting can also cause muscles to shorten and tighten up. Some people have muscles of differing strength and flexibility levels around the spine and other joints. If your spine-supporting musculature does not have a muscle balance that promotes good posture and body mechanics, you may have back pain or injury in the future.

Improper Posture and Body Mechanics Improper posture can lead to increased forces within the spine structures and eventually to back pain. Altered body mechanics resulting from improper posture puts you at risk for injury during all of your daily activities, but especially during exercise and sports activities.

Acute Trauma, Risky Occupations, and Medical Issues Acute trauma to the back can happen to anyone at any age. Trauma could be the result of a car accident, a sports and recreation injury, or any other accident that affects the spine. Avoiding risky sports and recreational activities will reduce your chance of trauma.

Jobs that involve a lot of bending, twisting, and repeated lifting of heavy objects put workers at especially high risk of developing back pain. Jobs that involve a great deal of sitting every day are also considered high risk. Occupations with a high incidence of back pain include truck driving, nursing, firefighting, construction, and some professional sports (e.g., football, power lifting, golf, and wrestling). Occupations that are highly stressful and require long hours also increase the risk of back pain. Stress is a risk factor for back injury, and long hours at work can reduce the time you have to exercise and relax, further increasing the risk of developing back pain.

Medical issues and individual health factors can also significantly increase your chance of developing lower-back pain. For instance, smokers have an increased risk of low-back pain due to vascular damage, which facilitates disc degeneration.[22] Obesity and weight gain during pregnancy can increase lower-back pain due to greater loads on the spine, misalignment of the pelvis and low back, and muscular weakness. Pain can also result from degenerative conditions such as arthritis or disc disease, osteoporosis or other bone diseases, congenital abnormalities, viral infections, and general conditions that cause irritation to joints or discs.[23]

Understand How the Back Is Supported

The back comprises bones, muscles, and other tissues that form the back side of your trunk. The trunk contains most of your essential organs and bears the weight of your upper body. It is also responsible for transmitting forces and movements from the upper limbs to the lower limbs, and vice versa. If something is amiss with your back or your trunk overall, any upper- or lower-body movement can be difficult. Your back and trunk are supported by the bony structures of the spine and by the core trunk muscles.

The Structure of the Spine

The spine or *spinal column* (also called the *vertebral column*) is the series of bones called *vertebrae* that connect the upper-body and lower-body skeleton and protect the spinal cord. Figure 5.5 shows the basic structure of the spine. Note that the spine has four distinct regions and curvatures: *cervical, thoracic, lumbar,* and *sacral*. The curvatures are an essential part of the force-absorbing capabilities of the spine.

Intervertebral discs are round, spongy pads of cartilage that act as shock absorbers. The discs have fibrous outer rings that are filled with gel and water-like substances that will distend slightly when compressed. That distention acts to absorb shock. The discs also ensure that there is adequate space between the vertebrae. When a change in body mechanics or posture occurs—or when an acute injury occurs—the resulting change to spinal alignment can damage the disc structures.

FIGURE **5.5** The spine has four distinct regions and curvatures (cervical, thoracic, lumbar, and sacral) made up of individual or fused vertebrae.

A permanent bulging of a disc out of the normal space is called a **disc herniation**. The disc can bulge toward the spinal column or nerves and cause pain or numbness in the back or other areas of the body. Disc herniations most often occur in the lower lumbar region, where most of the body weight and forces are applied.

Another problem that occurs with trauma or aging is dehydration, hardening, or degeneration of intervertebral discs. Without adequate fluid content and elasticity, discs cannot perform their shock-absorber role very well. The resulting smaller joint space between vertebrae applies pressure to the spinal nerves. This can cause back, hip, or leg pain and muscle weakness.

The Core Trunk Muscles The bones of the spinal column could not maintain their healthy curvatures and an upright posture without supporting muscles. Core trunk muscles support the trunk while you are standing, sitting, lying down, or moving. These muscles, located all around your body (Figure 5.6), are essential for supporting the spine and for performing sports, recreation, and everyday activities. **Core muscles** include back, abdominal, hip, gluteal, pelvis, pelvic floor, and lateral trunk muscles. Core muscles work together to effectively transmit forces between your upper and lower body. While weak core muscles can lead to back pain, strong core muscles can lead to increased performance levels in all of your activities.

Anterior view   **Posterior view**

- Trunk extensor muscles
- Trunk flexor muscles
- Hip flexor muscles
- Hip extensor muscles

FIGURE **5.6** Strengthening and stretching of the spine-supporting core muscles is essential for a healthy back. The core muscles include extensors of the trunk and hip and flexors of the trunk and hip.

Reduce Your Risk of Lower-Back Pain

You can reduce your risk of back pain by improving your body weight, muscle fitness, posture, and movement techniques. A review of multiple studies showed that exercise programs prevented back pain episodes in working-age adults, but other strategies, including shoe inserts and back supports, were not effective prevention measures.[24] Incorporating your new fitness knowledge from this course will help you gain strength and stability in your key spine-supporting muscles and reduce your risk of back pain.

Lose Weight The prevalence of lower-back pain rises with increases in body mass index or body weight and body fatness.[25] An increase in body weight puts extra strain and pressure on all the spinal structures. If the additional weight resides in the abdominal region, the pelvis may get pulled forward and result in a greater curvature of the lower back, causing back pain. Lowering your weight and body fat levels to within recommended ranges will reduce your risk of lower-back pain.

Strengthen and Stretch Key Muscles Most people's bodies have "weak" muscle areas, "tight" muscle areas, and areas that are both weak *and* tight.

- *Hip flexor muscles* tend to be tight in most people. This stems from extended sitting, resulting in shortened and inactive muscles. If you have tight hip flexor muscles, add hip flexor stretches (see Figure 5.3) to your weekly workout.

- *Hip extensor muscles* also tend to be tight and weak in many people and can benefit from stretching and strengthening.

- *Trunk flexor muscles* (abdominals) are often weak in individuals who are sedentary or overweight. Having a minimal level of strength in your abdominal muscles will help protect your spine and back and improve your exercise performance.

- *Trunk extensor muscles* are responsible for keeping your spine upright while sitting, standing, and moving.

If you do a lot of hunched-over sitting, these muscles are probably weak, and you should add safe back extensor strengthening exercises to your program.

The simplest prescription for back health is to maintain a healthy weight and an active lifestyle. If you are predisposed to back pain due to other reasons (e.g., hyperflexibility, sport history, occupation), try to add some specific back health exercises to your current exercise routine. Figure 5.7 illustrates back health exercises that will help you stretch or strengthen the key areas of the trunk and hips; Activate, Motivate, & Advance Your Fitness: A Back-Health Exercise Program at the end of the chapter (page 213) will help you develop a plan to get started.

FIGURE **5.7**

EXERCISES FOR A HEALTHY BACK

Perform 3 to 10 repetitions of the back health exercises, holding where appropriate for 10 to 30 seconds. (See Figure 4.8 on page 132 for a full-body muscle diagram.)

Videos for these exercises and more are available online at www.pearsonhighered.com/hopson and on MyFitnessLab.

1. Cat Stretch

Start on your hands and knees with a flat back. Looking at the ground, align your head with your spine. Drop your head and look back toward your knees while lifting your upper back toward the ceiling.

Muscles targeted:

12 Erector spinae

10 Trapezius; various neck muscles

2. Arm/Leg Extensions

Start on your hands and knees with a flat back. Looking at the ground, align your head with your spine. Extend your arm straight out in front of you while extending the opposite leg straight out behind you. Keep your arm and leg in a straight line with your spine. Do not lift them too high, because this causes too much arch in your lower back.

Muscles targeted:

12 Erector spinae

15 Gluteus maximus
16 Hamstrings

3 Rectus abdominis

(Continued)

3. Pelvic Tilt

Lie on your back with your knees bent and your feet flat on the floor. Relax in a comfortable posture, letting the natural curve of your spine bring your lower back off the mat. Breathe out as you tilt the bottom of your pelvis toward the ceiling, pulling your abdominals in and pressing your lower back flat against the floor.

Slight arch

Flat back

Muscles targeted:

12 Erector spinae

3 Rectus abdominis; various hip/pelvis stabilizers

4. Back Bridge

Lie on your back with your knees bent, your feet flat on the floor, and your arms extended straight along your sides. Lift your hips off the ground and press your pelvis toward the ceiling until your thighs and back are in a straight line. Look at the ceiling and keep your neck extended throughout the exercise (do not tuck your chin to your chest).

Muscles targeted:

12 Erector spinae

15 Gluteus maximus
16 Hamstrings

Other exercises that can help maintain back health include:

Plank (p. 145)

Side bridge (p. 145)

Knee-to-chest stretch (p. 184)

Hamstring stretch (p. 186)

Torso twist and hip stretch (p. 184)

Hip flexor stretch (p. 185)

Abdominal curl (p. 144)

Oblique curl (p. 145)

Maintain Good Posture and Proper Body Mechanics

If you have strong and flexible core trunk muscles, maintaining good posture and body mechanics is easier. The problem is that even with good muscular fitness, poor posture can become a habit. You might always hunch over at the computer and feel unnatural sitting up straight. Maybe you slouch back on the couch when you are watching TV. Over time, poor posture can create back problems.

Poor posture and poor muscle fitness can also lead to improper body mechanics while you perform everyday activities. Poor body mechanics put you at risk of muscle strain and back pain. **Lab 5.2** teaches you how to evaluate your posture, and Figure 5.8 illustrates proper postures for standing, walking, lifting, sitting, and lying down.

THINK! How long each day do you sit hunched over a pile of books, a laptop computer, or looking down at your smart phone?

ACT! Take a break every 20 minutes or so to do shoulder rolls, neck stretches, and dynamic hip and leg movements.

Properly Treat Lower-Back Pain

If you already experience regular back pain, you can do things to help manage your pain and prevent future recurrences. The box What Should I Do If I Already Have Back Pain? lists some strategies for back pain management.

Standing posture

Head centered between the shoulders and the crown of the head extended

Shoulders over the pelvis, level and relaxed

Knees over the ankles and not hyperextended

Chest elevated

Abdomen flat

Pelvis in a neutral position over the knees and hips level

Feet facing forward and weight distributed through heels

Improper postures include:

Kyphosis -lordosis

Flat-back

Sway-back

Walking posture

Shoulders relaxed, down, and back

Arms swing in opposition to legs and close to body; elbows relaxed or flexed to 90 degrees

Hips rotate naturally

Head balanced, chin parallel to ground

Chest lifted

Abdominals contracted and pelvis centered

Stride length is comfortable, not too short or long

Sitting posture

Top of monitor at eye level

If you have a "sway" back, elevate feet so knees are higher than hips; if you have a "flat" back, keep knees lower than hips

Chest elevated and back extended tall, not slumping

Elbows bent at 90°; use armrest if available

Hands in line with forearms (wrists straight); use wrist supports if necessary

Feet flat on the floor or foot rest

Low-back curvature supported by a back rest

Sleeping posture

Lying on one's back

Medium to firm mattress supports the spine

Head supported to maintain neck alignment, but avoiding a pillow that is too high

If needed, pillow or other lift placed under knees to reduce lumbar curvature and support the lower back

Lying on one's side

Hips and knees bent

Head and neck supported enough to maintain a straight spine

If needed, pillow placed between knees for additional support of the lower back, hips, and pelvis

Lifting and carrying posture

Get help if the weight is too much for you

Bend at the knees and hips; don't bend over at the waist

Use a wide straddle stance or a "stride" stance where one foot is forward and the other is back

Keep the weight close to your body when lifting and carrying

FIGURE **5.8** Proper posture is important for back health.

What Should I Do If I Already Have Back Pain?

While experiencing an acute episode of back pain, take the following treatment recommendations into account:

- Limit bed rest to 1 to 2 days at most. Bed rest alone may make back pain worse and may contribute to other problems such as muscle weakness and blood clots.

- Ice and heat may help with pain management, inflammation, and mobility. Apply cold treatments for 2 to 3 days after an acute event, and then add heat treatments as needed for increased muscle blood flow and relaxation.

- Engage in low-stress, back-healthy activities such as stretching, swimming, walking, and movement therapy as soon as you can.

- Check with a doctor before taking drugs for pain relief. Common medications include aspirin, ibuprofen, naproxen, topical muscle creams, and prescription muscle relaxers and pain medications.

- Spinal manipulation by a chiropractor or other qualified therapist can help some individuals with pain management and recovery.

- Nonconventional treatments (acupuncture, biofeedback, etc.) are considered by some patients when they are not responding to more traditional methods.

- Seek medical attention if you do not have a noticeable reduction in pain or if you experience continued inflammation after 72 hours of self-care.

Once you have your current episode of back pain under control, try to incorporate a back-health exercise routine into your weekly schedule (see the sample back-health exercise program at the end of this chapter). A strong and flexible core means you'll have less back pain. And take a look at your daily routine. Remember that sitting for long periods of time is one of the biggest culprits in back pain. If you spend a lot of time sitting, incorporate strategies to get up and move periodically. You might also re-think your workspace—make sure you have proper sitting posture (see Figure 5.8) and consider how you might stand and work for part of the day.

Source: National Institute of Arthritis and Musculoskeletal and Skin Diseases, *Back Pain* NIH Publication No. 09-5282 (Information Clearinghouse, National Institutes of Health: Bethesda, MD, 2010).

● ●

chapterin**review**

videos

Log on to **www.pearsonhighered.com/hopson** or MyFitnessLab to view these chapter-related videos.

Flexibility Exercises
Calf Stretch
Cat Stretch
Gluteal Stretch
Hamstrings Stretch (Seated)
Head Turn and Head Tilt
Hip Flexor Stretch
Inner-Thigh Butterfly Stretch
Low-Back Knee-to-Chest Stretch

Modified Hurdler Stretch
Outer-Thigh Stretch
Pectoral and Biceps Stretch
Quadriceps Stretch
Shin Stretch
Shoulder Stretch
Side Stretch
Torso Twist and Hip Stretch
Triceps Stretch

Upper Back Stretch
Core Strength Exercises
Abdominal Curl (Stability Ball)
Abdominal Tuck (Stability Ball)
Arm/Leg Extensions
Back Bridge
Back Extension (Stability Ball)
Bridge Leg Curl (Stability Ball)
Bridge Up (Stability Ball)

Oblique Curl
Oblique Side Crunch (Stability Ball)
Pelvic Tilt
Pike-Up (Stability Ball)
Plank (Forearm Position)
Plank (Push-Up Position)
Plank (Stability Ball)

Reverse Curl
Side Bridge (Beginner)
Side Bridge (Intermediate)
Side Bridge (Advanced)
Assessments
Posture Evaluation
Range-of-Motion Assessment

Sit-and-Reach Assessment (Box)
Sit-and-Reach Assessment
  (Yardstick)
Shoulder Flexibility Assessment
Trunk Rotation Assessment

Twist to Get Fit

onlineresources

Log on to **www.pearsonhighered.com/hopson** or MyFitnessLab for access to these book-related resources, and for links to other useful websites.

Audio case study
Audio PowerPoint lecture

Customizable 4-week flexibility training programs
Customizable 4-week back-health exercise programs
Behavior Change Logbook and Wellness Journal

Lab 6.1 Assess Your Flexibility
Lab 6.2 Assess Your Posture
Lab 6.3 Planning a Flexibility Program
Alternate Lab: Modified Sit-and-Reach Test
Alternate Lab: Chair Sit-and-Reach Test
Alternate Lab: Assessing Shoulder Flexibility
Alternate Lab: Assessing Trunk Rotation

Pre- and post-quizzes
Glossary flashcards

reviewquestions

1. _____a_____ is a measure of your overall joint stiffness during movement.
   a. Dynamic flexibility
   b. Static flexibility
   c. Passive flexibility
   d. Anatomical flexibility

2. Which of the following triggers a muscle to relax when there is too much force or tension in the muscle?
   a. Muscle spindle
   b. Baroreceptor
   c. Golgi tendon organ
   d. Reflex receptor

3. The intensity of each stretch should be stretching until you reach
   a. your toes.
   b. the point of tightness.
   c. moderate burning pain.
   d. your goal.

4. Stretching that involves voluntary muscle contractions to facilitate relaxation describes
   a. static stretching.
   b. dynamic stretching.
   c. ballistic stretching.
   d. PNF stretching.

5. Which of the following exercise styles uses a slow-moving series of forms to increase coordination, balance, and flexibility?
   a. Dance
   b. Pilates
   c. Yoga
   d. Tai chi

6. Which of the following is the primary underlying cause of low-back pain?
   a. Poor posture
   b. Sedentary living
   c. Muscle weakness
   d. Poor flexibility

7. The fluid of an intervertebral disc bulging outward and pressing on the nervous system structures in the spine is best described as disc
   a. dehydration.
   b. degeneration.
   c. herniation.
   d. hardening.

8. Which of the following sleep postures creates the most tension in your lower back and is not recommended?
   a. Lying on your side
   b. Lying on your stomach
   c. Lying on your back
   d. Sleeping in a chair

9. What approximate percentage of people will experience lower-back pain at some point in their lives?
   a. 25 percent
   b. 50 percent
   c. 70 percent
   d. 100 percent

10. Which of the following acute back pain self-care treatments is no longer recommended?
    a. Five days of bed rest
    b. Light exercise
    c. Pain relievers
    d. Cold and hot treatments

critical**thinking**questions

1. Explain how stretching can improve your posture and balance.
2. Describe how reducing the stretch reflex will enhance the effectiveness of your stretches.
3. Are the contraindicated stretches "off-limits" to everyone? Are there any sports, activities, or situations that would safely allow some of these movements and stretches? If so, which ones and which activities?
4. List three occupations that present high risk for low-back pain and explain why.

references

1. M. Nolan and others, "Age-related Changes in Musculoskeletal Function, Balance and Mobility Measures in Men aged 30–80 years," *Aging Male* 13, no. 3 (2010): 194–201.
2. M. J. Spink and others, "Foot and Ankle Strength, Range of Motion, Posture, and Deformity Are Associated with Balance and Functional Ability in Older Adults," *Archives of Physical Medicine and Rehabilitation* 92, no. 1 (2011): 68–75.
3. J. R. Pleis and others, National Center for Health Statistics, "Summary Health Statistics for U.S. Adults: National Health Interview Survey, 2009," *Vital Health Statistics* 10, no. 249 (2010).
4. H. B. Sun, "Mechanical Loading, Cartilage Degradation, and Arthritis," *Annals of the New York Academy of Science* 1211 (2010): 37–50; J. K. Cooney and others, "Benefits of Exercise in Rheumatoid Arthritis," *Journal of Aging Research* (2011): 681640; Y. Escalante, A. García- Hermoso, and J. M. Saavedra, "Effects of Exercise on Functional Aerobic Capacity in Lower Limb Osteoarthritis: A Systematic Review," *Journal of Science and Medicine in Sport* 14, no. 3 (2011): 190–8.
5. J. Peeler and J. E. Anderson, "Effectiveness of Static Quadriceps Stretching in Individuals with Patellofemoral Joint Pain," *Clinical Journal of Sport Medicine* 17, no. 4 (2007): 234–41.
6. F. Balagué and others, "The Association Between Isoinertial Trunk Muscle Performance and Low Back Pain in Male Adolescents," *European Spine Journal* 19, no. 4 (2010): 624–32 .

7. M. A. Jones and others, "Biological Risk Indicators for Recurrent Non-specific Low Back Pain in Adolescents," *British Journal of Sports Medicine* 39, no. 3 (2005): 137–40.
8. P. W. Marshall, J. Mannion, and B. A. Murphy, "Extensibility of the Hamstrings Is Best Explained by Mechanical Components of Muscle Contraction, Not Behavioral Measures in Individuals with Chronic Low Back Pain," *PM&R: The Journal of Injury, Function, and Rehabilitation* 1, no. 8 (2009): 709–18.
9. E. N. Johnson and J. S. Thomas, "Effect of Hamstring Flexibility on Hip and Lumbar Spine Joint Excursions during Forward-Reaching Tasks in Participants with and without Low Back Pain," *Archives of Physical Medicine and Rehabilitation* 91, no. 7 (2010): 1140–2.
10. N. Kofotolis and M. Sambanis, "The Influence of Exercise on Musculoskeletal Disorders of the Lumbar Spine," *Journal of Sports Medicine and Physical Fitness* 45, no. 1 (2005): 84–92.
11. R. J. Johns and V. Wright, "Relative Importance of Various Tissues in Joint Stiffness," *Journal of Applied Physiology* 17, no. 5 (1962): 824–8.
12. H. O. Kendall, F. P. Kendall, and G. E. Bennett, "Normal Flexibility According to Age Groups," *Journal of Bone and Joint Surgery* 30A, no. 3 (1948): 690–4; M. J. Alter, *The Science of Flexibility*, Human Kinetics, Champaign, IL, 2004.
13. I. G. Fatouros and others, "Resistance Training and Detraining Effects on Flexibility Performance in the Elderly Are Intensity-Dependent," *Journal of Strength and Conditioning Research* 20, no. 3 (2006): 634–42.
14. M. Amiri-Khorasani, N. A. Abu Osman, and A. Yusof, "Acute Effect of Static and Dynamic Stretching on Hip Dynamic Range of Motion during Instep Kicking in Professional Soccer Players," *Journal of Strength Conditioning Research* 25, no. 6 (2011): 1647–52.
15. J. R. Pleis and others, "Summary Health Statistics for U.S. Adults: National Health Interview Survey, 2009," 2010.
16. National Center for Health Statistics, Health Promotion Statistics Branch, CDC Wonder. *DATA2010...the Healthy People 2010 Database.* (Hyattsville, MD; Centers for Disease Control, 2010), http://wonder.cdc.gov/data2010/focus.htm (accessed May 2011).
17. Centers for Disease Control and Prevention, "Prevalence and Most Common Causes of Disability among Adults—United States, 2005," *Morbidity and Mortality Weekly Report* 58, no. 16 (2009): 421–6.
18. B. I. Martin, and others, "Expenditures and Health Status among Adults With Back and Neck Problems," *JAMA* 299, no. 6 (2008): 656–64.
19. Z. Heuscher and others, "The Association of Self-Reported Backpack Use and Backpack Weight with Low Back Pain among College Students," *Journal of Manipulative Physiological Therapy* 33, no. 6 (2011): 432–7.

20. C. Kennedy and others, "Psychosocial Factors and Low Back Pain among College Students," *Journal of American College Health* 57, no. 2 (2008): 191–5.

21. American College Health Association, *American College Health Association–National College Health Assessment II (ACHA-NCHA II) Reference Group Executive Summary Spring 2010* (Linthicum, MD: American College Health Association, 2010).

22. M. Iwahashi and others, "Mechanism of Intervertebral Disc Degeneration Caused by Nicotine in Rabbits to Explicate Intervertebral Disc Disorders Caused by Smoking," *Spine* 27, no. 13 (2002): 1396–401.

23. National Institute of Neurological Disorders and Stroke, *Low Back Pain Fact Sheet* NIH Publication No. 03-5161 (Office of Communications and Public Liaison, National Institutes of Health: Bethesda, MD, 2003).

24. S. J. Bigos and others, "High-quality Controlled Trials on Preventing Episodes of Back Problems: Systematic Literature Review in Working-Age Adults," *The Spine Journal: Official Journal of the North American Spine Society* 9, no. 2 (2009): 147–68.

25. D.M. Urquhart and others, "Increased Fat Mass Is Associated with High Levels of Low Back Pain Intensity and Disability," *Spine (Philadelphia, PA 1976)* 36, no. 16 (2011): 1320–5.

Name: _____   Date: _____

Instructor: _____   Section: _____

Materials: Exercise mat, yardstick or sit-and-reach box, a partner

Purpose: To assess your current level of lower-back, hip, and hamstring flexibility and your current level of joint mobility or range of motion.

SECTION I: THE SIT-AND-REACH TEST

This test measures the general flexibility of your lower back, hips, and hamstrings. The results are specific to those regions of your body and do not reflect your flexibility in other body areas. Choose the **box** or the **yardstick** test based upon equipment availability and/or your instructor's preference. You **need not** perform both assessments.

1. **Warm-up.** Complete 3 to 10 minutes of light cardiorespiratory activity to warm-up your body and then perform light range-of-motion exercises and stretches for the joints and muscles that you will be using.

2. **Prepare for the appropriate test.**

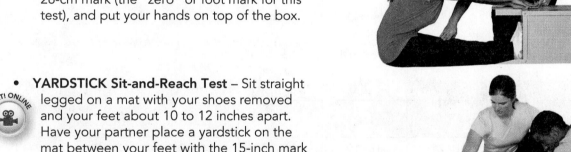

- **BOX Sit-and-Reach Test** – Place the sit-and-reach box against a wall to prevent it from moving during the test. Sit without shoes behind the box, place your feet flat against the box at the 26-cm mark (the "zero" or foot mark for this test), and put your hands on top of the box.

- **YARDSTICK Sit-and-Reach Test** – Sit straight legged on a mat with your shoes removed and your feet about 10 to 12 inches apart. Have your partner place a yardstick on the mat between your feet with the 15-inch mark at the edge of your heels. You can use a pre-placed and taped yardstick, tape the yardstick in place at the heels, or just have your partner hold the yardstick. Place your hands on top of the end of the yardstick.

3. **Properly perform the test.** Keep one hand on top of the other. It is important that fingertips remain together and that your hands remain in contact with the yardstick or box ruler at all times. Reach forward as far as you can by slowly bending forward, reaching with your arms, and sliding your fingertips out along the yardstick or box. Keep your legs straight, drop your head between your arms, and breathe out as you perform the test. Hold your ending position for at least two seconds. Your partner will watch to ensure that you have proper hand position and straight legs during the test.

4. **Find your reach distance.** Your *reach distance* is the most distant point reached with both fingertips. If you cannot keep your hands from separating, the most distant point reached by the fingertips of the *hand that is farthest back* should be considered the reach distance. Record the reach distance in inches, as measured by the yardstick, or centimeters, as measured by the box. Perform the test twice. Have your partner point to your reach distance for each trial. Record your best reach distance of the two trials in the RESULTS section on the next page.

FLEXIBILITY RESULTS

Box Sit-and-Reach Test: Reach Distance (cm): _____ Rating: _____

OR

Yardstick Sit-and-Reach Test: Reach Distance (in): _____ Rating: _____

5. **Find your flexibility rating by using the charts provided below.** Your rating tells you how you compare to others who have completed this test in the past. Record your rating in the RESULTS section above.

BOX Sit-and-Reach Test (centimeters)					
Men	**Excellent**	**Very Good**	**Good**	**Fair**	**Needs Improvement**
15–19 yrs	≥39	34–38	29–33	24–28	≤23
20–29 yrs	≥40	34–39	30–33	25–29	≤24
30–39 yrs	≥38	33–37	28–32	23–27	≤22
40–49 yrs	≥35	29–34	24–28	18–23	≤17
50–59 yrs	≥35	28–34	24–27	16–23	≤15
60–69 yrs	≥33	25–32	20–24	15–19	≤14
Women	**Excellent**	**Very Good**	**Good**	**Fair**	**Needs Improvement**
15–19 yrs	≥43	38–42	34–37	29–33	≤28
20–29 yrs	≥41	37–40	33–36	28–32	≤27
30–39 yrs	≥41	36–40	32–35	27–31	≤26
40–49 yrs	≥38	34–37	30–33	25–29	≤24
50–59 yrs	≥39	33–38	30–32	25–29	≤24
60–69 yrs	≥35	31–34	27–30	23–26	≤22

Source: From *Canadian Physical Activity, Fitness & Lifestyle Approach: CSEP-Health & Fitness Program's Health-Related Appraisal & Counseling Strategy.* 3rd edition © 2003. Reprinted with permission from the Canadian Society for Exercise Physiology.

YARDSTICK Sit-and-Reach Test (inches)							
Men	**Excellent**	**Good**	**Above Average**	**Average**	**Below Average**	**Poor**	**Very Poor**
18–25 yrs	22–28	20–21	18–19	16–17	14–15	12–13	2–11
26–35 yrs	21–28	19	17	15–16	13–14	11–12	2–9
36–45 yrs	21–28	18–19	16–17	15	13	9–11	1–7
46–55 yrs	19–26	16–18	14–15	12–13	10–11	8–9	1–6
56–65 yrs	17–24	15–16	13	11	9	6–8	1–5
>65 yrs	17–24	14–16	12–13	10–11	8–9	6–7	0–4
Women	**Excellent**	**Good**	**Above Average**	**Average**	**Below Average**	**Poor**	**Very Poor**
18–25 yrs	24–29	22	20–21	19	17–18	16	7–14
26–35 yrs	23–28	21–22	20	18–19	16–17	14–15	5–13
36–45 yrs	22–28	20–21	18–19	17	15–16	13–14	4–12
46–55 yrs	21–27	19–20	17–18	16	14	12–13	3–10
56–65 yrs	20–26	18–19	16–17	15	13–14	10–12	2–9
>65 yrs	20–26	18–19	17	15–16	13–14	10–12	1–9

Source: Adapted with permission from *YMCA Fitness Testing and Assessment Manual,* 4th edition. Copyright © 2000 by YMCA of the USA, Chicago. All rights reserved.

SECTION II: JOINT MOBILITY—RANGE-OF-MOTION TESTS

Range-of-motion tests assess your joints' ability to move through a normal range of motion. Follow the instructions for each of the tests shown below. Perform each test on both your right and left sides. Stop each movement when you feel resistance. To avoid injury, do not try to push past your normal range. Have a partner observe your movements, "eyeball" your estimated joint angle, and record your range-of-motion results on page 204.

1. Neck Lateral Flexion—
Sit or stand with your head neutral and looking forward. Tilt your head to the side and drop your ear toward your shoulder.

Average range 0–45°

2. Shoulder Flexion—
Starting with your arms at your sides, reach a straight arm forward and up toward your head.

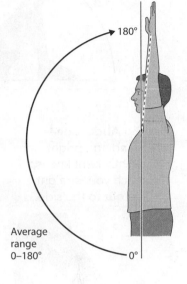

Average range 0–180°

3. Shoulder Extension—
With your arms at your sides, reach a straight arm behind you and up.

Average range 0–50°

4. Shoulder Abduction—
Reach your straight arm out to the side and up to your head.

Average range 0–180°

5. Shoulder Adduction—Reach your straight arm down and across your body in front.

Average range 0–50°

6. Trunk Lateral Flexion—
Standing upright with slightly bent knees and your arms at your sides, bend your torso sideways and reach your arm down your leg for support.

Average range 0–25°

7. **Hip Flexion**—Lying on your back, lift a straight leg up into the air while keeping the other leg bent with the foot flat on the ground.

Average range 0–90°

90°

0°

8. **Hip Extension**—Lying on your stomach with your head on the mat, reach your straight leg up behind you, keeping the other leg flat on the ground.

30°

Average range 0–30°

0°

9. **Hip Abduction**—Standing upright with slightly bent knees, reach your straight leg out to the side.

40°

0°

Average range 0–40°

10. **Ankle Dorsiflexion**—Sitting without shoes and your legs extended in front of you, flex your foot back toward your knee.

0°

20°

Average range 0–20°

11. **Ankle Plantar Flexion**—Sitting without shoes and your legs extended in front of you, point your foot toward the floor.

0°

40°

Average range 0–40°

Joint Mobility RESULTS			
Joint	**Movement and Average Range (degrees)**	**Full Average Joint Range?**	
		Right Side	*Left Side*
1. Neck	Lateral Flexion 0–45	_____ Yes _____ No	_____ Yes _____ No
2. Shoulder	Flexion 0–180	_____ Yes _____ No	_____ Yes _____ No
3. Shoulder	Extension 0–50	_____ Yes _____ No	_____ Yes _____ No
4. Shoulder	Abduction 0–180	_____ Yes _____ No	_____ Yes _____ No
5. Shoulder	Adduction 0–50	_____ Yes _____ No	_____ Yes _____ No
6. Trunk	Lateral Flexion 0–25	_____ Yes _____ No	_____ Yes _____ No
7. Hip	Flexion 0–90	_____ Yes _____ No	_____ Yes _____ No
8. Hip	Extension 0–30	_____ Yes _____ No	_____ Yes _____ No
9. Hip	Abduction 0–40	_____ Yes _____ No	_____ Yes _____ No
10. Ankle	Dorsiflexion 0–20	_____ Yes _____ No	_____ Yes _____ No
11. Ankle	Plantar Flexion 0–40	_____ Yes _____ No	_____ Yes _____ No

Sources: Adapted from American College of Sports Medicine, *ACSM's Health-Related Physical Fitness Assessment Manual.* 3rd ed. (Baltimore, MD: Lippincott Williams & Wilkins, 2009); American College of Sports Medicine, *ACSM's Resource Manual for Guidelines for Exercise Testing and Prescription.* 6th ed. (Baltimore, MD: Lippincott Williams & Wilkins, 2009).

Name: _____ Date: _____

Instructor: _____ Section: _____

Purpose: To evaluate your posture.

Before you begin: Wear clothing that will not interfere with the assessment of your posture. If it is comfortable, men should wear shorts only, and women should wear shorts and a tank top. Remove your shoes. If you have long hair, pull it back into a ponytail for the assessment.

Stand against a wall and have a partner evaluate your posture using the chart on page 206. Your partner should assign you a score of between 1 and 5 for each of the 10 areas of your body shown on the next page.

Posture Results	
Posture Score	Posture Rating
45 or higher	Excellent
40–44	Good
30–39	Average
20–29	Fair
19 or less	Poor

Source: Adapted from *New York State Physical Fitness Test for Boys and Girls Grades 4–12. A Manual for Teachers of Physical Education,* Division of Physical Education and Research, State University of New York. Albany, NY: New York State Education Dept., 1972.

	Good—5	Fair—3	Poor—1	Score
Head	Head erect, gravity passes directly through center	Head twisted or turned to one side slightly	Head twisted or turned to one side markedly	
Shoulders	Shoulders level horizontally	One shoulder slightly higher	One shoulder markedly higher	
Spine	Spine straight	Spine slightly curved	Spine markedly curved laterally	
Hips	Hips level horizontally	One hip slightly higher	One hip markedly higher	
Knees and Ankles	Feet pointed straight ahead, legs vertical	Feet pointed out, legs deviating outward at the knee	Feet pointed out markedly, legs deviated markedly	
Neck and Upper back	Neck erect, head in line with shoulders, rounded upper back	Neck slightly foward, chin out, slightly more rounded upper back	Neck markedly forward, chin markedly out, markedly rounded upper back	
Trunk	Trunk erect	Trunk inclined to rear slightly	Trunk inclined to rear markedly	
Abdomen	Abdomen flat	Abdomen protruding	Abdomen protruding and sagging	
Lower back	Lower back normally curved	Lower back slightly hollow	Lower back markedly hollow	
Legs	Legs straight	Knees slightly hyperextended	Knees markedly hyperextended	
			Total score	

LAB 5.3 • PLANNING A FLEXIBILITY PROGRAM

Name: _____   Date: _____

Instructor: _____   Section: _____

Materials: Results from Lab 5.1

Purpose: To learn how to set appropriate flexibility goals and create a personal flexibility program.

SECTION I: SHORT- AND LONG-TERM GOALS

Create short- and long-term goals for flexibility and back health. Be sure to use SMART goal-setting guidelines (specific, measurable, action-oriented, realistic, time-oriented). Select appropriate target dates and rewards for completing your goals.

Short-Term Goal for Flexibility (3 to 6 months)

_____

_____

Target Date: _____

Reward: _____

Optional: Short-Term Goal for Back Health (3 to 6 months)

_____

_____

Target Date: _____

Reward: _____

Long-Term Goal for Flexibility (12+ months)

_____

_____

Target Date: _____

Reward: _____

Optional: Long-Term Goal for Back Health (12+ months)

_____

_____

Target Date: _____

Reward: _____

SECTION II: FLEXIBILITY PROGRAM DESIGN

Complete one line for each exercise you have chosen to do in your program.

Stretching Exercises	Frequency (days/week)	Time (sec)	Reps (number)	Total Time (sec)
LOWER BODY				
1.				
2.				
3.				
4.				
5.				
6.				
7.				
8.				
UPPER BODY				
1.				
2.				
3.				
4.				
5.				
6.				
7.				
8.				

SECTION III: TRACKING YOUR PROGRAM AND FOLLOWING THROUGH

1. **Goal and Program Tracking:** Use the following chart to monitor your progress. Change the frequency, time, sets, and reps frequently to ensure continuing progress toward your goals.

2. **Goal and Program Follow-up:** At the end of the course or at your short-term goal target date, reevaluate your flexibility and answer the following questions:

a. Did you meet your short-term goal or your goal for the course?

b. If so, what positive behavioral changes contributed to your success? If not, which obstacles blocked your success?

c. Was your short-term goal realistic? After evaluating your progress during the course, what would you change about your goals or training plan?

Flexibility Training Log

DATE	Stretches Completed (with time/reps)	COMMENTS (e.g., stretches modified, stretches held longer, how you felt, etc.)

activate, motivate, & ADVANCE YOUR FITNESS

A FLEXIBILITY TRAINING PROGRAM

ACTIVATE!

Looking to improve your posture, circulation, and joint mobility? Follow these programs to gradually incorporate regular stretching into your weekly exercise routines.

What Do I Need for Flexibility Training?

GEAR: For flexibility training programs, you'll want a mat, towel, and something stable to hold onto for standing stretches. While you really don't need any other equipment for stretching, you may want to use a strap, foam roller, yoga block, or even a training partner.

CLOTHING: Wear comfortable clothing that allows for full range-of-motion movements.

How Do I Start a Flexibility Training Program?

TECHNIQUE: Safe and effective flexibility training depends on good body alignment and awareness. Read through each exercise description and take time to learn the proper form. If you need assistance, ask your instructor or a fitness specialist at your facility. Perform static stretches in a slow and controlled manner. Hold at the point of tightness but not pain. Exhale with the stretching exercise to help you relax and increase your flexibility.

ETIQUETTE: Most facilities will have mats, equipment, and a designated stretching area for you to use. Wipe down your mat or any other equipment after use.

STRETCHING BEFORE A WORKOUT: Dynamic stretching (stretching through movement) performed during your warm-up can prepare your body for the upcoming more intense activity. Incorporate slow and controlled movements that mimic the motions of your workout.

STRETCHING AFTER A WORKOUT: After your workout program your muscles are warm and ready to be stretched. Static or PNF stretching performed at this time will result in the biggest gains in flexibility, particularly after a cardiorespiratory workout.

Flexibility Training Warm-Up & Cool-Down

Warming up prior to stretching is crucial and should include gentle cardiorespiratory exercises for 5 to 10 minutes. After breaking a light sweat, add dynamic movements that increase your range of motion. Ease into the first repetition of each static or PNF stretching exercise. Ensure proper form, posture, and body alignment as you move into your full range of motion.

Flexibility Training Programs

If you are new to flexibility training or if you have not stretched for more than three months, start slowly and build gradually by beginning with Program A. If you already stretch two days a week, then start with Program B. Adjust intensity, volume and training days to suit your personal fitness level and schedule; visit the companion website for more options.

P R O G R A M **A** **GOAL:** Incorporate a full-body stretching routine into weekly schedule

Frequency	Intensity	Time	Number & Type of Stretches
2 non-consecutive days a week	Stretch to a point of mild tightness, not pain	Perform 2–3 repetitions of each stretch, holding for 10–20 seconds each time	8 static stretches

Order of Stretches

Side Stretch
Upper-Back Stretch
Pectoral and Biceps Stretch
Inner-Thigh Side Lunge

Quadriceps Stretch (Standing)
Hamstrings Stretch (Supine Lying)
Low-Back Knee-to-Chest Stretch (Two Knees)
Calf Stretch (Gastrocnemius Lunge)

P R O G R A M **B** **GOAL:** Improve full body range of motion and overall physical function

Frequency	Intensity	Time	Number & Type of Stretches
3 non-consecutive days a week	Stretch to a point of mild tightness, not pain	Perform 2–4 repetitions of each stretch, holding for 20–30 seconds each time	12 static stretches

Order of Stretches

Neck Stretches (Head Turn)
Side Stretch
Upper-Back Stretch
Shoulder Stretch
Pectoral and Biceps Stretch
Inner-Thigh Side Lunge

Outer-Thigh Stretch
Quadriceps Stretch (Lying)
Hamstrings Stretch (Supine Lying)
Low-Back Knee-to-Chest Stretch (Two Knees)
Gluteal Stretch
Calf Stretch (Heel Drop)

M O T I V A T E !

Create your own exercise log to track your flexibility training program—make note of days, actual stretches, type of stretch, repetitions, time—or use the log available through the companion website. Here are a few tips to keep you stretching.

FIND A PARTNER: With a stretching partner, you can keep each other accountable, help each other reach goals, and have greater options when incorporating PNF stretches, as well as a wider variety of both passive and active stretches. Bye-bye boredom!

TRY A NEW CLASS: Shorter classes specifically designed for stretching, foam rolling, core strength, and/or back health are popping up everywhere. You can also try a yoga or martial arts class and have exercises that increase flexibility built right in! Learn something new, meet new people, and keep "reaching" toward your goals.

STRESS? WHAT STRESS? Take a deep breath. Exhale. Slowly move into your stretch. Hold for at least 10 seconds. Repeat three more times. Before you know it you will feel refreshed and relaxed from head to toe. The simple act of performing your flexibility program can increase your circulation, decrease your blood pressure, and keep you calm and focused. Stretch more, stress less!

ADVANCE!

Now that you have established your flexibility program, you might find that you want more stretches that are specific to your sport or activity. Below are three more advanced flexibility programs specific for walkers/runners, cyclists, and swimmers. You can follow these or log onto the companion website to find more options or simply to personalize this program or any of the programs in this book.

PROGRAM C **GOAL:** Add stretches of specific use for walkers and runners

Frequency	Intensity	Time	Number & Type of Stretches
3 non-consecutive days a week	Stretch to a point of mild tightness, not pain	Perform 2–4 repetitions of each stretch, holding for 20–30 seconds each time	5 additional static stretches*

*Perform following a walking/running cardiorespiratory workout, and in addition to Flexibility Program B.

Stretches to Add

Hip Flexor Stretch (Standing for walkers and Low Lunge for runners)
Torso Twist and Hip Stretch (Seated Twist)

Hamstrings Stretch (Modified Hurdler)
Calf Stretch (Soleus Stretch)
Shin Stretch

PROGRAM D **GOAL:** Add stretches of specific use for cyclists

Frequency	Intensity	Time	Number & Type of Stretches
3 non-consecutive days a week	Stretch to a point of mild tightness, not pain	Perform 2–4 repetitions of each stretch, holding for 20–30 seconds each time	5 additional static stretches*

*Perform following a cycling cardiorespiratory workout, and in addition to Flexibility Program B.

Stretches to Add

Neck Stretches (Head Tilt)
Hip Flexor Stretch (Standing or Low Lunge)
Torso Twist and Hip Stretch (Seated Twist)

Calf Stretch (Soleus Stretch)
Shin Stretch

PROGRAM E **GOAL:** Add stretches of specific use for swimmers

Frequency	Intensity	Time	Reps	Number & Type of Stretches
3 non-consecutive days a week	Stretch to a point of mild tightness, not pain	20–30 sec per stretch	2–4	5 additional static stretches

*Perform following a swimming cardiorespiratory workout, and in addition to Flexibility Program B.

Stretches to Add

Neck Stretches (Head Tilt)
Triceps Stretch
Hip Flexor Stretch (Standing)

Torso Twist and Hip Stretch (Seated Twist)
Shin Stretch

activate, motivate, & ADVANCE YOUR FITNESS

A BACK-HEALTH EXERCISE PROGRAM

Want to avoid back pain or manage pain you may already have? Try the core stretching and strengthening exercise programs outlined on the next page. They are specifically designed to help you increase the strength of your core trunk muscles and decrease tightness. Combine programs A and B for a full-core back-health program. Together, these programs can stand alone; however, the exercises are designed to be incorporated into your current muscular fitness and flexibility programs. Visit the companion website to find more options or to personalize this or any of the programs in this book.

CORE PROGRAM **A**   **GOAL:** Increase core muscle endurance and strength

Frequency	Intensity	Time			Number & Type of Exercises
		Reps	Sets	Rest	
2 non-consecutive days a week	60% 1RM	12	2	2 minutes between sets	8 core muscle exercises

Core Strength Exercises

Arm/Leg Extensions
Plank (hold each plank for 15 to 30 seconds and complete 2 to 4 repetitions)
Back Extension
Abdominal Curl

Reverse Curl
Oblique Curl
Pelvic Tilt
Side Bridge (hold each side bridge for 15 seconds and complete 4 repetitions)

CORE PROGRAM **B**   **GOAL:** Decrease core muscle tightness

Frequency	Intensity	Time	Number & Type of Exercises
2 non-consecutive days a week	Stretch to a point of mild tightness, not pain	Perform 2–4 repetitions of each stretch, holding for 10–30 seconds each time	8 core stretch exercises

Core Stretches

Back Bridge
Low-Back Knee-to-Chest Stretch (Two Knees)
Gluteal Stretch
Hamstrings Stretch (Supine Lying)

Quadriceps Stretch (Lying)
Torso Twist and Hip Stretch (Seated Twist)
Cat Stretch
Hip Flexor Stretch (Low Lunge)

6

Understanding Body Composition

Learning Outcomes

1. Discuss how body composition is related to lifelong fitness and wellness.

   HEAR IT! ONLINE — Audio case study and audio PowerPoint lecture

   SEE IT! ONLINE — Normal weight obesity

2. Describe how the assessment of body size and shape differs from the assessment of body composition.

3. Evaluate your BMI and body circumferences and relate your scores to your overall health status.

   DO IT! ONLINE — Lab 6.1 How to Calculate Your BMI

   Lab 6.2 How to Measure and Evaluate Your Body Circumferences

4. Set and continually reevaluate goals to reach your healthy body fat percentage.

   DO IT! ONLINE — Lab 6.3 Estimate Your Percent Body Fat (Skinfold Test)

   SEE IT! ONLINE — Demonstration videos of body composition measurement techniques

   LIVE IT! ONLINE — Take Charge of Your Health worksheets and Behavior Change Logs for assessing body composition and creating a change plan

Pre- and post-quizzes and glossary flashcards — **REVIEW IT! ONLINE**

casestudy

JESSIE

"Hi, I'm Jessie. I started running and resistance training two months ago and feel great! I like the new muscle tone in my legs, and I've made a lot of friends from the running group I joined. The ironic thing is, I started working out mainly because I wanted to lose weight, but I actually weigh a little bit more right now than I did when I first started. It doesn't make any sense to me, because my clothes fit better and I look more 'toned.' I've heard that muscle weighs more than fat, but that doesn't make any sense, either—doesn't a pound of muscle weigh the same as a pound of fat?"

HEAR IT! ONLINE

How much of your body is composed of fat? It's impossible to get an exact answer to that question, but you can estimate it. Body fat is a component of your total **body composition**, along with the amount of lean tissue in your body. Although this health-related component of physical fitness is not measured by your physical performance on a task like the others, body composition is an important determinant of overall health. Estimating body composition involves determining your lean body mass, fat mass, and percent body fat. Your **lean body mass** is your body's total amount of lean or fat-free tissue (muscles, bones, skin, other organs, and body fluids). Your **fat mass** is body mass made up of fat (adipose) tissue. **Percent body fat** is the percentage of your total weight that is fat tissue—that is, the weight of fat divided by total body weight.

All fat tissue can be labeled as either essential fat or storage fat. **Essential fat** is necessary for normal body functioning; it includes fats in the brain, muscles, nerves, bones, lungs, heart, and digestive and reproductive systems. Men need a minimum of three percent essential body fat. Women need significantly more (12 percent essential body fat) because of reproductive system-related fat deposits in their breasts, uterus, and elsewhere (Figure 6.1). **Storage fat** is nonessential fat stored in tissue near the body's surface and around major body organs. Storage fat provides energy, insulation, and padding. Men and women have similar amounts of storage fat but may differ in the location of larger fat stores. Your individual amount of storage fat depends upon many factors, including your lifestyle and genetics.

In this chapter, you will learn why body size, shape, and composition are useful measurements of fitness and wellness. You'll also learn how each of these measurements is determined and how you can change or maintain your body composition. (In Chapter 8, you will combine your knowledge of physical activity, body composition, and diet to create your own weight-management plan.)

Why Do My Body Size, Shape, and Composition Matter?

You might think of body size, shape, and composition mainly in terms of your physical appearance, but they encompass more than how you look. They are important components (as well as measurements) of your overall fitness and wellness.

Knowing Your Body Composition Can Help You Assess Your Health Risks

From the mid-1970s to 2008, the number of overweight children and adolescents increased from a mere 5 percent to 17 percent of the U.S. population![1]

---

body composition The relative amounts of fat and lean tissue in the body

lean body mass Body mass that is fat-free (muscle, skin, bone, organs, and body fluids)

fat mass Body mass that is fat tissue (adipose tissue)

percent body fat Percentage of total weight that is fat tissue

essential fat Body fat that is essential for normal physiological functioning

storage fat Body fat that is not essential but does provide energy, insulation, and padding

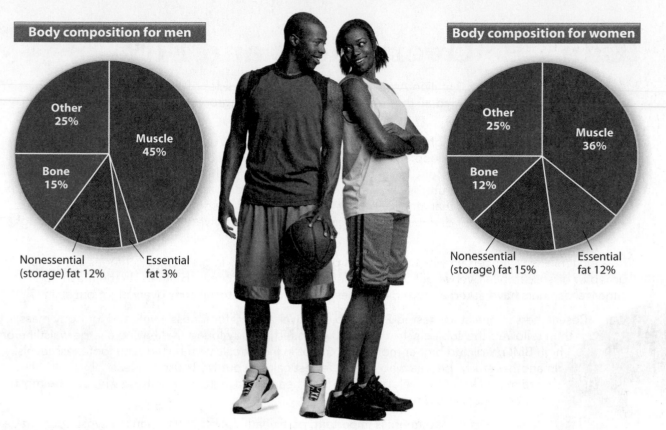

Body composition for men

Other 25%

Muscle 45%

Bone 15%

Nonessential (storage) fat 12%

Essential fat 3%

Body composition for women

Other 25%

Muscle 36%

Bone 12%

Nonessential (storage) fat 15%

Essential fat 12%

FIGURE **6.1**　The body compositions of typical 20- to 24-year-old men and women vary primarily in the amounts of muscle and essential fat.

Data from McArdle and others, *Exercise Physiology: Energy, Nutrition, and Human Performance.* 7th ed. (Baltimore, MD: Lippincott Williams & Wilkins, 2010).

This is a problem because childhood obesity significantly increases your risk for heart disease and premature death and disability in adulthood.[2,3] Over a ten year period (1999–2008), the number of overweight or obese adults in the United States grew from 64 percent to 68 percent of the population. Of those, 38 percent are classified as obese![4]

Studies of obesity, however, often rely on measurements of total body weight rather than measurements of body composition. While measurements of total body weight can be useful in studying large populations, they are less useful in assessing an individual's health risks and body changes. For individuals, estimates of body composition—specifically, of lean and fat mass—provide additional important information. By knowing your percent body fat, you can more effectively determine your risks for chronic disease and decide just how much weight you should try to lose (or gain).

Evaluating Your Body Size and Shape Can Help Motivate Healthy Behavior Change

If you are just beginning an exercise program for fitness, it is often more useful to assess changes in body size and shape as a measurement of your progress, rather than weighing yourself daily on a bathroom scale. The reason: Healthy increases in muscle tissue (achieved by exercise) may cause you to temporarily gain weight, until the process of body fat loss catches up with muscle tissue gains. This is a *good* thing, but you would not know it if you relied solely on the scale to determine your progress. By monitoring improvements in your body size and shape instead, you can get a more realistic sense of your achievement and stay motivated to stick with an exercise program. The box Can I Be Overweight and Fit? discusses overweight, disease, and fitness in more detail.

Can I Be Overweight and Fit?

A recent federal study of 2.3 million American adults analyzed decades of mortality data from people over age 25.[1] The study divided all the subjects into standard BMI groupings: underweight, normal weight, overweight, and obese.

The study found that underweight people had higher-than-standard death rates for non-cancer and non-CVD causes. Overweight people had higher rates for cancer, diabetes, and heart disease. Obese people had higher death rates for CVD and slightly higher rates for the cancers associated with body fat: colon, breast, esophagus, uterus, ovary, kidney, and pancreas. Overweight and obese people may even have lower death rates than normal-weight individuals for some non-cancer and non-CVD causes. However, when all causes of death were combined, their death rates were higher than in normal-weight individuals.

Researchers aren't yet certain why underweight people tend to die in greater percentages from one group of diseases while overweight and obese people tend to succumb to others. In the meantime, other researchers have asked a more direct question: Can you be technically overweight but still fit?

Researchers in one study tested 2,600 subjects over age 60 for fitness levels and for body mass, then followed the subjects' health for 20 years.[2] The study found that having a large waistline or high BMI predicted higher mortality, but not in individuals who tested high for fitness levels. In another study, people who ate the fewest calories but were also the least physically active were more likely to develop and die from heart disease than were those who ate the most calories but also did the most exercise.[3]

Research says that fitness is important, particularly for boys who want to avoid adult diabetes, but cardiorespiratory fitness has benefits, independent of fatness, on disease markers in all adolescents.[4,5] The evidence is strong that muscular and cardiovascular fitness helps protect us from illness and disease as we grow older, too. One study found that elasticity in large arteries is altered by fitness level but not obesity level. So, being fit can help offset some of the risks associated with obesity and blood vessel health.[6] And while BMI, according to another study, had the greatest effect on blood pressure results, even a moderate level of fitness was associated with the lowest blood pressure grouping.[7] Finally, exercise can have a positive effect on depression, no matter what your BMI.[8]

Fitness allows us to stay healthier, to maintain mobility, and to experience a higher quality of life. Do you feel energetic, get plenty of exercise, and have a high fitness level? If so, you can probably worry less about current definitions of "overweight" and "high BMI" and instead focus on continuing to maintain or increase your fitness level.

Sources:
1. K. M. Flegal and others, "Cause-Specific Excess Deaths Associated with Underweight, Overweight, and Obesity," *Journal of the American Medical Association* 298, no. 17 (2007): 2028–37.
2. X. Sui and others, "Cardiorespiratory Fitness and Adiposity as Mortality Predictors in Older Adults," *Journal of the American Medical Association* 298, no. 21 (2007): 2507–16.
3. J. Fang and others, "Exercise, Body Mass Index, Caloric Intake, and Cardiovascular Mortality," *American Journal of Preventative Medicine* 25, no. 4 (2003): 283–89.
4. D. M. Cummings and others, "Fitness versus Fatness and Insulin Resistance in U.S. Adolescents," *Journal of Obesity* (2010): 195729.
5. S. Kwon, T. L. Burns, and K. Janz, "Associations of Cardiorespiratory Fitness and Fatness with Cardiovascular Risk Factors among Adolescents: The NHANES 1999-2002," *Journal of Physical Activity and Health* 7, no. 6 (2010): 746–53.
6. K. Davison and others, "Relationships between Obesity, Cardiorespiratory Fitness, and Cardiovascular Function," *Journal of Obesity* (2010): 191253.
7. J. Chen and others, "Fitness, Fatness, and Systolic Blood Pressure: Data from the Cooper Center Longitudinal Study," *American Heart Journal* 160, no. 1 (2010): 166–70.
8. L. G. Perraton, S. Kumar, and Z. Machotka, "Exercise Parameters in the Treatment of Clinical Depression: A Systematic Review of Randomized Controlled Trials," *Journal of Evaluation in Clinical Practice* 16, no. 3 (2010): 597–604.

How Can I Evaluate My Body Size and Shape?

How do you determine whether your body size and shape are "healthy"? This is a much-debated topic, but there are three common methods of doing so: calculating your body mass index, measuring your body circumferences, and identifying the patterns of fat distribution on your body. (Evaluating your body composition is a somewhat more complicated process, which we discuss later in this chapter.)

Calculate Your Body Mass Index (BMI) But Understand Its Limitations

Body mass index (BMI) is one of the most common measurements that doctors and researchers use to assess risk of weight-related disease, death, and disability. BMI is a measurement based on your weight and height. You can calculate your BMI now, using the chart in Figure 6.2.

Weight (pounds)

Height (feet and inches)	100	110	120	130	140	150	160	170	180	190	200	210	220	230	240	250	260
4'6"	24	27	29	31	34	36	39	41	43	46	48	51	53	55	58	60	63
4'8"	22	25	27	29	31	34	36	38	40	43	45	47	49	52	54	56	58
4'10"	21	23	25	27	29	31	33	36	38	40	42	44	46	48	50	52	54
5'0"	20	22	23	25	27	29	31	33	35	37	39	41	43	45	47	49	51
5'2"	18	20	22	24	26	27	29	31	33	35	37	38	40	42	44	46	48
5'4"	17	19	21	22	24	26	28	29	31	33	34	36	38	40	41	43	45
5'6"	16	18	19	21	23	24	26	27	29	31	32	34	36	37	39	40	42
5'8"	15	17	18	20	21	23	24	26	27	29	30	32	33	35	37	38	40
5'10"	14	16	17	19	20	22	23	24	26	27	29	30	32	33	34	36	37
6'0"	14	15	16	18	19	20	22	23	24	26	27	29	30	31	33	34	35
6'2"	13	14	15	17	18	19	21	22	23	24	26	27	28	30	31	32	33
6'4"	12	13	15	16	17	18	20	21	22	23	24	26	27	28	29	30	32
6'6"	12	13	14	15	16	17	19	20	21	22	23	24	25	27	28	29	30
6'8"	11	12	13	14	15	17	18	19	20	21	22	23	24	25	26	28	29
6'10"	11	12	13	14	15	16	17	18	19	20	21	22	23	24	25	26	27
7'0"	10	11	12	13	14	15	16	17	18	19	20	21	22	23	24	25	26

Key:
- Underweight
- Normal weight
- Overweight
- Obese

FIGURE **6.2** Estimate your BMI by finding where your weight and height intersect.

BMI scores place individuals in categories as follows:[5]

Underweight (BMI of <18.5)

Normal weight (BMI of 18.5 to 24.9)

Overweight (BMI of 25.0 to 29.9)

Obese—Class I (BMI of 30.0 to 34.9)

Class II (BMI of 35.0 to 39.9)

Class III (BMI of >40.0)

Figure 6.3 on page 220 illustrates that very low and very high BMI scores are correlated with greater risk of death and disability.

The limitation with using BMI scores to assess "fitness" or "fatness" is that they do not differentiate between fat mass and lean mass. BMI is solely determined by height and weight. While BMI measurements can be helpful for individuals of average muscle and bone density, they can be misleading for athletes, bodybuilders, and short or petite individuals. For instance, someone who has an exceptionally heavy skeleton and larger-than-average muscle mass may have a BMI score that classifies him or her as "overweight," even if his or her percent body fat is in the "healthy" range. Because of BMI's limitations, it helps to also consider other factors, such as percent body fat, when assessing the overall picture of a person's fitness. **Lab 6.1** walks you through how to calculate your own BMI.

> **body mass index (BMI)**
> A number calculated from a person's weight and height that is used to assess risk for health problems

THINK! Do you think BMI will be a good predictor of body fitness and/or fatness for you? Why or why not?

ACT! Look at the ranges above and guess which BMI category you fall into. Why do you think you are in that range? Use the chart in Figure 6.2 or go to www.cdc.gov/healthyweight/assessing/bmi/index.html to check your estimate.

DO IT! ONLINE

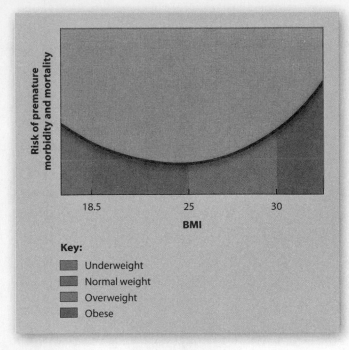

FIGURE **6.3** Extremely low or extremely high BMIs are associated with a greater risk of premature death and disability.

Data from Katherine Flegal and others, "Excess Deaths Associated with Underweight, Overweight, and Obesity," *Journal of the American Medical Association* 293, no. 15 (2005): 1861–67.

Key:
- Underweight
- Normal weight
- Overweight
- Obese

(chart axes: y = Risk of premature morbidity and mortality; x = BMI; 18.5, 25, 30)

Measure Your Body Circumferences

You can measure circumferences of various parts of your body to monitor your body's changes over time and to further assess your risk of disease. If you want to gain or lose weight, you can measure the circumference of your waist, hips, neck, upper arm, chest, thigh, and calf and then monitor changes in your body over time. You can also use waist and hip circumferences to assess disease risk. As shown in Table 6.1, waist circumference (a marker of abdominal fat) can indicate greater risk of diabetes, high blood pressure, and heart disease if it is greater than 102 cm in males or 88 cm in females.[6] As the table also shows, the people at greatest risk

waist-to-hip ratio (WHR) Waist circumference divided by hip circumference

android Body shape described as "apple-shaped," with excess body fat distributed primarily on the upper body and trunk

gynoid Body shape described as "pear-shaped," where excess body fat is distributed primarily on the lower body (hips and thighs)

subcutaneous fat Adipose tissue that is located just below the surface of the skin

visceral fat Adipose tissue that surrounds organs in the abdomen

are those with high waist circumferences *and* high BMIs.

You can also use waist and hip circumferences to determine your waist-to-hip ratio (WHR). **Waist-to-hip ratio** is your waist circumference divided by your hip circumference. A higher WHR is associated with more health risks. Young men with a WHR of 0.94 or more and young women with a WHR of 0.82 or more fall into a high-risk category.[7] **Lab 6.2** will walk you through the process of measuring your body circumferences and determining your WHR. Although waist circumference and WHR are both measures of disease risk, waist circumference is generally preferred because it is simpler, because of its relationship with abdominal fat, and because of its strong association to disease risk factors.[8]

DO IT! ONLINE

Identify Your Body's Patterns of Fat Distribution

Body fat distribution patterns are mostly genetically determined. You have probably noticed that people take after one parent in the way they "wear their fat." Some individuals tend to accumulate fat around their midsections; others collect it in the lower body or hips. These distributions contribute to an overall body shape that can be correlated to a higher or lower risk of disease.

The two most common body shapes are **android** ("apple-shaped") and **gynoid** ("pear-shaped") (Figure 6.4). A person with *android pattern obesity* has excess body fat on the upper body and trunk and has a greater risk of developing chronic disease than a person with *gynoid pattern obesity,* who carries excess body fat in the lower body. Higher waist circumferences due to excess abdominal fat are associated with higher levels of **subcutaneous fat** and **visceral fat**.[9] Although

TABLE 6.1 Waist Circumference, BMI, and Disease Risk

Weight Classification	BMI (kg/m²)	Waist Circumference and Disease Risk*	
		Smaller Waist Men ≤102 cm (40 in) Women ≤88 cm (35 in)	Larger Waist Men >102 cm (40 in) Women >88 cm (35 in)
Underweight	<18.5	—	—
Normal Weight	18.5–24.9	—	—
Overweight	25.0–29.9	Increased	High
Obese—I	30.0–34.9	High	Very High
Obese—II	35.0–39.9	Very High	Very High
Obese—III	>40.0	Extremely High	Extremely High

*Risk for type 2 diabetes, hypertension, and cardiovascular disease, relative to normal weight and waist circumference.

Source: Adapted from National Heart, Lung, and Blood Institute—Expert Panel on the Identification, Evaluation, and Treatment of Overweight in Adults, "Clinical Guidelines on the Identification, Evaluation, and Treatment of Overweight and Obesity in Adults: Executive Summary," *American Journal of Clinical Nutrition* 68 (1998): 899–917. Used with permission.

both are associated with metabolic diseases, fat in the abdominal cavity (visceral fat) has a stronger relationship to disease risk.[10] The good news is that a reduction in total body fat will result in reductions in subcutaneous fat, visceral fat, and disease risk.[11,12] While men tend to store fat in the abdomen and women tend to store it in the lower body, there are exceptions, and fat distribution is strongly influenced by genetics. If you have an "apple-shaped" body, understanding the health risks can help motivate you to keep your "apple" from getting too large and round!

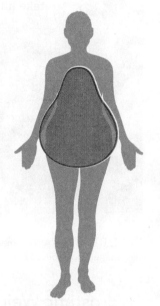

(a) Android ("apple-shaped") fat patterning

(b) Gynoid ("pear-shaped") fat patterning

FIGURE **6.4** (a) Android ("apple-shaped") fat distribution, associated with greater risk of heart disease and diabetes, is more common in men of all ages and postmenopausal women; (b) gynoid ("pear-shaped") fat distribution is more common in premenopausal women.

casestudy

JESSIE

"My friend Emily explained to me that I probably gained weight after starting my exercise program because I was building muscle faster than I was losing fat and that I shouldn't worry about it. She suggested that I check my body measurements instead of getting on the scale. I like that idea, and she offered to help, but now I am not sure which ones to do. My problem areas have always been my hips and thighs. Should I measure those areas and call it good?"

THINK! Why would body measurements/circumferences be a better way for Jessie to measure her progress than body weight? What body shape, gynoid or android, does Jessie most likely have? Does her shape increase or decrease her risk for disease?

ACT! Write out three of your "problem" body areas. Next to each indicate whether you want to increase or decrease your size.

What Methods Are Used to Assess Body Composition?

Unlike BMI and body circumference measurements, body composition (lean mass vs. fat mass) can only be estimated indirectly. A true, direct assessment of body composition requires dissection after death; in fact, researchers judge the accuracy of the indirect measures by comparing them with dissection results from cadavers.

Methods of estimating body composition range from assessments that trained fitness instructors can easily administer, such as skinfold measurements and bioelectrical impedance analysis, to sophisticated tests that must be conducted by clinicians in a lab or hospital setting. The most accurate estimates of body composition are body scans such as an MRI (magnetic resonance imaging) or a CT (computed tomography) scan. These are used in medical settings to diagnose injury and illness but are not often used for body composition analysis alone. In the next section, we discuss methods that are commonly used to assess body composition.

Skinfold Measurements

Skinfold measurements are an easy, inexpensive way to estimate your percent body fat. **Calipers** (shown in Lab 6.3) are used to measure the thickness of a fold of skin and subcutaneous adipose tissue. Skinfold measurements at specific sites around the body are recorded and entered into an equation that predicts percent body fat. This prediction of percent body fat has an error range of 3 to 4 percent;[13] for example, if your body fat measurement is 16 percent, the true value could be anywhere from about 12 to 20 percent.

More recent research has shown that current equations to predict body fat from skinfolds will underestimate percent body fat levels by about 1.3% in men and 3.0% in women (compared to DXA measured body fat levels), and may result in additional over- or underestimates for ethnically and racially diverse populations.[14] If you use this method to estimate your body

fat, remember it is just that—an estimate! **Lab 6.3** provides instructions for skinfold measurements. Performing an accurate skinfold assessment takes education and practice, so be sure to ask a qualified fitness instructor to help you.

Dual-Energy X-Ray Absorptiometry

Dual-energy X-ray absorptiometry (DXA) is the "gold-standard" reference method for body composition assessment in clinical and research settings (Figure 6.5). In a DXA scan, low-radiation X rays are used to distinguish fat, bone mineral, and bone-free lean components of the body. Measuring bone mineral (in addition to fat and lean mass) increases the accuracy of body fat estimates. In the medical setting, DXA scans are most often used to determine bone density for osteoporosis diagnosis. Body composition estimates can be obtained from whole body DXA scans that take less than 20 minutes. However, DXA tests are expensive, require a prescription for a medical X ray, and are not well designed to examine people who are extremely obese.

FIGURE **6.5** A DXA machine uses low-radiation X rays to determine body composition.

Hydrostatic Weighing

Hydrostatic weighing (also called *underwater weighing*) is widely used in research and college settings (Figure 6.6). In this method of body composition assessment, a person is first weighed outside a water tank and then weighed while completely submerged in the tank. Hydrostatic weighing is based on the concept that the more fat a person has, the more he or she will tend to float and the less weight he or she will exert against the bottom of the tank. From this process, a technician can assess total body volume and body density and use them to calculate

skinfold A fold of skin and subcutaneous fat that is measured with calipers to determine the fatness of a specific body area

calipers A handheld and spring-loaded instrument with calibrated jaws and a meter that reads skinfold thickness in millimeters

dual-energy X-ray absorptiometry (DXA) A technique using two low-radiation X rays to scan bone and soft tissue (muscle, fat) to determine bone density and to estimate percent body fat

hydrostatic weighing A technique that uses water to determine total body volume, total body density, and percent body fat

FIGURE **6.6** Hydrostatic (underwater) weighing uses total body water displacement to calculate estimated percent body fat.

an estimated percent body fat. The method is valid and reliable, but access to an equipped facility may be limited and not everyone is comfortable with being submerged.

Air Displacement (Bod Pod)

While hydrostatic weighing measures total body *water* displacement, the **Bod Pod** measures total body *air* displacement (Figure 6.7). The person being assessed puts on a swimsuit and then sits in the egg-shaped Bod Pod chamber while the air displacement is measured. The volume of air displaced is used together with other measures (such as weight) to determine total body volume and density and then to estimate percent body fat.

FIGURE **6.7** The Bod Pod uses total body air displacement to calculate estimated percent body fat.

Bod Pod percent body fat measurements are generally within 1–2% of hydrostatic weighing and DXA-measured levels of percent body fat.[15] Bod Pod measurements are available in many clinical and college settings, but availability in fitness settings is still somewhat limited.

> **Bod Pod** An egg-shaped chamber that uses air displacement to determine total body volume, total body density, and percent body fat
>
> **bioelectrical impedance analysis (BIA)** A technique that distinguishes lean and fat mass by measuring the resistance of various body tissues to electrical currents

Bioelectrical Impedance Analysis

In **bioelectrical impedance analysis (BIA)**, a machine measures the resistance of various body tissues to electrical currents. BIA machines send small electrical currents through the body via the hands, feet, or both (Figure 6.8). Fat does not conduct electricity very well, so fat tissues will demonstrate a resistance to the currents. Fat-free tissues have more body water and conduct electricity well; thus, fat-free tissues do not offer as much resistance to the currents. These resistance differences are used to estimate percent body fat. Higher resistance indicates higher levels of overall body fat. The error range of BIA is 3 to 4 percent, but accuracy depends upon the quality of the machine and upon the subject's following instructions, especially concerning his/her water intake.[16] Higher or lower levels of body water will significantly alter a BIA machine's results, so it is important to avoid drinking too much or too little prior to assessment.

FIGURE **6.8** Bioelectrical impedance analysis (BIA) machines measure the resistance of different body tissues to electrical currents. These measurements are then used to estimate percent body fat. A handheld BIA machine is shown here.

How Can I Change My Body Composition?

After you assess your body size, shape, and composition, the next steps are evaluation, goal setting, and (if your results are not within healthy ranges) planning for change.

Determine Whether Your Percent Body Fat Is within a Healthy Range

SEE IT! ONLINE

Normal
Weight
Obesity

Because people accumulate fat very differently and not all fat is the same, it is difficult to specify the exact level of body fat that is "healthy" or "unhealthy" for an individual. For instance, abdominal fat increases your risk for disease much more than fat on your calves does. Because of these differences, researchers do not agree upon desired body fat percentages for people of all ages, and you will find that research articles, books, and websites differ in their recommendations. Table 6.2 provides percent body fat norms.

Set Reasonable Body Composition Goals

You have many choices in setting body composition goals. If you are already in the healthy ranges, you can set additional goals for increasing lean mass or decreasing fat mass (within the low limits). Keep in mind that real body composition changes take time. Quick weight

casestudy

JESSIE

"A trainer at my gym gave me a skinfold test. I was amazed how much of my body is fat—50 lbs, wow! The trainer said that it sounds like a lot but it means my body fat is 31 percent and that is an okay number for my health. She did say she would help me with a program to reduce it though. We are planning to retest my skinfolds in three months to see how all of my exercise is paying off!"

THINK! What other methods could Jessie use to determine her body composition? What methods of assessing body composition are readily available to you?

ACT! Use one body composition measurement method to determine your body fat. Make a note in your calendar to get re-tested in 3 months to check your progress.

HEAR IT! ONLINE

· ·

loss is easier for those with more weight to lose, but most weight that is lost quickly consists of water and muscle—the very things you *don't* want to lose. To lose fat only, you have to be committed to exercise and slow, consistent weight loss. Aim for a body composition goal

TABLE 6.2 Percent Body Fat Norms for Men and Women*						
MEN						
Age	*Very Lean*	*Excellent*	*Good*	*Fair*	*Poor*	*Very Poor*
20–29	≤6%	7–10%	11–15%	16–19%	20–23%	≥24%
30–39	≤10%	11–14%	15–18%	19–21%	22–25%	≥26%
40–49	≤13%	14–17%	18–20%	21–23%	24–27%	≥28%
50–59	≤14%	15–19%	20–22%	23–24%	25–28%	≥29%
60–69	≤15%	16–20%	21–22%	23–25%	26–28%	≥29%
70–79	≤15%	16–20%	21–23%	24–25%	26–28%	≥29%
WOMEN						
Age	*Very Lean*	*Excellent*	*Good*	*Fair*	*Poor*	*Very Poor*
20–29	≤13%	14–16%	17–19%	20–23%	24–27%	≥28%
30–39	≤14%	15–17%	18–21%	22–25%	26–29%	≥30%
40–49	≤16%	17–20%	21–24%	25–28%	29–32%	≥33%
50–59	≤17%	18–22%	23–27%	28–30%	31–34%	≥35%
60–69	≤17%	18–23%	24–28%	29–31%	32–35%	≥36%
70–79	≤17%	18–24%	25–29%	30–32%	33–36%	≥37%

*Please note that there are no agreed-upon standards for recommended percent body fat; however, a range of 10–22% for men and 20–32% for women is considered healthy.

Adapted from American College of Sports Medicine, *ACSM's Guidelines for Exercise Testing and Prescription.* 8th ed. (Baltimore, MD: Lippincott Williams & Wilkins, 2010). Copyright © ACSM. Reprinted by permission of Wolters/Kluwer.

Will Spot Reduction Get Rid of My Belly Fat or Cellulite?

Have you ever thought, "I don't need to work on my whole body. I just need to lose some fat off my hips (or thighs or abdomen)!" Despite people's desire to spot-reduce and the multimillion-dollar industry it has spawned for ab-crunchers, thigh-slimmers, arm-toners, and cellulite creams, the answer is disappointingly simple: spot reduction doesn't work.

Researchers have punctured the spot-reduction myth with several carefully controlled studies and have verified that fat doesn't disappear through repeated exercise to one area. Instead, fat stores throughout the entire body dwindle when a negative caloric balance causes you to use up calories stored in fat tissue. In one study, researchers compared fat thickness in both arms of several tennis players. If anyone could work off fat selectively, it would be a tennis player, since he or she holds and swings a racquet thousands of times per week with the dominant hand and arm. The fat thickness, however, was identical in both arms.[1]

Research does show that laser therapy can spot-reduce fat and change body contours,[2] but in order to maintain such changes, the subject must make changes in diet and exercise. For most of us, it makes more sense to just go ahead and make the changes in diet and exercise and skip the time-consuming and expensive laser treatment!

You may be all too familiar with *cellulite*, a rippled appearance in the skin that typically appears around the buttocks and hips where fat deposits bulge. While no truly effective methods exist for getting rid of cellulite, tips for avoiding cellulite include:[3]

- Eating a healthy diet rich in fruits, vegetables, and fiber

- Staying hydrated with plenty of fluids

- Exercising regularly to keep muscles toned and bones strong

- Maintaining a healthy weight (no yo-yo dieting)

- Not smoking

The best strategy for reaching and maintaining a healthy body composition is still to exercise regularly—particularly with resistance training because you simultaneously strengthen and build lean tissue—and follow a structured diet.[4] If your calorie balance is also negative and you lose fat body-wide, your muscle definition will show more clearly, both in the offending spots and elsewhere as well!

Sources:
1. C. X. Bryant, "Why Is the Concept of Spot Reduction Considered a Myth?" *ACE FitnessMatters* 10, no. 1 (2004).
2. M. K. Caruso-Davis and others, "Efficacy of Low-Level Laser Therapy for Body Contouring and Spot Fat Reduction," *Obesity Surgery* 21, no. 6 (2010): 722–9.
3. National Library of Medicine, National Institutes of Health, Medline Plus, "Cellulite," www.nlm.nih.gov/medlineplus/ency/article/002033.htm, updated August 2011.
4. R. B. Kreider and others, "A Structured Diet and Exercise Program Promotes Favorable Changes in Weight Loss, Body Composition, and Weight Maintenance," *Journal of the American Dietetic Association* 111, no. 6 (2011): 828–43.

and a target weight that is healthy and that you can maintain for a lifetime. The box Will Spot Reduction Get Rid of My Belly Fat or Cellulite? discusses further the need for a whole-body approach to body composition.

Follow a Well-Designed Exercise and Nutrition Plan

Fad diets are just that: fads. Most of the time they do not work or only work for a short period of time. True body changes come from sticking with a carefully planned and executed nutrition and exercise program. This book will help you get started. For additional assistance, seek out qualified medical, nutrition, and fitness experts.

Monitor Your Body Size, Shape, and Composition Regularly

Stay motivated in your body change program by monitoring your progress regularly. Since body fat changes may take time, allow two to four months between body composition (percent body fat) assessments. Other types of

assessments can be done more frequently. Here is a suggested schedule:

- Body size/shape (mirror and fit of clothes)—assess daily or weekly
- Weight—assess weekly
- Circumferences—measure monthly (or less frequently)
- BMI—measure monthly (or less frequently)
- Percent body fat—measure every other month (or less frequently)

In addition to tracking these measurements, log how you're feeling. Remember, improving your body composition should help you feel good about yourself! The box Self-Esteem and Unhealthy Body Composition Behaviors talks about some problems to be watchful for.

Keep a separate log, journal, or notebook of your progress, but do not feel burdened by it. Some people are more motivated by journaling than others—find the monitoring system that works best for you, and use it consistently.

DIVERSITY

Self-Esteem and Unhealthy Body Composition Behaviors

Body composition can become a major problem for athletes in certain sports—not because they are too fat, but because they are too thin. This is true for both sexes, though the problem is more common in females, who are at risk of developing the female athlete triad (described below). Men may also develop disordered eating habits, as well as a body composition disorder known as muscle dysmorphia, in which men who are of normal weight and even unusually muscular think that they are "puny." (Muscle dysmorphia is discussed further in Chapter 8.) Some sports—gymnastics, figure skating, wrestling, ballet dancing, body-building—place a huge emphasis on appearance and having a lean body. The pressure to look lean and to weigh less can push athletes to cut back on what they eat and increase their workouts to the point where they lose too much weight.

An athlete's self esteem can make a big difference. Lower self esteem can lead to believing that life events are out of your control (external locus of control) and vice versa. One study has shown that if a female athlete has an internal locus of control (or belief that she has power

or control over her body and training), she will be more immune to coach and social pressures that can lead to disordered eating.[1] This can help her avoid the female athlete triad (see figure), a triangle of three interrelated problems: menstrual dysfunction, low bone density, and low energy availabilty as a result of disordered eating

Low energy availability

or eating disorders. In the triad, too little caloric intake coupled with too much exercise can lead to hormonal changes and the stopping of menstruation.[2] Improper nutrition, including too little calcium and vitamin D intake, can lead to altered hormones and to bone loss and a risk of fractures. Such changes taking place in adolescence or early adulthood can permanently reduce the size of a woman's skeleton and increase her lifelong risk for osteoporosis. In dancers, one study has shown that the triad negatively affects cardiovascular health.[3]

Athletes with low self-esteem and at high risk for the female athlete triad should carefully monitor their body composition, menstrual health, eating habits, and perhaps bone density. If the triad is suspected, the athlete should eat more nutritious food and/or exercise less, and may need to seek treatment for an eating disorder.

Sources:
1. S. Scoffier, Y. Paquet, and F. d'Arripe-Longueville, "Effect of Locus of Control on Disordered Eating in Athletes: The Mediational Role of Self-regulation of Eating Attitudes," *Eating Behaviors* 11, no. 3 (2010): 164–9.
2. A. M. McManus and N. Armstrong, "Physiology of Elite Young Female Athletes," *Medicine and Sport Science* 56 (2011): 23–46.
3. A. Z. Hoch and others, "Association between the Female Athlete Triad and Endothelial Dysfunction in Dancers," *Clinical Journal of Sport Medicine* 21, no. 2 (2011): 119–25.

chapterin**review**

videos

Log on to **www.pearsonhighered.com/hopson** or MyFitnessLab to view these chapter-related videos.

Measuring Hip-to-Waist Ratio   Skinfold Measurement   Normal Weight Obesity

onlineresources

Log on to **www.pearsonhighered.com/hopson** or MyFitnessLab for access to these book-related resources, and for links to other useful websites.

 Audio case study
Audio PowerPoint lecture

 Lab 6.1 How to Calculate Your BMI
Lab 6.2 How to Measure and Evaluate Your Body Circumferences
Lab 6.3 Estimate Your Percent Body Fat (Skinfold Test)

 Take Charge of Your Health! Worksheets
Behavior Change Log Book and Wellness Journal

 Pre- and post-quizzes
Glossary flashcards

reviewquestions

1. The proportion of your total weight that is fat is called
   a. body composition.
   b. lean mass.
   c. percent body fat.
   d. BMI.
2. Women have a greater amount of *essential fat* due to
   a. larger calves and thighs.
   b. their eating habits.
   c. less physical activity.
   d. reproduction-related fat deposits.

3. Which of the following statements about BMI is true?
   a. Your BMI is an estimate of your body fat percentage.
   b. BMI differentiates between lean mass and fat mass.
   c. Very low and very high BMI scores are associated with greater risk of mortality.
   d. BMI stands for "Basic Measure Indices."

4. Which of the following BMI ratings is considered "overweight"?
   a. 20 b. 25 c. 30 d. 35

5. Which of the following circumference measures indicates an increased risk of disease?
   a. A waist circumference over 100 cm for men and over 80 cm for women
   b. A waist circumference over 102 cm for men and over 88 cm for women
   c. A waist-to-hip ratio of 0.50 or higher
   d. A waist-to-hip ratio of 0.75 or higher

6. Which of the following body shapes or body fat distribution patterns is associated with an increased risk of heart disease and diabetes?
   a. Bell-shaped
   b. Android pattern obesity
   c. Pear-shaped
   d. Gynoid pattern obesity

7. Skinfold measurements are used to assess the amount of
   a. subcutaneous fat.
   b. visceral fat.
   c. essential fat.
   d. intramuscular fat.

8. Which of the following body composition measurement methods uses air displacement to estimate total body volume, density, and percent body fat?
   a. Bioelectrical impedance analysis
   b. Hydrostatic weighing
   c. The Bod Pod
   d. Skinfold measurement

9. Which body composition measurement method relies heavily on body water or hydration levels being normal (not too low or too high)?
   a. Bioelectrical impedance analysis
   b. Hydrostatic weighing
   c. The Bod Pod
   d. Skinfold measurement

10. The female athlete triad consists of the following interrelated issues:
    a. disordered eating, low bone density, and menstrual dysfunction.
    b. weak eyesight, poor nutrition, and brittle bones.
    c. low body weight, poor nutrition, and diabetes.
    d. excessive exercise, high blood pressure, and menstrual issues.

critical**thinking**questions

 REVIEW IT! ONLINE

1. Explain the usefulness and limitations of using BMI to determine fitness goals.

2. What factors should you consider when determining a healthy percent body fat range for yourself?

references

1. C. Ogden and M. Carroll, National Center for Health Statistics, Health E-Stats: "Prevalence of Obesity Among Children and Adolescents: United States, Trends 1963–1965 Through 2007–2008." www.cdc.gov, June 2010.

2. J. J. Reilly and J. Kelly, "Long-term Impact of Overweight and Obesity in Childhood and Adolescence on Morbidity and Premature Mortality in Adulthood: Systematic Review." *International Journal of Obesity (London)*. 35, no. 7 (2011): 891–8.

3. J. L. Baker, L. W. Olsen, and T. I. Sorensen, "Childhood Body-Mass Index and the Risk of Coronary Heart Disease in Adulthood," *New England Journal of Medicine* 357, no. 23 (2007): 2329–37.

4. K. M. Flegal and others, "Prevalence and Trends in Obesity Among US Adults, 1999–2008," *Journal of the American Medical Association* 303, no. 3 (2010): 235–41.

5. National Heart, Lung, and Blood Institute—Expert Panel on the Identification, Evaluation, and Treatment of Overweight in Adults, "Clinical Guidelines on the Identification, Evaluation, and Treatment of Overweight and Obesity in Adults: Executive Summary," *American Journal of Clinical Nutrition* 68, no. 4 (1998): 899–917.

6. Ibid.

7. V. H. Heyward, *Advanced Fitness Assessment and Exercise Prescription.* 6th ed. (Champaign, IL: Human Kinetics, 2010).

8. J. P. Reis and others, "The Relation of Leptin and Insulin with Obesity-Related Cardiovascular Risk Factors in U.S. Adults," *Atherosclerosis* 200, no. 1 (2008): 150–60.

9. A. Bosy-Westphal and others, "Measurement Site for Waist Circumference Affects Its Accuracy as an Index of Visceral and Abdominal Subcutaneous Fat in a Caucasian Population." *The Journal of Nutrition* 140, no. 5 (2010): 954–61.

10. C. S. Fox and others, "Abdominal Visceral and Subcutaneous Adipose Tissue Compartments: Association with Metabolic Risk Factors in the Framingham Heart Study." *Circulation* 116, no. 1 (2007): 39–48.

11. G. Fisher and others, "Effect of Diet with and without Exercise Training on Markers of Inflammation and Fat Distribution in Overweight Women." *Obesity (Silver Spring)* 19, no. 6 (2011): 1131–6.

12. B. H. Goodpaster and others, "Effects of Diet and Physical Activity Interventions on Weight Loss and Cardiometabolic Risk Factors in Severely Obese Adults: A Randomized Trial." *JAMA* 304, no. 16 (2010): 1795–802.

13. V. H. Heyward, *Advanced Fitness Assessment and Exercise Prescription* (2010).

14. A. S. Jackson and others, "Cross-validation of Generalised Body Composition Equations with Diverse Young Men and Women: The Training Intervention and Genetics of Exercise Response (TIGER) Study." *British Journal of Nutrition* 101, no. 6 (2009): 871–8.

15. D. A. Fields, M. I. Goran, and M. A. Mc-Crory, "Body-composition Assessment via Air-displacement Plethysmography in Adults and Children: A Review." *American Journal of Clinical Nutrition* 75, no. 3 (2002): 453–67.

16. V. H. Heyward, *Advanced Fitness Assessment and Exercise Prescription* (2010).

LAB 6.1 • HOW TO CALCULATE YOUR BMI

Name: _____ Date: _____

Instructor: _____ Section: _____

Purpose: To learn how to calculate your BMI.

Materials: Weight scale, measuring tape, calculator

SECTION I: CALCULATE YOUR BMI

1. Record your weight and height below:

Weight _____ lb   Height _____ inches

2. Convert your weight and height to metric units:

Weight _____ lb ÷ 2.2 = _____ kg

Height _____ inches × 2.54 = _____ cm ÷ 100 = _____ meters (m)

3. Calculate your BMI:

BMI = _____ ÷ [_____ × _____]
        (weight in kg)   (height in m)   (height in m)

BMI = _____ kg/m²

Note: Square the height (multiply by itself) before dividing into weight.

4. Indicate your BMI rating in the table below:

Weight Classification	BMI (kg/m2)
Underweight	_____ <18.5
Normal Weight	_____ 18.5–24.9
Overweight	_____ 25.0–29.9
Obese—I	_____ 30.0–34.9
Obese—II	_____ 35.0–39.9
Obese—III	_____ >40.0

SECTION II: REFLECTION

1. Is your BMI category what you thought it would be?

_____

2. Remember that BMI categories can be misleading for individuals with above-average muscle mass. Do you

fall into this category? _____

3. Monitoring changes to your BMI over time is one way to assess your progress with a fitness program. Two months after you begin a new exercise program, recalculate your BMI. Has it changed?

_____

LAB 6.2 • MEASURE AND EVALUATE YOUR BODY CIRCUMFERENCES

Name: _____   Date: _____

Instructor: _____   Section: _____

Purpose: To learn how to measure your body circumferences.

Materials: Measuring tape, partner

SEE IT! ONLINE

SECTION I: MEASURING CIRCUMFERENCES

Using a cloth or plastic tape measure, have a partner assist you with the following circumference measures. Be sure to mark your measurements (centimeters or inches) and record them to the nearest 0.5 cm or 0.25 inch.

Site	Description	Measurement
Waist	For those with a visible waist, measure at the narrowest part of the torso; for those with a larger torso, measure at the navel.	
Hip	Measure with the legs slightly apart. Measure where the hip/buttock circumference is the greatest.	
Upper Arm	Measure midway between the shoulder and elbow.	Right: Left:
Forearm	Measure at the greatest circumference between the wrist and elbow.	Right: Left:
Thigh	Measure with your leg on a bench or chair (knee at 90 degrees). Measure half way between the crease in your hip and your knee.	Right: Left:
Calf	Measure at the greatest circumference between the knee and ankle.	Right: Left:
Neck	Measure midway between the head and shoulders.	

Source: Adapted from American College of Sports Medicine, *ACSM's Guidelines for Exercise Testing and Prescription.* 8th Ed. (Baltimore, MD: Lippincott Williams & Wilkins, 2010).

SECTION II: EVALUATING CIRCUMFERENCES AND DISEASE RISK

1. Calculate your waist-to-hip ratio (WHR):

WHR = _____ ÷ _____

      (waist circumference)   (hip circumference)

WHR = _____

2. Evaluate your WHR using the table below:

Disease Risk and WHR				
Age (years)	Low	Moderate	High	Very High
<u>Men:</u> 20–29	<0.83	0.83–0.88	0.89–0.94	>0.94
30–39	<0.84	0.84–0.91	0.92–0.96	>0.96
40–49	<0.88	0.88–0.95	0.96–1.00	>1.00
50–59	<0.90	0.90–0.96	0.97–1.02	>1.02
60–69	<0.91	0.91–0.98	0.99–1.03	>1.03
<u>Women:</u> 20–29	<0.71	0.71–0.77	0.78–0.82	>0.82
30–39	<0.72	0.72–0.78	0.79–0.84	>0.84
40–49	<0.73	0.73–0.79	0.80–0.87	>0.87
50–59	<0.74	0.74–0.81	0.82–0.88	>0.88
60–69	<0.76	0.76–0.83	0.84–0.90	>0.90

Source: Reprinted with permission from V. H. Heywood, 2010, ADVANCED FITNESS ASSESSMENT AND EXERCISE PRESCRIPTION, 6th Edition. (Champaign: IL: Human Kinetics), 222.

Evaluate your waist circumference using the table below:

Waist Circumference (WC)		
Disease Risk Category	Women	Men
Very Low	<70 cm (<28.5 in)	<80 cm (<31.5 in)
Low	70–89 cm (28.5–35.0 in)	80–99 cm (31.5–39.0 in)
High	90–109 cm (35.5–43.0 in)	100–120 cm (39.5–47.0 in)
Very High	>110 cm (>43.5 in)	>120 cm (>47.0 in)

Source: From "Don't Throw the Baby Out with the Bath Water," George A. Bray, American Journal of Clinical Nutrition, 2004, Vol. 70, No. 3, pp. 347–349, by permission of the American Society for Nutrition.

3. Record your disease risk from WHR and waist circumference below:

Disease rating for WHR: _____

Disease rating for WC: _____

SECTION III: REFLECTION

1. Do your ratings for disease risk based upon circumferences surprise you? _____

2. Which of your circumference measures are you most interested in changing and why?

_____

LAB 6.3 • ESTIMATE YOUR PERCENT BODY FAT (SKINFOLD TEST)

Name: _____ Date: _____

Instructor: _____ Section: _____

Materials: Skinfold calipers, appropriate clothing (shorts, tank top, sports bra for women)

Purpose: To assess your current percent body fat.

Directions: Complete the sections below with a trained instructor.

SECTION I: SKINFOLD MEASUREMENT

You will need an experienced, trained instructor to complete your measurements. Note the time of day of your measurements and perform any follow-up measurements at the same time of day.

1. Identify the correct skinfold locations. If you are male, locate the chest, abdomen, and thigh locations (see photos below). If you are female, locate the triceps, suprailiac, and thigh locations (see photos). Your instructor should mark these locations on the right side of the body with a pen before using the caliper.

Chest	A diagonal fold measured midway between the shoulder/armpit crease and the nipple.	
Abdomen	A vertical fold measured one inch to the right of the navel.	

Thigh	A vertical fold measured midway between the crease in your hip and the top of your knee.	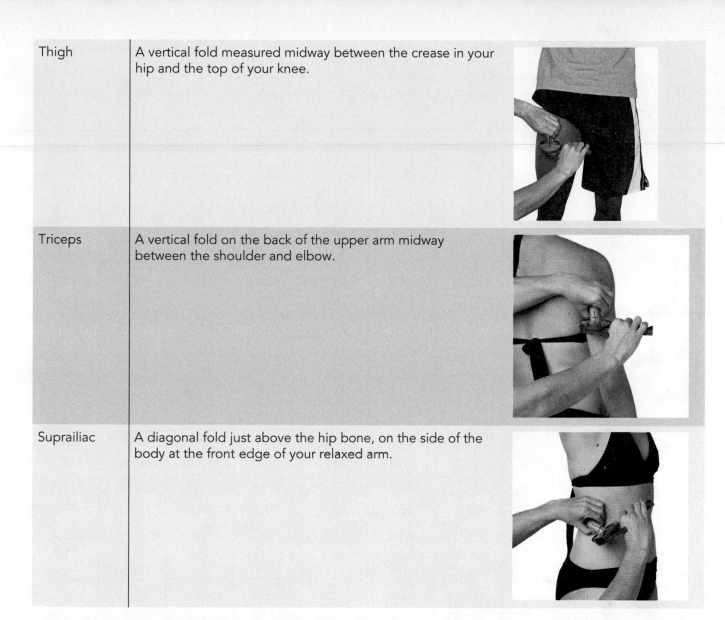
Triceps	A vertical fold on the back of the upper arm midway between the shoulder and elbow.	
Suprailiac	A diagonal fold just above the hip bone, on the side of the body at the front edge of your relaxed arm.	

Source: Adapted from American College of Sports Medicine, *ACSM's Guidelines for Exercise Testing and Prescription.* 8th ed. (Baltimore, MD: Lippincott Williams & Wilkins, 2010).

2. Your instructor will measure each skinfold location using the technique below. Record the results below and then add up the numbers for the three skinfold sites to obtain your overall skinfold sum.

Skinfold measurement technique: After locating the correct sites, grab a double fold of skin on both sides of the skinfold location. Open your fingers about three inches when lifting the fold (> than three inches is required for larger individuals). Holding the fold in place, pick up the calipers with your other hand. While still holding the fold, place the caliper jaws on the skinfold location, measuring halfway between the crest and the base of the fold. You should measure perpendicular to the fold and about one cm away from your fingers. Read the measurement two to three seconds after placing the calipers and record the skinfold numbers to the nearest 0.5 mm. For accuracy, measure each site three times and average the two closest numbers.

MEN			WOMEN		
Chest	_____	mm	Triceps	_____	mm
Abdomen	_____	mm	Suprailiac	_____	mm
Thigh	_____	mm	Thigh	_____	mm
Sum of 3 =	_____	mm	Sum of 3 =	_____	mm

3. Using the sum of three skinfolds, find your estimated percent body fat in the tables for women and men.

Sum of Skinfolds (mm)	Percent Body Fat Estimates for WOMEN (from triceps, suprailiac, and thigh skinfolds)								
	AGE (years)								
	Under 22	23–27	28–32	33–37	38–42	43–47	48–52	53–57	Over 57
23–25	9.7	9.9	10.2	10.4	10.7	10.9	11.2	11.4	11.7
26–28	11.0	11.2	11.5	11.7	12.0	12.3	12.5	12.7	13.0
29–31	12.3	12.5	12.8	13.0	13.3	13.5	13.8	14.0	14.3
32–34	13.6	13.8	14.0	14.3	14.5	14.8	15.0	15.3	15.5
35–37	14.8	15.0	15.3	15.5	15.8	16.0	16.3	16.5	16.8
38–40	16.0	16.3	16.5	16.7	17.0	17.2	17.5	17.7	18.0
41–43	17.2	17.4	17.7	17.9	18.2	18.4	18.7	18.9	19.2
44–46	18.3	18.6	18.8	19.1	19.3	19.6	19.8	20.1	20.3
47–49	19.5	19.7	20.0	20.2	20.5	20.7	21.0	21.2	21.5
50–52	20.6	20.8	21.1	21.3	21.6	21.8	22.1	22.3	22.6
53–55	21.7	21.9	22.1	22.4	22.6	22.9	23.1	23.4	23.6
56–58	22.7	23.0	23.2	23.4	23.7	23.9	24.2	24.4	24.7
59–61	23.7	24.0	24.2	24.5	24.7	25.0	25.2	25.5	25.7
62–64	24.7	25.0	25.2	25.5	25.7	26.0	26.2	26.4	26.7
65–67	25.7	25.9	26.2	26.4	26.7	26.9	27.2	27.4	27.7
68–70	26.6	26.9	27.1	27.4	27.6	27.9	28.1	28.4	28.6
71–73	27.5	27.8	28.0	28.3	28.5	28.8	29.0	29.3	29.5
74–76	28.4	28.7	28.9	29.2	29.4	29.7	29.9	30.2	30.4
77–79	29.3	29.5	29.8	30.0	30.3	30.5	30.8	31.0	31.3
80–82	30.1	30.4	30.6	30.9	31.1	31.4	31.6	31.9	32.1
83–85	30.9	31.2	31.4	31.7	31.9	32.2	32.4	32.7	32.9
86–88	31.7	32.0	32.2	32.5	32.7	32.9	33.2	33.4	33.7
89–91	32.5	32.7	33.0	33.2	33.5	33.7	33.9	34.2	34.4
92–94	33.2	33.4	33.7	33.9	34.2	34.4	34.7	34.9	35.2
95–97	33.9	34.1	34.4	34.6	34.9	35.1	35.4	35.6	35.9
98–100	34.6	34.8	35.1	35.3	35.5	35.8	36.0	36.3	36.5
101–103	35.3	35.4	35.7	35.9	36.2	36.4	36.7	36.9	37.2
104–106	35.8	36.1	36.3	36.6	36.8	37.1	37.3	37.5	37.8
107–109	36.4	36.7	36.9	37.1	37.4	37.6	37.9	38.1	38.4
110–112	37.0	37.2	37.5	37.7	38.0	38.2	38.5	38.7	38.9
113–115	37.5	37.8	38.0	38.2	38.5	38.7	39.0	39.2	39.5
116–118	38.0	38.3	38.5	38.8	39.0	39.3	39.5	39.7	40.0
119–121	38.5	38.7	39.0	39.2	39.5	39.7	40.0	40.2	40.5
122–124	39.0	39.2	39.4	39.7	39.9	40.2	40.4	40.7	40.9
125–127	39.4	39.6	39.9	40.1	40.4	40.6	40.9	41.1	41.4
128–130	39.8	40.0	40.3	40.5	40.8	41.0	41.3	41.5	41.8

Source: A. S. Jackson and M. L. Pollock, "Practical Assessment of Body Composition," *The Physician and Sportsmedicine* 13, no. 5 (1985): 76–90. Copyright © 1985 JTE Multimedia, LLC. Used with permission.

Sum of Skinfolds (mm)	Percent Body Fat Estimates for MEN (from chest, abdomen, and thigh skinfolds)								
	AGE (years)								
	Under 22	23–27	28–32	33–37	38–42	43–47	48–52	53–57	Over 57
8–10	1.3	1.8	2.3	2.9	3.4	3.9	4.5	5.0	5.5
11–13	2.2	2.8	3.3	3.9	4.4	4.9	5.5	6.0	6.5
14–16	3.2	3.8	4.3	4.8	5.4	5.9	6.4	7.0	7.5
17–19	4.2	4.7	5.3	5.8	6.3	6.9	7.4	8.0	8.5
20–22	5.1	5.7	6.2	6.8	7.3	7.9	8.4	8.9	9.5
23–25	6.1	6.6	7.2	7.7	8.3	8.8	9.4	9.9	10.5
26–28	7.0	7.6	8.1	8.7	9.2	9.8	10.3	10.9	11.4
29–31	8.0	8.5	9.1	9.6	10.2	10.7	11.3	11.8	12.4
32–34	8.9	9.4	10.0	10.5	11.1	11.6	12.2	12.8	13.3
35–37	9.8	10.4	10.9	11.5	12.0	12.6	13.1	13.7	14.3
38–40	10.7	11.3	11.8	12.4	12.9	13.5	14.1	14.6	15.2
41–43	11.6	12.2	12.7	13.3	13.8	14.4	15.0	15.5	16.1
44–46	12.5	13.1	13.6	14.2	14.7	15.3	15.9	16.4	17.0
47–49	13.4	13.9	14.5	15.1	15.6	16.2	16.8	17.3	17.9
50–52	14.3	14.8	15.4	15.9	16.5	17.1	17.6	18.2	18.8
53–55	15.1	15.7	16.2	16.8	17.4	17.9	18.5	19.1	19.7
56–58	16.0	16.5	17.1	17.7	18.2	18.8	19.4	20.0	20.5
59–61	16.9	17.4	17.9	18.5	19.1	19.7	20.2	20.8	21.4
62–64	17.6	18.2	18.8	19.4	19.9	20.5	21.1	21.7	22.2
65–67	18.5	19.0	19.6	20.2	20.8	21.3	21.9	22.5	23.1
68–70	19.3	19.9	20.4	21.0	21.6	22.2	22.7	23.3	23.9
71–73	20.1	20.7	21.2	21.8	22.4	23.0	23.6	24.1	24.7
74–76	20.9	21.5	22.0	22.6	23.2	23.8	24.4	25.0	25.5
77–79	21.7	22.2	22.8	23.4	24.0	24.6	25.2	25.8	26.3
80–82	22.4	23.0	23.6	24.2	24.8	25.4	25.9	26.5	27.1
83–85	23.2	23.8	24.4	25.0	25.5	26.1	26.7	27.3	27.9
86–88	24.0	24.5	25.1	25.7	26.3	26.9	27.5	28.1	28.7
89–91	24.7	25.3	25.9	26.5	27.1	27.6	28.2	28.8	29.4
92–94	25.4	26.0	26.6	27.2	27.8	28.4	29.0	29.6	30.2
95–97	26.1	26.7	27.3	27.9	28.5	29.1	29.7	30.3	30.9
98–100	26.9	27.4	28.0	28.6	29.2	29.8	30.4	31.0	31.6
101–103	27.5	28.1	28.7	29.3	29.9	30.5	31.1	31.7	32.3
104–106	28.2	28.8	29.4	30.0	30.6	31.2	31.8	32.4	33.0
107–109	28.9	29.5	30.1	30.7	31.3	31.9	32.5	33.1	33.7
110–112	29.6	30.2	30.8	31.4	32.0	32.6	33.2	33.8	34.4
113–115	30.2	30.8	31.4	32.0	32.6	33.2	33.8	34.5	35.1
116–118	30.9	31.5	32.1	32.7	33.3	33.9	34.5	35.1	35.7
119–121	31.5	32.1	32.7	33.3	33.9	34.5	35.1	35.7	36.4
122–124	32.1	32.7	33.3	33.9	34.5	35.1	35.8	36.4	37.0
125–127	32.7	33.3	33.9	34.5	35.1	35.8	36.4	37.0	37.6

Source: A. S. Jackson and M. L. Pollock, "Practical Assessment of Body Composition," *The Physician and Sportsmedicine* 13, no. 5 (1985): 76–90. Copyright © 1985 JTE Multimedia, LLC. Used with permission.

4. Record your estimated percent body fat and rating.

% body fat = _____

Indicate your body fat rating below:

Body Fat Rating	WOMEN	MEN
Athletic/Low	14–20%	6–13%
Fitness	21–24%	14–17%
Acceptable	25–31%	18–25%
Obese	>32%	>26%

Source: From "Percent Body Fat Norms for Men and Women" in ACE LIFESTYLE AND WEIGHT MANAGEMENT COACH MANUAL. Reprinted with permission from the American Council on Exercise® (ACE®), www.acefitness.org.

SECTION II: REFLECTION

1. Did your estimated percent body fat or rating surprise you? _____

2. How does your percent body fat rating compare with your other disease risk ratings from Lab 6.2?

_____

7 Improving Your Nutrition

Learning Outcomes

1. Describe ways to maintain a healthy diet during the college years and throughout your lifetime.

  Audio case study and audio Power-Point lecture

2. Identify the main nutrients in food and their roles in the body.

  How Much Sugar?

3. Discuss the role of portion size, food labels, food groups, and whole foods in maintaining a balanced diet.

 Lab 7.1 Reading a Food Label

  Going Green

4. Describe the special dietary needs of elite athletes, women, children, adults over 50, and vegetarians.

5. Examine your own specific nutritional needs.

6. Assess your current diet.

 Lab 7.2 Keeping a Food Diary and Analyzing Your Daily Nutrition

7. Create a plan for improved nutrition.

 Lab 7.3 Improving Your Nutrition

 Take Charge of Your Health! worksheets and Behavior Change Logs for logging eating habits and creating a change plan

  You Are What You Eat?

Pre- and post-quizzes and glossary flashcards

237

casestudy

CHAU

"Hi, I'm Chau. I'm a freshman and I live on campus in a dorm with my roommate, Tom. I moved here to Connecticut from Chicago. Living away from home for the first time has been quite an experience! I've been studying hard, taking a full load of classes, and trying to figure out if I want to major in history or political science. Plus, I'm in a few clubs and I'm playing a lot of soccer. I'm not on the team, but I like to play for fun. I'll jump into just about any pick-up game if I have time. I'm always rushing, though, and then I realize I'm starving! When I lived at home, there was always food around. My meal plan at the cafeteria covers 60 meals a month. For the others, I'm often scrambling at the last minute to find something to eat."

HEAR IT! ONLINE

H unger is one of our basic motivators. Eating—seeing, smelling, and tasting foods—is one of life's great pleasures. Hunger compels us to seek and consume the food that will supply our bodies with energy and raw materials. The pleasure of eating compels us to find the foods we enjoy or even crave. Our challenge is to eat a healthy balance of foods we need and foods we want to eat.

Food contains **nutrients**, chemical compounds that supply the energy and raw materials for

survival. Our cells break down food molecules and, in the process, change their shapes and release energy stored in their chemical bonds. The energy becomes available to drive the activities within our cells, tissues, and organs. The breakdown of nutrients also liberates raw materials that cells can take in, modify, and use in repair and growth.

Nutrition is the study of how people consume and use the nutrients in food. Nutrition researchers explore some of the basic questions about what we should be eating and how food affects our long-term health and disease. Is it better to eat butter or margarine? Should you drink tea, coffee, both, or neither? Should you take a daily vitamin pill? Is red meat okay? How much salt is too much?

Nutritional findings are sometimes contradictory. Since the 1970s, consumers have been advised to throw away butter and use margarine instead; then to do just the reverse; then to avoid almost all fats; then to avoid almost all carbohydrates, and so on. Understandably, some people have grown skeptical about nutritional information. As in every area of science, new studies in nutrition occasionally contain data that appear to invalidate older studies. Nevertheless, the field has made tremendous advances toward understanding our daily **diets**—the foods and drinks we select—as well as what we *should* be eating, what we should be *avoiding*, and why. The kinds of healthy diets we discuss in this chapter can help you stay fit and well. Keep in mind:

- A balanced diet helps sustain desirable body mass and weight and helps keep your fat-to-lean ratios within a recommended range. This, in turn, can improve appearance, make you more comfortable in your body, and reduce the risk of chronic illnesses related to excess weight and obesity.

- A good diet can help alleviate feelings of stress and depression, while a poor diet can contribute to them.

- A good diet can help prevent chronic diseases, frequent colds and infections, and the effects of vitamin deficiency. Conversely, poor diet is one of the biggest contributors to cardiovascular disease, diabetes, obesity, arthritis, osteoporosis, and several types of cancers.

If you are young and currently well, any of the above conditions may seem improbable and remote. However, the dietary habits you establish now either diminish or promote your later risk for all types of chronic illness. Optimal fitness and wellness—both now and in your future—requires good nutrition and good **eating habits**. This chapter shows you how to analyze and improve both.

---

nutrients Chemical compounds in food that are crucial to growth and function; include proteins, carbohydrates (starches and sugars), lipids (fats and oils), vitamins, and minerals

nutrition The study of how people consume and use the nutrients in food

diets The foods and drinks we select to consume

eating habits When, where, and how we eat; with whom we eat; what we choose to consume; and our reasons for choosing it

---

Why Are My College Years a Nutritional Challenge?

If you are like most college students, you often reach for cheap snacks and fast food to save time and money. You grab something tasty. You eat it quickly, maybe even while you walk or drive to the next class, job, study session, or social event. You may worry about calories and weight. But most students don't think much about vitamins, minerals, and other nutrients or worry much about the challenge of eating well during the college years.

The typical student's diet resembles the typical American diet: nearly one-third of Americans' total calories come from chips, cookies, donuts, desserts, French fries, candy bars, sugary drinks, beer, wine, and other alcoholic beverages.[1] The number-one takeout food is pizza, followed by Chinese food and fast food (burgers, fries, and so on). Other favorite "staples" of the American diet are coffee drinks, tacos, burritos, sandwiches, and salads. The most frequently eaten vegetables in America are iceberg lettuce and potatoes.[2]

Most Students Have Less-than-Optimal Eating Habits

Eating habits describe when, where, and how we eat; with whom we eat; what we choose to consume; and our reasons for choosing it. Like most Americans, college students, in general, have poor eating habits. Examples of poor eating habits are eating fast food and eating while driving or watching television. Good eating habits include sitting down to a relaxed meal and consuming fresh fruits and vegetables every day. How are your eating habits? Figure 7.1 can help you find out.

Less healthy eating habits	More healthy eating habits
Consuming sugary soft drinks with and between meals	Drinking water with and between meals
Skipping meals then gorging once or twice per day	Eating three meals plus one or two small, nutritious snacks at regular times
Eating large amounts of red meats, fatty meats, or fried meats	Choosing fish, lean poultry, tofu, or other proteins that are low in saturated fats
Choosing processed foods	Choosing whole foods such as fruits, vegetables, whole grains, nuts, seeds, and lean sources of protein
Hurriedly bolting down food on the run, in a car, on a bike	Sitting down to eat a relaxed meal with friends or family
Finishing the large portions served at restaurants	Eating half of a large restaurant portion and taking the rest home
Snacking before bed	Eating earlier in the evening
Eating heartily to be social, regardless of appetite	If you're not very hungry, drinking a low-cal beverage or eating a piece of fruit to be social
Eating out of habit or boredom, for example, while watching TV	Sitting down at a table to eat only when hungry, finding another outlet for boredom
Reaching for food when feeling stressed or angry	Learning stress reduction techniques

FIGURE **7.1** You can examine your own eating and snacking habits by comparing what, when, where, and how much you eat and drink to the sliding scale for each habit. You can also get ideas here for improving your daily diet.

Adapted from U.S. Department of Agriculture and U.S. Department of Health and Human Services, *Dietary Guidelines for Americans, 2010*, 7th Edition, "Chapter 5: Building Healthy Eating Patterns" (Washington, DC: U.S. Government Printing Office, 2010): 43–54.

Results of the American College Health Association's 2010 annual survey of nearly 96,000 students from colleges and universities throughout the United States highlighted the dietary deficiencies of today's students.[3] Taking produce as an example, only about 6 percent consumed the recommended five servings of fruits and vegetables each day. Fifty-eight percent reported eating only one to two servings each day, and 30 percent consumed three to four servings. Like their older counterparts, young adults report that they are interested in improving their health, yet they fall far short of the mark in meeting national dietary guidelines. It is no wonder that the term "Freshman 15" has become common language among students to describe the excess weight gain they often experience freshman year.

Good information and understanding can make a measurable difference in students' nutritional wellness, including the amount of weight they gain. The information throughout this book, especially in this chapter and in our discussion of weight management, can help you in the same ways.

THINK! How many servings of fruits and vegetables do you eat per day? One? Two? Five or more?

ACT! If you eat fewer than five servings a day, what specific things can you do to increase that number?

College Life Presents Obstacles to Good Nutrition

Food is easy to find in the many vending machines, cafeterias, bars, restaurants, and markets on campus and off. But nutritious foods—low in saturated fat, salt, and sugars, for instance, and high in fiber and vitamin content—are much harder to find on and near campus. Food choice is an important obstacle to student nutrition. There are other obstacles as well: time and money pressures, lack of home-cooking facilities, personal habits and attitudes, and the emotional stresses college can present.

Fast food and takeout appear to solve both time and money issues, but the food at these restaurants often provides poor nutrition. Even when students cook for themselves, however, nutritional misconceptions and a tight budget can still impede a good diet. If you do shop and cook, a few simple steps can help you achieve a healthy affordable diet: Buy fruits and vegetables that are in season. Watch for sales, use coupons, and shop at discount stores. Make a shopping list and stick to it. Buy

more plant proteins (e.g., beans and tofu) and less meat, fish, or poultry. And if possible, double your recipes and freeze portions for later.

Another obstacle to good nutrition is our natural human craving for sweet, fatty, salty, and high-protein foods. We love those treats! Students sometimes come to college with preexisting preferences and eating habits and then, away from parental influence for the first time, tip over into unhealthy dietary routines such as regularly eating junk food, skipping breakfast, snacking frequently, and limiting fruit and vegetable consumption.

Meal skipping or protein loading can also be an offshoot of body dissatisfaction at a time when social interaction and physical attractiveness are emphasized. Three-fifths of female college students and half of males are dissatisfied with their body size and

casestudy

CHAU

"I like eating in the dorm cafeteria but I have to take care of about 30 meals on my own each month. The idea was that I'd eat two meals a day in the dorm—probably breakfast and dinner—and grab lunch somewhere between classes. So far, though, it's not quite working out that way. On days when I don't have an early class, I tend to sleep through breakfast. Then, I've got to rush to my 11:00, which means grabbing donuts and coffee in the campus store. Sometimes I manage to get back to the dorm for lunch, but if I don't, I usually eat something on the run at the food court. The good thing is that my dorm has a late night café that accepts my meal plan. So if I'm up late studying, I can grab a pizza or bowl of cereal. I don't pay much attention to my diet or how many calories I'm eating. I figure at my age, it's more about getting enough calories then eating a 'balanced meal.' Doesn't it all kind of balance out naturally?"

THINK! What aspects of college life are influencing Chau's dietary choices? How does your own living situation and schedule affect your efforts to eat right?

ACT! Make a list of small lifestyle changes you could make to improve your diet and try to incorporate at least one in the coming week, another the following week.

Tips for Ordering at Restaurants

No matter what type of cuisine you enjoy, there will always be healthier and less healthy options on the menu. To help you order wisely, here are lighter options and high-fat pitfalls. "Best" choices contain fewer than 30 grams of fat, a generous meal's worth for an active, medium-sized woman. "Worst" choices have up to 100 grams of fat.

Cuisine	Best	Worst	Tips
Italian	Pasta with red or white clam sauce Spaghetti with marinara or tomato- and meat sauce	Eggplant parmigiana Fettucine Alfredo Fried calamari Lasagna	Stick with plain bread instead of garlic bread made with butter or oil. Avoid cream- or egg-based sauces. Try vegetarian pizza, and don't ask for extra cheese.
Mexican	Bean burrito (no cheese) Chicken fajitas with lots of vegetables	Beef chimichanga, deep fried Chile relleno, battered and fried	Choose soft tortillas (not fried) with fresh salsa, not guacamole. Order grilled shrimp, fish, or chicken. Ask for black or pinto beans made without lard or fat. Avoid cheeses and sour cream or ask for them on the side.
Chinese	Hot- and-sour soup Stir-fried vegetables Shrimp with garlic sauce Szechuan shrimp Wonton soup	Crispy chicken Kung pao chicken Moo shu pork Sweet-and-sour pork	Share a stir-fry. Request brown rice instead of white. Ask for vegetables steamed or stir-fried with less oil. Avoid fried rice, breaded dishes, egg rolls and spring rolls, and items loaded with peanuts or cashews. Avoid high-sodium sauces.
Japanese	Steamed rice and vegetables Tofu as a meat substitute Broiled or steamed chicken and fish	Fried rice dishes Miso Tempura	Avoid soy sauces. Avoid deep-fried dishes such as tempura. Eat sashimi and sushi (raw fish) only where the food is freshly made to avoid possible bacteria or parasites.
Thai	Clear broth soups Stir-fried chicken and vegetables Grilled meats	Coconut milk soup with chicken Peanut sauces for satay Deep-fried or batter-fried meats and vegetables	Avoid coconut-based soups and curries. Ask for steamed, not fried, rice. Try for brown rice rather than white. Avoid Thai iced tea, which is filled with sugar and high-fat evaporated milk.
American Breakfast	Hot or cold cereal with nonfat or one percent milk Pancakes or French toast with syrup Scrambled eggs with hash browns and plain toast	Belgian waffle with sausage Sausage and eggs with biscuits and gravy Ham-and-cheese omelet with hash browns and toast	Ask for whole-grain cereal or shredded wheat with two percent milk. Ask for whole wheat toast without butter or margarine. Order omelets without cheese. Order fried eggs without bacon or sausage.
Sandwiches	Veggies and tofu spread Roast beef Turkey	Tuna salad Reuben Submarine	Ask for mustard. Hold the mayonnaise and high-fat cheese.
Seafood	Broiled bass, halibut, or snapper Grilled scallops Steamed crab or lobster	Fried seafood platter Blackened catfish	Order fish broiled, baked, grilled, or steamed—not pan fried or sautéed. Ask for lemon instead of tartar sauce. Avoid creamy and buttery sauces.
Fast Food	Grilled chicken sandwich Lean roast beef sandwich Entrée salad, dressing on the side Water, nonfat or one percent milk, unsweetened iced tea Fresh fruit and yogurt	Extra-large or double-patty sandwiches Added cheese French fries and onion rings Fried chicken Fish fillets Chicken nuggets Apple pie Colas	Order sandwiches without mayo or special sauce. Avoid deep-fried items.

● ● ● ● **TOOLS FOR CHANGE** ●

shape.[4] Most students want to lose weight, while a few want to gain weight or add muscle. Body dissatisfaction leads some students to skip meals; avoid particular classes of foods such as fats or carbohydrates; go on drastic very-low-calorie diets; or take other measures that can cause an imbalance of nutrients, vitamins, and minerals.

Stress and social eating are additional contributors to poor diet. Stress itself can cause people to eat more, especially high-calorie "comfort" foods. Stress can also reduce sleep, which can lead to using food, caffeine, sugar, and alcohol to alter mood and energy levels. People under stress also tend to seek out the relief of socializing for relaxation, and when people get together, they eat and drink. The box Tips for Ordering at Restaurants describes healthy and unhealthy food items on a wide variety of menus.

Research shows that when nutritious foods are readily available in a cafeteria setting, many students will choose them. For example, in one study male students chose more fruits and vegetables and leaner meats in dormitory dining halls than did males eating in apartments, in restaurants, and so on.[5] Female students eating in dining halls chose amounts of fruit closer to USDA recommendations. However, although free choice in cafeteria lines does seem to encourage better nutrition for many students, it can still lead to consuming too many calories. There are several keys to overcoming the food obstacles of college life:

- Learn about nutrition and what your body needs to maintain maximum wellness.

- Learn to distinguish good food choices from poor ones and good eating habits from bad ones.

- As often as possible, frequent those restaurants, stores, and cafeterias that offer a wide selection of healthy foods.

- Improve your eating habits and hang out with other students who care about nutritious eating.

What Are the Main Nutrients in Food?

We humans share the need to "refuel" with every other kind of animal, from soaring eagles to drifting sea cucumbers. Our bodies can't originate energy-containing raw materials for activity, growth, and repair. Like all animals, we must obtain these compounds from foods and liquids in sufficient quantities to supply our daily needs. Our required nutrients are water, proteins, carbohydrates (starches and sugars), lipids (fats and oils), vitamins, and minerals (Figure 7.2). Within each class of nutrients, the three-dimensional molecular shapes of the individual kinds of sugars, fats, and so on, determine the

FIGURE **7.2** The six groups of essential nutrients in our foods provide energy, facilitate vital activities, and supply needed fluid for cells and tissues.

nutrients' unique chemical properties and in turn, their roles in the body.

Nutritionists use the term **essential nutrients** for those compounds we must get from foods in order to maintain normal body functioning. Our bodies chemically modify and use nutrients to build the thousands of components we need to allow our muscles to contract, our nerves to conduct, our cells to divide, and so on. Consuming nutrients keeps our internal "production line" efficiently manufacturing cell parts and usable energy compounds.

Nutritionists can measure the nutrients in individual foods—the natural sugars and starches in an apple, for example. They can measure the energy stored within those carbohydrates. And they can study the way our bodies release that stored energy during the digestion process. They measure the released energy in **calories**. One calorie (with a lowercase *c*) is the amount of energy required to raise the temperature of 1 gram of water 1 degree Celsius. When they refer to specific foods, nutritionists usually apply the larger measure **kilocalories (kcal)** or **Calories (C)**. One kilocalorie or Calorie (spelled with a capital *C*) equals 1,000 calories. A small-sized apple, for example, about the size of a tennis ball might have about 50 or 60 C.

To avoid confusion, this book will use "calories" when referring to food energy in general as well as when designating the energy in a specific food. Active adults need about 2,000 to 2,500 calories of food energy per day.

Proteins Are Building Blocks of Structure and Function

About 50 to 60 percent of your body weight is water; of the remainder, about half is protein. At 150 pounds, your body would contain about 75 pounds of water and about 37.5 pounds of protein, depending on your muscle mass. **Proteins** are major structural components of nearly every cell and are especially important to the building and repairing of bone, muscle, skin, and blood cells. Proteins are also critical to cell and body functioning: They make up the antibodies that protect us from disease, the enzymes that control all chemical reactions in the body, and many types of hormones that regulate body activities. Proteins also help transport oxygen, carbon dioxide, and various nutrients to body cells. When the body runs low on fats and carbohydrates as sources of ready energy, it can break down its own proteins as well. Protein supplies four calories of energy per gram.

Protein molecules are chains of subunits called *amino acids.* Sometimes called the "building blocks of life," amino acids contain carbon, hydrogen, oxygen, and nitrogen arrayed in particular ways. There are 20 different kinds of amino acids, each with a different three-dimensional shape. Your body uses the 20 types of amino acids to build tens of thousands of kinds of proteins. Many of these are *structural proteins* that make up parts of cells, tissues, and organs. Many kinds of structural proteins enable cells to move, to divide, and to transport materials around internally. Other structural proteins make up your hair strands, your fingernails and toenails, and the lenses of your eyes. A steady supply of amino acids in the diet allows your body to continuously build, repair, and replace its own structural proteins.

Proteins that perform crucial functions (rather than make up physical structures) are called *functional proteins* and include **enzymes**. Enzymes are proteins that enable thousands of kinds of chemical reactions to occur simultaneously within each body cell every second, including the enzyme reactions that break down food, absorb nutrients, and build new cell parts.

Proteins in the Diet Our bodies can manufacture only 11 of the 20 kinds of amino acids. Nutritionists call the other nine, which we must consume in food, the **essential amino acids**. Dietary protein that supplies all the essential amino acids is called *complete protein,* or *high-quality protein.* Typically, protein from animal products is complete. *Incomplete proteins* lack some of the essential amino acids and therefore some of the building blocks we need to produce the full spectrum of proteins for growth, repair, and activity.

essential nutrients Nutrients necessary for normal body functioning that must be obtained from food

calories A measure of the amount of chemical energy that foods provide. One calorie (lowercase *c*) can raise 1 gram of water 1 degree Celsius.

kilocalories (kcal) or **Calories (C)** A measure of energy equal to one thousand calories; also designated kilocalorie (kcal); nutritionists use kcal or C when they refer to specific foods.

proteins Biological molecules composed of amino acids. Proteins serve as crucial structural and functional compounds in living organisms.

enzymes Proteins that facilitate chemical reactions but are not permanently altered in the process; biological catalysts

essential amino acids Collectively, the nine of the 20 types of amino acids, or building blocks, that our bodies cannot manufacture and that we must consume in our foods

Proteins from plant sources are often incomplete, lacking one or two of the essential amino acids. Nevertheless, it is fairly easy for a vegetarian to combine plant foods to obtain *complementary proteins* from plant sources (Figure 7.3). Eating peanut butter on whole grain bread is one good example of combining plant foods to get all the essential amino acids. Eating corn and beans together is another.

Daily Protein Needs Nutritionists typically recommend that you get about 10 percent of your calories (or about 200 calories or more) from protein in a 2,000-calorie diet. Over a billion of the world's people face daily protein deficiency, but few Americans suffer it. The average American consumes between 60 and 100 grams (250 to 400 calories or more) of protein daily,

with as much as 70 percent of it coming from animal parts and products and dairy products high in saturated fats. Consuming too much protein, particularly animal protein, can place added stress on the liver and kidneys and can cause a painful disease called *gout*. An overload of protein may also increase calcium excretion in urine, which can increase your risk of bone loss and bone fractures.[6]

Use Figure 7.4 to calculate your daily protein needs. Here's an example: A healthy young woman weighing 132 pounds (60 kg) would need about 48 grams (60 × 0.8). One gram is equal to 0.035 ounce; therefore, she would need about 1.68 ounces of protein (0.035 × 48 = 1.68), which she could get, for example, by consuming 1 cup of skim milk, 3 ounces of chicken breast, and 3 ounces of salmon during the course of a day.

In recent years, millions of people have tried the Atkins diet and similar diets that nearly eliminate carbohydrates and prescribe large quantities of protein. While these diets *can* lead to weight loss, the dieter is losing weight due to total calorie reduction, not due to some magical property of dietary protein itself. Diets that are not nutritionally balanced are almost always flawed. People with fluid imbalances, kidney or liver problems, or cardiovascular disease should avoid these diets altogether, as they raise risk factors for various chronic diseases. Others who choose to try such unbalanced diets should limit the length of time they follow them.

Protein and Fitness It is fairly common for athletes and fitness buffs to load up on animal protein under the misguided notion that eating more protein will cause them to build bigger muscles. But muscles grow in response to being worked: you must use them to grow them! The many vegetarian Olympic athletes are proof that training and effort—not mountains of animal protein—are the crucial ingredients. Research has also shown that 1.0 gram/kg of protein is enough for all but the top athletes, most of whom can get all they need for heavy endurance and strength training in 1.5 to 1.6 g/kg/day.[7]

It's true that under some circumstances, you may need extra protein for cellular repair and replacement, such as when you are fighting off a serious infection, or if you are a pregnant woman. Most of us, though, need to be much more concerned with getting *low-fat* proteins than with meeting our daily protein needs.

Legumes and grains

+

Legumes and nuts and seeds

+

Green leafy vegetables and grains

+

Green leafy vegetables and nuts and seeds

FIGURE **7.3** Combining plant foods from different groups (for example, grains and legumes) on the same day can provide complementary proteins and all the necessary amino acids, even without eating meat or other animal foods.

Group	Daily protein requirement (g/kg body weight)		Calculating your daily protein requirement	Example (for average adult)
Most adults	0.8 g/kg		① Determine your body weight	① Weight = 132 lb
Recreational athletes	1.0 –1.1 g/kg		② Convert pounds to kilograms: lb ÷ 2.21 lb/kg = kg	② 132 lb ÷ 2.21 lb/kg = about 60 kg
Elite athletes in training	1.2 –1.6 g/kg		③ Multiply by 0.8 g/kg for average adult to get requirement in grams per day	③ 60 kg × 0.8 g/kg = 48 g Result: a 132 lb adult would need 48 grams of protein a day

FIGURE **7.4**   Use these formulas to determine your daily protein requirements, depending on your activity level.

Carbohydrates Are Major Energy Suppliers

Carbohydrates, including the sugars and starches, have ring- and chain-like three-dimensional structures that allow them to store and supply much of the energy we need to sustain normal daily activity. The **simple carbohydrates** or **sugars** are common in whole, unprocessed foods such as beets, sugarcane, carrots, other vegetables, and fruits such as grapes (Figure 7.5a). The **complex carbohydrates** include the starches found abundantly in grains (such as rice and wheat); cereals (such as oats); some fruits and vegetables (such as bananas and squash); and many root vegetables (such as potatoes, yams, and turnips) (Figure 7.5b).

Our cells can rapidly break down sugar molecules and release energy stored in their chemical bonds. For this reason, sugars such as glucose, sucrose (table sugar), and lactose (milk sugar) are a source of immediate energy for the body. Your muscle cells and your brain and nerve cells are particularly dependent on a steady supply of glucose, whether from fruits and vegetables or from the starches in grains. This dependence is the reason low blood sugar, or *hypoglycemia*, can leave you feeling foggy-headed, weak, and shaky. According

carbohydrates A class of nutrients containing sugars and starches; supply most energy for daily activity

simple carbohydrates or **sugars** Carbohydrates made up of one or two sugar subunits that deliver energy in a quickly usable form

complex carbohydrates Energy-storing and structural compounds made up of long chains of sugar molecules; most deliver energy slowly

Glucose, a simple sugar

(a)

Starch, a complex carbohydrate

(b)

FIGURE **7.5**   (a) Grapes are rich in glucose, a simple sugar. (b) Bananas contain starch, a complex carbohydrate.

Sweeteners: A Health Primer

Full-Calorie Sweeteners

The average American consumes more than 355 calories (more than 22 teaspoons per day) of sugars such as honey, corn syrup, or sucrose (table sugar) added to their foods and beverages. Most of this is in processed foods. Sweeteners can boost flavor, texture, and bulk. However, added sugars have health consequences: they add calories but virtually no other nutrients. They promote tooth decay. They tend to replace more nutritious foods in the diet such as fruits, vegetables, seeds, nuts, and whole grains. And they raise triglyceride levels in the blood; this, in turn, can contribute to cardiovascular disease.[1] The American Heart Association recommends a maximum daily limit of 100 calories of added sugars (the equivalent of six teaspoons of sugar) for most women, and 150 calories (equivalent to nine teaspoons) for most men.[2]

SEE IT! ONLINE
How Much Sugar?

Reduced-Calorie Sweeteners

Many products that claim to be "low in sugar" or "sugar free" include sugar alcohols: carbohydrates with a sweet flavor and a particular type of chemical structure. Examples of these ingredients include mannitol, sorbitol, xylitol, and hydrogenated starch hydrolysates. The products sometimes contain non-nutritive sweeteners, as well (see below). These "dietetic" foods do provide fewer calories—only about half of the calories in regular sweeteners—but can still be significant calorie and carbohydrate sources, depending on how much you consume.[3] They typically cost more, and to make them taste good, the manufacturers often add fat. Be sure to scan such food labels for these sweeteners as well as for *trans* fats and saturated fats.

Non-nutritive Sweeteners

Artificial sweeteners contain synthetic compounds or chemicals derived from naturally occurring herbs or sugars. The products in this class are intensely sweet and provide essentially no calories. Most "sugar free" gums and beverages, for example, contain an artificial sweetener such as aspartame (Equal, NutraSweet); sucralose (Splenda); neotame; acesulfame potassium (Sunett, Sweet One), or saccharin (Sugar Twin, Sweet'N Low). A recently released product, Truvia, contains the sweet-tasting nonnutritive compound rebiana derived from the leaves of the stevia plant. In addition to rebiana, Truvia contains a sugar-alcohol (see above). Despite some concerns about the safety of nonnutritive sweeteners based on experiments feeding animals with saccharin, health agencies including the National Cancer Institute find no sound scientific evidence that artificial sweeteners raise cancer risk or promote other serious health problems. Some researchers, however, have suggested an association between weight gain and artificial sweetener use, for unknown reasons.[4]

Sources:
1. Mayo Clinic Staff, "Added Sugar: Don't Get Sabotaged by Sweeteners," MayoClinic Online, www.mayoclinic.com/health/added-sugar/MY00845 (November 2010).
2. American Heart Association, "Sugars and Carbohydrates," www.heart.org /HEARTORG/GettingHealthy/NutritionCenter/HealthyDietGoals/Sugars-and-Carbohydrates_UCM_303296_Article.jsp (updated October 2010).
3. American Diabetes Association, "Sugar Alcohols," www.diabetes.org/food-and-fitness/food/what-can-i-eat/sugar-alcohols.html (accessed September 2011).
4. Mayo Clinic Staff, "Artificial Sweeteners: Understanding These and Other Sugar Substitutes," Mayo Clinic Online, www.mayoclinic.com/health/artificial-sweeteners /MY00073 (October 2010).

• •

to research outlined in the USDA's *2010 Dietary Guidelines for Americans*, most of us consume a diet that is too heavy in added sugars and other sweeteners. The box Sweeteners: A Health Primer explains how to recognize the many kinds of sweeteners listed on food labels and why we should limit our consumption of sweetened food.

Starches and other complex carbohydrates (also called *polysaccharides*, meaning "many sugars") can be a source of "timed release"

fiber Indigestible carbohydrates in the diet that speed the passage of partially digested food through the digestive tract

energy. The body's cells must break starch molecules down into sugar subunits before releasing the chemical bond energy contained in those sugars. This slower breakdown makes most starches important energy-storage compounds and structural building materials in plants and animals.

Fiber Horses and cows can survive on grass and hay alone because their digestive systems break down and derive energy from *cellulose* (a structural carbohydrate that makes up the cell walls of plants). In humans, cellulose acts as indigestible **fiber** in one of two forms. _Insoluble fiber,_ found in bran, whole grain breads and cereals, and in most fruits and vegetables, speeds the passage of foods and reduces bile acids and certain bacterial enzymes. _Soluble fiber,_ which is in oat bran, dried beans, and some fruits and vegetables, attaches to water molecules. Soluble fiber appears to help lower blood cholesterol levels and the risk of cardiovascular disease. Both kinds of fiber assist the passage of partially digested food through the digestive tract. They also help control appetite and body weight by creating a feeling of fullness without adding extra calories.

While the evidence of a link between fiber consumption and reduced cancer risk is weak, eating fiber-rich foods is still recommended because they contain other nutrients that may help reduce cancer risk and have other health benefits.[8] Fiber also helps prevent constipation by absorbing moisture like a sponge and producing softer, bulkier stools that are easily passed. Fiber-induced gas may also initiate bowel movements. Reducing constipation helps protect against diverticulosis—the formation of tiny pouches in the colon that bulge out through the intestinal wall like bubbles protruding through holes in a tire. These pouches tend to get inflamed and can cause intestinal pain, bloating, bleeding, blockages, and other symptoms.

The USDA's _2010 Dietary Guidelines for Americans_ recommends that we make at least half of our daily consumption of grains whole grain foods such as whole oats, whole wheat, and brown rice, and decrease our consumption of refined carbohydrates such as white flour, white bread and sandwich buns, and white rice. Table 7.1 lists many whole and refined grains. For tips on how to increase the fiber in your diet, see the box Tips for Eating More Fiber.

TABLE 7.1 Whole Grains and Refined Grains

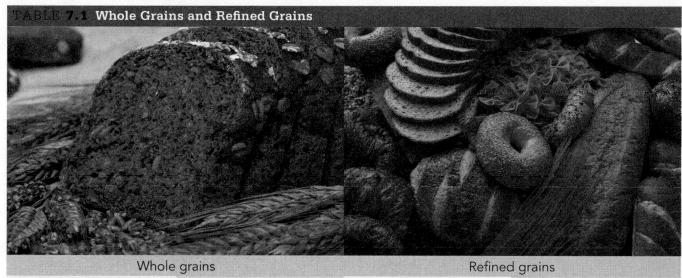

Whole grains		Refined grains	
brown rice	whole wheat bread	cornbread*	pitas*
buckwheat	whole wheat crackers	corn tortillas*	pretzels
bulgur (cracked wheat)	whole wheat pasta	couscous*	white bread
oatmeal	whole wheat sandwich	crackers*	white sandwich buns and
popcorn	buns and rolls	flour tortillas*	rolls
whole grain barley	whole wheat tortillas	grits	white rice
whole grain cornmeal	wild rice	noodles*	
whole rye		pasta*	_Ready-to-eat breakfast_
	Less common whole		_cereals:_
Ready-to-eat breakfast	_grains:_		corn flakes
cereals:	amaranth		
whole wheat cereal flakes	millet		
muesli	quinoa		
	sorghum		
	triticale		

*Most of these products are made from refined grains. Some are made from whole grains. Check the ingredient list for the words "whole grain" or "whole wheat" to decide whether they are made from a whole grain. Some foods are made from a mixture of whole and refined grains.

Source: USDA, "Food Groups: Grains," www.choosemyplate.gov/foodgroups/grains.html (modified June 2011).

Tips for Eating More Fiber

Most Americans should double their daily fiber intake. To increase the fiber in your diet, think "whole" and "traditional" foods instead of refined foods and choose more of these:

- Whole grains, including stone-ground wheat, bulgur wheat, wheat bran, wheat berries, whole barley, whole millet, whole quinoa, oatmeal, oat bran, popcorn, barley, cornmeal, whole rye, brown rice, and rice bran

- Peas, beans, nuts, and seeds

- Leafy greens such as baby spinach, endive, radicchio, arugula, mizuna, watercress, or dandelion greens

- Bran or flaxseed

- Fresh fruits and vegetables including, when edible, their cleanly scrubbed skins

- Plenty of liquids each day

At the same time, choose fewer of these:

- White bread, buns, or flour tortillas

- Cereals that list "enriched" flour as the main ingredient

- Cookies, pastries, desserts, candies

The daily recommended amount of fiber for an adult is 25 to 30 grams, but most Americans get less than that amount.[9] Some professional groups believe the requirements should be higher, perhaps even double the recommended amount. Food labels must list the fiber contents of foods and often break that number down into insoluble and soluble fiber.

The Glycemic Index of Foods Nutritionists use a tool called the **glycemic index** to measure the rate at which foods raise levels of glucose in the blood. If you eat food with a high glycemic index, especially in large portions, your bloodstream becomes flooded with glucose, and this, in turn, leads to an upsurge of the hormone insulin. The combination of glycemic index plus portion size is called *glycemic load*. Over time, this flooding and surging can contribute to being overweight and to type 2 diabetes, heart disease, and obesity.[10]

Using the glycemic index of foods to control the amount of sugar in your bloodstream requires some practice. A glycemic index chart can help you predict the effect a given food will have on your blood sugar levels. Note that not all sweet foods have a high index and many starchy or fatty foods do. See this book's website for links to these charts. The glycemic index of foods can help you plan a healthy diet, but it is just one factor to consider because some low–glycemic index foods are poor nutritional choices overall (i.e., premium ice cream, sausages) and some high–glycemic index foods are good choices overall (i.e., bran flakes, watermelon). The best approach to control your sugar intake is to develop a habit of reading food labels before you buy or eat something to discover the amount of dietary sugars in foods. Then, use glycemic index and glycemic load charts to help you get a feel for which foods raise your blood sugar levels quickly and which do not.

"Low-Carb" Foods In recent years, food manufacturers have introduced thousands of "low-carb" foods, influenced, in part, by the popularity of high-protein weight loss diets. As we've seen, however, whole grain foods are packed with healthful nutrients and fiber. The culprit is not the "carbs" themselves but the quantity most people eat and the refining of the carbohydrates. Whole fruits and vegetables, and foods made with whole grains, seeds, and nuts, are nutrient-dense and retain the fibrous cellulose in their skins and husks. Most "low-carb" foods are highly processed and contain substitute sugars such as mannitol, sorbitol, and dextrose. There is no solid evidence that "low-carb" products made with sweeteners protect you from diseases, and they cost much more than simple fruits, vegetables, whole grains, nuts, seeds, and beans.

glycemic index A measurement of the rate at which foods raise levels of glucose in the blood and, in turn, trigger the release of insulin and other blood-sugar regulators

Fats Are Concentrated Energy Storage

The "low-carb" diet craze was preceded by a "low-fat" craze that labeled all fats and oils as harmful. In fact, fats play vital roles in maintaining healthy skin and hair, padding the body organs against shock, insulating us against temperature extremes, storing energy to fuel muscle activity, and promoting healthy cell function. Although they are widely misunderstood nutrients, fats make foods taste better, carry the fat-soluble vitamins A, D, E, and K to cells, and provide certain essential compounds we can't get from other foods or manufacture in our own cells. They also provide a concentrated form of energy and raw materials that can stand in whenever carbohydrates are in short supply.

Types of Fats *Fat* is a common term for **lipids**, a class of molecules that includes fats and oils. **Fats**, such as butter, lard, and bacon grease, are solid at room temperature. **Oils** are usually liquid at room temperature; examples are corn and olive oils. Lipids also include *waxes*, such as beeswax, and *steroids*, such as steroid hormones, cholesterol, and certain vitamins.

Structurally, fats and oils are made up of long chains of carbon atoms, usually an even number between 4 and 28 linked in a chain. These chains are called **fatty acids**. The fatty acids in most foods and in the body occur in the form of **triglycerides**, molecules that have a "head," which contains the compound glycerol, and three tails (Figure 7.6a). The "tails" are made up of fatty acid chains of various lengths.

In lipid molecules of all types, the chemical bonding of carbon atoms is the key to whether the chains remain straight and form solid fats, or kink and form liquid oils. (Figure 7.6 b) Carbon atoms can form four bonds to other atoms. Where carbons are linked to each other in a chain (—C—C—), each carbon has two bonds left over,

$$
\begin{array}{cccc}
| & | & | & \\
C & -C & -C & -C \\
| & | & | &
\end{array}
$$

and these often link to hydrogen atoms:

$$
\begin{array}{cccc}
H & H & & \\
| & | & | & \\
C & -C & -C & -C \\
| & | & & \\
H & H & &
\end{array}
$$

In a fatty acid chain where every available carbon bond is *saturated* or filled with hydrogen atoms, the fat itself is called a **saturated fat**. Saturated chains remain straight and can pack solidly against each other. This explains why butter, beef fat, and lard—all saturated fats—occur as solids at room temperature (Figure 7.6c).

In an oil, there are also chains of carbon atoms, but at certain spots, the carbons have two bonds to other carbons (—C=C—). As a result, they have fewer bonds left over and can't be saturated or filled with hydrogen molecules at these points. The chains are said to be **unsaturated**. These double-bonded spots also cause the chains to kink and bend. Because the chains can't pack tightly together, they create a liquid oil rather than a solid fat. Fatty acid chains containing just one kinked (unsaturated) region are called **monounsaturated fatty acids (MUFAs)** (*mono* means "one"). Olive oil, canola oil, and cashew oil are all high in monounsaturated fatty acids. Chains containing two or more linked regions are called **polyunsaturated fatty acids (PUFAs;** *poly* means "many"). Corn oil, safflower oil, and cottonseed oil are all high in polyunsaturated fatty acids (Figure 7.6d).

Food manufacturers sometimes alter the properties of oils by adding hydrogen atoms to liquid oils, a process called hydrogenation. This results in partially hydrogenated oils that contain some *trans* fatty acids or **trans fats**. These have cooking properties of solid fats as well as their potentially negative effects on

lipids A category of compounds including fats, oils, and waxes that do not dissolve in water

fats Lipids, such as butter, lard, and bacon grease, which are usually solids at room temperature

oils Lipids, such as corn and olive oil, which are usually liquid at room temperature

fatty acids The most basic units of triglycerides

triglycerides Lipid molecules made up of three fatty acid chains or "tails" attached to one glycerol "head" containing a three-carbon backbone; common form of fats in foods and in organisms

saturated fat A lipid, usually a solid fat such as butter, in which most of the chains of carbon atoms are loaded (or "saturated") with as many hydrogen atoms as the chain can carry

unsaturated fat A lipid, usually a liquid oil, in which most carbon chains lack the maximum load of hydrogen atoms

monounsaturated fatty acids (MUFAs) Lipids whose fatty acid chains have just one kinked (unsaturated) region

polyunsaturated fatty acids (PUFAs) Lipids whose fatty acid chains have two or more kinked (unsaturated) regions

trans fats Unsaturated lipids or oils with hydrogen atoms added to cause more complete saturation and make the oil function as a solid

Triglyceride

Glycerol (head) — Fatty acid chains (tails)

(a)

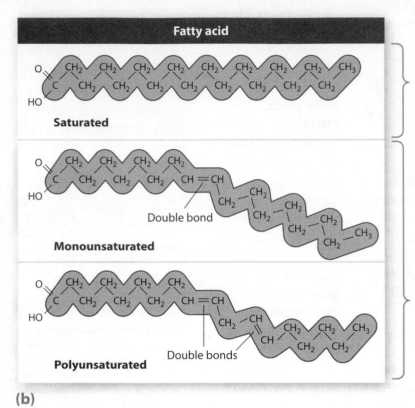

Fatty acid

Saturated

Double bond

Monounsaturated

Double bonds

Polyunsaturated

(b)

Long-chain saturated fatty acids lack double bonds and have straight carbon chains. They pack together to make solid forms at room temperature.

(c)

Mono- and polyunsaturated fatty acids can kink and bend at the double bond in the chain. Kinked chains slide past each other and act as liquid oils.

(d)

FIGURE **7.6** (a) Structure of triglyceride. (b) The chemical makeup of fatty acid chains in fats and oils helps explain why saturated fats (c) such as lard or butter are usually solid, and why mono- and polyunsaturated fats (d) such as olive and corn oil are usually liquids.

Adapted from NUTRITION: AN APPLIED APPROACH, 1st Edition, by Janice Thompson and Melinda Manore, © 2005. Reprinted by permission of Pearson Education, Inc., Upper Saddle River, NJ.

health. Margarines, shortenings, and many processed foods contain *trans* fats. Nutritionists often recommend that you eliminate or decrease foods containing *trans* fats from your diet. The *trans* fat content of foods is now indicated on food labels. We will discuss the health consequences of eating *trans* fats later.

All of our food sources of fats and oils contain both saturated and unsaturated fats, in different ratios (Figure 7.7). For example, a tablespoon of safflower oil contains 0.8 gram saturated fat, 10.2 grams of monounsaturated fat, and 2 grams polyunsaturated fat. A tablespoon of butter typically contains 7.2 grams saturated fat, 3.3 grams monounsaturated fat, and a trace of polyunsaturated fat. In general, lipids high in saturated fats are unhealthy for you, especially if you eat them frequently. While animals tend

to make saturated fats and plants tend to make unsaturated fats, some plants generate oils that are very high in saturated fats. Cocoa butter, palm kernel oil, and coconut oil contain more saturated fat per tablespoon than butter, beef fat, or lard! Since lipids high in mono- and polyunsaturated fats are much healthier for you than those high in saturated fat, it pays to learn about the types of oils so you can choose wisely. Figure 7.7 shows the oils containing the widest purple and red bands (which designate mono- and polyunsaturated fatty acids) are the healthiest. The fats and oils with the widest blue bands (designating saturated fatty acids) are the least healthy.

Omega-3 and Omega-6 Fatty Acids There are some types of fatty acids that our cells cannot construct and therefore we must consume in our diet. These fatty

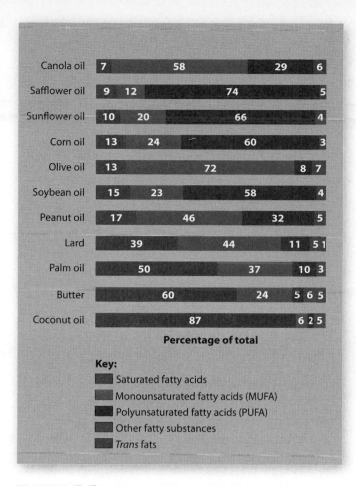

FIGURE **7.7** Common fats and oils have varying percentages of saturated and unsaturated fats, making them more or less healthful in the diet.

Key:
- Saturated fatty acids
- Monounsaturated fatty acids (MUFA)
- Polyunsaturated fatty acids (PUFA)
- Other fatty substances
- *Trans* fats

acids are called **essential fatty acids**. They include *linoleic acid,* an omega-6 fatty acid, and *linolenic acid,* an omega-3 fatty acid. An **omega-6 fatty acid** is polyunsaturated and has double-bonded carbons at two sites, including one at the sixth carbon along the carbon chain. An **omega-3 fatty acid** has double-bonded carbons at three sites, including one at the third carbon along the chain. Other omega-3 fatty acids include EPA and DHA, which the human body can modify into linolenic acid. Polyunsaturated oils such as canola oil, corn oil, soybean oil, and sunflower oil all contain high levels of omega-6 fatty acids. Polyunsaturated oils such as flaxseed oil, walnut oil, and, to a lesser degree, certain fish oils, canola oil, and soybean oil contain relatively high percentages of omega-3 fatty acids. The body can modify both types of essential fatty acids into various fats we need for blood clotting, building cell membranes in the brain, protecting against heart disease by contributing to healthy blood vessel walls, and by helping to prevent inflammatory bowel disease and other autoimmune diseases.[11]

Dietary Fats and Your Health As your body breaks down the fats and oils in the food you eat, it packages the lipids into particles called **lipoproteins** that can move along easily in the bloodstream. Lipoproteins contain lipid and protein portions, and carry both triglycerides and **cholesterol**, the most common steroid in the body (recall that steroids are one structural class of fats). Our cells need and make cholesterol to keep membranes pliable and use it as a building block for making steroid hormones and other substances. In common usage, lipoproteins carrying cholesterol are simply called *cholesterol.*

Eating saturated fat and *trans* fat raises the level of **low-density lipoproteins** (also called **LDLs** or "bad cholesterol") in your bloodstream. Over time, elevated levels of LDLs can lead to plaque deposits inside the blood vessels. These plaques can constrict blood flow, raise blood pressure, and lead to heart disease, heart attacks, and strokes. Eating saturated fat also raises the level of **high-density lipoproteins** (HDLs or "good cholesterol") in the blood, but to a lesser degree. HDLs prevent and reduce plaque deposits in the blood vessels and therefore help protect against cardiovascular disease, strokes, and heart attacks.

You may be wondering how something the human body makes

essential fatty acids Lipid components, including linolenic acid, EPA, DHA, and linoleic acid, which the body cannot manufacture and which we must obtain in polyunsaturated oils

omega-6 fatty acid A polyunsaturated fatty acid that has double-bonded carbons at two sites, including one at the sixth carbon along the chain

omega-3 fatty acid A polyunsaturated fatty acid that has double-bonded carbons at three sites, including one at the third carbon along the chain

lipoproteins Lipid-plus-protein transport particles that can move along easily in the bloodstream; carry triglycerides or cholesterol

cholesterol A waxy lipid in the steroid class that is an important component of cell membranes and is transported in the blood by carriers called *LDL* and *HDL*

low-density lipoproteins (LDLs) A form of lipoprotein sometimes called "bad cholesterol;" LDL levels rise in response to saturated fats in the diet and can contribute to plaque deposits inside blood vessels

high-density lipoproteins (HDLs) A form of lipoprotein sometimes called "good cholesterol;" HDL levels rise in response to polyunsaturated fats and prevent and reduce plaque deposits in the blood vessels and needs for its own cell membranes and hormones can be harmful in the diet. When some people consume cholesterol, their body cells make less cholesterol and their overall level stays constant. In other people, however, that "leveling mechanism" works inefficiently, and they tend to accumulate the extra dietary cholesterol in blood-vessel-narrowing plaques.[12] To be safe, the USDA recommends that you consume less cholesterol in the diet by cutting back on fatty meats, egg yolks, high-fat dairy products, and all sources of saturated or trans fats.

Research shows that *trans* fatty acids can be even more damaging than saturated fats. *Trans* fats increase LDLs and simultaneously lower HDLs, a doubly negative effect. A person who gets just two percent of his or her calories from *trans* fats would be raising his or her risk for heart disease by 23 percent and for sudden cardiac death by 47 percent.[13] The USDA recommends choosing products with little or no *trans* fats.[14] In fact, the USDA's ChooseMyPlate.gov website—which provides specific daily food recommendations based on your sex, size, age, and activity level—now classifies *trans* fats along with saturated fats and sugars as "empty calories." The site suggests you restrict your overall daily consumption of such empty calories to 260 per day (if you are a woman between 19 and 30) and to 330 per day (if you are a man in that same age group).

Trans fats also raise triglyceride levels. After a meal, the liver takes cholesterol and triglycerides that we don't use immediately in our tissues, packages them into HDLs and LDLs, and sends them through the blood to be stored in fat cells.[15] Coincidentally, consuming large quantities of refined starches, sugars, and/or alcohol also raises blood triglycerides. This helps explain why eating big helpings of such starches and sugars, as so many Americans do, can lead to obesity, diabetes, and heart disease.

Eating mono- and polyunsaturated fats lowers LDLs and raises HDLs, a doubly positive effect. As Figure 7.7 showed, most kinds of cooking oil are high in mono- and polyunsaturated fats and low in saturated fats, but there are exceptions, such as palm kernel oil and coconut oil. That's one reason it is important to read food labels rather than make assumptions about the fats in particular foods.

Some nutritionists encourage people to consume more oils. A popular plan called the Mediterranean diet encourages people to use olive oil liberally in cooking and at the table. Nutritionists from Harvard Medical School also encourage people to eat healthful plant oils at most meals.[16] The USDA ChooseMyPlate.gov website recommends a daily consumption of 6 teaspoons of mono- and polyunsaturated oils per day for women aged 19 to 30 and 7 teaspoons for men of the same age.

A Healthy Plan for Fats in Your Diet Most of us need to cut down on saturated fats while getting more heart-healthy fats into our diet. Here are some ideas:

LIVE IT! ONLINE

Worksheet 24 Cutting Out the Fat

- Always read food labels, looking at both the amount of saturated fat and the percentage it represents of your daily recommended maximum for saturated fat and total fat.

- Don't be fooled into thinking that cookies, crackers, or chips are healthy foods because they are labeled "low-fat." Watch out for high levels of added sugars, refined flour, salt, and *trans* fats (the label may read "vegetable shortening" or "partially hydrogenated vegetable oil").

- For salad dressings, sautéing, and other cooking needs, choose oils such as canola, soy, olive, and safflower that contain high levels of mono- and polyunsaturated fats.

- Whenever possible, instead of butter or margarine, use soft, buttery spreads that list "0 *trans* fats" on the label. For topping bread and crackers, alternatives to butter include all-fruit jams (no sugar added), fat-free cream cheese, tomato salsa, olive oil, or low-fat salad dressing.

- For protein, choose beans, nuts, seeds, tofu, lean meats, fish, or poultry instead of fatty meats such as bacon, sausages, hot dogs, bologna, pepperoni, or organ meats. Remove skin. Avoid frying. Drain off fat after cooking.

- Choose dairy products that have zero or one percent fat, such as skim milk, nonfat yogurt, and fat-free cottage cheese. Avoid reduced-fat dairy products (two percent fat) and whole-milk dairy products (four percent fat) whenever possible. Choose nonfat or low-fat frozen yogurt or sorbet rather than ice cream.

- Cook with chicken broth, wine, vinegar, low-calorie salad dressings, or unsaturated oils (mono- and polyunsaturated) rather than butter, margarine, sour cream, mayonnaise, and creamy salad dressings.

- Eat fatty fish (i.e., salmon, tuna, bluefish, herring, or sardines) one or two times per week. However, be aware of high mercury levels in some types of fish (see the box Is It Safe to Eat Fish?).

SEE IT! ONLINE

Which Fish Is Safest to Eat?

- Add green, leafy vegetables, walnuts, walnut oil, and milled flaxseed to your diet.

- Limit processed and convenience foods. These often contain refined carbohydrates in addition to *trans* fats.

Is It Safe to Eat Fish?

You may have heard that eating too much of certain kinds of fish can pose health hazards, especially to women of childbearing age and to children. At the same time, there are many nutritional benefits to eating fish, including high levels of healthy omega-3 fatty acids. So what's safe and what's not?

The problem is that mercury (either released in the air due to industrial pollution, or naturally occurring) can accumulate in bodies of water, where it becomes methylmercury and contaminates fish. People who eat fish containing high amounts of methylmercury can, in turn, accumulate mercury in their bloodstream. Women of reproductive age and children should be careful about their fish consumption because mercury can damage the brain and nervous systems in developing fetuses and young children.

The EPA advises women and children to avoid four types of fish altogether: tilefish, swordfish, shark, and King mackerel,[1] as these fish tend to contain exceptionally high levels of mercury. They also advise the two groups to limit consumption of fish containing low-levels of mercury—such as salmon, canned light tuna, and catfish—to 12 ounces (two average meals) per week. Other seafood containing low levels of mercury include anchovies, clams, codfish, crab, herring, lobster, and North Atlantic mackerel.[2]

Sources:
1. Environmental Protection Agency, "What You Need to Know about Mercury in Fish and Shellfish,"www.epa.gov/waterscience/fishadvice/advice.html (accessed July 2011).
2. U.S. Food and Drug Administration, "Mercury Levels in Commercial Fish and Shellfish, 1990–2010,"www.fda.gov/Food/FoodSafety/Product-SpecificInformation/Seafood/Food bornePathogensContaminants/Methylmercury/ucm115644.htm (updated May 2011).

Don't demand daily nutritional perfection from yourself. Try to balance your intake of different foods over a few meals and a couple of days at a time. If you have a high-fat breakfast or lunch, balance it with a low-fat dinner. If you forget to eat at least five servings of fruits and vegetables today, eat extra servings tomorrow. And closely monitor your diet to avoid consuming more than the small daily allotment the USDA recommends for empty calories such as sugars and saturated fats (no more than about 10 percent of daily calories).

Vitamins Are Vital Micronutrients

Vitamins are organic compounds that we need in tiny amounts to promote growth and help maintain life and health. Vitamins take part in the minute-by-minute cellular reactions that help maintain our nerves and skin, contribute to the production of blood cells, help us build bones and teeth, assist in wound healing, and help convert food energy to accessible fuel for cellular activities. Some vitamins are toxic in high doses, and for many vitamins, time spent on the shelf, the heat from cooking, and certain other environmental conditions can diminish their potency in foods.

Some vitamins can dissolve only in water and some only in fat. *Water-soluble vitamins,* including vitamin C and the B vitamins, dissolve easily in water and can be absorbed directly into the bloodstream.[17] Excess water-soluble vitamins are usually excreted in the urine and cause few toxicity problems. Because they are not stored in the liver, body fat, or other tissues, we must consume water-soluble vitamins on a regular basis in our foods. *Fat-soluble vitamins*, including vitamins A, D, E, and K, must associate with fat molecules in order to be absorbed through the intestinal tract. Excess, unused quantities of the fat-soluble vitamins tend to be stored in the body. High levels can accumulate in the liver

vitamins Organic compounds in foods that we need in tiny amounts to promote growth and help maintain life and health and cause damage. Table 7.2 lists 13 vitamins, their food sources, their chief functions in the body, and the symptoms caused by consuming too little or too much of each.

Vitamin vendors often make various claims about the benefits of taking vitamin supplements to augment what we consume in foods. For the most part, a careful diet will provide your vitamin needs, but because many people eat too few fruits and vegetables, they don't get optimal levels. In addition, certain groups of people, and all of us at certain life stages, do have special vitamin needs. People over 50, for example, must be careful to get enough vitamin B_{12} since absorption of certain nutrients,

TABLE 7.2 Guide to Vitamins				
Vitamin RDI	Best Food Sources	Main Functions in Body	Deficiency Symptoms	Toxicity Symptoms
Water-Soluble Vitamins				
B_1 (Thiamin) 1.5 milligrams (mg)	Meat, pork, liver, fish, poultry, whole grain and enriched breads and cereals, pasta, nuts, legumes	Energy harvest and use from nutrients; normal appetite; nervous system function	Poor appetite, heart irregularities, mental confusion, muscle weakness, poor growth	None known
B_2 (Riboflavin) 1.7 mg	Dairy products, dark green vegetables, liver, meat, whole grain and enriched breads and cereals	Energy harvest and use from nutrients; healthy skin, normal vision, normal growth	Eye problems, skin cracking around nose and mouth	None known
Niacin 20 mg	Meat, eggs, poultry, fish, milk, whole grain and enriched breads and cereals, nuts, legumes, yeast, all protein foods	Energy harvest and use from nutrients; healthy skin, nervous system function, digestion	Skin rash, loss of appetite, dizziness, weakness, irritability, fatigue, mental confusion, indigestion	Flushing, blurred vision, glucose intolerance, abnormal liver function
B_6 (Pyridoxine) 2.0 mg	Meat, poultry, fish, shellfish, legumes, whole grain foods, leafy greens, bananas	Breakdown of proteins and fats, formation of red blood cells and antibodies, conversion of niacin	Nervous disorders, skin rash, muscle weakness, anemia, convulsions, kidney stones	Sensory nerve damage, skin lesions
Folate 0.4 mg	Leafy greens, liver, legumes, seeds	Forming red blood cells, breakdown of proteins, cell division, proper formation of neural tube in embryo	Anemia, heartburn, diarrhea, smooth tongue, poor growth and development	Nerve damage; high levels may mask a vitamin B_{12} deficiency
B_{12} 6 micrograms (mcg)	Meat, fish, poultry, shellfish, milk, cheese, eggs, yeast	Nerve cell maintenance, red blood cell formation, building of new genetic material	Anemia, smooth tongue, fatigue, nerve degeneration progressing to paralysis	None known

TABLE **7.2** *(Continued)*

Vitamin RDI	Best Food Sources	Main Functions in Body	Deficiency Symptoms	Toxicity Symptoms
Pantothenic acid 10 mg	Widespread in foods	Crucial factor in energy harvest and use	Rare; sleep disturbances, nausea, fatigue	None known
Biotin 0.3 mg	Widespread in foods	Crucial factor in energy harvest and use, building fat molecules, energy storage in muscles	Loss of appetite, nausea, depression, muscle pain, weakness, fatigue, rash	None known
C (Ascorbic acid) 60 mg	Citrus fruits, cabbage-type vegetables, tomatoes, potatoes, dark green vegetables, peppers, cantaloupe, strawberries, mangos, papayas	Helps heal wounds; maintains connective tissue, bones, and teeth; strengthens blood vessels; antioxidant; boosts immunity; aids absorption of iron	Scurvy, anemia, blood vessel damage, depression, frequent infections, loose teeth, bleeding gums, bleeding, muscle wasting, rough skin, weak bones, poor wound healing	Nausea, abdominal cramps, diarrhea, red blood cell breakdown in some people, kidney stones in people with kidney disease. Upon withdrawing from high doses, deficiency symptoms may appear

Fat-Soluble Vitamins

Vitamin RDI	Best Food Sources	Main Functions in Body	Deficiency Symptoms	Toxicity Symptoms
A 5000 international units (IU)	Milk, cream, cheese, butter, eggs, liver, dark leafy greens, broccoli, deep orange fruits and vegetables	Healthy vision, growth and repair of tissues, formation of bones and teeth, immunity, building hormones, cancer protection	Night blindness; rough skin; frequent infections; impaired growth, especially of bones and teeth; eye problems leading to blindness	Miscarriage, birth defects, red blood cell breakage, nosebleeds, abdominal cramps, nausea, blurred vision, bone pain, dry skin, rashes, hair loss
D 200 IU	Sunlight on skin; fortified milk and margarine, eggs, liver, fish	Healthy bones and teeth; aids absorption of calcium and phosphorus	Rickets in children, weakened bones and bone problems in adults, abnormal growth, joint pain, soft bones	Raised blood calcium, constipation, weight loss, irritability, weakness, nausea, kidney stones, mental and physical retardation, calcium deposits
E 30 IU	Vegetable oils, leafy greens, wheat germ, whole grains, butter, liver, egg yolk, milk, nuts, seeds, fortified cereals, soybeans, avocado	Healthy red and white blood cells, healthy cell membranes in lungs and elsewhere, antioxidant activity	Muscle wasting, weakness, damage to red blood cells, anemia, bleeding, fibrocystic breast disease	Interference with anticlotting medication, intestinal discomfort, increased risk of stroke
K	Liver, milk, leafy greens, cabbage-type vegetables, vegetable oils	Aids digestion, blood clotting, regulation of calcium in blood, builds bone tissue	Bleeding	None known

Do I Have Special Vitamin and Mineral Needs?

Most nutritionists agree that you should try to get your daily vitamins and minerals from a healthful diet rather than eating carelessly and relying on supplements. People in a number of population groups, however, are at risk for vitamin deficiencies. If you belong to one of these groups, you should pay extra attention to your diet and perhaps consider taking a multivitamin.[1]

- Women of reproductive age who could become pregnant need 400 micrograms of folate per day to prevent potential neurological defects in a developing fetus. Pregnant women need 600 micrograms per day.

- Premenopausal women, especially those with heavy menstrual bleeding, need 18 milligrams of iron per day in foods or in total from foods and a multivitamin. They must also get enough vitamin C to help them absorb iron from foods. Men and postmenopausal women need 10 milligrams per day and should be careful not to get too much.

- Everyone needs a good supply of calcium each day from low-fat dairy products, fortified juices, and other sources. The daily value for people under 50 is 1,000 milligrams. Pregnant women, nursing mothers, teens, and older adults need extra calcium (1,200 to 1,500 milligrams per day) for the development and maintenance of bones and to lower the risk of osteoporosis.

- Older adults need sufficient potassium for normal muscle contraction and nerve transmission and sodium within a healthy range to supply cellular needs but lower the risk of high blood pressure.

- Older adults, dark-skinned individuals, and people who do not get regular exposure to sunlight have a special need for vitamin D. The government currently recommends that people under 50 consume 200 IU (International Units) of vitamin D per day, people between 50 and 70 consume 400 I.U. per day, and people over 70 consume 600 I.U. per day.

- People over 50 naturally produce less stomach acid and absorb less vitamin B_{12} from foods. Older adults should be careful to get at least 2.4 micrograms of B_{12} per day or more, especially if they take stomach acid blockers.

- Cigarette smoking decreases bone density and interferes with the body's normal use of vitamin C. Smokers therefore need to consume higher levels of calcium (1,200 mg per day) and of vitamin C (110 mg in women, 125 mg per day in men) compared to 90 mg for nonsmoking adults.

- People with diseases that disrupt normal metabolism or nutrient absorption (diabetes and certain cancers, for example) can develop vitamin or mineral deficiencies. Physicians often recommend special diets or multivitamins as part of their treatment.[2]

- The USDA dietary guidelines provide specific pointers for parents and guardians to help kids and teens get the balance of nutrients they need to support their growth and development.

- Details about the special nutritional needs of vegetarians and diabetics are covered on pages 272–273.

If you plan to take a multivitamin, apply common sense. There is no need to get more than the RDI for vitamins and minerals. Doses exceeding 100 percent can lead to serious side effects. Since fat-soluble vitamins and certain minerals can build up in the body, be sure a multivitamin has less than the RDI for vitamins A, D, E, and K and for magnesium, chromium, selenium, and zinc.[3] To be safe, people in high-risk groups should consult a doctor before taking supplements regularly.

Sources:
1. Center for Science in the Public Interest, "The Multivitamin Maze" and "How to Read a Multi Label," *Nutrition Action Healthletter* (March 2006): 6–7.
2. U.S. Department of Agriculture and U.S. Department of Health and Human Services, *Dietary Guidelines for Americans, 2010*, 7th Edition (Washington, DC: U.S. Government Printing Office, 2010).
3. National Institutes of Health, "NIH State of the Science Panel Urges More Informed Approach to Multivitamin/Mineral Use for Chronic Disease Prevention," www.nih.gov/news/pr/may2006/od-17.htm (May 2006).

including B$_{12}$, declines naturally with age. The box Do I Have Special Vitamin and Mineral Needs? discusses both the vitamin needs of specific groups and the issue of taking vitamin supplements versus getting vitamins from food alone. Few Americans suffer from true vitamin deficiencies if they eat a fairly balanced diet. Taking very high levels of certain vitamins can even lead to a toxic condition know as *hypervitaminosis*.

Minerals Are Elemental Micronutrients

The micronutrients called **minerals** allow our nerves to transmit impulses, our hearts to beat, oxygen to reach our tissue cells, and our digestive tracts to absorb vitamins from food. They are usually not toxic, and we excrete excess quantities of most minerals from the body. The **major minerals** (also called *macrominerals*) are elements that the body needs in relatively large amounts. We need smaller amounts of the **trace minerals** (also called *microminerals*). Table 7.3 lists most of the major and trace minerals, their functions, food sources, and symptoms of deficiency and/or toxicity. We discuss three minerals—sodium, calcium, and iron—in more detail because of their crucial roles in the body and their excesses or deficiencies in many students' diets.

Sodium We need sodium, the Na in sodium chloride (NaCl), or table salt, for regulating the water contents of blood and body fluids; for the transmission of nerve impulses; for muscle contraction, including the heartbeat; and for several metabolic functions inside cells. However, most of us consume much more than we need.[18] The average adult at rest and not sweating profusely needs only 500 mg of sodium (about one-quarter teaspoon) per day. Nutritionists estimate, however, that the average American man consumes 3,100 to 4,700 mg per day and the average woman 2,300 to 3,100 mg per day in salted snacks and processed foods! The *2010 Dietary Guidelines for Americans* recommends that everyone restrict sodium to less than 2,300 mg per day, and that certain groups (those over 51 years old, African Americans, and people with hypertension, diabetes, or chronic kidney disease) reduce their sodium consumption to under 1,500 mg per day. Pickles, salty snack foods, processed cheeses, many breads and bakery products, and smoked meats and sausages often contain several hundred milligrams of sodium per serving. Many fast-food entrées and convenience entrées pack 500 to 1,000 mg of sodium per serving.

Many experts believe that there is a link between excessive sodium intake and hypertension (high blood pressure).[19] Researchers began recommending several years ago that people with hypertension cut back on sodium to reduce their risk of cardiovascular disorders.[20]

You can shake your own salt habit by choosing low-sodium or salt-free food products. For example, order popcorn without salt. Switch to kosher salt—it has 25% less sodium than regular table salt. Instead of adding salt to food you prepare, try using fresh or prepackaged herb blends to season foods. These small changes can add up to a significant reduction in unneeded sodium.

Calcium High sodium intake may also increase calcium loss in urine, which increases your risk for debilitating fractures as you age.[21] The element calcium (Ca) is crucial for the development and maintenance of bones and teeth, for blood clotting, muscle contraction, nerve transmission, and fluid balance between the cell's interior and its environment. Nevertheless, most Americans consume less than the 1,000 mg to 1,300 mg of calcium per day recommended by government guidelines.[22]

Osteoporosis is a disease of thinning, weakened, porous bones that affects more than 44 million Americans (women and men) over age 50. The risk for it climbs if you consume too little calcium during childhood and adolescence when bones are developing, if you have a small skeleton (or "frame"), and/or if you consume too little calcium during adulthood. Bone weakness can lead to pain, stooped posture, and fractures, and can diminish mobility and independence. Forty to 50 percent of women and 13 to 22 percent of men will break a bone as a result of osteoporosis.[23]

Dairy products are among the richest dietary sources of calcium, but calcium-fortified orange juice and soy milk are also good sources, as are leafy green vegetables and many other foods (see Table 7.3). Be aware that the added phosphoric acid (phosphate) in carbonated colas and possibly other soft drinks can cause you to excrete calcium

minerals Elements such as calcium or sodium that allow vital physiological processes including nerve transmission, heartbeat, oxygen delivery, and absorption of vitamins

major minerals Elements needed in relatively large amounts, including sodium, calcium, phosphorus, magnesium, potassium, and chloride

trace minerals Elements the body needs in very tiny amounts; includes iron, zinc, copper, iodine, selenium, fluoride, and chromium

osteoporosis A disease of thinning, weakened, porous bones during which too little calcium is deposited or retained in the bones

TABLE **7.3** Guide to Selected Minerals

Mineral RDI	Best Food Sources	Main Functions in Body	Deficiency Symptoms	Toxicity Symptoms
Calcium 1.0 g	Milk and dairy products, small fish with bones, tofu, leafy greens, legumes	Building bones and teeth, muscle contraction and relaxation, nerve function, blood clotting, blood pressure	Stunted growth in children, bone weakness and thinning in adults	Mineral imbalances, shock, kidney failure, fatigue, mental confusion
Phosphorus 1.0 g	All animal tissues	Component of every cell, helps regulate pH balance	Unknown	Can unbalance calcium; can lead to calcium deficiency, spasms, convulsions
Magnesium 400 mg	Nuts, legumes, whole grains, deep leafy greens, seafood, chocolate	Bone hardening, protein synthesis, enzyme activity, normal function of muscles and nerves	Weakness, confusion, poor growth, impaired hormone production, muscle spasms, disturbed behavior	Mega-doses can lead to nausea, cramps, dehydration, death
Sodium 2400 mg	Salt, soy sauce, processed foods, cured, canned, pickled foods	Helps maintain normal fluid balance and pH within body	Muscle cramps, mental apathy, loss of appetite	Hypertension, water retention, increased calcium loss
Chloride 2300 mg	Salt, soy sauce, processed foods, cured, canned, pickled foods	Component of stomach acid and needed for digestion, helps maintain normal fluid balance	Dangerous changes in pH, irregular heartbeat	Vomiting
Potassium 3500 mg	Meats, fruits, milk, vegetables, grains, legumes	Involved in biochemical reactions that help build protein, maintain fluid balance, transmit nerve impulses, contract muscles	Muscle weakness, paralysis, confusion; accompanies dehydration; can cause death	Muscular weakness, vomiting, irregular heartbeat; can stop heart
Iodine 150 mcg	Iodized salt, seafood	Component of thyroid hormone, helps regulate metabolism	Goiter; mental and physical retardation due to thyroid deficiency	Goiter or enlargement of thyroid gland
Iron 18 mg	Beef, fish, poultry, shellfish, eggs, legumes, dried fruits	Crucial component of hemoglobin in red blood cells, myoglobin in muscles; takes part in oxygen transfer, energy use	Anemia, weakness, pallor, headaches, frequent infections, difficulty concentrating	Nausea, vomiting, dizziness, rapid heartbeat, damage to organs, death
Zinc 15 mg	Meats, fish, poultry, grains, vegetables	Component of insulin and many enzymes; takes part in DNA, protein synthesis, immune response, taste, wound healing, normal development, sperm production, vitamin A transport	Growth failure in children, delayed sexual development, loss of taste, poor wound healing	Fever, nausea, vomiting, diarrhea, headaches, depressed immune function

TABLE **7.3** (Continued)

Mineral *RDI*	Best Food Sources	Main Functions in Body	Deficiency Symptoms	Toxicity Symptoms
Copper *2 mg*	Meats, drinking water	Absorption of iron, component of several enzymes	Anemia, bone changes (rare)	Liver damage if toxicity is due to certain diseases; nausea, diarrhea, vomiting
Fluoride *10 mg*	Drinking water (natural or fluoridated), tea, seafood	Formation and maintenance of bones and teeth	Susceptibility to tooth decay and bone loss	Discoloration of teeth, joint pain, stiffness
Selenium *400 mcg*	Seafood, meats, grains	Helps protect body compounds from oxidation	Muscle pain and possible deterioration, possible damage to nails and hair	Vomiting, nausea, rash, brittle hair and nails, cirrhosis of liver
Chromium *30 mcg*	Meats, whole foods, fats, vegetable oils	Associated with insulin, needed for breakdown and use of glucose	Diabetes-like condition with poor glucose utilization	Unknown. Occupational overexposure damages skin and kidneys

and thus deplete needed calcium from your bones.[24] Calcium/phosphorus imbalance may lead to kidney stones and bone spurs and to the deposits or plaques inside blood vessels that contribute to cardiovascular diseases.

Vitamin D improves absorption of calcium; that's why dairies are required by law to add it to milk. Sunlight shining on your skin also increases your body's own manufacture of vitamin D, so a moderate amount of sunlight helps improve calcium absorption. The best way to obtain calcium, like all nutrients, is to consume it as part of a balanced diet, but certain people do need calcium supplements (see the Diversity box on page 256).

Iron Each of us needs the element iron (Fe) for producing healthy blood, for muscle function, and for normal cell division. Females aged 15 to 50 need about 18 mg/day; males aged 19 to 50 need about 10 mg/day. Worldwide, iron deficiency is the most common nutrient deficiency, affecting more than one billion people. In developing countries, more than one-third of the children and women of childbearing age suffer from **iron-deficiency anemia**, in which the body fails to produce enough of the red hemoglobin pigment in the blood, leading to unusually low oxygen levels and unusually high carbon dioxide levels and resulting in mental and physical fatigue. About five percent of all Americans get too little iron in their food.[25] Among toddlers, adolescent girls, and women of childbearing age, about 10 percent show iron-deficiency anemia. Table 7.3 lists good dietary sources of iron.

Getting the right amount of iron is important. Researchers have linked iron deficiency to a host of problems, including poor immune system functioning and a propensity toward certain cancers. Some research has also suggested a link between too much iron in the diet and/or stored in the body and a higher risk for cardiovascular disease.

Acute iron toxicity due to ingesting too many iron-containing supplements remains the leading cause of accidental poisoning in small children in the United States. Dozens of children have died from overdoses of as few as five iron tablets.[26]

Water Is Our Most Fundamental Nutrient

Imagine you are stranded on a desert island for a reality TV show and you can take along just one provision. Would you choose food, water, or a cell phone? We hope you said water!

Humans are mostly water—close to 60 percent. Watery fluids bathe each of our internal cells. They help maintain a proper balance of salts within our blood and tissues, help maintain pH balance, and help facilitate the transport of substances throughout the body. Human blood plasma (the fluid portion of blood exclusive of red and white blood cells and other solid components) is approximately 91.5 percent water.[27] This proportion must remain fairly constant for blood to efficiently carry oxygen and nutrients to the cells and carry away carbon dioxide and other wastes.

iron-deficiency anemia A disease in which the body takes in too little iron and makes too little oxygen-carrying hemoglobin

dehydrated Depleted of normal, necessary levels of body fluids

Even under the most severe conditions, the average person can live for weeks on the energy stored in body fat. You can also get along without certain vitamins and minerals from foods for an equal amount of time before experiencing serious deficiency symptoms. Without water, however, you would become **dehydrated**, or depleted of normal levels of body fluids, within hours. Within one day without drinking water, you would probably begin to feel sluggish, dizzy, and nauseated, and would experience headaches, muscle cramps, or weakness. After a few days without water, your tongue would be parched and swollen, your heart would be racing, and you'd very likely go into shock and die.

A person's need for water varies dramatically based on age, size, diet, exercise, overall health, and environmental temperature and humidity levels. Most of us get enough water through foods and beverages just by satisfying our thirst.[28] People with certain diseases such as diabetes or cystic fibrosis, however, excrete extra fluid and must generally take in a higher volume. On a hot day, especially if exercising, you need to consciously replace fluids lost to sweat and exhalation. It is possible, though,

to take in too much water and become nauseated, confused, or weak or even to lose consciousness from excess hydration leading to *hyponatremia* (sometimes called water intoxication). This condition results from too much water in the blood and therefore a salt concentration that is too low due to dilution. It often occurs in conjunction with heavy perspiration. If your intake is high enough that you gain water weight during an active exercise session, you are probably imbibing too much.

Commercial energy drinks can help exercisers replenish water lost through sweat and to restore salt and sugar. Some energy drinks, however, include ingredients that are ineffectual or that can be harmful in large quantities. For example, researchers have failed to confirm any health benefit for ingredients such as taurine, bee pollen, and ginkgo biloba.[29] High concentrations of added sugars can boost energy in the short term but can create sluggishness later. Added vitamins C and B are unnecessary in a balanced diet. If overused, energy drinks containing the stimulants caffeine and/or ginseng can speed bone loss, raise blood pressure, and increase the risk of cardiovascular diseases.

casestudy

CHAU

"I kind of understand that your body uses different nutrients for different things. But I've never had a weight problem, so I've been more concerned with quantity than quality. I realize I'm eating a lot more carbs than I used to, mostly cereal and white bread. And Tom's girlfriend is always baking him cookies, so I load up on those. I also eat cheese and pepperoni pizzas in the cafeteria. Still, I don't worry about eating fat or being fat. Everyone in my family is thin!"

THINK! Chau often eats meals prepared on campus, where he has no access to nutrition labels. How could Chau estimate the amount of protein, carbohydrate, and fat in his diet? Given what you know about Chau's diet, which nutrients might he be deficient in? Which nutrients might he be consuming too much of?

ACT! Analyze your own diet. What nutrients, if any, are you deficient in? Calculate how much protein you need each day. Are you taking in more protein than you really need?

HEAR IT! ONLINE

How Can I Achieve a Balanced Diet?

The average American adult consumes about 1,000 calories more per day than the average citizen worldwide and yet still gets unbalanced nutrition. To counter these trends toward overeating and substandard nutrition, the U.S. government:

- Sets guidelines for minimum and recommended levels of nutrients, vitamins, and minerals

- Publishes an interactive website called ChooseMyPlate.gov to help individuals manage their daily nutrition, including calorie counting and energy expenditure through exercise

- Requires standardized nutrition labels on most packaged and processed foods

- Determines appropriate portion sizes, and

- Regulates the safety of our food supply

This massive effort is designed to improve our national wellness, and the many tools the USDA, FDA, National Academy of Sciences, and other governmental agencies provide can help you achieve a better diet, maintain a healthy weight, and help prevent several chronic diseases.

Follow Guidelines for Good Nutrition

There are so many parts to the government's nutritional advice to the public that they publish an overview—think of it as a cheat sheet for nutrition—called the *Dietary Guidelines for Americans*. The latest version came out in 2010 from the USDA and U.S. Department of Health and Human Services. We discuss the government's nutritional guidelines for specific sex, age, and ethnic groups later in the chapter. Here, we summarize the major recommendations in the 2010 version:

- *Balance calories to maintain weight.*
  - Balance the calories you take in from food with the calories your burn through activity and exercise. For most people, this means eating less and exercising more.
  - Learn about standard portion sizes so you can avoid oversized portions.

- *Increase certain foods and nutrients in your diet.*
  - Make at least half of your plate fruits and vegetables and eat a variety of produce types.
  - Consume at least half of your daily grains as whole grains and reduce refined grains.
  - Switch to fat-free or low-fat (one percent) dairy products.
  - Eat proteins low in solid (saturated) fats such as eggs, beans, seeds, soy, fish, lean meats, and poultry.
  - Eat more vegetables, whole grains, and fat-free or low-fat dairy products to increase potassium, dietary fiber, calcium, and vitamin D.

- *Decrease consumption of certain foods and components.*
  - Compare sodium in foods such as soup, bread, and frozen meals—and choose the foods with the lower numbers.
  - Drink water instead of sugary drinks.
  - Avoid *trans* fats and reduce saturated fat. Increase mono- and polyunsaturated oils to recommended levels for your sex, age, size, and activity level.
  - Reduce cholesterol.
  - Reduce added sugars and count the calories as "empty."
  - Reduce refined grains to less than half of your daily grains.
  - Limit alcohol consumption.

- *Build healthy eating patterns.*
  - Eat so that you can balance your nutrient and caloric needs over time.
  - Keep track of what you eat and drink and make sure they fit your long-term pattern.
  - Follow safety rules for food preparation and eating to avoid foodborne illnesses.

Several government scientific advisory boards serve up an "alphabet soup" of specific recommended daily minimum and maximum intakes for each type of nutrient (fat, carbohydrates, proteins), and for the various types of vitamins and minerals. The box What Do All Those Acronyms on the Food Label Mean? offers a short introduction to these **RDAs (Recommended Daily Allowances), DRVs (Daily Reference Values)**, and other daily intake recommendations. Sorting them out can be challenging, but it's easier if you keep in mind the simplified general guidelines just listed and concentrate on the **DVs (Daily Values)** listed on food labels.

RDAs (Recommended Dietary Allowances) A listing of the average daily nutrient intake level for a list of vitamins and minerals that meets most people's daily needs

DRVs (Daily Reference Values) Set of general intake guidelines of total fat, saturated fat, cholesterol, carbohydrates, protein, fiber, sodium, and potassium

DVs (Daily Values) A listing of all the important nutrients from two less inclusive government lists—the RDIs (Reference Daily Intakes) and the DRVs (Daily Reference Values); DVs are printed on all nutrition labels

What Do All Those Acronyms on Food Labels Mean?

- *DRI (Dietary Reference Intake)* is a listing of 26 nutrients essential to maintaining health. The DRI listing identifies recommended and maximum safe intake levels of the nutrients for healthy people, and identifies minimum levels needed to prevent deficiencies and diseases. DRIs are an umbrella category for several older classifications. The National Academy of Sciences Food and Nutrition Board publishes DRIs.

- *RDAs (Recommended Dietary Allowances)* are a listing of the average daily nutrient intake levels of vitamins and minerals that meet most people's daily needs. The National Academy of Sciences introduced RDAs in 1941 and updates the list periodically.

- *RDIs (Reference Daily Intakes)* are a listing of needed daily nutrients based on the National Academy of Science's RDAs. Tables 7.2 and 7.3 list the current RDIs for various vitamins and minerals.

- *DRVs (Daily Reference Values)* cover some nutrients the RDIs left out that proved to be important for daily dietary monitoring. They cover fat (including saturated fat and cholesterol), carbohydrates (including fiber), protein, sodium, and potassium. Table 7.4 lists the current DRVs for these nutrients.

- *DVs (Daily Values)* are the RDIs and the DRVs as printed on food labels. American consumers need to know what's in their food and what they should be eating without sorting through a bunch of confusing acronyms. Therefore, the U.S. Food and Drug Administration (FDA) invented a simpler term, DV, for all the important nutrients from the RDI and DRV lists to include on food labels. If you look on any food label, you will see a column labeled "% Daily Value."

You will probably come across the above-mentioned listings the most often. However, when looking into calorie requirements and safe levels of vitamins and minerals, you may also see references to a few other daily intakes:

- *EAR (Estimated Average Requirement)* is a listing of the intake that meets the requirement of half the healthy people of a certain gender at a certain life stage, such as adolescence, young adulthood, and so on.

- *AIs (Adequate Intakes)* are recommendations for daily nutrient intake where actual RDIs aren't known. Some of the values for vitamins and minerals are AIs because scientists have yet to discover exact daily requirements for those nutrients.

- *ULs (Tolerable Upper Intake Levels)* are recommendations for the highest levels that pose no risk when too much of a particular vitamin or mineral could be harmful.

- *EERs (Estimated Energy Requirements)* are calorie intake levels based on age, gender, height, weight, and activity level.

- *AMDRs (Acceptable Macronutrient Distribution Ranges)* are ranges of percentages for carbohydrate, fat, and protein consumption that provide adequate nutrition and reduces the risk of chronic diseases. For example, the AMDR for fat is 20 to 35 percent of total calories. For carbohydrate, it is 45 to 65 percent of total calories. For protein, it is 10 to 35 percent.

Reading Food Labels The U.S. government requires nutrition labels on the packages of most food products, including the familiar panel entitled "Nutrition Facts" (Figure 7.8). Reading and understanding these labels can help you judge both appropriate portion sizes and the nutritional merits of the foods you eat. By law, every food package must

- prominently identify the product, such as "multigrain cereal" or "fat-free milk";

- state the quantity of food product in the package by weight, volume, or number of pieces so you can judge the value of what you are buying;

- list all the ingredients by common name in order of amount from most to least by weight;

- give contact information for the food company in case you want more information;

- supply nutritional information in a standardized panel so you can compare and judge the dietary merits of the product before you buy it.

The Nutrition Facts panel provides the greatest concentration of information; it identifies a serving size and how many servings you'll get in a package. For example, the serving size of the soup in Figure 7.8 is 1 cup. The panel tells you how many calories each serving provides and how many of those calories come from fat. It lists daily recommended values (DVs) for nutrients that people should limit in their diets, including total fat, saturated fat, cholesterol, carbohydrates, and sodium. It also lists nutrients that many people should increase in their diets, such as vitamins A and C, calcium, and iron, giving the % Daily Value for each nutrient.

In 2010, First Lady Michelle Obama launched the "Nutrition Keys" front-of-package nutrition labeling initiative. She requested that the U.S. food industry create a new system of simplified front-of-package food labels that would act as a kind of "CliffsNotes" for quickly scanning and judging a food's nutrient content. In early 2011, some manufacturers responded by using streamlined front labels that highlight calories-per-serving information and the values per serving for three nutrients of interest for that type of food (Figure 7.9). A package of cookies, for example, might include calories, grams of saturated fat and sugar, and milligrams of sodium per serving. Other foods might highlight calories per serving

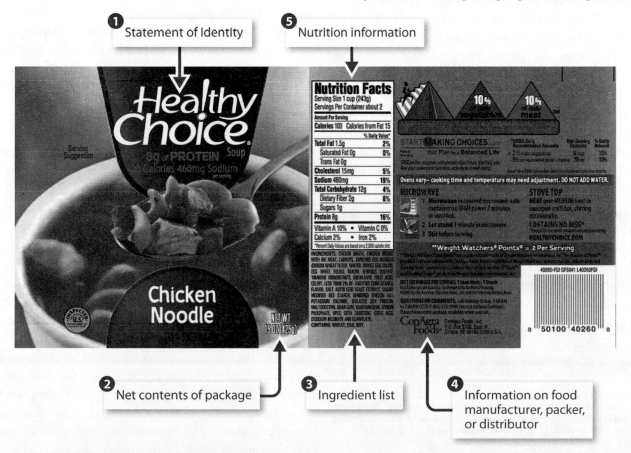

FIGURE 7.8 An important part of improving personal nutrition is reading food labels and understanding the information they provide.

Image © ConAgra Foods, Inc. Used with permission.

| 450 CALORIES | 5g SAT FAT | 360mg SODIUM | 14g SUGARS | 500mg POTASSIUM | 3g FIBER |
| | 25% DV | 15% DV | | 14% DV | 12% DV |

FIGURE **7.9** One serving of this imaginary product has a whopping 450 calories, contains one-quarter of a day's saturated fat, one-sixth of a day's sodium, and the gram equivalent of three teaspoons of sugar. It does, however, also provide some potassium and fiber.

and three other types of nutrients such as vitamins A, C, or D; calcium; fiber; or protein content.

Without simplified front "keys" and more detailed side label panels, it would be easy for a consumer to eat half of a large bag of potato chips and think of that as one serving. Or to pick out a box of sweetened granola with 250 calories in one-half cup and mistakenly consider that food to be the nutritional equivalent of high-fiber, low-sugar multigrain flakes with only 100 calories in three-quarters of a cup. Individual consumers then must then provide the effort to read those labels, understand the issues behind the various values, and make intelligent choices.

Determining Your Calorie Needs If you read the fine print near the bottom of any nutrition label, you will see that the listings of nutrients are based on diets of either 2,000 or 2,500 calories per day. The U.S. government chose a 2,000 calorie-per-day diet as the basis for recommending the daily values of 65 grams of fat, 300 grams of carbohydrates, and 50 grams of protein (see Table 7.4). Does that mean you should be eating 2,000 calories per day regardless of whether you are 4' 9" tall and weigh 90 pounds, or 6' 9" and weigh 230 pounds? And does it mean that you

TABLE **7.4** Daily Reference Values (DRVs)	
Food Component	DRV
Fat	65 grams (g)
Saturated fatty acids	20 g
Cholesterol	300 milligrams (mg)
Total carbohydrate	300 g
Dietary fiber	25 g
Protein*	50 g

(Based on 2,000 calories a day for adults and children over 4 only)
* DRV for protein does not apply to certain populations; Reference Daily Intake (RDI) for protein has been established for these groups: children 1 to 4 years: 16 g; infants under 1 year: 14 g; pregnant women: 60 g; nursing mothers: 65 g.

Adapted from U.S. FDA Food Labeling Guide, www.fda.gov/FoodLabelingGuide; (revised October 2009).

should adhere to those daily values regardless of your activity level? No, on both counts.

A round number like 2,000 calories makes it easy to extrapolate your actual calorie needs and serving sizes. It is also a maintenance level of energy input for a medium-sized person—about 150 pounds—who expends a medium amount of energy such as 30 minutes of moderate activity a few times per week. Food labels usually also provide a second level, 2,500 calories, as a calculation base for larger or more active people. Your actual calorie needs are determined by your size, age, gender, activity level, and medical conditions and your basal metabolic rate (BMR), which is partly inborn and partly activity-based.

Your BMR, the amount of energy your body uses in a given time period while resting or sleeping, accounts for 50 to 70 percent of your calorie consumption each day and allows you to maintain a steady heartbeat, a temperature of about 98.6°F, and so on. You use another 20 percent of your calories moving around and doing physical work such as walking, talking, carrying things, running, or sweeping the floor. Finally, eating and digesting food itself uses up about 5 to 10 percent of the calories you burn each day.

In determining calorie needs, the big variables are body size, BMR, and energy expenditure through physical activity. Larger people, more muscular people, and those who do hard physical work or exercise burn extra calories. You can get a specific calorie estimate using diet analysis tools such as www.ChooseMyPlate.gov. Use your own personal calorie estimate to calculate appropriate serving sizes and numbers when reading food labels and planning your diet.

Understanding Portion Sizes One reason that Americans eat an average of nearly 3,500 calories per day rather than the world average of 2,400 to 2,600 is that our typical food portions are too big. The U.S. government recommends that each of us eat a certain number of servings each day from each food group based on standard serving sizes. Most Americans, however, don't know how to recognize standard portions. It helps to have some visual aids for estimating proper serving sizes and recognizing the right amount of food. Figure 7.10 illustrates various foods, healthy serving sizes in cups and ounces, and visual devices for remembering proper portions. For example, one serving of cooked whole-wheat pasta or brown rice is half a cup, about the size of half a baseball. This figure puts into startling perspective the servings we receive at most restaurants: the mountains of pasta, the big wedges of pie, the stacks of plate-sized pancakes, the

1 Serving Looks Like ...	1 Serving Looks Like ...
Grain Products	**Vegetables and Fruit**
1 cup of cereal flakes = fist	1 cup of salad greens = baseball
1 pancake = compact disc	1 baked potato = fist
¹/₂ cup of cooked rice, pasta, or potato = ¹/₂ baseball	1 medium fruit = baseball
1 slice of bread = cassette tape	¹/₂ cup of fresh fruit = ¹/₂ baseball
1 piece of cornbread = bar of soap	¹/₄ cup of raisins = large egg

1 Serving Looks Like ...	1 Serving Looks Like ...
Dairy and Cheese	**Meat and Alternatives**
1¹/₂ oz cheese = 4 stacked dice or 2 cheese slices	3 oz meat, fish, and poultry = deck of cards
¹/₂ cup of ice cream = ¹/₂ baseball	3 oz grilled or baked fish = checkbook
Fats	2 Tbsp peanut butter = Ping-Pong ball
1 tsp margarine or spreads = 1 die	

FIGURE **7.10** One of the challenges of following a healthy diet is judging how big a portion size should be and how many servings you are really eating. The comparisons on this card can help you recall what a standard food serving looks like. For easy reference, photocopy or cut out this card, fold on the dotted line, and keep it in your wallet. You can even laminate it for long-term use.

Source: National Heart, Lung and Blood Institute, "Serving Size Card," http://hp2010.nhlbihin.net/portion/servingcard7.pdf (accessed April 2010).

bucket-sized soft drinks, and the other servings we accept and expect as normal.

Using Food Guides The USDA has issued Food Guides since the 1940s to help Americans select healthy diets as defined by contemporary nutritionists. They have used wheels, rectangles, pyramids, and most recently a divided plate to summarize and illustrate their recommendations simply for the public.[30] The plate icon introduced in 2011 uses segments of certain colors and sizes to symbolize the kinds and relative amounts of foods

FIGURE **7.11** The ChooseMyPlate.gov icon shows the proper proportion of each food group in a healthy diet. The supporting website provides each visitor with an individualized recommendation for daily servings and portion sizes of each food type.

and nutrients (fruits, vegetables, grains, dairy, protein) consumers should select each day (Figure 7.11). The supporting website (www.ChooseMyPlate.gov) provides specific personalized diet analysis and recommendations based on your sex, age, size, and activity level.

Nongovernment nutritionists have published several alternative food plans. A pyramid published by Harvard Medical School's Department of Nutrition recommends that you minimize all sugars and refined or low-fiber carbohydrates such as white flour, white rice, pasta, and peeled potatoes. It also discourages the consumption of red meat, butter, cheese, and other sources of saturated fat. At the same time, it encourages consumption of vegetables, whole grains, nuts, beans, and unsaturated fats from plant oils. On the Internet, you can find alternative pyramids for Mediterranean, Asian, Latin American, and vegetarian eating patterns.

Acquire Skills to Improve Your Nutrition

Do you know the nutritional value of your diet? Do you know how to find out? A few simple skills will help you analyze and improve your diet. Developing a habit of quickly checking seven items from the typical food label can greatly improve your daily nutrition. **Lab 7.1** will encourage this habit. Here are the seven you should look for on a regular basis:

- *What is the normal serving size?* Let's say you bought a bag of corn chips and were planning to eat the whole thing. The label, however, says it contains 8.5 servings. That provides a valuable hint about the calorie density of that food, not to mention the amount of fat and sodium in the whole bag. If you decide to eat just one serving, you can count out your seven or eight chips and enjoy them—slowly!

- *What is the main ingredient?* If it is water, corn syrup, or enriched (translation, "white") flour, are you getting your money's worth—and good nutrition?

- *How do the total fats and saturated fats compare to the listed daily values?* Just 1 tablespoon of butter, for example, will provide one-third of your DV for saturated fat. Do you really want to consume that much fat in one pat?

- *What is the* trans *fat content?* Reduce or eliminate *trans* fats because of their potentially negative health consequences.

- *How does the sodium compare to % Daily Value?* People diagnosed with high blood pressure, diabetes, kidney disease, and certain other conditions must limit sodium levels. Others should limit sodium to within recommended levels.

- *Does the food provide any fiber?* If not, could you substitute something that does—for example, baby spinach leaves instead of iceberg lettuce in a salad, or a fresh apple instead of canned pineapple, or brown rice instead of white?

- *Finally, what is the % Daily Value of sugars?* Technically, there is no DV for sugars or other sweeteners, but you can see the content in grams listed on food labels. Sugars are common in cereals, sauces, and other processed foods and add empty calories that you could devote to more filling and nutritious foods. For example, instead of eating a cup of raisin bran with 19 grams of sugar and 188 calories of food energy, try choosing one cup of bran flakes with only 5 grams of sugar and 122 calories, and then adding a cup of sliced, fresh strawberries (high in volume, flavor, vitamin C, and fiber and containing only 55 calories).

Keeping a Food Diary Did you have three servings of fruit yesterday or two? 200 calories of fats and sugars or 600? If you are like most people, you can only remember a highlight or two from yesterday's meals, and not much of what you ate the other days of the week. To get an accurate idea of whether your diet is nutrient rich or

Worksheet 19
Food Log

poor and whether it provides enough fiber, try to record snacks and meals for a few days. This is best done immediately after eating, not hours later when you have discarded wrappers with nutrient labels or lost count of serving sizes.

One way to track your diet is to fill in a food diary. Keeping a food diary helps you learn to judge serving sizes. It requires you to read and apply the information on nutrition labels, learn the value of your typical foods, and substitute healthier items for the foods you usually choose.

Using Diet Analysis Software An online program such as www.ChooseMyPlate.gov is a powerful tool for keeping track of what you eat, analyzing its nutrient content, and making needed changes in your diet. It is just one of several such programs that can streamline your efforts to achieve better nutrition. Many smart phone "apps" help you keep track of calories, as well.

To use this USDA website and its personalized features, visit www.ChooseMyPlate.gov. Find the box "I want to…," and click on "Get a Personalized Plan." Enter your age, sex, weight, height, and general activity level. The next screen will present you with the number of daily calories you should consume; the number of servings you should eat from each of the five food groups (grains, vegetables, fruits, dairy, and protein foods); pointers for eating enough whole grains and for varying your vegetables each week so you include some dark green ones, some orange ones, some legumes, some starchy vegetables, and others; a reminder to consume enough healthful oils; and advice on limiting the calories in fats and sugars. You can then print out a personalized food plan based on your individual information. Beyond the personalized plan, the site also provides these features:

- You can use a meal tracking worksheet to keep tabs on each food you ate on a given day and save this for comparison with additional days.

- You can use the ChooseMyPlate Tracker to assess the nutrients—calories, fats, carbohydrates, vitamins, and so on—in specific foods such as a tuna fish sandwich or a slice of pizza (see **Lab 7.2**).

- You can make a data bank of nutritional information for foods or meals you eat routinely—say, your typical breakfast of cereal, juice, and toast—so you don't have to enter them individually each time.

- You can do a more detailed analysis of your physical activities to get an estimate of calories burned as you do a particular exercise for a certain period of time.

- Finally, you can keep track of trends in your diet and physical activity over time if you are making changes to benefit your fitness and wellness.

Choose the method—online or on paper—that works best for you, as that's the one you'll stick with.

Adopt the Whole Foods Habit

Analyzing your daily foods for calories and nutrients can help you achieve nutritional wellness. So can a simpler approach: making each bite you take more nutritious by choosing primarily **whole foods**, or dietary items produced with the minimum of refining, preservatives, or processing for quick preparation.

SEE IT! ONLINE

Going Green

LIVE IT! ONLINE

Worksheet 18 Grocery Shopping List

Decades ago, virtually all food was "whole," or real and unchanged. Many packaged foods today, however, have long lists of ingredients and additives that reduce the cost of ingredients, extend shelf life, intensify flavor, and make food preparation easier. People have learned to like the taste and convenience of processed foods, but these products tend to contain hidden fats and sugars, relatively large amounts of sodium, and various additives and preservatives. They also tend to have less naturally occurring fiber and fewer vitamins. Let's compare a medium-sized fresh apple, for example, with one cup of processed, preserved, and dried apple slices. The fresh apple contains about 95 calories, 17 grams of carbohydrates, 3 grams of fiber, and 13 grams of sugars. The cup of dried apple slices (derived from two or more whole apples) contain 209 calories, 51 grams of carbohydrates, 7 grams of fiber, and 49 grams of sugars, and may contain added sucrose or corn syrup and preservatives such as sulfur.

Shifting from a diet heavy in processed foods to one rich in whole foods doesn't mean you have to sacrifice good taste or feel hungry or dissatisfied. In fact, you will probably find snacks and meals very filling and delicious if you choose as many foods as possible that are nutrient-dense, high in volume but low in calories, high in fiber, and rich in antioxidants.

Nutrient-Dense Foods You may have heard people talk about foods—sugar, for example—that provide only "empty calories." What they mean is that such foods provide calories for energy without supplying other healthful nutrients. By contrast, **nutrient-dense foods** provide rich sources of vitamins, minerals, antioxidants, and fiber and minimize saturated fat, added sugars, sodium, and refined carbohydrates. Choosing nutrient-dense foods means striving to maximize the food value of each and every meal and snack you consume.

To see what this means in a practical way, compare two small meals—a glass of cola and a hot dog versus a glass of low-fat milk and a small serving of salmon. The cola provides 105 calories, all from refined carbohydrates. In about the same number of calories, the milk provides 8 grams

whole foods Dietary items produced and consumed with the minimum of processing (refining, adding preservatives, or altering form for quick preparation)

nutrient-dense foods Foods or beverages that provide a high level of nutrients and thus maximize the nutritional value of each meal and snack consumed of protein along with vitamin D and calcium. The cola is nutrient-poor; the milk is nutrient-dense.

Now compare the hot dog and salmon. A hot dog on a white-bread bun supplies 420 calories. It contains more than a whole day's recommended amount of saturated fat, 9 grams of protein, most of a day's allotted sodium, and refined white flour lacking much fiber. In contrast, a serving of salmon provides fewer than 200 calories, 10 grams of heart-healthy omega-3 fatty acids, twice as much protein, and a small fraction of the sodium. The hot dog has fewer healthful nutrients while the salmon is nutrient-dense.

Learning to reach for nutrient-dense foods every time you get hungry will greatly benefit your lifelong fitness and wellness. If your diet consists primarily of processed foods such as pastries, coffee drinks, pizza, hamburgers, and cola, you may not even know what wellness feels like! Why should you care about eating too many calories, too much saturated fat, too many refined carbohydrates, and too much sodium? Because dietary excesses can affect your appearance, energy level, athletic performance, social life, ability to fight off infections, and overall sense of well-being. Try shifting toward nutrient-dense foods and away from empty calories, and watch for positive changes in those short-term measures. Focus on establishing habits, including the whole foods habit, that keep you looking and feeling vibrantly well today and your lifelong wellness will improve, too.

High-Volume, Low-Calorie Foods

We eat for many reasons, but the primary one is *satiety*: a feeling of fullness and the physical and emotional pleasure it brings. Nutrition researchers have discovered that each of us has a characteristic weight of food that we eat in a day. You can eat that weight of food in candy bars, potato chips, steak, and ice cream, but you will be getting too few nutrients and too many calories and you probably wouldn't feel full for very long between meals. You could eat that same weight of food in celery, iceberg lettuce, and bran and still get too few nutrients, but the volume would help keep you full. The proper goal is somewhere in between: a filling, calorie-appropriate diet

antioxidants Compounds in foods that help protect the body against the damaging effects of oxygen derivatives called *free radicals*

that also emphasizes nutrient density. Relatively recent nutritional research has shown that eating nutritious foods with more volume due to higher air or water content can help people feel full and satisfied longer.[31] This is especially helpful for dieters or for people who want to maintain their weight and not gain more.

Foods with high contents of water, fiber, or protein tend to keep you full and satisfied longer, while those with high contents of fat, sugar, or refined carbohydrates leave you feeling hungry sooner. However, the water must be in the food (as in soups, fruits, and vegetables) and not just in a glass accompanying your meal. Apparently, your brain's satiety center knows the difference and isn't fooled by drinking water. Figure 7.12 compares two sandwiches with approximately the same number of calories, but very different ingredients. Table 7.5 lists familiar foods by calorie density.

High-Fiber Foods

Fiber adds bulk and, often, a chewy quality to food. Both help satisfy hunger better and for longer periods. Soluble fiber such as that in oats, barley, and apples, for example, lowers LDL cholesterol. Grains that are intact (like brown rice or bulgur wheat) instead of finely ground (as in whole wheat flour) have a lower glycemic index. High-fiber foods also improve the passage of digested material through the digestive tract.

Antioxidant-Rich Foods

Free radicals are molecules with unpaired electrons that the body produces in excess when it is overly stressed. Free radicals can damage or kill healthy cells, cell proteins, or genetic material in cells. **Antioxidants** produce enzymes that scavenge free radicals, slow their formation, and actually repair oxidative stress damage. Thus, the theory goes that if you

(a)   **(b)**

FIGURE **7.12**   These two sandwiches have approximately the same number of calories (300), but one (a) is small and filled with saturated fat. It contains mayonnaise, butter, cheese, and bacon on a white roll. The other sandwich (b) is large, high-volume, and rich in fiber and vitamins. It contains whole wheat bread, tomato, lettuce, green and red peppers, and cheese.

TABLE 7.5 Comparing Calorie Density in Common Foods

Examples of Foods with Low Calorie Density	Examples of Foods with Medium Calorie Density	Examples of Foods with High Calorie Density
Raw celery (1250 grams = 200 calories)	Brown rice, cooked (179 grams = 200 calories)	Hot dog, Oscar Meyer beef (61 grams = 200 calories)
Watermelon (666 grams = 200 calories)	Enriched spaghetti, cooked (126 grams = 200 calories)	French fries, McDonald's (59 grams = 200 calories)
Raw broccoli (588 grams = 200 calories)	Chicken breast, roasted (121 grams = 200 calories)	Potato chips, plain salted (37 grams = 200 calories)
Red or green grapes (290 grams = 200 calories)	Salmon, cooked, Alaskan wild (110 grams = 200 calories)	Peanut butter, smooth salted (34 grams = 200 calories)

Data from U.S. Department of Agriculture, Agricultural Research Service. 2007. USDA National Nutrient Database for Standard Reference, Release 20. Nutrient Data Laboratory Home Page, http://www.ars.usda.gov/ba/bhnrc/ndl

consume lots of antioxidants, you will nullify or greatly reduce the negative effects of oxidative stress. Among the more commonly cited nutrients touted as providing a protective effect are vitamin C, vitamin E, beta-carotene and other carotenoids, and the mineral selenium.

How valid is the theory? To date, many claims about the benefits of antioxidants in reducing the risk of heart disease, improving vision, and slowing the aging process have not been fully investigated; conclusive statements about their true benefits are difficult to make. Large, longitudinal epidemiological studies support the hypothesis that antioxidants in foods, mostly fruits and vegetables (Figure 7.13), help protect against cognitive decline and risk of Parkinson's disease. However, because of problems with study design and difficulties in isolating dietary effects from supplement effects, it is difficult to assess overall benefits of antioxidants.[32]

Some studies indicate that when people's diets include foods rich in vitamin C, they seem to develop fewer cancers, but other studies detect no effect from dietary vitamin C.[33] Recent studies indicate that high-dose vitamin C given intravenously, rather than orally, may be effective in treating cancer and providing protection from diseases affecting the central nervous system.[34] Early studies seemed to show that vitamin E had antioxidant effects that could help prevent heart disease and cancer. Large trials involving hundreds of people

taking vitamin E supplements, however, have shown very mixed results, with some indicating no benefit.[35] The vitamin E in foods does seem to help protect the cell membranes of red blood cells and the delicate surface lining our lungs.

Phytochemicals Plants make thousands of compounds collectively called *phytochemicals* (meaning literally "plant chemicals"), many of which have antioxidant properties. Fruit, flowers, and plant leaves form a bright palette of colors, in part because plants can generate pigments with antioxidant properties such as *beta-carotene* (yellow and orange pigments), *lycopene* (red

FIGURE **7.13** Fruits and vegetables such as blueberries and kale are high in antioxidants.

pigments), and *lutein,* found in various green, red, yellow, and orange foods.[36]

Most people love the idea of "magic bullets"—pills that will quickly solve their health problems with no other effort. Many people have begun taking antioxidant supplements despite a lack of evidence for their effectiveness in supplement form. Most nutrition researchers recommend getting your antioxidants from nutrient-dense foods or from multivitamin supplements.[37]

Foods Containing Folate In 1998, the U.S. Food and Drug Administration (FDA) started requiring food manufacturers to fortify all bread, cereal, rice, and macaroni products sold in the United States with **folate** (also called *folic acid*). Folate is a form of vitamin B that participates in the development of the spinal cord. Folate also helps break down the compound homocysteine, which is produced as the body digests meat and other high-protein foods. By helping break down homocysteine, folate may also protect against cardiovascular disease, heart attacks, and strokes.[38]

Do I Need Special Nutrition for Exercise?

Fitness requires physical activity, but does it also require a special diet? Active people may need some extra nutrients—a little more protein, perhaps, and some extra carbohydrates for fast energy and endurance. But big imbalances in the major nutrients, such as those caused by a high-protein diet or a low-carbohydrate regimen, cannot support improved fitness.

Most Exercisers Can Follow General Nutritional Guidelines

Exercisers often look for an "edge" and wonder what they can eat, drink, or swallow in pill form that will help them get into shape faster or better. Significantly, sports physiologists and nutritionists have conducted hundreds of studies of recreational, collegiate, and professional athletes, trying to determine optimal energy and nutrient levels for peak performance. Their findings may surprise and disappoint many fitness enthusiasts: they closely follow general nutritional guidelines with only a few minor adjustments.

folate A form of vitamin B that is vital for spinal cord development and helps break down homocysteine as the body digests proteins

Carbohydrates
The best source of energy before and during exercise is carbohydrates; they

should provide up to about 55 to 65 percent of daily calories.[39] Restricting carbohydrates can impede your fitness efforts by leaving you energy-deprived. Sugars can give a little energy boost but can also cause a rise in insulin and a drop in blood sugar that produces fatigue.

Proteins For moderate strengthening and endurance exercise, most of us need about 0.75 to 0.8 gram of protein per kilogram of body weight per day. Protein does not in itself help build muscle. Only activity, including weight training, adds new muscle.

Elite Athletes Have Extra Nutritional Needs

While most exercisers can get complete nutrition from a balanced diet of nutrient-dense foods, some elite athletes—those with the potential for intercollegiate, Olympic, or professional sports—do need to modify their eating patterns for better training and performance.

Calories People in regular training for competitive sports need extra calories. Athletes often have greater muscle mass than the average person, and muscle tissue consumes more calories than fat tissue, even at rest. A tall young man training with a football or basketball team, for example, could require 5,000 calories or more daily. High activity levels sustained for long periods—the running during a soccer match, for example—also require extra fuel. About 55 to 65 percent of that extra athletic fuel should come from complex carbohydrates—bread, pasta, cereals, grains, vegetables, and fruits.[40] Some nutritionists recommend up to 70 percent carbohydrates for sustained high-level activities.

Endurance events requiring heavy exertion for more than 90 minutes use two types of internal body fuels, glycogen and fat. Your muscles can store about 90 minutes' worth of glycogen, and additional storage in your liver can fuel a few more minutes of exercise. After that, your body uses its own fat to fuel activity (Figure 7.14). Endurance athletes such as marathon runners, swimmers, and soccer players often consume 60 or 70 percent of their diet in complex carbohydrates starting two to three days before an athletic event to store sufficient glycogen and fat. Consuming five to seven grams of carbohydrates per kilogram of body weight per day is usually enough for general training, while seven to 10 grams/kilogram/day will fuel endurance training and strenuous one-time events.

Pre- and Post-event Meals Trainers usually instruct athletes to drink plenty of water, to eat complex carbohydrates three or four hours before an event, and to avoid

Types of metabolic fuels:

■ Muscle glycogen
■ Blood glucose
■ Fatty acids from adipose triglycerides
■ Muscle triglycerides

During first hour of exercise · During second hour of exercise · During third hour of exercise · During fourth hour of exercise

FIGURE **7.14** If you exercise for less than one hour, your body uses mostly glycogen and fatty acids (triglycerides) stored in your muscles. If you exercise for four hours, the fuel ratios shift dramatically and your activity is mainly powered by blood sugar and the breakdown of fat (adipose) tissue.

proteins, fats, refined sugars, caffeine, and gas-producing foods in the pregame meal. They recommend avoiding protein, because protein takes more time to digest and can lead to increased urination and dehydration. Likewise, fats and oils are slow to digest. Sugar is on the list because it induces a surge of insulin in the blood and later, during the event, can cause an energy dip. Caffeine can lead to increased urination and dehydration and to an accelerated heartbeat. Gas-producing foods can upset digestion.

Most athletes need water and additional carbohydrates during the event, and many choose sports drinks diluted with water to sustain energy and provide sufficient hydration. You can learn more about this by visiting the American College of Sports Medicine's website (www.acsm.org) to view their guidelines on exercise and fluid replacement.[41]

Selecting foods for post-performance meals is also important to help restore the muscles' energy supply. After a training or performance session you should eat simple and complex carbohydrates as soon as possible.

Is the popular practice of carbo-loading necessary? If you define *carbo-loading* as eating one huge starch meal the night before an athletic event, then no, it is not necessary or desirable. This kind of consumption can cause the body to retain water, the muscles to feel stiff the next day, and the athlete to feel slow and sluggish when the event starts.

If you define *carbo-loading* as eating 55 to 65 percent of your calories as complex carbohydrates at every meal for two to three days before an event, then it is desirable because it can load the muscles with glycogen for sustained activity if previous carbohydrate intake was low. Manipulating the pre-exercise diet with more or less sugar, fat, or protein seems to have little effect on most people's performance.[42]

Vitamins and Minerals The body's energy production and use requires B vitamins; bone- and blood-building require iron and calcium; sweating causes the loss of sodium and potassium that must be replenished during or after events. A balanced diet provides most athletes with enough vitamins and minerals to meet recommended intakes.

Supplements Optimal muscle growth and strength gain do not require nutritional supplements. Most competitive athletes in high school and college do take various kinds of supplements, including mega-doses of certain vitamins and minerals as well as purported muscle builders.[43] Where there is no deficiency to start with, these mega-doses provide little or no benefit to performance.[44] The popular creatine monohydrate is chemically related to a natural substance called *creatine phosphate*, which helps fuel muscle contraction. Vendors claim creatine monohydrate helps build muscle, increases energy to improve performance, and delays muscle fatigue. Objective scientific studies suggest that taking creatine orally may cause muscles to temporarily retain more water, and this may boost short-term performance under anaerobic conditions. Thus, it may pump up the muscles a bit so they feel bigger, but it is not helpful for endurance events. And it does not do what many athletes are hoping for: build permanently bigger muscles. This requires regular physical strength training.

Also popular are individual, concentrated amino acid supplements such as taurine, arginine, glutamine, and leucine. Eating protein-rich foods provides these very same building blocks but in safe concentrations and in naturally occurring mixtures of multiple amino acids. In contrast, supplements provide artificially high concentrations of individual amino acids that may block your body's absorption of the full amino acid spectrum.

What's more, amino acid supplements can become contaminated and are far more expensive than eating protein-rich foods. Most importantly, vendors claim that amino acid supplements will help build muscle and sustain muscle contraction, but there is no good evidence of these benefits.

Meal Timing People use the term *meal timing* in various ways, and some trainers claim that *when* you eat fats, proteins, and carbohydrates will determine how quickly you can build muscles in the gym or how well you can sustain activity during a long bike ride. Carbo-loading and pre- and post-event meals are all forms of meal timing. So are regimens that instruct you to eat proteins early in the day, carbohydrates at lunch, and so on.

Research shows that the most significant thing about meal timing is the effect on your appetite. Skipping meals, getting ravenously hungry, then "gorging" most of your day's calories at dinner is far more likely to cause fat accumulation than "grazing" on five or six small meals throughout the day. Sumo wrestlers deliberately apply this principle to put on hundreds of pounds

. . . .

casestudy

CHAU

"I'm not an 'athlete,' but I do like sports. I've never worried too much about supplementing my diet with extras. I figure as long as I eat enough to feel satisfied, my body's getting what it needs. Some of my friends—like Tom, who's a cross-country runner—are always drinking sports drinks and eating energy bars. I've also noticed Tom often has a pasta dinner two days before a big run, and then he will eat a lighter meal the night before the race. He's also pretty strict about taking a multivitamin every day. It makes me wonder if I should start taking vitamins too."

THINK! How do Chau's and Tom's nutritional needs differ? Should Chau begin taking vitamin supplements? Why would Tom eat pasta two nights before a big run, instead of the night before the race?

ACT! Analyze your own physical activity. Could you benefit from consuming more or fewer calories? Do you need to add nutrients to your diet, and if so which ones?

HEAR IT! ONLINE

of fat. If they spread their daily 6,000 calories into five or six meals instead of two, they would weigh up to 25 percent less![45]

Do I Have Special Nutritional Needs?

In its *Dietary Guidelines for Americans*, the USDA highlights several groups with special nutritional needs and concerns, including children, teens, adults over 50, vegetarians, and diabetics. We review the needs of vegetarians and diabetics here.

Vegetarians Must Monitor Their Nutrient Intake

More and more people today are choosing partial or strict vegetarian diets. Between five and 15 percent of all Americans claim to be one of the following, arranged in order from the strictest and most exclusive of animal products to the least: Strict *vegetarians* (also called *vegans*) avoid all foods of animal origin, including dairy products and eggs; *lacto-vegetarians* avoid animal flesh but eat dairy products; *ovo-vegetarians* avoid animal flesh and dairy products but eat eggs; *lacto-ovo-vegetarians* consume both dairy products and eggs; or *semi-vegetarians,* consume fish and/or poultry but no red meat.

Vegetarian diets have certain benefits.[46] Most people who follow a balanced vegetarian diet weigh less than non-vegetarians of similar height. Most also have healthier cholesterol levels, less constipation and diarrhea, and a lower risk of heart disease. Research indicates that vegetarians may also have a lower risk for colon and breast cancers.[47] It is not clear whether these lower risks are due to their vegetarian diets per se or to some combination of lifestyle factors such as eating less saturated fat, avoiding smoking, and exercising more.

Despite their benefits, vegetarian diets can have deficiencies; with careful food choices, however, vegetarians can avoid deficiencies. Lacto-ovo vegetarians who eat dairy products and small amounts of chicken or fish are seldom nutrient-deficient. Vegans can get enough essential amino acids through complementary combinations of plant products (review Figure 7.3 on page 244). Lacto-vegetarians usually get enough vitamins D and B$_{12}$ from dairy products, while strict vegans can develop deficiencies. Fortified products such as soy milk can usually provide enough of these vitamins. Vegans are sometimes deficient in vitamin B$_2$ (riboflavin) since

Daily Beverage Recommendations:
6 glasses of water

Alcohol in moderation

Eggs & sweets — Weekly

Egg whites, soy milk & dairy — Daily

Nuts & seeds

Plant oils

Whole grains

Fruits & vegetables

Legumes & beans

At every meal

Daily physical activity

FIGURE **7.15**   Vegetarians must be careful to get enough protein, calcium, B vitamins, and other nutrients; they can do this by following this pyramid as a food guide.

Source: Oldways' Vegetarian Diet Pyramid. Copyright © 2000 Oldways Preservation and Exchange Trust. Used by permission, www.oldwayspt.org.

it is found mainly in meat, eggs, and dairy products. They can get enough B_2, however, by eating generous amounts of broccoli, asparagus, almonds, and fortified cereals. Because meat is rich in iron and dairy products are rich in calcium, vegans who avoid both can develop deficiencies of these minerals. Solutions include choosing mineral-rich plant foods (see Table 7.3) and/or taking multivitamin/mineral supplements.

In general, vegans can stay in excellent health by eating a wide variety of grains, legumes, fruits, vegetables, and seeds each day. Figure 7.15 shows a vegetarian food pyramid.

Those with Diabetes Must Reduce Carbohydrates

Anyone diagnosed with type 1 or type 2 diabetes will receive specific information from medical providers about both necessary drug treatments and dietary changes. Because diabetes is a disorder of blood-sugar regulation, patients usually must cut back on sweets and desserts, both to reduce surges of sugar in the blood and to control obesity, which can lead to and intensify diabetes. Choosing foods with a lower rather than higher glycemic index (see page 248) is also beneficial, and this usually means less-processed foods and reduced fat content. The American Diabetes Association advises diabetics to eats lots of non-starchy vegetables and fruits, to choose whole grains over processed grain products, to include beans and lentils in the diet, to eat fish two to three times per week, to choose lean meats and nonfat dairy products, to drink water and diet drinks instead of sugary drinks, to avoid saturated fats and *trans* fats during cooking, and to watch portion sizes.[48]

Good Food Safety Practices Are for Everyone

Sometimes people think they have the flu when it is actually "food poisoning." Food-borne illnesses usually cause diarrhea, nausea, cramping, and vomiting. They usually occur five to eight hours after eating and last only a day or two. For many of us, food poisoning is unpleasant and inconvenient. For the very young, the elderly, or people with cancer, diabetes, AIDS, or other severe illnesses, it can be fatal.

Every year, millions of Americans become sick from unclean or poorly handled foods, sometimes with life-threatening consequences. The CDC estimates that every year 48 million Americans are sickened, 128,000 are hospitalized, and 3,000 die from food-borne illnesses.[49]

A rise in imports of fresh fruits and vegetables from developing countries, as well as increased urbanization, industrialization, travel, and restaurant dining raise the risk of unsafe food handling and resulting illness. Here are some tips for avoiding foodborne illness:

• Be aware of cleanliness in stores and restaurants. When purchasing food, be aware of the expiration dates on perishable foods.

- Use proper at-home techniques for storing and handling food.
  - Keep hands and cooking surfaces clean.
  - Separate raw foods from cooked foods during storage and cooking.
  - Scrub and thoroughly rinse produce before eating it.
  - Heat foods to high enough temperatures to kill germs.
  - Refrigerate perishable foods.
  - Safely handle the most common sources of foodborne illness: raw eggs, meat, poultry, and fish; unwashed or outdated bean or alfalfa sprouts; and unpasteurized milk and juices.

Some people have concerns about the safety of foods produced with the use of genetically modified organisms or their products, or foods that are irradiated to kill microorganisms and prolong shelf life. You can learn more about these issues by visiting the web links listed on this book's website.

How Can I Create a Behavior Change Plan for Nutrition?

You've no doubt heard the famous phrase, "You are what you eat." But did you know that its origin was a book written in 1825 by Anthelme Brillat-Savain—a French lawyer who loved the pleasures of the table above all else? What he actually wrote was, "Tell me what you eat and I shall tell you what you are." We could modify that slightly to make it perfectly relevant to this book and to you, the reader: tell us what you eat and we'll tell you how fit and well you're likely to be now and in the future!

SEE IT! ONLINE

You Are What You Eat?

Assess Your Current Diet

Would you benefit from changes to your current diet? The most successful way to change long-ingrained eating habits is to break the task into steps and keep track of your progress.

Recording What You Eat If you filled in Lab 7.2 using either a manual food diary or the food tracker found at www.ChooseMyPlate.gov, then you are on your way to a better diet. Self-awareness is the necessary starting point for change, followed by your own actions for self-improvement.[50]

LIVE IT! ONLINE

Worksheet 20 Your Eating Habits

You should get a pretty clear idea of how many calories your daily diet provides and whether your diet meets, exceeds, or falls short of the daily values for carbohydrates, fats, proteins, fiber, vitamins, and minerals. If there are gaps in your food diary, keep track of your hour-by-hour food consumption for another day or two so you have a clear picture of your typical nutritional profile.

Identifying Your Patterns Go through your food diary and analyze your reasons for eating each meal and snack. Was it primarily hunger? Primarily socializing? Primarily boredom? If it is hunger, are you satisfying that need with nutrient-dense foods? If it is primarily socializing, are you even hungry at the time? Does peer pressure persuade you to eat an after-dinner snack of pizza and frozen yogurt when you could be happy with a salad, an apple, or a low-cal beverage? If you are eating out of boredom or stress—snacking on chips and cola while studying, for example—could you find a more nutritious alternative such as carrot sticks, whole wheat crackers, unsalted peanuts, popcorn, or grapes?

By reflecting on and identifying your own reasons for food preferences and eating habits, you can start to understand your patterns and perhaps change them for the better. It is seldom easy or automatic to improve your diet because it means breaking long-standing habits. But new behaviors become somewhat simpler if you realize when and why you reach for certain foods and that the resistance to change may come from within yourself or your family and friends.

Review Your Behavior Change Skills

Examining your current eating patterns is just one part of applying behavior change skills to improve your nutrition. Here are some other ways you can incorporate the behavior change model:

- *Look at your motivation.* Do you really want a different and better diet? What do you see as the immediate benefits of improved nutrition? What do you expect over the long term? Solidifying your motivation can help you get ready for change.

- *Identify barriers to a better diet.* What are some of the difficulties you foresee in achieving better nutrition? Time? Money? Eating in less-than-optimal ways with friends and family? Naming some of those barriers and coming up with alternatives can help you on the path to change. If you have trouble brainstorming solutions, the student health service or counseling center may be able to help you.

- *Make a commitment to learning about better nutrition.* Based on what you learn, list ways in which an improved diet will benefit your life. What could eating more whole grain fiber do for you? How about consuming more fruits and vegetables? Listing these will help you stick with your plan for change.

- *Choose a target behavior by identifying your biggest nutritional concern.* What is the most pressing issue with your current diet? Review your food diary. If you see that you're getting too much saturated fat every day, outline an approach for getting less saturated fat in your meals and snacks. If you discover that fried meats and cheese (on hamburgers, nachos, pizzas, etc.) are pushing up your daily total, think of lower-fat alternatives from those same menus, or try new places to eat.

- *Note where you stand in the typical stages of change.* Are you contemplating change? If so, gathering more information or talking more with friends and family might help. Are you planning for change and getting ready to take action?

- *Have you noticed any helpful role models?* Do you know people with good eating habits and a nutritious diet? Observing their food choices and talking to them about your nutritional issues may help you learn to counter your current habits with others based on better food choices, more successful eating patterns, and solid nutritional information.

Get Set to Apply Nutritional Skills

With this chapter, you've already begun to learn and apply nutritional skills. Review your use of them and look for ways to improve those skills and call upon them daily.

Examine food guides to compare your daily servings of various food groups with the amounts that nutritionists recommend from governmental agencies or from academic institutions. Read food labels more often and watch for those nutrients you've identified as problematic in your own diet. For example, watch for hidden fats and sugars and look for opportunities to increase fiber.

Recognize proper portion sizes and note when the helping you are served in a restaurant or cafeteria is way too big (three cups of pasta instead of half

a cup, for example) or way too small (a side salad the size of a golf ball, for example, instead of a softball). Use www.ChooseMyPlate.gov or other kinds of diet software to get an individual analysis of the daily calories and nutrients you consume and how they compare with the recommended daily intakes of each.

Both behavior-change skills and nutritional tools can help you plan your own program for improved nutrition. Working this plan can give you practice at recognizing nutrient-dense foods. You can start to choose high-volume, low-density alternatives to high-density, high-calorie foods. You may find that you now prefer whole grains to refined ones. And you may start to savor the colors, flavors, and textures of fruits and/or vegetables with every snack and meal.

Your plan may be your first deliberate application of nutritional tools and behavioral-change skills for nutrition. In time, however, it should become a continual and automatic part of each day. The goal is to balance nutrients and control calories naturally as part of your long-term efforts for fitness and wellness and your ongoing management of body mass and weight.

Create a Nutrition Plan

Begin planning your own program using **Lab 7.3**. As you work through the lab, write down your own notes and observations and swap them with others in your class, perhaps during a class discussion or in a small discussion group.

Keep track of calories for your new plan. Are you on track? Where could you cut or add without increasing saturated fats or sugars?

After two weeks, discuss the plan and your results with your fitness/health instructor, and revise if necessary. Again, if possible, discuss your experiences with others in your class to exchange successful ideas and get support for your efforts.

For several weeks, continue tracking your daily diet, either manually or using www.ChooseMyPlate.gov—at least for the number of servings of the main food groups. This helps you eat sufficient amounts of the foods you needed to increase (for example, whole grains, fruits, vegetables, beans, nuts) and helps you cut back on those that are already overrepresented (for example, saturated fat or refined carbohydrates). Be sure to continue applying nutritional skills such as reading labels and comparing serving sizes to the portions in Figure 7.10 (on page 265).

Don't try for perfection! Approach your diet in sets of two or three days at a time. When you have a day with too few fruits and vegetables, increase them the next day. When you have a day with too little protein, have more the next day. If you get too much protein one day, eat less the next or eat less-concentrated protein foods such as tofu, beans, or skim milk.

chapterin**review**

videos

Log on to **www.pearsonhighered.com/hopson** or MyFitnessLab to view these chapter-related videos.

How Much Sugar?   Going Green   You Are What You Eat?
Which Fish Is Safest to Eat?

onlineresources

Log on to **www.pearsonhighered.com/hopson** or MyFitnessLab for access to these book-related resources, and for links to other useful websites.

 Audio case study
Audio PowerPoint lecture

 Lab 7.1 Reading a Food Label
Lab 7.2 Keeping a Food Diary and Analyzing Your Daily Nutrition
Lab 7.3 Improving Your Nutrition

 Take Charge of Your Health! Worksheets:
Worksheet 18 Grocery Shopping List
Worksheet 19 Food Log
Worksheet 20 Your Eating Habits and Extra Calories
Worksheet 24 Cutting out the Fat
Behavior Change Log Book and Wellness Journal

 Pre- and post-quizzes
Glossary flashcards

reviewquestions

1. Which of the following would be considered a healthy, nutrient-dense food?
   a. Cheddar cheese
   b. Soft drink
   c. Potato chips
   d. Fat-free milk

2. Essential amino acids are
   a. found only in animal proteins.
   b. found only in plant proteins.
   c. best taken as supplements.
   d. protein building blocks your body can't produce.

3. Simple carbohydrates
   a. are important amino acid compounds.
   b. act as structural compounds in plants.
   c. provide fiber in the diet.
   d. deliver energy in a quickly usable form.

4. Using the glycemic index, one can determine
   a. the percentage of glucose in a food.
   b. the percentage of glycine in a food.
   c. how quickly a food will boost your blood sugar levels.
   d. the caloric content of a food.

5. What do nutritionists sometimes call "bad cholesterol"?
   a. Saturated fat
   b. Butter
   c. HDLs
   d. LDLs

6. Which of these is a poor source of essential fatty acids?
   a. Omega-3 fatty acids
   b. Omega-6 fatty acids
   c. Polyunsaturated oils
   d. Saturated oils such as palm kernel or coconut

7. Vitamins can
   a. act as structural components of bones and teeth.
   b. act as hormones that help regulate the body's use of glucose.
   c. help us convert food molecules into cellular fuel.
   d. delay wound healing.

8. Calcium can
   a. cause osteoporosis (brittle bones).
   b. delay blood clotting.
   c. prevent proper nerve impulse transmission.
   d. play an important role in muscle contraction.

9. An example of an antioxidant would be
   a. vitamin C.
   b. vitamin B 12.
   c. selenium.
   d. iron.

10. For proper food handling and safety
   a. use all produce straight from the garden or market without washing.
   b. avoid pasteurized milk and juices.
   c. observe expiration dates on food packaging.
   d. store raw and cooked foods together in airtight containers.

11. By law, a food label must
   a. tell the exact number of items in the package.
   b. give the manufacturer's business address.
   c. calculate the percentage of calories from fat.
   d. provide a recommended serving size.

critical**thinking**questions

 REVIEW IT! ONLINE

1. Write out a healthy menu for yourself for one breakfast, one lunch, and one dinner, including portion sizes for each type of food you select.
2. Excluding water, what are the major types of nutrients in food? What are the main roles of each?
3. Name several protective functions of dietary fiber.

4. Differentiate *trans* fat and saturated fat. Name two dietary sources of each. Which is worse, and why?
5. How do antioxidants protect the body against the damaging effects of free radicals?
6. Describe the requirements for calcium and vitamin D in children, women of childbearing age, and people over 50.

references

1. U.S. Department of Agriculture, Agriculture Research Service, "What We Eat in America, NHANES 2003–2004," 2006.
2. U.S. Department of Agriculture, Agricultural Marketing Service, *How to Buy Fresh Vegetables*, Home and Garden Bulletin No. 258, 1994.
3. American College Health Association, *ACHA-National College Health Assessment Survey II: Reference Group Data Report Spring 2010* (Linthicum, MD: American College Health Association, 2010).
4. W. D. Hoyt, S. B. Hamilton, and K. M. Rickard, "The Effects of Dietary Fat and Caloric Content on the Body-Size Estimates of Anorexic Profile and Normal College Students," *Journal of Clinical Psychology* 59, no. 1 (2003): 85–91.
5. L. B. Brown, R. K. Dresen, and D. L. Eggett, "College Students Can Benefit by Participating in a Prepaid Meal Plan," *Journal of the American Dietetic Association* 105, no. 3 (2005): 445–8.
6. P. W. Lemon, "Is Increased Dietary Protein Necessary or Beneficial for Individuals with a Physically Active Lifestyle?" *Nutrition Review* 54, no. 4 pt. 2 (1996): S 169–75.
7. S. M. Phillips, "Protein Requirements and Supplementation in Strength Sports," *Nutrition* 20, nos. 7–8 (2004): 689–95.

8. American Cancer Society, "ACS Guidelines on Nutrition and Physical Activity for Cancer Prevention: Common Questions about Diet and Cancer," www.cancer.org /Healthy/EatHealthyGetActive /ACSGuidelinesonNutritionPhysical ActivityforCancerPrevention /acs-guidelines-on-nutrition-and-physical-activity-for-cancer-prevention-diet-cancer-questions (revised May 2011).
9. U.S. Food and Drug Administration, "How to Understand and Use the Nutrition Facts Label," www.fda.gov/food/labelingnutrition /consumerinformation/ucm078889.htm (updated March 2011).
10. J. Higdon, "Micronutrient Information Center: Glycemic Index and Glycemic Load," Linus Pauling Institute, Oregon State University, http://lpi.oregonstate.edu /infocenter/foods/grains/gigl.html (updated April 2010).
11. F. Sacks, "Ask the Expert: Omega-3 Fatty Acids," The Nutrition Source, Harvard School of Public Health, www.hsph .harvard.edu/nutritionsource/questions /omega-3/index.html (accessed February 2011); N. D. Riediger and others, "A Systemic Review of the Roles of n-3 Fatty Acids in Health and Disease," *Journal of the American Dietetic Association* 109, no. 4 (2009): 668–79.

12. J. Thompson and M. Manore, *Nutrition: An Applied Approach* 3rd Edition (San Francisco: Pearson, 2012).
13. W. Willett and D. Mozaffarian, "*Trans* Fats in Cardiac and Diabetes Risk: An Overview," *Current Cardiovascular Risk Reports* 1, no. 1 (2007): 16–23.
14. United States Department of Agriculture, "Empty Calories: What Are 'Solid Fats'?" www.choosemyplate.gov/foodgroups /emptycalories_fats.html (modified June 2011).
15. American Heart Association, "What Are Triglycerides?," American Heart Association internet publication, www.americanheart .org.
16. F. B. Hu and W. C. Willett, "Optimal Diets for Prevention of Coronary Heart Disease," *Journal of the American Medical Association* 288, no. 20 (November 2002): 2569–78.
17. J. May, "Ascorbic Acid Transporters in Health and Disease," paper given at Linus Pauling Diet and Optimum Health Annual Conference, Portland, OR, May, 2007.
18. L. J. Appel and C. A. M. Anderson, "Compelling Evidence for Public Health Action to Reduce Salt Intake," *New England Journal of Medicine* 362, no. 7 (2010): 650–2.
19. H. W. Cohen and others, "Sodium Intake and Mortality in the NHANES II Follow-Up Study," *American Journal of Medicine* 119, no. 3 (2006): 275.e7–14; J. Feng and others,

"Salt Intake and Cardiovascular Mortality," *American Journal of Medicine* 120, no. 1 (2007): e5–e7; H. Karppanen and E. Mervaala, "Sodium Intake and Hypertension," Progress in Cardiovascular Diseases 49, no. 2 (2006): 59–75.

20. J. Midgley and others, "Effects of Reduced Dietary Sodium on Blood Pressure: A Meta-Analysis of Randomized Controlled Trials," *The Journal of the American Medical Association* 275, no. 20 (1996): 1590–7.

21. Robert P. Heaney, "Role of Dietary Sodium in Osteoporosis," *Journal of the American College of Nutrition* 25, no. 3 suppl (2006): 271S–276S.

22. J. Ma, R. Johns, and R. Stafford, "Americans Are Not Meeting Current Calcium Recommendations," *American Journal of Clinical Nutrition* 85, no. 5 (2007): 1361–6.

23. I. A. Dontas and C.K. Yiannakopoulos, "Risk Factors and Prevention of Osteoporosis-Related Fractures," *Journal of Musculoskeletal and Neuronal Interactions* 7, no. 3 (2007): 268–272.

24. K. Tucker and others, "Colas, but Not Other Carbonated Beverages, Are Associated with Low Bone Mineral Density in Older Women: The Framingham Osteoporosis Study," *American Journal of Clinical Nutrition* 84, no. 4 (2006): 936–42.

25. World Health Organization, "Micronutrient Deficiencies: Iron Deficiency Anaemia," www.who.int/nutrition/topics/ida/en/index.html (accessed February 2011).

26. Office of Dietary Supplements, National Institutes of Health, "Dietary Supplement Fact Sheet: Iron," (Reviewed August 2007).

27. J. Postlethwait and J. Hopson, *Explore Life* (Pacific Grove, CA: Brooks/Cole, 2003): 400–1 .

28. Institute of Medicine of the National Academies, Food and Nutrition Board, *Dietary Reference Intakes for Water, Potassium, Sodium, Chloride, and Sulfate* (Washington, DC: The National Academies Press, 2004).

29. Consumers Union, "A Guide to the Best and Worst Drinks," *Consumer Reports on Health* (July 2006): 8–9.

30. USDA, Center for Nutrition Policy and Promotion, "A Brief History of USDA Food Guides," www.choosemyplate.gov/downloads/MyPlate/ABriefHistoryOfUSDAFoodGuides.pdf (June 2011).

31. B. J. Rolls, E. A. Bell, and B. A. Waugh, "Increasing the Volume of a Food by Incorporating Air Affects Satiety in Men," *American Journal of Clinical Nutrition* 72, no. 2 (2000): 361–8.

32. A. Asherio, "Dietary Antioxidant Intakes and Neurological Disease Risks," Paper presented at the Linus Pauling Diet and Optimum Health Annual Conference (Portland, OR: May 2007).

33. J. Thompson and M. Manore, *Nutrition: An Applied Approach* 3rd Edition, 2012.

34. J. May, "Ascorbic Acid Transporters in Health and Disease," 2007.

35. E. R. Miller III and others, "Meta-Analysis: High-Dosage Vitamin E Supplementation May Increase All-Cause Mortality," *Annals of Internal Medicine* 142, no. 1 (2005): 37–46.

36. W. Willett, *Eat, Drink, and Be Healthy: The Harvard Medical School Guide to Healthy Eating* (New York: Free Press, 2003).

37. B. Frei, "Closing Remarks Summary, 2001," Paper presented at the Linus Pauling Institute International Conference on Diet and Optimum Health (Portland, OR: May, 2001).

38. Ibid.

39. M. Gonzalez-Gross and others, "Nutrition in the Sport Practice: Adaptation of the Food Guide Pyramid to the Characteristics of Athletes Diet," *Archives of Latino American Nutrition* 51, no. 4 (2001): 321–31.

40. L. M. Burke and others, "Carbohydrates and Fat for Training and Recovery," *Journal of Sports Science* 22, no. 1 (2004): 15–30.

41. M. N. Sawka, "American College of Sports Medicine Position Stand: Exercise and Fluid Replacement," *Medicine and Science in Sports and Exercise* 39, no. 2 (2007): 377–90.

42. W. H. Saris and L. J. van Loon, "Nutrition and Health: Nutrition and Performance in Sports," [article in Dutch] *Nederlands Tijdschrift voor Geneeskunde* 148, no. 15 (2004): 708–12.

43. J. J. Crowley and C. Wall, "The Use of Dietary Supplements in a Group of Potentially Elite Secondary School Athletes," *Asia-Pacific Journal of Clinical Nutrition* 13, suppl. (2004): S39.

44. R. Maughan, "The Athlete's Diet: Nutritional Goals and Dietary Strategies," *Proceedings of the Nutritional Society* 61, no. 1 (2002): 87–96.

45. J. B. Anderson and others, *Eat Right! Healthy Eating in College and Beyond* (San Francisco: Benjamin Cummings, 2007).

46. American Dietetic Association, "Position of the American Dietetic Association: Vegetarian Diets," *Journal of the American Dietetic Association* 109, no. 7 (2009): 1266–82.

47. S. Loft, "Diet, Oxidative DNA Damage, and Cancer," Paper presented at the Linus Pauling Institute International Conference on Diet and Optimum Health (Portland, OR: May, 2001).

48. American Diabetes Association, "Making Healthy Food Choices," www.diabetes.org/food-and-fitness/food/what-can-i-eat/making-healthy-food-choices.html (accessed September 2011).

49. Centers for Disease Control and Prevention, "CDC Estimates of Foodborne Illness in the United States: CDC 2011 Estimates: Findings," www.cdc.gov/foodborneburden/2011-foodborne-estimates.html (updated April 2011).

50. J. Kurman, "Self-Enhancement, Self-Regulation, and Self-Improvement Following Failures," *British Journal of Social Psychology* 45, pt 2. (2006): 339–56.

LAB 7.1 • READING A FOOD LABEL

Name: _____ **Date:** _____

Instructor: _____ **Section:** _____

Purpose: To learn how to read food labels and analyze the nutritional content of a packaged food.

Directions: Select any packaged food item from your kitchen or from a grocery store. Find the "Nutrition Facts" panel on the package and answer the following questions.

1. What is the name of the packaged food you are examining?

_____

2. What is the "serving size" stated on the Nutrition Facts panel?

_____

Does this "serving size" match the portion you typically consume of this food in one sitting? Is it bigger or smaller than the amount that you typically consume?

_____

3. Examine the ingredients. What are the main ingredients (i.e., which items are listed first)?

_____

Does this list of main ingredients surprise you? How nutritious are the main ingredients?

_____

4. Complete the following table for your chosen food, listing amounts and % Daily Value (% DV) for various nutrients:

Calories (per serving)	Total Fat	Saturated Fat	*Trans* Fat	Sodium	Dietary Fiber	Sugars	Vitamins/ Minerals
	Amount:	Amount:	Amount:	Amount:	Amount:	Amount:	Amount:
	% DV:	% DV:	% DV:	% DV:	% DV:	% DV:	% DV:

Examine your data. Is this food excessively high in fat, saturated fat, *trans* fat, or sodium? Does it provide any dietary fiber? How much sugar is in this food? Does this food supply any vitamins and minerals?

_____

_____

_____

5. What is your overall assessment of the nutritional value of the packaged food you have examined?

_____

_____

LAB 7.2 • KEEPING A FOOD DIARY AND ANALYZING YOUR DAILY NUTRITION

Name: _____ Date: _____

Instructor: _____ Section: _____

Purpose: To get an initial assessment of your current nutrition and identify areas to be improved.

Directions: Follow the instructions below. You will need Internet access to complete this lab.

1. Log on to www.mypyramidtracker.gov.

2. Click "Assess Your Food Intake."

3. If you are accessing this site for the first time, click the link for New Users to set up your personalized login and password. When prompted, enter your age, gender, height, and weight. Then click "Proceed to Food Intake."

4. Enter all of the food items you have eaten today. (It's best to complete this at the end of the day, when you have finished all of your meals.) Enter each food individually by entering the name of the food in the search field, clicking "Search," and then clicking "Add." If you cannot find the exact food you are looking for, select the food that is the most similar. After you have "added" a food, it should pop up on the right side of the screen. Click "Select Quantity" and select a serving size from the drop-down menu. Enter the number of servings you consumed. Click "Enter Foods" to enter additional foods. Repeat until you have entered all of the foods you consumed today. (Don't forget to include any snacks and beverages!)

5. When your list of foods consumed is complete, click "Save and Analyze" or "Analyze Your Food Intake."

6. You will see a screen with several links to analyzed data. Click on "Calculate Nutrient Intakes from Foods." This screen will illustrate how your nutrient intake compares to the "recommended or acceptable range." Print this page.

    a. Does your intake of any nutrient fall short of the "recommended or acceptable" range? If so, which nutrient(s)?

    _____

    _____

    b. Does your intake of any nutrient exceed the "recommended or acceptable" range? If so, which nutrient(s)?

    _____

    _____

7. Click "Analyze Your Food Intake" to return to the main screen containing links to analyzed data. This time, click on "MyPyramid Recommendation." Print this page.

    How does your food intake compare to the recommendations?

    _____

    _____

Note: For more accurate results, record your intake for at least three consecutive days, and then analyze your data again.

Name: _____ Date: _____

Instructor: _____ Section: _____

Purpose: To create a detailed plan for improving your personal nutrition.

Materials: Results from Lab 7.2.

SECTION I: PLANNING CHANGES TO YOUR DIET

1. Look back at your results for Lab 7.2. Which nutrients do you consume too little of?

_____

_____

List at least three foods you could add to your diet in order to increase your consumption of these nutrients:

Food:_____   Rich in: _____

Food: _____   Rich in: _____

Food: _____   Rich in: _____

2. Do you consume too much protein, fat, saturated fat, cholesterol, or sodium? If so, what foods high in these substances could you reduce or eliminate from your diet? List at least 3:

Food: _____   High in: _____

Food: _____   High in: _____

Food: _____   High in: _____

3. How closely did your diet match up with the USDA recommendations? Fill in the blanks below.

Current Milk Intake: _____ cups   Recommended Milk Intake: _____ cups

Current Meat and Beans Intake: _____ oz.   Recommended Meat and Beans Intake: _____ oz.

Current Vegetables Intake: _____ cups   Recommended Vegetables Intake: _____ cups

Current Fruits Intake: _____ cups   Recommended Fruits Intake: _____ cups

Current Grains Intake: _____ oz.   Recommended Grains Intake: _____ oz.

How can you adjust your diet to more closely meet recommended intake levels for each food group?

- I would like to increase/decrease my milk intake by _____ cups.
- I would like to increase/decrease my meat and beans intake by _____ oz.
- I would like to increase/decrease my vegetables intake by _____ oz.
- I would like to increase/decrease my fruits intake by _____ cups.
- I would like to increase/decrease my grains intake by _____ oz.

SECTION II: SHORT- AND LONG-TERM GOALS

Create short- and long-term goals for your healthy eating plan. Be sure to use SMART (specific, measurable, action-oriented, realistic, time-limited) goal-setting guidelines and the information obtained from Section I of this lab and all of your Lab 7.2 materials. Choose appropriate target dates and rewards for completing your goals.

1. Short-Term Goal (3–6 Months)

    a. Goal:_____

    _____

    b. Target Date:_____

    c. Reward:_____

2. Long-Term Goal (12+ Months)

    a. Goal: _____

    _____

    b. Target Date:_____

    c. Reward: _____

SECTION III: BARRIERS TO GOOD NUTRITION; STRATEGIES FOR OVERCOMING THEM

1. What barriers or obstacles might hinder your plan for nutrition changes? Indicate your top three nutritional barriers here:

    a. _____

    b. _____

    c. _____

2. Overcoming these barriers to change will be an important step in reaching your goals. List three strategies for overcoming the obstacles listed:

    a. _____

    b. _____

    c. _____

SECTION IV: GETTING SUPPORT

List resources you will use to help you change your nutritional behavior and how each of these resources will support your goals:

Friend/partner/relative: _____

School-based resource: _____

Community-based resource: _____

Other: _____

8 Managing Your Weight

Learning Outcomes

1. Explain why obesity is both a worldwide trend and a serious concern in America.
    Audio case study and audio Power-Point lecture

2. Discuss the effects of body weight on wellness.

3. Identify several effective tools for successful weight management.
     Lab 8.1 Calculating Energy Balance and Setting Energy Balance Goals
   Miscounting Calories

4. List reasons why some diets work but most fail.
    Food Diary Diet Writing
   Diet Dream Drug

5. Describe the major eating disorders.
     Extreme Healthy Eating

6. Choose a realistic target weight based on your metabolic rate, activity level, eating habits, and environment.

7. Create a behavior change plan for long-term weight management.
     Lab 8.2 Your Diet IQ
   Lab 8.3 Your Weight Management Plan
      Customizable 4-week starter weight loss fitness programs

Pre- and post-quizzes and glossary flashcards

283

casestudy

MARIA

"My name is Maria. I'm 25 and a full-time student in southern Florida, finishing a BA in child development. I was halfway through college when my daughter, Anna, was born. Now that she's in preschool, I'm back to taking a full load of classes and hope to finish college in two more years. I love being a mom. The only thing I'd like to change is my weight! Ever since Anna was born, I've been trying to get back into my pre-pregnancy clothes. I've tried lots of ways to lose the extra pounds—diet pills, liquid diets, Atkins, South Beach—you name it, I've tried it! Sometimes it works for a while, but eventually the weight always comes back. I'm willing to try again, but how do I find a plan that will stick?"

HEAR IT! ONLINE

• •

Weight is a serious and growing health issue in America. While introducing a new campaign to combat obesity, First Lady Michelle Obama warned, "The surge in obesity in this country is nothing short of a public health crisis that is threatening our children, our families, and our future."[1] Over one-third of American adults (34.2 percent) are **overweight** (see Figure 8.1), meaning that their body weight is more than 10 percent over the recommended range and their body mass index, or BMI, is over 25.[2] Another one-third of adults (33.8 percent) are **obese**, with a BMI of 30 or above.[3] Only about 1.6 percent of Americans older than age 20 are **underweight**, with a BMI below 18.5 or a weight 10 percent below recommended range.[4]

Part of the First Lady's concern comes from the alarming trend in children: In the past 25 years, obesity rates for young children have more than doubled; for kids aged 6 to 11, the rates have nearly tripled; and for adolescents, they have more than tripled (Figure 8.2).[5]

College students have historically been in better shape than other adult populations. Until fairly recently, only about 25 percent of college students were overweight or obese, a much smaller percentage than the 66 percent of overweight and obese people in the population as a whole.[6,7] However, there is evidence that overweight is increasing in college populations. A recent study of nearly 10,000 college students in Minnesota indicated that over 39 percent of students were overweight, obese, or extremely obese.[8] A similar study of students at the University of New Hampshire indicated that over one-third of students were overweight or obese, and nearly 60 percent of male students had high blood pressure.[9] Results from a recent national survey by the National College Health Association also indicate a rise in overweight to 21.9 percent of the students surveyed; in obesity (to 11.6 percent of respondents); and in self-reports of disordered eating.[10]

Regardless of your age and stage of life, you should keep several key points in mind as you assess your own diet, exercise, and weight management strategies:

- The changes you make in your diet and exercise habits cannot be short-term fixes; they must become a new way of life. No diet program, product, or service will magically make weight melt away. Successful weight loss takes time, effort, motivation, and the commitment to change habits permanently.

- Recognize that your overall percentage of body fat is more important than your weight or the amount of weight you lose.

- Understand that fast weight loss usually involves a temporary decrease in tissue fluids and often a loss in lean muscle mass, as well. "Healthy weight loss" means the slow, sustained loss of fat, coupled with increases in muscle mass and the preservation and maintenance of lean body mass.

- Learn how long-term weight management balances calories consumed in foods with calories expended through metabolism, activity, and exercise—an equation called **energy balance**.

---

overweight In an adult, a BMI of 25 to 29 or a body weight more than 10 percent above recommended levels

obese In an adult, a BMI of 30 or more or a body weight more than 20 percent above recommended levels

underweight In an adult, a BMI below 18.5 or a body weight more than 10 percent below recommended levels

energy balance The relationship between the amount of calories consumed in food and the amount of calories expended through metabolism and physical activity

---

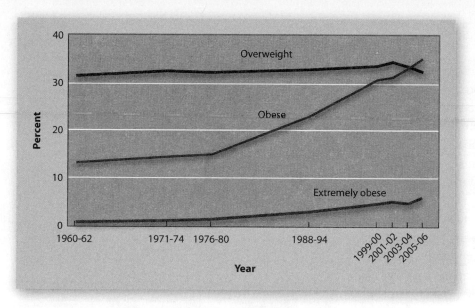

FIGURE **8.1** For the past half century, one-third of Americans have been overweight despite massive government campaigns and personal efforts at weight reduction. During that same period, the percentages of obese Americans have more than doubled.

Source: NCHS E-Stat: Prevalence of Overweight, Obesity and Extreme Obesity among Adults: United States, Trends 1960–1962 through 2007–2008, National Health and Nutrition Examination Survey (2010).

FIGURE **8.2** In the past 30 years, obesity rates for children aged 2 to 5 years have more than doubled, going from 5% to 10.4%, while rates for those aged 6 to 11 years went from 6.5% to 19.6%. The biggest increase was in adolescents aged 12 to 19 years, whose obesity rates more than tripled from 5% to 18.1%!

Data from NCHS E-Stat: Prevalence of Obesity among Children and Adolescents: United States, Trends 1963–1965 through 2007–2008, National Health and Nutrition Examination Survey (2010).

This chapter presents the tools and techniques you need to determine a healthy target weight and create a sound plan for reaching and maintaining it. Incorporating **weight management** into your ongoing wellness program will allow you to realize the significant benefits—physiological, social, and emotional—of sustaining your body mass and body composition within recommended ranges throughout adult life.

Why Is Obesity on the Rise?

In 2011, the World Health Organization (WHO) estimated that 1.6 billion of the world's people were overweight and that the number could increase to 2.3 billion by 2015. Obese adults number over 400 million worldwide and this number could grow to 900 million by 2015. The WHO coined the new term "globesity" to describe this trend. Obesity is a problem in high-income industrialized countries as well as in low- and middle-income developing countries.[11] Diets high in processed fats, meats, sugars, and refined starches provide excess calories while labor-saving devices and sedentary lifestyles reduce energy expenditure. In developing countries, entire cultures are moving away from traditional diets—rich in fruits, vegetables, grains, and low-fat proteins—as well as from manual labor. As a result, they are experiencing the same gain in body fat percentages and weight that Americans did three decades ago. Only the poorest countries of sub-Saharan Africa do not reflect this worldwide trend.[12]

Several Factors Contribute to Overweight and Obesity in America

In the last quarter century, the number of overweight Americans has risen slowly while the number of obese adults has more than doubled.[13] The maps in Figure 8.3 reveal that the rapid increase is distributed unevenly: the southern and upper Midwestern states show the highest

> **weight management** A lifelong balancing of calories consumed and calories expended through exercise and activity to control body fat and weight

rates of obesity in the nation. Several factors contribute to the rapid increase.

Overconsumption Americans consume an average of 523 calories more per day now than they did in 1970 according to the U.S. Department of Agriculture.[14] Without additional exercise, this imbalance leads to weight gain. Many societal factors encourage overeating: "portion distortion," the constant availability of food, advertising, and price.

Food portions in restaurants and supermarkets have grown steadily over the past half-century (Figure 8.4). Researchers have also found that people don't read their own "fullness signals," or feelings of *satiety*, very well. So, the bigger the portions, the more they will eat overall.[15]

Easy access to food and food choices also encourages overeating.[16] Today, most drugstores, gas stations, schools, and public buildings sell packaged food. People eat more treats if they are available in plain sight than if the same food is less accessible.[17] Too, the more food choices people have, the more they tend to eat. People will eat more total food at a four-course meal than at a two-course meal—and even more at a buffet.[18]

Advertising also contributes to overeating. Amazingly, one third of our daily calories come from just a few categories of highly-advertised, empty-calorie foods: sweets, sodas and fruit drinks, alcoholic beverages, and salty snacks.[19] Food price also influences consumption: When experimenters lowered the price of snacks in vending machines, the sales grew immediately.[20]

Too Little Exercise The ease of our modern life is an improvement over the hard physical labor of past generations. Yet the exertion we are spared amounts to hundreds of calories per day that we *don't* burn off as we sit at our desks or change channels with a remote control.[21] Even the layout of modern towns and cities contributes to reduced energy expenditure. The majority of Americans live in suburbs—environments that encourage driving. The greater the urban or suburban sprawl, the less people walk, the more they weigh, and the more likely they are to have high blood pressure, heart disease, cancer, diabetes, and other diseases.[22]

Hereditary Factors With all these overconsumption factors in play, why isn't *everyone* overweight or obese? Part of the answer lies in heredity. If most of your relatives are overweight or obese, you are more likely to gain weight during adulthood yourself. If most of your relatives are thin, you are more likely to be thin as well.

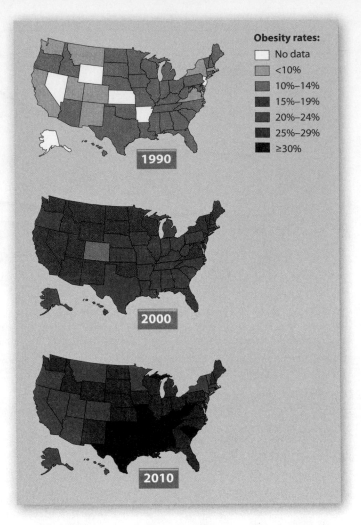

FIGURE **8.3** Obesity rates have risen dramatically over recent decades. Rates are highest in the upper Midwest and in the South.

Source: Centers for Disease Control, "U.S. Obesity Trends," www.cdc.gov/obesity /data/trends.html (updated July 2011).

Researchers have learned that dozens—perhaps hundreds—of genes help determine your weight.[23] Genes control whether our metabolism is fast, burning off most of our excess calories, or "thrifty," tending to conserve food energy.

"Non-Exercise" Activity Uses Energy In recent years, researchers have discovered another factor with hereditary underpinnings: our tendencies to save or use energy during rest and activity. Some people tend to conserve energy by sitting quietly for long stretches and being generally less active all day. Others tend to use energy by being fidgety, jiggling their head, hands, and feet, and getting up to walk around every few minutes. James Levine and colleagues at the Mayo Clinic have demonstrated that lean people burn 279 to 477

20 years ago	Today
333 kcal	590 kcal
210 kcal	610 kcal

FIGURE **8.4** Today's serving portions are significantly larger than those of past decades. A 25-ounce prime-rib dinner served at one local steak chain contains nearly 3,000 calories and 150 grams of fat. That's twice as many calories and more than three times the fat that most adults need in a whole day, and it's just the meat part of the meal!

Data are from National Heart, Lung, and Blood Institute, "Portion Distortion," http://hp2010.nhlbihin.net/portion (accessed September 2011).

more calories per day than obese people through this type of **non-exercise activity**—an expenditure that can significantly affect fat storage and body weight.[24]

The box Get Up from Your Chair! explores how even small, deliberate breaks from sitting can assist in weight management.

LIVE IT! ONLINE

Worksheet 23 Why Do You Eat?

Demographic and Lifestyle Factors A mix of demographic factors both biological and non-biological—including sex, race/ethnicity, culture, education, and economic level—all influence weight. As the box Race/Ethnicity, Gender, and Weight explains, your body weight and likelihood of overweight or obesity vary by race/ethnic group as well as by sex. Biological and cultural factors interact, of course: Our family and ethnic group influences what, when, and how much we eat, as well as how much we exercise and participate in other activity. The choice of high-fat, high-calorie foods, for instance, is partly based on family upbringing, habit, and preference. And 25 percent of Americans engage in no exercise, sports, or other physical activity at all during their leisure time.[25] Education and income make a difference: The higher a person's education level, and the more money he or she makes, the more likely the individual is to be physically active and make healthy food choices. Tough economic times inspire many to choose less expensive foods which, in turn, tend to have more calories and be more highly processed.[26]

TOOLS FOR **CHANGE** •

Get Up from Your Chair!

Researchers have discovered that sitting for long periods day after day can negatively impact your health—even if you exercise on those same days. Several studies have shown that people who spend the most time sitting also have the highest mortality rates from cardiovascular disease and other illnesses.[1]

Conversely, recent research shows that people who interrupt sedentary time with movement "breaks" have narrower waistlines and lower risk of cardiovascular disease. Scientists in Australia interpreted data from a large American study sponsored by the Centers for Disease Control and Prevention. They found

correlations with a trimmer waistline and less risk for cardiovascular diseases in 4,750 participants who wore devices that monitored movement and recorded breaks in sedentary time.[2]

The team recommends that people take a "whole day approach" to increasing physical

(Continued)

activity, adding physical exercise but also breaking up sedentary time to benefit wellness.

First Lady Michelle Obama's "Let's Move!" campaign shares a similar goal, encouraging parents to walk with their families after dinner and kids to "Move everyday!" by getting one hour or more of active play time plus breaking up TV viewing with jumping jacks and other non-sitting activities.[3]

THINK! How much time do you spend sitting each day as you study, attend class, drive your car, and so on?

ACT! List ways you can break up that sitting time with exercise and movement of various types.

Sources:
1. N. Owen, A. Bauman, and W. Brown, "Too Much Sitting: A Novel and Important Predictor of Chronic Disease Risk?" *British Journal of Sports Medicine* 43, no. 2 (2009): 81–83
2. G. Healy, and others, "Sedentary Time and Cardio-Metabolic Biomarkers in U.S. Adults; NHANES 2003–06," *European Heart Journal* (2011) DOI: 10.1093/eurheartj/ehq451.
3. Let's Move!, "Move Everyday!" www.letsmove.gov/move-everyday (accessed September 2011).

DIVERSITY

Race/Ethnicity, Gender, and Weight

Body weight varies by racial/ethnic groups to some degree, based on genes as well as on cultural preferences for food and exercise. Hispanic males, African American males and females, Native American males and females, Pacific Islander males, and white males have the highest percentages of overweight (68 to 72 percent of adults in these groups). Hispanic females, Pacific Islander females, and white females have somewhat lower rates of overweight (51 to 62 percent). Asian Americans have the lowest percentages of overweight (men 46 percent, women 28 percent).

Some ethnic groups appear to have "thrifty genes" that helped their ancestors survive during extended periods of famine by slowing down metabolism to conserve food energy. In a modern environment of plentiful food, widespread mechanization, and diminished activity, however, "thrifty genes" can lead to easy weight gain. This helps explain, for example, why today, 90 percent of Pima Indians are overweight and 75 percent are obese.

Women have a tendency to burn fewer calories than men due to their higher level of essential body fat and lower ratio of lean body mass to fat mass. Because muscle cells burn more energy, and because men usually have more muscle tissue than women,

men burn 10 to 20 percent more calories than women do, even at rest. Monthly hormonal cycles and pregnancy also increase the likelihood of weight fluctuation and gain. Significantly, though, adult men are more likely to be overweight than adult women.

Sources: C. A. Schoenborn and P. F. Adams, National Center for Health Statistics, "Health Behaviors of Adults: United States, 2005–2007," *Vital and Health Statistics* 10, no. 245 (2010).

casestudy

MARIA

"I was never overweight as a kid, and I gained a normal amount of weight during my pregnancy, but now I'm considered overweight. My parents, grandparents, and two older sisters are all on the heavy side, so I wonder if my "heavy" gene just decided to kick in! While I was pregnant, I got used to eating more food than before, and after giving birth to Anna, I guess I just didn't cut back. I spend a lot of time running around after Anna, but otherwise, I drive everywhere and don't set aside special time to exercise. Anna is a picky eater right now—she'll only eat macaroni and cheese, chicken strips, and pizza—so we end up eating those most of the time. That makes it really hard to diet!"

THINK! Do you share any of Maria's eating and exercise habits? Is she like any of your friends?

ACT! Write down your current BMI. Does it represent underweight, healthy weight, overweight, or obesity? List aspects of your lifestyle that may have contributed to your current BMI.

HEAR IT! ONLINE

. . . .

How Does My Body Weight Affect My Wellness?

A leading nutritionist has written that body weight sits at the center of an intricate web of health and disease.[27] Indeed, research shows: You are more likely to remain healthy throughout life if (1) your BMI is between 21 and 23 for women and 22 and 24 for men; (2) you maintain approximately the same BMI and the same waist size throughout your adult life; and (3) your body's fat deposits tend to occur around the hips and thighs rather than the abdomen. High BMIs and abdominal fat (indicated by a large waist size) are associated with higher risk for several chronic diseases.[28]

Being underweight is an important but far less common problem. Fewer than five percent of Americans have a BMI under 18.5.[29] Underweight carries its own significant health risks and can be the result of an unusually fast metabolism, excessive dieting, extreme levels of exercise, eating disorders, smoking, or illness.

Body Weight Can Promote or Diminish Your Fitness

A stable, healthy-range BMI goes hand in hand with regular exercise. Maintaining weight and BMI within recommended ranges leads to increased energy and reduced likelihood of injury during fitness activities.

Overweight and under-weight can contribute to poor fitness. Overweight can lead to a downward fitness spiral: An over-accumulation of body fat can strain bones, joints, and muscles and make exercising harder and injury more likely. Resulting stiffness and pain in the hands, feet, knees, and back, in turn, make exercising even more difficult. They also make work, employment, and activities of daily living—walking up stairs, carrying books or grocery bags, shoveling snow, getting in and out of automobiles, and so on—harder.

Underweight can lead to muscle wasting as the body breaks down muscle tissue for energy when fat stores are low. Muscle wasting, in turn, can lead to weakness and declining ability to exercise and accomplish daily tasks. These inevitably reduce both fitness and wellness.

Body Weight Can Have Social Consequences

Being overweight can subject a person to significant discrimination in education, employment, health care, and social interactions, starting in childhood.[30] "Weight stigma," or prejudice against overweight and obese people, is widespread in society and often starts with parents and teachers of overweight youngsters. Researchers have discovered, for example, that parents spend less money sending their overweight children to college than they do their thinner children, even when money isn't a limiting factor and the children have equivalent grades.[31] Adoption agencies and prospective parents are less likely to choose an overweight child for adoption than a thin one.[32] And adult attitudes rub off on children. Preschoolers are more likely to describe overweight kids their own age as "mean, ugly, or stupid."[33]

Weight stigma is also quite common among employers. Overweight job applicants suffer discrimination, get hired less often, and get fired more often than thinner individuals with similar qualifications.[34] In one study, job applicants standing near obese people were less likely to get hired, even if they were strangers![35] Weight stigma is even pronounced among health professionals, including specialists who treat the obese.[36]

Negative self-images and beliefs can lead to discouragement, shame, hopelessness, and in many, to eating "comfort foods" that temporarily boost mood but cause more weight gain.[37] Weight stigma scholars consider anti-fat bias to be a serious societal issue in need of more study and creative solutions. Awareness is a good starting place.

• •

THINK! Do you say or do things that reveal weight stigma?

ACT! If so, think of substitute thoughts and actions that you could choose and have them ready.

• •

Body Weight Can Influence Your Risk for Chronic Disease

Researchers have confirmed that people with excess body fat have higher levels of several serious chronic diseases (Figure 8.5).[38] Specific cancers linked to high BMI include cancers of the prostate, colon, rectum, esophagus, pancreas, kidney, gallbladder, ovary, cervix, liver, breast, uterus, and stomach.[39]

Fat accumulation around the waist (a 40-inch waistline or higher for a man, or a 35-inch waistline or higher for a woman) increases the risk for developing *metabolic syndrome*. This serious medical condition is a combination of high blood cholesterol, high blood pressure, abdominal fat deposits, and insulin resistance or full-fledged type 2 diabetes.[40] A weight loss of just 10 pounds can bring measurable health benefits, even to an obese individual.[41]

Body Weight Can Affect Your Life Expectancy

You can expect to live longer if your body weight and BMI are within recommended ranges than you can if they fall under the categories for obesity or underweight.

Negative health effects
• Increased risk of stroke
• Increased risk of sleep apnea and asthma
• Increased risk for kidney cancer
• Increased risks for gallbladder cancer and gallbladder disease
• Increased risks for type 2 diabetes and pancreatic cancer
• Higher rates of sexual dysfunction
• Increased risks for prostate, endometrial, ovarian and cervical cancer
• Increased risk of breast cancer in women

Negative health effects
• Higher triglyceride levels and decreased HDL levels
• High blood pressure and increased risk for all forms of heart disease
• Increased risks for stomach and esophageal cancer
• Increased risks for colon and rectal cancer
• Increased risk of osteoarthritis, especially in weight-bearing joints, such as knees and hips
• In pregnant women, increased risks of fetal and maternal death, labor and delivery complications, and birth defects

FIGURE **8.5** Body weight can influence the risks for chronic disease.

As Figure 8.6 shows, being fit significantly reduces mortality risk, especially when combined with healthy weight. Being obese (having a BMI of 30 or above) cuts an average of six to seven years from the life of a non-smoker and 13 to 14 years from a smoker.[42] Research indicates that Americans' average life expectancy may begin to decline because obesity is so prevalent and can shorten life so dramatically.[43]

Underweight people have a shorter life expectancy than normal-weight or overweight people.[44] In fact, some studies indicate that underweight people may have more than 18 times the risk of dying of cancer, and four times the risk of CVD death.[45] Only obese people have a shorter life expectancy. The statistics for early deaths among the underweight reflect the fact that a low BMI is characteristic of patients with illnesses such as cancer, uncontrolled diabetes, and disordered eating. People who are underweight but *not* ill and who are careful to get complete daily nutrition may actually realize greater longevity.[46] Underweight associated with poor nutrition, however, can lead to life-shortening conditions such as anemia, susceptibility to disease and infection, slower recovery from illness, muscle wasting and weakness, and osteoporosis and bone fractures.

Why Don't Most Diets Succeed?

Food Diary
Diet Writing

Overweight or obese Americans face a discouraging cultural phenomenon. Most media images, such as television and magazines, show slim people or buffed up athletes. This leads to high levels of body dissatisfaction and in turn, fuels a $30 billion per year diet industry. Many people are convinced that they will successfully lose weight if they can simply find the right diet. They bounce from one highly publicized diet to another: low-fat, high carbohydrate; low carbohydrate, high protein and so on. Experts tend to agree that any calorie-cutting diet can produce weight loss in the short-term, often through water-weight loss. They also acknowledge that most diets are ineffective and that most people's attempts at weight loss will fail over the long run unless they change their eating habits permanently and make sustained exercise and activity part of their daily lives. Let's look more closely at dieting and why most diets fail.

Diets Often Lead to Weight Cycling

Do you know someone who is dieting? The Centers for Disease Control and Prevention estimates that about one-quarter of women aged 18 to 45 dieted in a recent six-month period.[47] Dismayingly, three-quarters of dieters will regain their weight within two years (or sooner) after a major diet. Most will wind up in a process called **weight cycling**—a pattern of repeatedly losing and regaining weight.

Weight experts refer to this pattern as **yo-yo dieting** (Figure 8.7). Yo-yo dieting may have significant health consequences. Some studies show a link to high blood pressure and other chronic diseases, but experts are not sure whether weight cycling in itself leads to physical health problems.[48] It is a common misconception that yo-yo dieting slows your metabolism and makes each new diet harder and less likely to succeed.[49] Studies of weight cycling do not reveal increases in fat

weight cycling The pattern of repeatedly losing and gaining weight, from illness or dieting

yo-yo dieting A series of diets followed by eventual weight gain

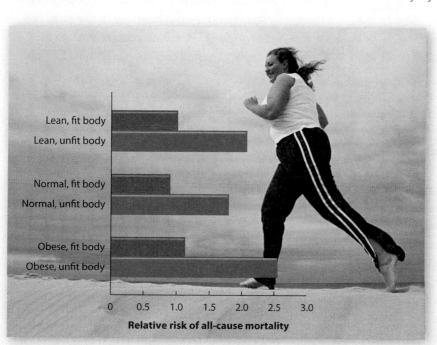

FIGURE **8.6** Being fit significantly reduces your mortality risk in any given year, regardless of your degree of body fat.

From "Cardiorespiratory fitness, body composition and all-cause and cardiovascular disease mortality in men," Chong Do Lee, et al., American Journal of Clinical Nutrition, 1999, Vol. 69, No. 3, pp. 373-380, by permission of the American Society for Nutrition.

Relative risk of all-cause mortality

Lean, fit body
Lean, unfit body
Normal, fit body
Normal, unfit body
Obese, fit body
Obese, unfit body

0   0.5   1.0   1.5   2.0   2.5   3.0

FIGURE **8.7** Actress Kirstie Alley, who was recently a contestant on *Dancing with the Stars,* has long struggled with "yo-yo dieting" or weight cycling.

tissue, decreases in muscle tissue, or decreased metabolic rate as a result of weight cycling. Weight cycling can, however, lead to feelings of depression or failure.

Marketers of diet plans, books, and foods often promise quick weight loss with no hunger and very little effort. These diets usually backfire. One major reason they do is that they are rigid. **Rigid diets** specify rules like "eat only cabbage soup and grapefruit," or "never eat after 6:00 PM." Because rigid diets are unpleasant and restrictive, people seldom stick with them. People on rigid diets tend to have a higher percentage of body fat than people on more flexible plans.[50] The followers of rigid diets tend to exhibit more depression, anxiety, and binge eating as well.

In contrast to rigid diets, **flexible diets** are based on energy balancing of calories eaten and burned. They focus on portion size and make allowances for variations in daily routine, appetite, and food availability. For example, if you go to a party and overeat, a flexible diet allows you to cut extra

LIVE IT! ONLINE

Worksheet 21
All-or-Nothing Thinking

rigid diets Weight-loss regimens that specify strict rules on calorie consumption, types of foods, and eating patterns

flexible diets Weight-loss regimens that focus on portion size and make allowances for variations in daily routine, appetite, and food availability

calories tomorrow and increase your exercise regimen to compensate. As a result, people tend to stay on flexible diets longer and in the process, learn better long-term eating habits.

Everyone who diets will experience some degree of lowered metabolism during a period of calorie restriction as the body "defends" its fat stores. That's why even in a sensible diet, weight loss tends to slow down after an initial quick drop. It's also part of the reason why successful weight maintenance requires permanent changes to your old eating habits.

Our Built-In Appetite Controls Make Diets Less Effective

Our bodies have a complicated set of internal chemical signals and control mechanisms that tell us when to eat, how much to eat, how much fat our bodies should store, and how we should respond when those fat stores start to shrink.[51] Researchers have learned, for example, that we produce powerful appetite stimulants such as leptin and ghrelin. Fat cells make the hormone leptin. The levels of this hormone fall when your body uses stored fat. This stimulates your appetite—and contributes to the difficulty of dieting. Before a meal, your stomach and small intestines make more of a hormone called ghrelin that stimulates food consumption. When leptin levels fall or ghrelin levels climb, your nervous system stimulates food seeking and eating behaviors.

Our bodies do make natural compounds that suppress appetite and signal a feeling of fullness. These compounds help diminish our appetites and get us to stop eating when full. They are less powerful than the factors that increase appetite, though, so they are much easier for most people to tolerate or ignore.[52] Thus, the biology of appetite control works against dieting.

Most Diet Products and Plans Are Ineffective

Most over-the-counter products—"fat burners," "starch blockers," muscle stimulators, diet books, diet supplements, weight-loss

SEE IT! ONLINE

Diet Dream Drug

program memberships, meal replacements, and other diet aids—are ineffective, and some are even dangerous. In 2004, the U.S. Food and Drug Administration banned the popular supplement ephedra (also called *ma huang*) after it caused heart attacks, seizures, and strokes in more than 16,000 people and precipitated more than 100 deaths. Even prescription diet drugs are only modestly effective and can have serious side effects.[53] As the box Do Drastic Weight Loss Methods Work? explains, prescription diet drugs and surgery are a viable option for only a small minority of overweight and obese people.

What about commercial diet plans and programs? One comprehensive study revealed that none of the nationally known programs—Weight Watchers, Jenny Craig, Optifast, eDiets.com, and Overeaters Anonymous—really deliver.[54] For example, after two years, people who joined Weight Watchers had lost an average of just 6.4 pounds. Equally ineffective are diet books that promise easy, permanent weight loss; invoke spurious factors such as your blood type or food allergies; or prescribe extreme diets (very low-calorie or based on eliminating whole categories of nutrients such as carbohydrates or fats).

What, then, should a would-be dieter do? If you are buying a book, look for one that advocates balanced nutrients and regular exercise. If you are joining a program, low-cost support groups are probably the best alternative for most people. They provide one important component: encouragement and support, either in person, through weekly groups, or online. Campus health centers can usually help students find group support for dieting. It's also important to enlist the personal encouragement of friends, roommates, and family members. If people undermine your diet efforts, tell them firmly that you need a different approach. We consider more tools for effective weight loss and management later in the chapter.

What Are Eating Disorders?

Skipping meals, going on diet after diet, and binging on junk food are all forms of **disordered eating**: atypical, abnormal food consumption that is common in the general public. Disordered eating diminishes your wellness but is usually neither long-lived nor disruptive to everyday life. **Eating disorders** are long-lasting, disturbed patterns of eating, dieting, and perceptions of body image that have psychological, environmental, and possibly genetic underpinnings.

Eating disorders can disrupt relationships, emotions, and concentration and can lead to physical injury, hospitalization, and even death. They require diagnosis and treatment from a psychiatrist or other physician.

SEE IT! ONLINE

Extreme Healthy Eating?

Recognizing an eating disorder in yourself or a loved one can lead to treatment that improves or stops the behavior. The statements in Figure 8.8 can help you recognize abnormal or disordered thoughts about food and body image. People with eating disorders often believe they look fat even when they are rail thin. This unrealistic and negative self-perception can be part of a related syndrome called **body dysmorphic disorder** (BDD), in which a person becomes obsessed with a physical "defect" such as nose size or body shape.

The three most common types of eating disorders are anorexia nervosa, bulimia nervosa, and binge eating disorder. About eleven million Americans—ten million of whom are young women—meet the criteria for one of these disorders.[55]

Eating Disorders Have Distinctive Symptoms

LIVE IT! ONLINE

Worksheet 25 Out of Control or Overcontrol?

Anorexia nervosa is a persistent, chronic eating disorder characterized by deliberate food restriction and severe, life-threatening weight loss (Figure 8.9, page 296). People with anorexia first restrict their intake of high-calorie foods, then of almost all foods, and then purge what they do eat through vomiting or using laxatives. They sometimes fast or exercise compulsively as well. The symptoms of anorexia include refusal to maintain a BMI of 18.5 or more; intense fear of gaining weight; disturbed body perception; and in teenage girls and women, amenorrhea (cessation of menstruation) for three

disordered eating Atypical, abnormal food consumption that diminishes wellness but is usually neither long-lived nor disruptive to everyday life

eating disorders Disturbed patterns of eating, dieting, and perceptions of body image that have psychological, environmental, and possibly genetic underpinnings and that lead to consequent medical issues

body dysmorphic disorder A psychological syndrome characterized by unrealistic and negative self-perception focusing on a perceived physical defect

anorexia nervosa A persistent, chronic eating disorder characterized by deliberate food restriction and severe, life-threatening weight loss

Do Drastic Weight Loss Methods Work?

Millions of people think to themselves, "I hate diets and exercise, and they don't work for me, anyway. Why can't I just take drugs or have surgery to get thin?" Unfortunately, prescription diet drugs are expensive, relatively ineffective, and have side effects. Over-the-counter diet drugs can be dangerous and are even less effective. And weight loss surgical procedures carry significant risks and are generally reserved for the severely obese or those with uncontrolled weight-related diseases like diabetes or high blood pressure.

Users of the prescription drug Xenical (orlistat), which partially blocks digestion of fats, lose an average of 13 pounds in a year (about 4 ounces per week), but side effects include oily stools and spotting, gas with fecal discharge, and urgent elimination. The prescription drugs Phentride (phentermine) and Tenuate (diethylpropion) suppress appetite.[1] However, these drugs are addictive and are prescribed only for short periods. For long-term success, people who take prescription diet drugs must still change their eating and exercise habits permanently. Without these changes, virtually all will regain the weight after the prescription ends.

The FDA has banned many other drugs and supplements (for example, drugs containing ephedra or phenylpropanolamine, also called *fen-phen*) and discouraged the use of others (such as Meridia) because of harmful side effects.[2] Over-the-counter diet remedies have not proven to be effective and can be harmful as well. *Hoodia gordonii* is widely advertised and sold but lacks convincing evidence for effectiveness. Other unproven supplements include St. John's wort, herbal laxatives, bitter orange, ginseng and ginkgo, and green tea extracts.

Surgery for weight loss (known as bariatric surgery) has grown more than ten-fold, from about 16,000 procedures per year in the 1990s to an estimated 220,000 in 2008. During gastric banding, the surgeon partitions the stomach into two parts using an inflatable band that acts like a belt. The patient then eats far less before feeling full and stays full longer. This procedure is surgically reversible. In gastric bypass, the surgeon creates a permanent small stomach pouch that connects to the small intestine. This drastically reduces the amount a person can eat as well as the nutrients he or she can absorb—vitamins and minerals as well as calories. This irreversible surgery poses many medical risks but it has been shown to improve type 2 diabetes in obese patients and can lead to significant weight loss.[3] The high cost of bariatric surgery ($15,000 and up) and its on-going medical risks restrict access for most people. Fifteen percent of those who have had bariatric surgery regain all of their original weight.[4] About half experience medical complications or nutrient deficiencies.[5] This discouraging picture could change with future medical research and development.

Sources:
1. D. Rucker and others, "Long-Term Pharmacotherapy for Obesity and Overweight: Updated Meta-Analysis," *British Medical Journal* 335, no. 7631 (2007): 1194–99.
2. A. Pollack, "Abbot Lab Withdraws Meridia, It's Diet Drug, From the Market," *New York Times*, October 9, 2010.
3. F. Rubino and others, "Metabolic Surgery to Treat Type 2 Diabetes: Clinical Outcomes and Mechanisms of Action," *Annual Review of Medicine* 61 (2010): 393–411.
4. D. Grady, "Operation for Obesity Leaves Some in Misery," *New York Times,* May 4, 2004.
5. G.J. Service and others, "Hyperinsulinemia Hypoglycemia with Nesidioblastosis after Gastric-Bypass Surgery," *New England Journal of Medicine* 353, no. 3 (2005): 249–54.

Eating disordered
- I regularly stuff myself and then exercise, vomit, use diet pills or laxatives to get rid of the food or calories.
- My friends/family tell me I am too thin.
- I am terrified of eating fat.
- When I let myself eat, I have a hard time controlling the amount of food I eat.
- I am afraid to eat in front of others.

Disruptive eating patterns
- I have tried diet pills, laxatives, vomiting or extra time exercising in order to lose or maintain my weight.
- I have fasted or avoided eating for long periods of time in order to lose or maintain my weight.
- I feel strong when I can restrict how much I eat.
- Eating more than I wanted to makes me feel out of control.

Food preoccupied/obsessed
- I think about food a lot.
- I feel I don't eat well most of the time.
- It's hard for me to enjoy eating with others.
- I feel ashamed when I eat more than others or more than what I feel I should be eating.
- I am afraid of getting fat.
- I wish I could change how much I want to eat and what I am hungry for.

Concerned well
- I pay attention to what I eat in order to maintain a healthy body.
- I may weigh more than what I like, but I enjoy eating and balance my pleasure with eating with my concern for a healthy body.
- I am moderate and flexible in goals for eating well.
- I try to follow Dietary Guidelines for healthy eating.

Food is not an issue
- I am not concerned about what others think regarding what and how much I eat.
- When I am upset or depressed I eat whatever I am hungry for without any guilt or shame.
- Food is an important part of my life but only occupies a small part of my time.

Body hate/dissociation
- I often feel separated and distant from my body—as if it belongs to someone else.
- I don't see anything positive or even neutral about my body shape and size.
- I don't believe others when they tell me I look OK.
- I hate the way I look in the mirror and often isolate myself from others.

Distorted body image
- I spend a significant amount of time exercising and dieting to change my body.
- My body shape and size keeps me from dating or finding someone who will treat me the way I want to be treated.
- I have considered changing or have changed my body shape and size through surgical means so I can accept myself.

Body preoccupied/obsessed
- I spend a significant time viewing my body in the mirror.
- I spend a significant time comparing my body to others.
- I have days when I feel fat.
- I am preoccupied with my body.
- I accept society's ideal body shape and size as the best body shape and size.

Body acceptance
- I base my body image equally on social norms and my own self-concept.
- I pay attention to my body and my appearance because it is important to me, but it only occupies a small part of my day.
- I nourish my body so it has the strength and energy to achieve my physical goals.

Body ownership
- My body is beautiful to me.
- My feelings about my body are not influenced by society's concept of an ideal body shape.
- I know that the significant others in my life will always find me attractive.

FIGURE **8.8** Thought patterns associated with healthy and disordered eating habits exist on a continuum, as do thought patterns associated with positive and negative body image.

Adapted from Smiley/King/Avery: Campus Health Service. Original continuum, C. Schislak: *Preventive Medicine and Public Health.* Copyright 1997 Arizona Board of Regents. Used with permission.

months or more. Five to twenty percent of anorexics eventually die from medical conditions brought on by vitamin or mineral deficiencies or physiological results of starvation. This gives anorexia the highest death rate of any psychological illness.[56]

Bulimia nervosa is characterized by frequent bouts of binge eating followed by purging (self-induced vomiting), laxative abuse, or excessive exercise. Bulimics tend to consume much more food than most people would during a given time period and feel a loss of control over it. Binging and purging are often done secretly. A medical diagnosis includes binging and purging at least twice a week for three months. People with bulimia are also obsessed with their bodies, weight gain, and how they appear to others. Unlike those with anorexia, however, people with bulimia are often normal weight. Treatment appears to be more effective for bulimia than for anorexia.

Binge eating disorder, a variation of bulimia, involves binge eating but usually no purging, laxatives, exercise, or fasting. Individuals with BED often wind up significantly overweight or obese but tend to binge much more often than does the typical obese person.

bulimia nervosa An eating disorder characterized by frequent bouts of binge eating followed by purging (self-induced vomiting), laxative abuse, or excessive exercise

binge eating disorder A variation of bulimia that involves binge eating but usually no purging, laxatives, exercise, or fasting

FIGURE **8.9** Anorexia nervosa is characterized by severe, life-threatening weight loss.

Eating Disorders Can Be Treated

Because eating disorders have complex physical, psychological, and social causes that unfold over many years, there are no quick or simple solutions for them. Still, eating disorders *are* treatable. The primary goal of treatment is usually to reduce the threat to the patient's life posed by his or her eating behaviors and the physical damage they can cause to the bones, teeth, throat, esophagus, stomach, intestines, heart, and other organs. Once the patient is stabilized medically, long-term therapy can begin. Often, the affected individual comes from a family that places undue emphasis on achievement, body weight, and appearance. Genetic susceptibility can also play a role.[57] Therapy focuses on the psychological, social, environmental, and physiological factors that have contributed. Therapy is aimed at helping the patient develop new eating behaviors, build self-confidence, deal with depression, and find constructive ways of dealing with life's problems. Eating disorder support groups can be pivotal as well.

What Concepts Must I Understand to Achieve My Weight Goals?

Understanding the role of metabolic rates, recognizing your body's set point, and understanding the energy balance equation are all important weight management tools. Taking lessons from successful weight maintainers can help you set and achieve realistic weight goals. And balancing your energy equation by keeping track of your calorie intake and by adding or continuing a regular exercise program can help you maintain a healthy weight over time.

Recognize the Role of Your Metabolic Rate

As much as 60 to 70 percent of your daily calorie intake—typically between 900 and 1,800 calories per day—is consumed as your body sustains functions such as heartbeat, breathing, and maintenance of body temperature.[58] The rate at which your body consumes food energy to sustain these basic functions is your **basal metabolic rate (BMR)**. Your **resting metabolic rate (RMR)** is slightly higher, because it includes the energy you expend to digest food. BMR can be influenced by your activity level and your body composition. The more lean tissue you have, the greater your BMR; the more fat tissue you have, the lower your BMR. The higher your fitness level, the greater your ratio of lean tissue to fat mass is likely to be, and the more energy you will burn while exercising and at rest. Cardiovascular and strength-building exercises contribute most directly to speeding up BMR.

Recognize Your Body's Set Point

Perhaps you've noticed that your body is programmed around a certain weight or **set point** that it returns to fairly easily when you gain or lose a few pounds. Many dieters reach a plateau after a certain amount of weight loss and can't seem to trim off more pounds. This plateau is due, in part, to a downshifted metabolism balancing out lower calorie intake: the person's energy balance is now at a weight-maintenance, not a weight-loss, level. To "outsmart" and reset one's set point, a dieter must lose weight slowly and increase exercise.

Balance Your Energy Equation

Long-term weight management relies on balancing your energy equation—that is, reaching a balance where the calories you eat equal the calories you burn over time. To lose or gain weight, you must deliberately "unbalance" that equation for a while. If you expend more calories than you consume over time, you'll lose weight due to a **negative caloric balance** (Figure 8.10). Consume more calories than you expend

(a) Energy intake < Energy expenditure ⟶ Weight loss

(b) Energy intake > Energy expenditure ⟶ Weight gain

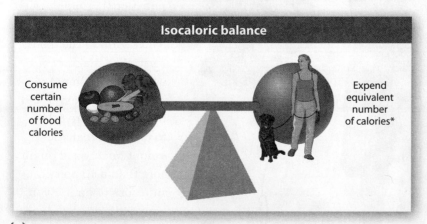

(c) Energy intake = Energy expenditure ⟶ Weight maintenance

basal metabolic rate (BMR) Your baseline rate of energy use, dictated by your body's collective metabolic activities

resting metabolic rate (RMR) Basal metabolic rate plus the energy expended in digesting food

set point A pre-programmed weight that your body returns to easily when you gain or lose a few pounds

negative caloric balance A state in which the amount of calories consumed in food falls short of the amount of calories expended through metabolism and physical activity

FIGURE **8.10** On any given day, each of us has a personal energy equation with either a negative caloric balance, a positive caloric balance, or an isocaloric balance. Over time, this equation helps determine our body weight.

*Calories are expended through metabolism, activity, and exercise.

and you'll gain weight due to a **positive caloric balance**. Consume and expend approximately the same number of calories over a period of time and you'll reach an **isocaloric balance**—and with it, be able to maintain your weight.

There are several ways to approximate your daily calorie consumption and expenditure. You can calculate your current energy balance and set goals for a better balance in **Lab 8.1.** Another approach is logging on to the ChooseMyPlate website at www.ChooseMyPlate.gov to get a target number for calorie consumption based on your age, sex, and level of daily moderate or vigorous activity. This website provides calorie counts for specific foods and portions so you can keep track of how many calories you consume each day. You can also get calorie-counting programs for smart phones, or find them online at websites such as www.caloriecontrol.org.

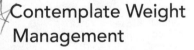
DO IT! ONLINE

> **positive caloric balance** A state in which the amount of calories consumed in food exceeds the amount of calories expended through metabolism and physical activity
>
> **isocaloric balance** A state in which the amount of calories consumed in food is approximately the same as the amount of calories expended through metabolism and physical activity

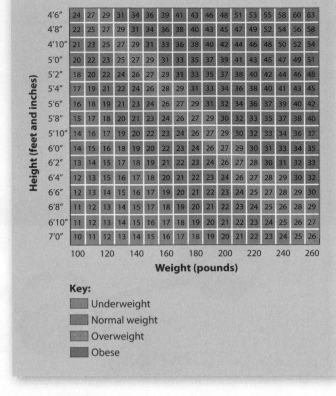

FIGURE **8.11** Locate your height, read across to find your weight, and then read up to determine your BMI. Note that BMI values have been rounded to the nearest whole number.

How Can I Create a Behavior Change Plan for Weight Management?

Let's look at the steps you can take to manage your weight.

Assess Your Current Weight and Choose a Realistic Goal

Figure 8.11 shows healthy weight and BMI ranges based on height. If your body fat percentage is low and your muscle development is high, your healthy weight and your BMI will be on the higher end of the range. The same is also true if your frame size is large. If your body fat percentage is high and your muscle development is low, your healthy weight will be in the middle-to-low end of the range. This is also true if your frame size is medium or small. Knowing these factors will help you calculate a realistic weight goal.

Contemplate Weight Management

If you are satisfied with your current weight, you can simply pursue and refine your application of good nutritional principles and regular exercise. If you are in the dissatisfied majority, use the assessment of your current weight and BMI from Figure 8.11 to choose a realistic weight goal based on no more than a 10 percent initial loss or gain. Even if you don't need weight change now, you can use the specifics in this section to stabilize your current weight and maintain it for the next few decades. Readiness requires motivation, commitment, goals, and a positive attitude. **Lab 8.2** at the end of this chapter helps you assess your readiness for weight change—your diet IQ.

Prepare for Better Weight Management

- *Think about your beliefs and attitudes.* Do you see yourself as a hopeless victim of "bad genes," overwork, or low budget? Think you are too young to worry about deliberate weight management? Believe that you can take effective control of your body composition and weight largely through eating intelligently, limiting your calorie intake, and establishing a program of regular exercise? Talk with others or write in your journal to clarify your attitudes in preparation for making an effective weight management plan.

- *Consider your goals.* Motivating goals are usually personal and extended, such as looking good, feeling fit and capable, and staying well over a period of years. Avoid short-term goals that can lead to weight cycling. If one of your reasons is a specific upcoming event (a beach trip or a sports match, for example), find additional reasons with longer time frames. Long-term goals help you see beyond poorly designed quick-fix diet remedies. You can write out your specific goals in **Lab 8.3.**

- *Identify barriers to change.* What keeps you from changing or maintaining your weight? A lack of information about good weight management techniques? Poor nutrition and eating habits? Eating triggers that encourage overconsumption? Lack of social

TOOLS FOR **CHANGE** •

Tips for Weight Management

Try these ideas for reframing weight loss in your mind, rather than jumping right in to a diet regimen unprepared:

- Think substitution. Instead of cookies or ice cream at snack time, substitute fresh fruit. Instead of chips or fries, substitute unbuttered popcorn, nuts, or vegetable sticks and low-fat dip.

- Consider yourself successful if you lose 1/2 to 1 pound per week. Faster weight loss stimulates too much hunger, slows metabolism, and loses lean tissue.

- Avoid feeling famished by choosing high-volume, nutrient-dense foods. Items such as clear soups, light salads, whole grains, fruits, vegetables, and beans fill you more quickly and control hunger longer.

- Avoid rigid dieting. Strictly limiting calorie counts or forbidding yourself certain foods can trigger binging and weight gain, not loss. Flexible dieting works better and emphasizes portion control and lower-calorie, higher-volume foods.

- Don't drink "empty" calories. Drinks sweetened with sugar or corn syrup contribute disproportionately to weight gain. Alcoholic drinks pack a lot of calories and stimulate the appetite.

Worksheet 22 It Doesn't Last If You Fast

- Sleep well. Get seven to nine hours of sleep each night. Sleep deprivation triggers greater levels of hunger and eating.

- Increase the physical activity in your life. Take the stairs instead of the elevator. Walk the last mile to class instead of riding in a car or bus. Turn off the TV and go play Frisbee with a friend.

- Join a support group. Support groups help most people lose at least a small amount of weight and keep it off.

- Use an online or smartphone application to track calories, keep food diaries, calculate body fat and fat grams in foods, log in your weight to a social site, and so on. These high tech tools can't substitute for your own motivation and adherence, but they can make tracking your information and getting support easier and more fun!

or emotional support? Lack of exercise? Identify your barriers and brainstorm solutions to them.

- *Visualize new behaviors.* What specific new behaviors will you adopt to improve your BMI and body composition? Here are some good choices: Choosing only nutritious foods. Avoiding foods filled with saturated fats, sweeteners, or sodium. Tracking the numbers of servings you eat from each food group. Planning for exercise most days of the week. Keeping a log of your daily and weekly exercise. Asking friends for support.

Take Action

- *Commit to your goals.* Behavior change requires commitment. Thinking and talking about your commitment with friends is helpful; so is writing it down and showing it to someone.

- *Set up support.* Solicit the help of people you can trust to support your efforts. Let's say it is 9:30 PM, you've finished studying and you're hungry, but you've already eaten the 1,800 calories on your day's food plan. A supportive friend might say, "Well, you can always have some raw vegetables to fill up. You'll be glad you stuck with your program. Just think, once you've lost weight, you can add back some extra calories each day—and that won't be so long from now!" The box Tips for Weight Management tells more.

Establish a Regular Exercise Program

Along with monitored and controlled eating, physical activity is crucial both to weight change (loss or gain) and to weight maintenance. In addition to following a healthy diet, you may need to be active for more than an hour per day in order to lose weight, while sixty minutes per day will sustain weight at current levels. These figures are cumulative: Add seven minutes of stair-climbing here, plus eleven minutes of brisk walking across campus there, plus twenty minutes of stationary biking, and so on. Aerobic exercise is the best calorie burner.

The greater the frequency, intensity, and time spent on an activity, the more energy you use and the more calories you burn. There are other considerations for choosing types of fitness exercise as well. The larger the muscle groups you use, the more you boost your metabolism and, in turn, your calorie expenditure. Kick boxing, for example, uses the thigh, calf, and gluteus muscles as well as those that move and support your torso. By contrast, lifting small hand weights works mainly the smaller muscles

of the hand, wrist, and lower arms. Table 8.1 lists the caloric expenditures for several popular activities, sports, and exercises for adults of different weight levels.

Achieve Weight Maintenance

Weight management and weight change are similar in principle. The tools are the same; your daily calorie goal for weight management will simply be isocaloric while your daily goal for weight loss or gain will have a negative or positive caloric balance. Some degree of

TABLE 8.1 Calories Burned through Activity			
Activity, Sport, or Exercise	Calories You Expend per Minute If You Weigh...		
	110 lb	150 lb	190 lb
Aerobics, 10" step	7.0	9.5	12.0
Basketball, pick-up	7.0	9.5	12.0
Biking, slow	5.3	7.1	9.0
Bowling	2.6	3.6	4.5
Dancing, moderate pace	4.2	5.7	9.0
Downhill skiing, moderate pace	5.5	7.5	9.5
Driving	1.8	2.4	3.0
Frisbee, casual	2.6	3.6	4.5
Golf, walking and pulling clubs	4.4	6.0	7.5
Grocery shopping	3.1	4.2	5.3
Hiking, hills	5.3	7.1	9.0
Jogging, moderate pace	5.3	7.1	9.0
Kickboxing	8.8	12.0	14.7
Office work	1.3	1.8	2.3
Ping-Pong	3.5	4.8	6.0
Reading	0.9	1.2	1.5
Soccer, noncompetitive	6.1	8.3	10.5
Softball	4.4	6.0	7.5
Stair climbing, 40 stairs/minute	6.1	8.3	10.2
Stretching	3.5	4.8	5.8
Swimming	~8	~10	~13
Tennis, singles, recreational	7.0	9.5	12.0
Watching TV	1.0	1.4	1.8

Source: Adapted from *Calorie Expenditure Charts*, by Frank I. Katch, Victor L. Katch, and William D. McArdle (Ann Arbor, Michigan: Fitness Technologies Press, 1996).

casestudy

MARIA

"We moved to a new apartment recently, and after living there for a month, it's gotten easier to climb up and down the three flights of stairs. I guess I'm getting used to it! I know this isn't enough exercise to make me lose weight, but at least I'm a little more active. I can see that I need to change daily habits—eating and exercising—instead of just 'going on a diet.' Because I'll regain everything I lose as soon as I go off of it, right? So I need to figure out more ways to be active—ways that feel natural, like taking the stairs; not forced, like doing push ups!

"I weigh 155 right now. I need to lose 35 pounds to get back to my prepregnancy weight of 120. For now, I'm just going to try losing 10 pounds, at least to start off with. I've heard about weight-loss groups that help you plan meals, control how much you eat, and get regular exercise. I think a group might be a good approach for me."

THINK! You've just read about several tools for effective weight management. Which tools is Maria considering? Which tools do you already use? Which others could you use?

ACT! Write down some steps you can take to begin a regular exercise program, to improve the one you already have, or just to fit more physical activity into your day.

· ·

calorie-tracking is usually involved in both maintenance and change, and a weekly weigh-in is important. If you have lost or gained ten percent of your body weight, you will need to maintain that level for a few months before

resuming more weight change. The skills you employ during an interim phase of weight maintenance will be excellent practice for the rest of your life! Once weight management skills, good nutrition, and daily exercise and activity become second nature, both change and maintenance become relatively easy for most people.

Take Lessons from Successful Weight Maintainers

Most people who sustain a normal, healthy weight over years or decades engage in a physically active lifestyle, averaging an hour per day of moderate to vigorous physical activity.[59] They don't skip meals; they eat breakfast every day. They eat a nutritious diet that is low in fats and high in complex carbohydrates, has moderate levels of protein, and has a high volume but a low calorie density—even on weekends! They avoid sodas and juice drinks sweetened with sugar or corn syrup.

Successful weight maintainers also stay conscious of situations that trigger overeating and they apply strategies to prevent overeating. They are motivated to stay at a healthy weight, and they respond quickly by cutting back calories and increasing activity when their weight starts to creep up.[60]

People who are successful at maintaining a healthy weight typically have tools for coping with problems and handling life stresses. They assume responsibility for their lifestyle behaviors, know where to seek help, and tend to be self-reliant. They have a good social support system, both for their weight maintenance and their lives in general.[61]

Maintaining recommended weight and BMI confer so many benefits upon your appearance, energy level, and overall wellness that once you master the needed skill set, you'll rarely miss the junk food you used to eat, nor will you miss the few minutes it will take each day to track energy consumed and expended. The rewards in lifelong wellness are fully worth the trade-off!

chapterin**review** ·

Log on to **www.pearsonhighered.com/hopson** or MyFitnessLab to view these chapter-related videos.

Diet Dream Drug
Miscounting Calories

Food Diary Diet Writing

Extreme Healthy Eating

onlineresources

Please visit this book's website at **www.pearsonhighered.com/hopson** to access links related to topics in this chapter.

 Audio case study
Audio PowerPoint lecture

 Lab 8.1 Calculating Energy Balance and Setting Energy Balance Goals
Lab 8.2 Your Diet IQ
Lab 8.3 Your Weight Management Plan

 Take Charge of Your Health! Worksheets:
　　Worksheet 21 All-or-Nothing Thinking and
　　　"Safe Foods" versus "Forbidden Foods"
　　Worksheet 22 It Doesn't Last If You Fast
　　Worksheet 23 Why Do You Eat?
　　Worksheet 25 Out of Control or Overcontrol?
　　Behavior Change Log Book and Wellness
　　Journal

 Pre- and post-quizzes
Glossary flashcards

reviewquestions

1. The World Health Organization coined the term "globesity" to promote an understanding of
   a. global hunger.
   b. rising obesity rates in underdeveloped countries.
   c. rising obesity rates in developed countries.
   d. the epidemic of obesity in the global population.

2. Excess body weight can affect body systems negatively. Indicate the one least likely to be affected negatively.
   a. Cardiovascular system (heart and lungs)
   b. Digestive system (gallbladder, kidneys, colon)
   c. Musculoskeletal system (bones and joints)
   d. Integumentary system (skin and hair)

3. At more than 20 percent above the recommended weight range, a person who is 5'8" tall is considered
   a. overweight.
   b. obese.
   c. at ideal weight.
   d. at his/her set point.

4. A BMI of 16 in a woman indicates
   a. overweight.
   b. underweight.
   c. normal weight.
   d. obesity.

5. Getting up, walking around, and jiggling your feet when seated are all examples of
   a. energy conservation.
   b. appetite control.
   c. non-exercise activity.
   d. depression.

6. To lose weight, you must establish a(n)
   a. negative caloric balance.
   b. isocaloric balance.
   c. positive caloric balance.
   d. set point.

7. Weight cycling is
   a. a pattern of repeatedly losing and regaining weight.
   b. characterized by rigid diets.
   c. characterized by flexible diets.
   d. uncommon.

8. Anorexia nervosa is characterized by
   a. frequent bouts of binge eating followed by self-induced vomiting.
   b. deliberate food restriction and severe, life-threatening weight loss.
   c. the use of laxatives.
   d. obesity.

9. The rate at which your body consumes food energy to sustain basic functions is your
   a. basal metabolic rate.
   b. resting metabolic rate.
   c. BMI.
   d. set point.

10. Successful weight maintainers are most likely to do which of the following?
    a. Indulge in junk food on weekends
    b. Skip meals
    c. Drink diet sodas
    d. Eat a nutritious diet that is low in fats, with high volume but low calorie density

critical**thinking**questions

1. How do height, physical build, and musculature affect recommended weight and BMI?
2. What do you see as the greatest contributor to "globesity"? Defend your answer.
3. List several effective tools for successful weight management. Is one more important than the others? If so, discuss.
4. Why do most diets fail?

references

1. First Lady Michelle Obama, Introduction of New Plan to Combat Overweight and Obesity, Press Conference, Alexandria, Virginia, January 28, 2010.
2. K. M. Flegal and others, "Prevalence and Trends in Obesity among U.S. Adults, 1999–2008," *Journal of the American Medical Association* 303, no. 3 (2010): 235–41.
3. Ibid.
4. C. D. Fryar and C. L. Ogden, "NCHS Health E-Stat: Prevalence of Underweight Among Adults Aged 20 Years and Over: United States, 2007–2008." National Health and Nutrition Examination Survey, www.cdc.gov/nchs/data/hestat/underweight/underweight_adults.htm (updated May 2009).
5. M. Ogden and M. Carroll, "NCHS E-Stat: Prevalence of Obesity among Children and Adolescents: United States, Trends 1963–1965 through 2007–2008," National Health and Nutrition Examination Survey, www.cdc.gov/nchs/data/hestat/obesity_child_07_08/obesity_child_07_08.htm (updated June 2010).
6. American College Health Association, *American College Health Association–National College Health Assessment II (ACHA-NCHA II) Reference Group Executive Summary Spring 2010* (Linthicum, MD: American College Health Association, 2010).
7. Charlotte A. Schoenborn and others, "Body Weight Status of Adults: United States, 1997–1998." *Advance Data from Vital and Health Statistics* no. 330 (2002).
8. University of Minnesota, Boynton Health Service, "News Release: First Ever Comprehensive Report on the Health of Minnesota College Students Looks at Mental Health, Obesity, Financial Health, Sexual Health and More," www1.umn.edu/news/news-releases/2007/UR_RELEASE_MIG_4318.html (November 2007).
9. University of New Hampshire, "College Students Face Obesity, High Blood Pressure, Metabolic Syndrome." *ScienceDaily* www.sciencedaily.com/releases/2007/06/070614113310.htm (June 2007).
10. American College Health Association, *ACHA-NCHA II Reference Group Executive Summary Spring 2010,* 2010.
11. World Health Organization, "Fact sheet no. 311: Obesity and Overweight," www.who.int/mediacentre/factsheets/fs311/en/index.html (updated March 2011).
12. International Union of Nutritional Sciences, "The Global Challenge of Obesity and the International Obesity Task Force," September 2002, www.iuns.org/features/obesity/obesity.htm (accessed March 2011).
13. M. Ogden and M. Carroll, "NCHS E-Stat: Prevalence of Overweight, Obesity, and Extreme Obesity among Adults: United States, Trends 1960–1962 through 2007–2008," National Health and Nutrition Examination Survey, www.cdc.gov/nchs/data/hestat/obesity_adult_07_08/obesity_adult_07_08.htm (updated June 2011).
14. U.S. Department of Agriculture Economic Research Service, "U.S. Food Consumption Up 16 Percent Since 1970," *Amber Waves,* November 2005, www.ers.usda.gov/AmberWaves/November05/findings/usfoodconsumption.htm.
15. B. Wamsink, J. E. Painter, and J. North, "Bottomless Bowls: Why Visual Cues of Portion Size May Influence Intake," *Obesity Research* 13, no. 1 (2005): 93–100.
16. J. C. Spence and others, "Relation between Local Food Environments and Obesity among Adults," *BMC PublicHealth* 9 (2009): 192; M. Wang and others, "Changes in Neighbourhood Food Store Environment, Food Behaviour, and Body Mass Index, 1981–1990," *PublicHealth Nutrition* 11, no. 9 (2008): 963–70.
17. B. Wansink, "Environmental Factors that Increase the Food Intake and Consumption Volume of Unknowing Customers," *Annual Review of Nutrition* 24 (2004): 455–79.
18. B. Wansink, J. E. Painter, and J. North, "Bottomless Bowls: Why Visual Cues of Portion Size May Influence Intake," 2005.
19. G. Block and others, "Foods Contributing to Energy Intake in the U.S.: Data from NHANES III and NHANES 1999–2000," *Journal of Food Chemistry and Analysis* 17, no. 3–4 (2004): 439–47.
20. S. A. French, "Public Health Strategies for Dietary Change: Schools and Workplaces," *Journal of Nutrition* 135, no. 4 (2005): 91–92.
21. National Center for Health Statistics, "NCHS Health E-Stat: Prevalence of Sedentary Leisure-Time Behavior among Adults in the United States," www.cdc.gov/nchs/data/hestat/sedentary/sedentary.htm (updated February 2010); M. S. Treuth and others, "A Longitudinal Study of Sedentary Behavior and Overweight in Adolescent Girls," *Obesity* 17, no. 5 (2009): 1003–08.
22. M. Papas and others, "The Built Environment and Obesity," *Epidemiological Reviews* 29, no. 1 (2007): 129–43; M. Rao and others, "The Built Environment and Health," *The Lancet* 370, no. 9593 (2007): 1111–13.
23. I. S. Farooqi and S. O'Rahilly, "Genetic Factors in Human Obesity," *Obesity Reviews* 8, Suppl 1 (2007): 37–40.
24. J. A. Levine and others, "Interindividual Variation in Posture Allocation: Possible Role in Human Obesity," *Science* 307, no. 5709 (2005): 584–86.
25. Centers for Disease Control and Prevention, U.S. Physical Activity Statistics, "1988–2008 No Leisure-Time Physical Activity Trend Chart," www.cdc.gov/nccdphp/dnpa/physical/stats/leisure_time.htm (updated February 2010).
26. M. Beydoun, L. Powell, and Y. Yang, "The Association of Fast Food, Fruit, and Vegetable Prices with Dietary Intakes among U.S. Adults: Is There Modification by Family Income?" *Social Science and Medicine* 66, no. 11 (2008): 2218–29.
27. W. Willett, *Eat, Drink, and Be Healthy: The Harvard Medical School Guide to Healthy Eating* (New York: Free Press, 2003): 35.
28. D. Canoy and others, "Body Fat Distribution and Risk of Coronary Heart Disease in Men and Women in the European Prospective Investigation into Cancer and Nutrition in Norfolk Cohort: A Population-Based Prospective Study," *Circulation* 116, no. 25 (2007): 2933–43.
29. C. D. Fryar and C. L. Ogden, "Prevalence of Underweight among Adults Aged 20 Years and Over: United States, 2007–2008," 2009.
30. R. Puhl and K.D. Brownell, "Bias, Discrimination, and Obesity," *Obesity Research* 9, no. 12 (2001): 788–805.
31. D. R. Musher-Eizenman and others, "Body Size Stigmatization in Preschool Children: The Role of Control Attributions," *Journal of Pediatric Psychology* 29, no. 8 (2004): 613–20; S. H. Thompson and S. Digsby, "A Preliminary Survey of Dieting, Body Dissatisfaction, and Eating Problems among High School Cheerleaders," *Journal of School Health* 74, no. 3 (2004): 85–90.
32. R. Puhl and K.D. Brownell, "Bias, Discrimination, and Obesity," 2001.
33. D. R. Musher-Eizenman and others, "Body Size Stigmatization in Preschool Children," 2004.
34. R. Puhl and K.D. Brownell, "Bias, Discrimination, and Obesity," 2001; M. R. Hebl and L. M. Mannix, "The Weight of Obesity in Evaluating Others: A Mere Proximity Effect," *Perspectives in Social Psychology Bulletin* 29, no. 1 (2003): 28–38.
35. M. R. Hebl and L. M. Mannix, "The Weight of Obesity in Evaluating Others," 2003.
36. M. B. Schwartz and others, "Weight Bias among Health Professionals Specializing in Obesity," *Obesity Research* 11, no. 9): 1033–39.
37. S. S. Wang and others, "The Influence of the Stigma of Obesity on Overweight Individuals," *International Journal of Obesity* 28, no. 10 (2004): 1333–37.

38. C. O'Neil and T. Nicklas, "State of the Art Reviews: Relationship between Diet/Physical Activity and Health," *American Journal of Lifestyle Medicine* 1, no. 6 (2007): 457–81.

39. E. Calle and others, "Overweight, Obesity, and Mortality from Cancer in a Prospectively Studied Cohort of U.S. Adults," *New England Journal of Medicine* 348, no. 17 (2003): 1625–38.

40. N. Pandey and V. Gupta, "Trends in Diabetes," *Lancet* 369, no. 9569 (2007): 1256–57.

41. Mayo Clinic Staff, "Metabolic Syndrome," www.mayoclinic.com/health/metabolic%20syndrome/DS00522 (November 2009).

42. C. C. Mann, "Provocative Study Says Obesity May Reduce U.S. Life Expectancy," *Science* 307, no. 5716 (2005): 1716–17.

43. S. J. Olshansky and others, "A Potential Decline in Life Expectancy in the United States in the 21st Century," *New England Journal of Medicine* 352, no. 11 (2005): 1138–45.

44. K. Flegal and others, "Excess Deaths Associated with Underweight, Overweight, and Obesity," *Journal of the American Medical Association* 298, no. 17 (2007): 2028–37; K. M. Flegal and B. I. Graubard, "Estimates of Excess Deaths Associated with Body Mass Index and Other Anthropometric Variables," *American Journal of Clinical Nutrition* 89, no. 4 (2009): 1213–19.

45. Y. Takata and others, "Association between Body Mass Index and Mortality in an 80-Year-Old Population," *Journal of the American Geriatric Society* 55, no. 6 (2007): 913–17.

46. L. Fontana and others, "Long-Term Calorie Restriction Is Highly Effective in Reducing the Risk for Atherosclerosis in Humans," *Proceedings of the National Academy of Sciences* 101, no. 17 (2004): 6659–63.

47. S. L. Boulet and others, "Folate Status in Women of Childbearing Age, by Race/Ethnicity—United States, 1999–2000, 2001–2002, and 2003–2004," *Morbidity and Mortality Weekly Report*, 54, no. 38 (2005): 8.

48. U.S. Department of Health and Human Services, National Institute of Diabetes and Digestive and Kidney Diseases (NIDDK), "Weight Cycling," NIH Publication No. 01-3901, www.win.niddk.nih.gov/publications/PDFs/wtcycling2bw.pdf (May 2008).

49. NIDDK, "Weight Cycling," 2008.

50. C. F. Smith and others, "Flexible versus Rigid Dieting Strategies: Relationship with Adverse Behavioral Outcomes," *Appetite* 32, no. 3 (1999): 295–305.

51. S. Stock and others, "Ghrelin, Peptide YY, Glucose-Dependent Insulinotropic Polypeptide, and Hunger Responses to a Mixed Meal in Anorexic, Obese, and Control Female Adolescents," *Journal of Clinical Endocrinology and Metabolism* 90, no. 4 (2005); E. T. Poehlman, "Reduced Metabolic Rate after Caloric Restriction," *Journal of Clinical Endocrinology and Metabolism* 88, no. 1 (2003): 14–15.

52. D. Rucker and others, "Long-Term Pharmacotherapy for Obesity and Overweight: Updated Meta-Analysis," *British Medical Journal* 335, no. 7631 (2007): 1194–99; ConsumerSearch, "Diet Pills: Reviews," www.consumersearch.com/diet-pills (updated August 2009).

53. Ibid.

54. A. Tsai and T. Wadden, "Systematic Review: An Evaluation of Major Commercial Weight Loss Programs in the U.S.," *Annals of Internal Medicine* 142, no. 1 (J2005): 56–66.

55. National Eating Disorder Association, "Statistics: Eating Disorders and Their Precursors," www.nationaleatingdisorders.org/information-resources/general-information.php#facts-statistics (2005).

56. K. Beals and A. Hill, "The Prevalence of Disordered Eating, Menstrual Dysfunction, and Low Bone Mineral Density among US Collegiate Athletes," *International Journal of Sport Nutrition and Exercise Metabolism* 16, no. 1 (2006): 1–23; American Psychiatric Association, "DSM-5 Development: Proposed Revision: 307.1 Anorexia Nervosa," www.dsm5.org/ProposedRevisions/Pages/proposedrevision.aspx?rid=24 (updated October 2010).

57. C. M. Bulik and others, "The Genetics of Anorexia Nervosa," *Annual Review of Nutrition* 27 (2007): 263–75.

58. Mayo Clinic Staff, "Metabolism and Weight Loss: How You Burn Calories," www.mayoclinic.com/health/metabolism/WT00006 (October 2009).

59. R. R. Wing and S. Phelan, "Long-Term Weight Loss Maintenance," *American Journal of Clinical Nutrition* 82, no. 1 (2005): 222S–25S.

60. K. Elfhag and S. Rossner, "Who Succeeds in Maintaining Weight Loss?" *Obesity Review* 6, no. 1 (2005): 67–85.

61. Ibid.

LAB 8.1 • CALCULATING ENERGY BALANCE AND SETTING ENERGY BALANCE GOALS

Name: _____ **Date:** _____

Instructor: _____ **Section:** _____

Materials: Calculator, access to Internet (optional)

Purpose: To learn how to calculate energy balance and set realistic goals for calorie intake and energy expenditure.

Directions: Complete the following sections.

SECTION I: CALCULATING BMR AND ENERGY EXPENDITURE

Your **basal metabolic rate (BMR)** is the rate at which you burn calories to sustain life functions at rest at a normal room temperature. Your activities, fitness level, stress level, and many other things will affect your BMR.

1. Calculate your BMR (the method shown here uses the Harris-Benedict formula):

Men

1. BMR = 66 + (6.3 × weight in pounds) + (12.9 × height in inches) − (6.8 × age in years)

2. BMR = 66 + (   ) + (   ) − (   )

3. BMR = _____ calories

Women

1. BMR = 655 + (4.3 × weight in pounds) + (4.7 × height in inches) − (4.7 × age in years)

2. BMR = 655 + (   ) + (   ) − (   )

3. BMR = _____ calories

2. Estimate your total energy expenditure (EE):

Total energy expenditure takes into account your amount of activity within a 24-hour period. You can calculate your energy expenditure by keeping an activity log and adding up the calories expended during any nonsleep time. To do this, use the physical activity tracking tool on the ChooseMyPlate website (www.choosemyplate.gov). Another way to estimate total energy expenditure is to use the following calculations. Choose your level of activity on *average* and use that formula to calculate your energy expenditure (EE).

Multiply your BMR by the appropriate activity factor, completing ONE equation below:

- If you are **sedentary** (little or no exercise):
  EE = _____(BMR) × **1.2** = _____ calories
- If you are **lightly active** (light exercise/sports 1–3 days/week):
  EE = _____(BMR) × **1.375** = _____ calories
- If you are **moderately active** (moderate exercise/sports 3–5 days/week):
  EE = _____(BMR) × **1.55** = _____ calories
- If you are **very active** (hard exercise/sports 6–7 days/week):
  EE = _____(BMR) × **1.725** = _____ calories
- If you are **extra active** (very hard daily exercise/sports & physical job or 23-day training):
  EE = _____(BMR) × **1.9** = _____ calories

SECTION II: CALCULATING ENERGY BALANCE

1. Estimated **calorie INTAKE**

_____ calories

2. Estimated **calorie EXPENDITURE** (EE from Section I)

_____ calories

3. Subtract your EXPENDITURE (#2) from your INTAKE (#1) to get:

Out of balance calories = _____ calories

SECTION III: TOOLS FOR YOUR WEIGHT MANAGEMENT PLAN

1. What was your caloric intake from your dietary analysis? _____ What was your energy
expenditure? _____ What was your overall energy balance? _____

- **Energy balance** (+/− 200 calories): You are supplying your body with its energy needs and maintaining
  current weight.
- **Negative energy balance** (−201 calories): You are expending more energy than you are eating and
  should be losing weight.
- **Positive energy balance** (+201 calories): You are eating more energy than you are expending and
  should be gaining weight.

2. Do you want or need to lose body fat? **YES or NO**

3. What is your **goal** for your body fat percentage? _____

4. Complete the following calculations to figure out how many **pounds of fat** you need to lose in order to
reach this goal:

- Find your **current fat weight:**

  _____ (current weight, lb) × _____ (current % body fat, expressed as a decimal) =
  _____ current fat weight (lb)

- Find your **lean body mass**

  (LBM): _____ (weight, lb) − _____ (fat weight, lb) = _____ LBM (lb)

- Find your **target body weight:**

  _____ (LBM) ÷ (1 − goal % body fat expressed as a decimal) = _____ target body weight (lb)

- Find the **lb of fat loss** needed to reach your body fat percentage goal:

  _____ (current weight, lb) − _____ (target weight, lb) = _____ fat loss needed (lb)

5. If you lose 1 pound of fat per week (500 calorie deficits per day), how many weeks will it take you to lose
your desired fat weight? _____

6. Brainstorm ways that you can get to a −500 calorie deficit per day through diet and exercise/activity changes.

DIET CHANGE (−250 calories)   **ACTIVITY CHANGE (−250 calories)**

_____   _____

_____   _____

_____   _____

_____   _____

LAB 8.2 • YOUR DIET IQ

Name: _____ Date: _____

Instructor: _____ Section: _____

Purpose: To encourage students to think critically about their dieting history, ways of controlling food consumption, and readiness for weight changes.

Directions: Complete the following sections to analyze your dieting patterns.

SECTION I: DIET HISTORY

1. How many times have you been on a diet?

_____0 times _____1–3 times _____4–10 times _____11–20 times _____more than 20

2. How much weight did you lose?

_____0 lb. _____1–5 lb. _____6–10 lb. _____11–20 lb. _____more than 20 lb.

3. How long did you stay at the new lower weight?

_____Under 1 mo. _____2–3 mos. _____4–6 mos. _____6 to 12 mos. _____Over 1 yr.

4. Put a check mark by each dieting method you have tried:

_____skipping breakfast _____skipping lunch or dinner

_____cutting out all snacks _____counting calories

_____cutting out most fats _____cutting out most carbohydrates

_____increasing regular exercise _____taking "weight loss" supplements

_____taking appetite suppressants _____using meal replacements such as Slim Fast

_____taking laxatives _____inducing vomiting

_____taking prescription appetite suppressants

_____other _____

SECTION II: READINESS TO START A WEIGHT-LOSS PROGRAM

If you are thinking about starting a weight-loss program, answer questions A–F:

A. How motivated are you to lose weight?

1	2	3	4	5
Not at all motivated	Slightly motivated	Somewhat motivated	Quite motivated	Extremely motivated

B. How certain are you that you will stay committed to a weight-loss program long enough to reach your goal?

1	2	3	4	5
Not at all certain	Slightly certain	Somewhat certain	Quite certain	Extremely certain

C. Taking into account other stresses in your life (school, work, and relationships), to what extent can you tolerate the effort required to stick to your diet plan?

1	2	3	4	5
Cannot tolerate	Can tolerate somewhat	Uncertain	Can tolerate well	Can tolerate easily

D. Assuming you should lose no more than 1 to 2 pounds per week, have you allotted a realistic amount of time for weight loss?

1	2	3	4	5
Very unrealistic	Somewhat unrealistic	Moderately realistic	Somewhat realistic	Realistic

E. While dieting, do you fantasize about eating your favorite foods?

1	2	3	4	5
Always	Frequently	Occasionally	Rarely	Never

F. While dieting, do you feel deprived, angry, upset?

1	2	3	4	5
Always	Frequently	Occasionally	Rarely	Never

Total your scores from questions A–F, circle your score category, and answer any questions below:
6 to 16: This may not be a good time for you to start a diet. Inadequate motivation and commitment and unrealistic goals could block your progress. Think about what contributes to your unreadiness. What are some of the factors? Consider changing these factors before undertaking a diet. How could you alter the most important ones?

17 to 23: You may be nearly ready to begin a program but should think about ways to boost your readiness. Regardless of readiness level, what are a few additional things you could do at this time to prepare?
24 to 30: The path is clear—you can decide how to lose weight in a safe, effective way.
Section II Comments:

SECTION III: HUNGER, APPETITE, AND EATING

Think about your hunger and the cues that stimulate your appetite or eating, and then answer parts A–C.

A. When food comes up in conversation or in something you read, do you want to eat, even if you are not hungry?

1	2	3	4	5
Never	Rarely	Occasionally	Frequently	Always

B. How often do you eat for a reason other than physical hunger?

1	2	3	4	5
Never	Rarely	Occasionally	Frequently	Always

C. When your favorite foods are around the house, do you succumb to eating them?

1	2	3	4	5
Never	Rarely	Occasionally	Frequently	Always

Total your scores from questions A–C, circle your score category, and answer any questions below:

3 to 6: You might occasionally eat more than you should, but it is due more to your own attitudes than to temptation and other environmental cues. Controlling your own attitudes toward hunger and eating may help you. What are some of these attitudes, and how could you control or change them?

7 to 9: You may have a moderate tendency to eat just because food is available. Losing weight may be easier for you if you try to resist external cues and eat only when you are physically hungry. What are some ways you could better resist external cues?

10 to 15: Some or much of your eating may be in response to thinking about food or exposing yourself to temptations to eat. Think of ways to minimize your exposure to temptations so you eat only in response to physical hunger.

Section III Comments:

SECTION IV: CONTROLLING EATING

How good are you at controlling overeating when you are on a diet? Answer parts A–C.

A. **A friend talks you into going out to a restaurant for a midday meal instead of eating a brown-bag lunch. As a result, you:**

1	2	3	4	5
Would eat much less	Would eat much less	Would make no difference	Would eat somewhat more	Would eat much more

B. **You "break" your diet by eating a fattening, "forbidden" food. As a result, for the day, you:**

1	2	3	4	5
Would eat much less	Would eat much less	Would make no difference	Would eat somewhat more	Would eat much more

C. **You have been following your diet faithfully and decide to test yourself by taking a bite of something you consider a treat.** As a result, for the day, you:

1	2	3	4	5
Would eat much less	Would eat much less	Would make no difference	Would eat somewhat more	Would eat much more

Sum your scores from questions A–C, circle your score category, and answer any questions below:

3 to 7: You recover rapidly from mistakes. However, if you frequently alternate between out-of-control eating and very strict dieting, you may have a serious eating problem and should get professional help. Does that kind of alternation describe your pattern? If so, where on your college campus could you turn for professional guidance?

8 to 11: You do not seem to let unplanned eating disrupt your program. This is a flexible, balanced approach. Do "flexible" and "balanced" describe your dieting? How could you achieve even more flexibility and balance?

12 to 15: You may be prone to overeating after an event breaks your control or throws you off track. Your reaction to these problem-causing events could use improvement. What are some ways you could try to more effectively control an overeating reaction?

Section IV Comments:

SECTION V: REFLECTION

1. Were your previous dieting patterns successful? Why or why not? Was it hard to be consistent with these dieting methods?

2. Which dieting methods were challenging or did not work for you at all? Why were these methods more difficult? What would be the ideal dieting method for you?

LAB 8.3 • YOUR WEIGHT MANAGEMENT PLAN

Name: _____   Date: _____

Instructor: _____   Section: _____

Materials: None

Purpose: To create an appropriate weight management goal, you must apply behavior change tools and make a plan to implement your goals.

Directions: Complete the following sections.

SECTION I: SHORT- AND LONG-TERM GOALS

1. Short-Term Goals

- My 3-month *or* 6-month (circle one) % body fat goal is _____%.
- My 3-month *or* 6-month (circle one) weight goal is _____ lb.
- My 3-month *or* 6-month (circle one) BMI goal is _____ kg/m².

2. Long-Term Goals

a. Based on my current weight, BMI, % body fat, and the tools gained in Lab 8.2:

- My 1-year % body fat goal is _____%.
- My 1-year weight goal is _____ lb.
- My 1-year BMI goal is _____ kg/m².

b. I plan to reach that goal by consuming about _____ calories per day and adding

_____ activity calories per day.

SECTION II: DIET OBSTACLES AND STRATEGIES

1. Negative Food and Eating Triggers

Eating and food preferences can be triggered by emotions, social situations, and the sights and smells around you.

a. Fill out the following table exploring your negative food and eating triggers. For example, a situational trigger for you eating sugary foods may be "attending holiday parties."

Diet Behavior	Emotional Triggers	Social Triggers	Situational Triggers
Eating More Food			
Eating Late at Night			
Eating More Often			
Eating Sugary Foods			
Eating Fatty Foods			
Eating Fast Foods			
Eating Out			
Others:			

b. List three strategies to overcome or manage your food and eating triggers:

(1) _____

(2) _____

(3) _____

2. **Changing Food Patterns**

a. I will eat LESS of the following foods and beverages:

_____

_____

b. For good nutrition and weight management goals, I will replace the above foods and beverages with the following:

_____

_____

SECTION III: EXERCISE AND ACTIVITY OBSTACLES AND STRATEGIES

1. **Reducing Sedentary Behaviors**

a. Evaluate your sedentary activities in the space below. List your top three sedentary activities (not including time spent in class), the number of days per week you do them, and how many minutes per day.

	Sedentary Activity	Days/wk	Min/day
1			
2			
3			

b. Which sedentary activity could you replace with physical activity or even supplement with physical activity (such as exercising while you watch TV, or stretching while on your cell phone)? Write down three ideas for replacing sedentary activities with more active ones.

(1) _____

(2) _____

(3) _____

2. **List a few of the obstacles to replacing sedentary activity with more energy-intensive physical activity, along with strategies for overcoming these obstacles.**

Activity Obstacle	Strategy to Overcome
(1) _____	_____
(2) _____	_____
(3) _____	_____

SECTION IV: GETTING SUPPORT

1. I feel supported in my weight goals by these people:

_____

Here's what they do that assists me:

_____

2. I need additional support from these people:

_____

Here's what I need to ask for:

_____

3. **If I need group or medical support,** here are a few places to seek it: student health service, family physician, local hospital, local Weight Watchers chapter, online groups. If needed, I would be inclined to use _____ for support.

SECTION V: REWARDS

1. When I make the **short-term** behavior change described above, my reward will be:

_____

Target date _____

2. When I make the **long-term** behavior change described above, my reward will be:

_____

Target date _____

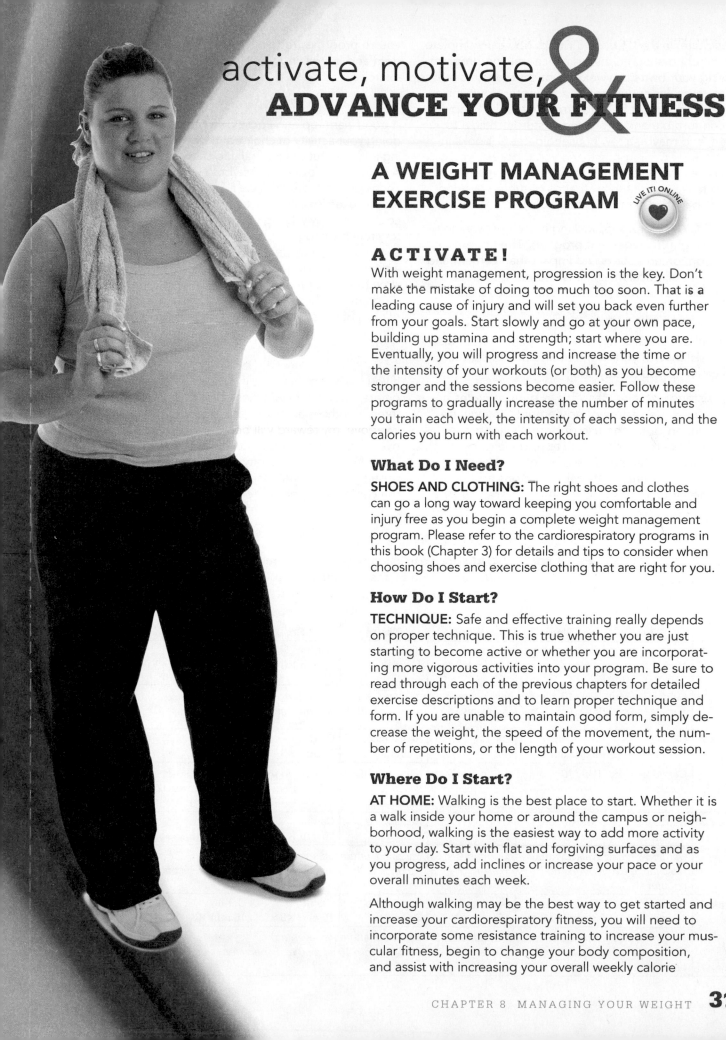

activate, motivate, & ADVANCE YOUR FITNESS

A WEIGHT MANAGEMENT EXERCISE PROGRAM

ACTIVATE!

With weight management, progression is the key. Don't make the mistake of doing too much too soon. That is a leading cause of injury and will set you back even further from your goals. Start slowly and go at your own pace, building up stamina and strength; start where you are. Eventually, you will progress and increase the time or the intensity of your workouts (or both) as you become stronger and the sessions become easier. Follow these programs to gradually increase the number of minutes you train each week, the intensity of each session, and the calories you burn with each workout.

What Do I Need?

SHOES AND CLOTHING: The right shoes and clothes can go a long way toward keeping you comfortable and injury free as you begin a complete weight management program. Please refer to the cardiorespiratory programs in this book (Chapter 3) for details and tips to consider when choosing shoes and exercise clothing that are right for you.

How Do I Start?

TECHNIQUE: Safe and effective training really depends on proper technique. This is true whether you are just starting to become active or whether you are incorporating more vigorous activities into your program. Be sure to read through each of the previous chapters for detailed exercise descriptions and to learn proper technique and form. If you are unable to maintain good form, simply decrease the weight, the speed of the movement, the number of repetitions, or the length of your workout session.

Where Do I Start?

AT HOME: Walking is the best place to start. Whether it is a walk inside your home or around the campus or neighborhood, walking is the easiest way to add more activity to your day. Start with flat and forgiving surfaces and as you progress, add inclines or increase your pace or your overall minutes each week.

Although walking may be the best way to get started and increase your cardiorespiratory fitness, you will need to incorporate some resistance training to increase your muscular fitness, begin to change your body composition, and assist with increasing your overall weekly calorie expenditure. In the beginning weeks, you can complete your weight management resistance training program by using your own bodyweight against gravity to increase muscular endurance and strength. However, a few key items might help your motivation by keeping you comfortable and interested: a sturdy chair, a towel or mat, and maybe a few household items (books in your backpack, for instance). As you progress, you can add pieces of equipment to provide more resistance and increase your intensity (bands or tubing, a good stability ball, and even medicine balls).

AT THE GYM: Here, too, walking is the best way to start a weight management program. The treadmill is a great option and offers less impact than cement and asphalt. An elliptical machine is another good option that reduces the stress placed on hips, knees, ankles, and feet. If your gym has a pool, make use of it. Water walking (shallow or deep) is a great way to move your body without placing stress on your joints. Water also adds resistance to your workout and of course, the pool can help you to stay cool!

For resistance training sessions, a gym provides access to the wide variety of equipment. You will be able to incorporate the use of barbells (long bars with weights attached or slots to add weight plates), dumbbells (smaller, hand-held weights), benches (flat, incline, decline), plus cable stations and the latest the industry has to offer. All of these will help

you to progress, reducing your chances of boredom and increasing your likelihood of continued exercise.

Warm-Up and Cool-Down

A good warm-up and cool-down consists of simply doing your activity of choice at a slower pace and easing into and out of your training session. Break a light sweat as you slowly increase both your respiratory rate and your heart rate. Include a few dynamic range-of-motion exercises. After you finish your workout session, cool-down slowly, bringing your heart rate and respiratory rate back to your starting point. Once you have cooled down, include a few more dynamic moves or try a bit of foam rolling. Then begin to perform your static stretches for improved flexibility. (Be sure to review the programs in Chapter 5 for more ideas and descriptions of each of the stretches.)

Four-Week Weight Management Programs

If you are just beginning, if you have a BMI of 30 or greater, or if you have taken a lay-off of more than three months, start slowly and build gradually with Program A. Doing this will help you increase your overall calorie expenditure while helping to keep you injury free! Adjust intensity, volume, and training days to suit your personal fitness level and schedule; visit the companion website for more options.

PROGRAM A

LIVE IT! ONLINE

GOAL: Increase cardiorespiratory exercise frequency to 3 days a week and time to 15 minutes continuously, 100+ minutes/week; also incorporate resistance training 2 days a week.

	Mon	Tue	Wed	Thurs	Fri	Sat	Sun
Week 1	Cardio, 10 min ×3	Resistance, 1 circuit	Cardio, 10 min ×3	Resistance, 1 circuit	Cardio, 10 min ×3		
	Cardio workout: Walk 10 minutes continuously 3× (morning, afternoon, evening) *Resistance circuit workout: Do each exercise for 60 seconds with 15-second rests between exercises*						
Week 2	Cardio, 10 min ×3	Resistance, 2 circuits	Cardio, 10 min ×3	Resistance, 2 circuits	Cardio, 10 min ×3	Cardio, 10 min ×3	
	Cardio workout: Walk 10 minutes continuously, 3× (morning, afternoon, evening) *Resistance circuit workout: Do each exercise for 60 seconds with 15-second rests between exercises, 60-second rests between circuits*						
Week 3	Cardio, 15 min ×3	Resistance, 2 circuits	Cardio, 15 min ×3	Resistance, 2 circuits	Cardio, 15 min ×3		
	Cardio workout: Walk 15 minutes continuously, 3× (morning, afternoon, evening) *Resistance circuit workout: Do each exercise for 60 seconds with no rest between exercises, 60-second rests between circuits*						
Week 4	Cardio, 15 min ×3	Resistance, 3 circuits	Cardio, 15 min ×3	Resistance, 3 circuits	Cardio, 15 min ×3	Cardio, 15 min ×3	
	Cardio workout: Walk 15 minutes continuously, 3× (morning, afternoon, evening) *Resistance circuit workout: Do each exercise for 45 seconds with 10-second rests between exercises, 60-second rests between circuits*						

Order of Resistance Circuit Exercises for Home Workout

Squat
Push-Up or Modified Push-Up
Lunge
Plank or Modified Plank
Row with Resistance Band or dumbbell
Lat Pull-Down with Resistance Band
Side Bridge (each side)
Back Extension

Order of Resistance Circuit Exercises for Facility Workout

Chest Press
Squat or Leg Press Machine
Upright Row
Leg Extension
Rows
Overhead Press
Lat Pull-Down
Biceps Curl
Triceps Extension
Plank

MOTIVATE!

Create an exercise log to track your own weight management exercise program—make note of days, actual exercises, sets, reps, load amounts, rest intervals—or use the one on the companion website. Here are a few tips to get you moving:

MOTIVATING MEASUREMENTS: Whether you use a scale, a tape measure, or simply your favorite jeans, be sure to check your progress each week. This can encourage and motivate you, and it will serve as a good catch to help you get back on track if you are not maintaining your nutrition and exercise program.

BAN THE FAT TALK: Stop your negative self-talk and start anew! Surround yourself with only positive comments, upbeat training partners, and true supporters of your new healthy behaviors and lifestyle. Stay focused. Remember your goals. Be patient with yourself and be sure to acknowledge how much you have already accomplished!

TAKE A LITTLE "YOU" TIME: Make fitness and nutrition a priority. Take time for you—schedule your favorite fitness activity (a stroll, your yoga DVD, pool time) and keep the appointment as you would for any other priority.

KEEP A DIGITAL PHOTO LOG: Take a "before" picture, and take a new picture each week. It may sound like the last thing you want to do at first. However, it can remind you of just how far you've come and keep you motivated to continue. This also works for your meals (especially when you eat out). Take pictures of your meals and gain a different perspective on what you are eating, how much, and when.

ADVANCE!

Now that you have established your exercise and weight management program, challenge yourself. Follow Program B if you already exercise at least two days a week, if you have a BMI of 25 to 29, or if you simply want to take your weight management program to the next level. Visit the companion website to find more options or to personalize this or any of the programs in this book.

PROGRAM B

LIVE IT! ONLINE

GOAL: Increase cardiorespiratory exercise frequency to 5 days a week and time to 30 minutes continuously, 300+ minutes/week; also incorporate resistance training 3 days a week.

	Mon	Tue	Wed	Thurs	Fri	Sat	Sun
Week 1	Walk/jog 15 min continuously, ×3 (morning, afternoon, evening)	Resistance, 2 circuits	Walk/jog 15 min continuously, ×3 (morning, afternoon, evening)	Resistance, 2 circuits	Walk/jog 15 min continuously, ×3 (morning, afternoon, evening)	Walk/jog 20 min continuously, ×2 (morning, evening)	
	Resistance circuit workout: Do each exercise for 60 seconds with 10-second rests between exercises, 60-second rests between circuits						

	Mon	Tue	Wed	Thurs	Fri	Sat	Sun
Week 2	Walk/jog 20 min continuously, ×3 (morning, afternoon, evening)	Walk/jog 15 min + Resistance, 2 circuits	Walk/jog 20 min continuously, ×3 (morning, afternoon, evening)	Walk/jog 15 min + Resistance, 2 circuits	Walk/jog 20 min continuously, ×3 (morning, afternoon, evening)	Walk/jog 25 min continuously, ×2 (morning, evening)	
	Resistance circuit workout: Do each exercise for 60 seconds with 10-second rests between exercises, 60-second rests between circuits						
Week 3	Walk/jog 25 min continuously, ×3 (morning, afternoon, evening)	Walk/jog 15 min + Resistance, 3 circuits	Walk/jog 25 min continuously, ×3 (morning, afternoon, evening)	Walk/jog 15 min + Resistance, 3 circuits	Walk/jog 25 min continuously, ×3 (morning, afternoon, evening)	Walk/jog 30 min continuously, ×2 (morning, evening)	
	Resistance circuit workout: Do each exercise for 60 seconds with 10-second rests between exercises, 60-second rests between circuits						
Week 4	Walk/jog 30 min continuously, ×3 (morning, afternoon, evening)	Walk/jog 15 min + Resistance, 3 circuits	Walk/jog 30 min continuously, ×3 (morning, afternoon, evening)	Walk/jog 15 min + Resistance, 3 circuits	Walk/jog 30 min continuously, ×3 (morning, afternoon, evening)	Walk/jog 15 min + Resistance, 3 circuits	
	Resistance circuit workout: Do each exercise for 60 seconds with 10-second rests between exercises, 60-second rests between circuits						

Order of Resistance Circuit Exercises for Home Workout

Squat + Overhead Press with Resistance Band or Dumbbells
Push-Up or Modified Push-Up
Lunge + Biceps Curl with Resistance Band or Dumbbells
Row with Resistance Band or Dumbbells
Lat Pull-Down with Resistance Band
Triceps Extension with Resistance Band or Dumbbells
Oblique Curl
Plank or Modified Plank
Back Extension

Order of Resistance Circuit Exercises for Facility Workout

Squats or Leg Press Machine
Chest Press
Leg Extension
Overhead Press
Leg Curl
Upright Row
Lunge + Biceps Curl with Resistance Band or Dumbbells
Rows
Lat Pull-Down
Pullover
Plank
Abdominal Curl
Back Extension

9

Managing Stress

Learning Outcomes

1. Define stress.

HEAR IT! ONLINE — Audio case study & audio PowerPoint lecture

2. Describe how your body responds to stress.

3. Explain how stress can harm your body.

4. List the kinds of harm stress can cause to your cardiovascular, immune, and other body systems.

5. Identify the major sources of stress.

SEE IT! ONLINE — Stress at Work and Home

DO IT! ONLINE — Lab 9.1 How Stressed Are You?

6. Describe effective tools for stress management.

LIVE IT! ONLINE — Customizable 4-week starter and intermediate meditation programs

DO IT! ONLINE — Lab 9.2 Managing Your Time

SEE IT! ONLINE — The Multi-Tasking Myth

7. Create your own stress management plan.

DO IT! ONLINE — Lab 9.3 Your Personal Stress Management Plan

Pre- and post-quizzes and glossary flashcards

REVIEW IT! ONLINE

casestudy

CORY

"Hi, I'm Cory. I'm a junior, majoring in biology. I'm from Denver, Colorado, and just transferred schools in August to be closer to my dad, who lives alone and has diabetes. I take five classes, I work part-time as a lab assistant, and I'm up late every night studying so that I can keep up my grades for applying to medical school. I've always been able to work under pressure, but I have to admit, these past few months have been rough. I am constantly worn out, worried about my dad, and I can barely stay awake in class sometimes. I know that medical school will be even harder, so maybe I should just get used to living like this! But I am so tired of feeling dragged out."

HEAR IT! ONLINE

Everyone feels stress at least some of the time, be it from traffic, competition for the courses you need, job hunting, fast-changing technology, or a hectic pace that seems to accelerate yearly. Over time, stress can diminish not just our enjoyment of life, but our health and well-being, too.[1] Thus, learning effective stress-management techniques is an important part of any complete wellness program.

This chapter explains the stress response, details the ways accumulated stress can affect your health, and proposes several helpful strategies you can use to counteract stress. Using the stress-management tools in this chapter, you can better face the pressures of college life and beyond.

What Is Stress?

In a recent national survey, college students reported stress as the biggest impediment to their academic success, with a greater impact on achievement than colds, flu, sleep difficulty, relationship issues, and all other concerns.[2] But what, exactly, *is* stress?

Stress is a term that is commonly used in many different ways. In this book, we'll define stress as the disturbed physical and/or emotional state that a person experiences as a result of an event. The event may be physical, social, or psychological, such as a threat, aggravation, or excitement that disturbs an individual's "normal" physiological state and to which the body must try to adapt. Any event that disrupts your body's "normal" state is a **stressor**. A stressor can be physical, such as an uncomfortably heavy backpack. It can also be emotional, like the anxiety you feel before a major exam. The term for the physical effect of a stressor is the **stress response**: the set of physiological changes initiated by your body's nervous and hormonal signals. The stress response prepares the brain, heart, muscles, and other organs to respond to a perceived threat or demand.

A more traditional view of stress includes the concepts of both positive stress and negative stress. Positive stress, or **eustress**, presents an opportunity for personal growth, satisfaction, and enhanced well-being. Eustress can invigorate us and motivate us to work harder and achieve more. Entering college, starting a job, and developing a new relationship are all challenges that can produce eustress. Negative stress, or **distress**, can result from negative stressors such as academic pressures, relationship discord, or money problems. It can even result from an overload of positive stressors such as graduating from college, getting married, moving to a new state, and starting a new job all in the same week. Distress can reduce wellness by promoting cardiovascular disease, impairing immunity, or causing mental and emotional dysfunction.

How Does My Body Respond to Stress?

As you sit down in the lecture hall to take your hardest midterm exam, you realize your heart is pounding, your breathing has quickened, your hands are sweating, you have "butterflies" in your stomach, and you feel a sense

> **stress** The disturbed physical or emotional state experienced as a result of a physical, social, or psychological event or circumstance that disturbs the body's "normal" state and to which the body must try to adapt
>
> **stressor** A physical, social, or psychological event or circumstance to which the body tries to adapt; stressors are often threatening, unfamiliar, disturbing, or exciting
>
> **stress response** A set of physiological changes initiated by your body in response to a stressor
>
> **eustress** Stress based on positive circumstances or events; can present an opportunity for personal growth
>
> **distress** Stress based on negative circumstances or events, or those perceived as negative; can diminish wellness

of dread. You are experiencing a stress response: a reaction involving nervous and hormonal activities that prepare both body and mind to deal with the disturbance to your normal state.

The Stress Response

Here's what happens during the seconds that the body initiates a stress response and in the minutes and hours as the response continues (Figure 9.1):

1. Your senses perceive and your brain interprets something as a threat; in the example above, an exam that will determine half your grade.

2. The threat triggers a region of your brain called the *hypothalamus* to release a hormone that in turn triggers your pituitary gland to secrete **adrenocorticotropic hormone (ACTH)** into your blood.

3. ACTH travels through the bloodstream and reaches the outer zone of each adrenal gland (located on top of each kidney). ACTH causes the adrenal glands to secrete **cortisol**, your body's main stress hormone.

adrenocorticotropic hormone (ACTH) A hormone secreted by the pituitary gland that causes adrenal glands to secrete cortisol

cortisol The body's main stress hormone, secreted by the cortex or outer layer of the adrenal glands located on top of the kidneys; stimulates the sympathetic nervous system; can also damage or destroy neurons.

At the same time, nerve signals from your brain and spinal cord reach and stimulate the central zone of each adrenal gland. Both adrenals respond

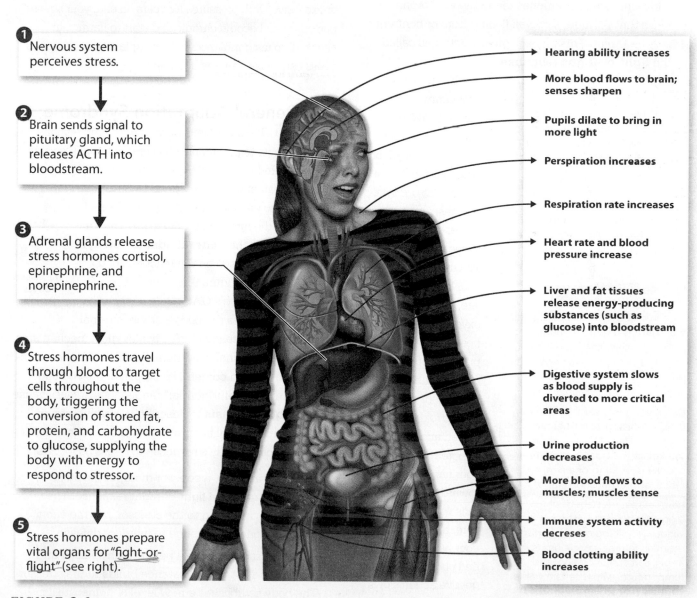

❶ Nervous system perceives stress.

❷ Brain sends signal to pituitary gland, which releases ACTH into bloodstream.

❸ Adrenal glands release stress hormones cortisol, epinephrine, and norepinephrine.

❹ Stress hormones travel through blood to target cells throughout the body, triggering the conversion of stored fat, protein, and carbohydrate to glucose, supplying the body with energy to respond to stressor.

❺ Stress hormones prepare vital organs for "fight-or-flight" (see right).

→ **Hearing ability increases**

→ **More blood flows to brain; senses sharpen**

→ **Pupils dilate to bring in more light**

→ **Perspiration increases**

→ **Respiration rate increases**

→ **Heart rate and blood pressure increase**

→ **Liver and fat tissues release energy-producing substances (such as glucose) into bloodstream**

→ **Digestive system slows as blood supply is diverted to more critical areas**

→ **Urine production decreases**

→ **More blood flows to muscles; muscles tense**

→ **Immune system activity decreases**

→ **Blood clotting ability increases**

FIGURE **9.1** The stress response.

by releasing two additional stress hormones that ready the body for quick action: **epinephrine** (also called **adrenaline**) and **norepinephrine** (or **noradrenaline**).

4. Traveling inside the bloodstream, cortisol reaches specific *target cells* within the body fat and within several organs, including the liver and intestines. Cortisol quickly triggers target cells to convert stored fat, protein, and carbohydrate molecules into glucose. Soon, more glucose is circulating in the blood, supplying the whole body—especially the brain and skeletal muscles—with the extra energy needed to respond to the stressor.

5. The epinephrine and norepinephrine released into the blood rapidly reach target cells in the heart, lungs, stomach, intestines, sense organs, and muscles. Along with signals from sympathetic nerves, these additional stress hormones ready the vital organs in ways that promote survival: fleeing from or confronting the threat. This physiological reaction is called the **fight-or-flight response**.

---

epinephrine (adrenaline) One of two stress hormones released by adrenal glands that readies your body for quick action by stimulating sympathetic nerves

norepinephrine (noradrenaline) One of two stress hormones secreted by adrenal glands that readies your body for quick action by increasing arousal

fight-or-flight response A physiological reaction induced by nervous and hormonal signals that readies the heart, lungs, brain, muscles, and other vital organs and systems in ways that promote survival: fleeing from or confronting a threat

general adaptation syndrome (GAS) A historical model proposed by Hans Selye; it attempts to explain the body's stress response consisting of alarm, resistance, and exhaustion stages.

homeostasis A state of physiological equilibrium wherein various physiological mechanisms maintain internal conditions (such as pH, salt concentration, and temperature) within certain viable ranges

---

If you have ever jammed on the brakes to avoid an accident, you have probably felt a jolt of epinephrine. As part of the fight-or-flight response, your pupils dilate, enabling you to see more clearly. The air passages in your lungs also dilate, allowing more oxygen to enter. Your heart beats faster and pumps more blood to your muscles and brain. Your sweat glands release more sweat, and blood is directed away from your hands and feet toward your large muscles and body core; this can make your hands feel cold and clammy. Your digestive action slows or stops, and your

bladder function slows, since neither process is crucial to short-term survival. Primed in all these ways, your body is ready to handle the stressor, at least in the short term.

After a perceived stressor subsides, your nervous system returns the body to its "normal" state with slower heartbeats, normal breathing rate, normal digestion, and so on. The stress-reduction techniques you will learn later deliberately encourage the body's return to this more relaxed state.

Why Does Stress Cause Harm?

Why is chronic stress harmful? After all, if a truck is speeding toward you, your fight-or-flight response could save your life. However, if you are faced with financial hardship or excessive work pressures for years on end, your stress response can become chronic and start to harm your health. Two insightful models help explain how *sustained* stress can cause damage over time.

The General Adaptation Syndrome

In the 1930s, biologist Hans Selye studied the response of laboratory rats to painful physical or emotional stressors. He discovered that a wide variety of stressors—such as extreme heat, extreme cold, forced exercise, or surgery—all seemed to provoke the same general set of changes in the rats' bodies. Selye proposed a model he called the **general adaptation syndrome (GAS)**, based on the reactions of the rats he observed (Figure 9.2).[3]

LIVE IT! ONLINE

Worksheet 8 Stress Reaction

Central to Selye's GAS model is the idea that stress disrupts the body's stable internal environment, or *steady state*. Physiological mechanisms work to keep internal conditions (such as body temperature, blood-oxygen content, blood pH, and blood sugar levels) within certain "normal" ranges. Life scientists use the term **homeostasis** to describe the body's steady state. Selye's general adaptation syndrome characterizes the stages of the body's response to stress as follows:

1. In the *alarm stage*, a stressor disrupts the steady state and triggers a fight-or-flight response. The body starts adapting to the stressor, but the effort can lower one's resistance to injury or disease.[4]

2. In the *resistance stage*, a person's physiology and behavior adjust, and resistance builds to the stressor. The body establishes a new level of homeostasis, despite the continued presence of the stressor.

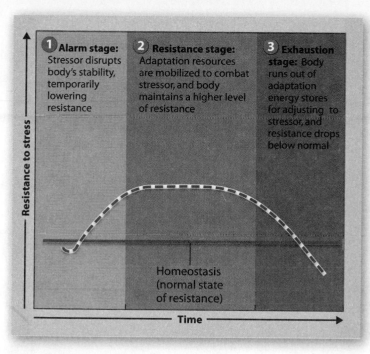

① **Alarm stage:** Stressor disrupts body's stability, temporarily lowering resistance

② **Resistance stage:** Adaptation resources are mobilized to combat stressor, and body maintains a higher level of resistance

③ **Exhaustion stage:** Body runs out of adaptation energy stores for adjusting to stressor, and resistance drops below normal

Resistance to stress

Homeostasis (normal state of resistance)

Time

FIGURE **9.2** Hans Seyle's general adaptation syndrome.

3. In the hypothetical *exhaustion stage,* the body runs out of resources to successfully adapt to the stressor, resulting in physiological harm in the form of reduced immunity and increased susceptibility to physical or mental illness.

The general adaptation syndrome recognized that sustained stress can take a toll on wellness. However, scientists have since modified Selye's concept of an "exhaustion stage" and the idea that illness results from running out of resources to adapt to a stressor. Rather, they now believe that over time, the stress response *itself* can damage the body and increase one's risk of developing illness, as we will see in the next section.

Allostatic Load

Today's stress researchers use the term **allostasis** to describe the many simultaneous changes that occur in the body to maintain homeostasis, and they use the term **allostatic load** to refer to the long-term wear and tear on the body that is caused by prolonged allostasis.[5]

Allostatic load can result if your body's ability to shut off the stress response (after a stressor has disappeared) is impaired, allowing high levels of stress hormones to remain in the bloodstream. It can also develop when your body releases too *few* stress hormones and cannot mount an adequate stress response.[6] And it can build up if you experience a sustained string of stressful events over a long period of time. A classic example of a consequence

of allostatic load is the development of stress-induced high blood pressure (hypertension.) As you will see shortly, chronically high blood pressure can damage arteries and increase one's risk of developing cardiovascular disease.[7]

A person's behavior and choices can also result in allostatic load. For example, some people respond to stress by exercising more, meditating, getting extra sleep, and avoiding drugs and alcohol—all behaviors that can help minimize allostatic load. Others respond by exercising less, staying up late, drinking more, or starting to smoke or take drugs. Such counterproductive measures can result in allostatic load and increase one's susceptibility to developing illness.

allostasis The many simultaneous changes that occur in the body to maintain homeostasis

allostatic load The long-term wear and tear on the body that is caused by prolonged allostasis

casestudy

CORY

"I knew this year was going to be a challenge—transferring to a new school and taking upper-level classes. The first month actually went okay. I liked my classes, my dad seemed to be doing better, and I got used to getting by on five hours of sleep each night. Then sometime in September I caught a cold that didn't go away for four weeks! I was coughing all night, could barely pay attention in class, and did badly on one of my midterms. Now I have to work even harder to make up for the bad grade."

THINK! List Cory's main sources of stress. Which would you classify as *eustress* and which would you classify as *distress*? How might the allostatic load model explain what is happening with Cory?

ACT! Make a list of your own major sources of stress, organizing them into eustress and distress. How does stress affect your body and mind? What do you do when you feel stressed out? If you typically choose unhealthy responses to stress, list some alternative healthy responses you'd like to try.

HEAR IT! ONLINE

What Kinds of Harm Can Stress Cause?

Studies indicate that 40 percent of deaths and 70 percent of disease in the United States are related, in whole or in part, to stress.[8] The list of ailments related to chronic stress includes heart disease, diabetes, cancer, headaches, ulcers, low back pain, depression, and the common cold.

Stress and Cardiovascular Disease

Perhaps the most studied and documented health consequence of unresolved stress is cardiovascular disease (CVD). Research on this topic has demonstrated the impact of chronic stress on heart rate, blood pressure, heart attack, and stroke.[9] Historically, the increased risk of CVD from chronic stress has been linked to increased plaque buildup due to elevated cholesterol, hardening of the arteries, alterations in heart rhythm, and increased and fluctuating blood pressure. Recent research also points to metabolic abnormalities, insulin resistance, and inflammation in blood vessels as major contributors to heart disease.[10] In the past 15 to 20 years, researchers have identified direct links between the incidence and progression of CVD and stressors such as job strain, caregiving, bereavement, and natural disasters.[11] Whatever the mechanism, the evidence is clear that stress is a significant contributor to CVD morbidity and mortality.

Stress and the Immune System

A growing area of scientific investigation known as **psychoneuroimmunology (PNI)** explores the intricate relationship between the mind's response to stress and the immune system's ability to function effectively. Research suggests that too much stress over a long period can negatively regulate various aspects of the cellular immune response.[12] Whereas a short-term fight-or-flight response is usually protective, prolonged stress depresses the immune system. During prolonged stress, elevated levels of adrenal hormones (such as cortisol) destroy or reduce the ability of certain white blood cells, known as killer T cells, to aid the immune response.[13] When killer T cells aren't working correctly, the body becomes more susceptible to illness.

psychoneuroimmunology (PNI) Science of the interaction between the mind and the immune system

post-traumatic stress disorder (PTSD) An acute stress disorder caused by experiencing an extremely traumatic event

Stress and Other Physical Effects

Prolonged periods of stress can have other physical effects, as well:

- *Weight gain* Evidence from animal and human studies shows that stress hormones can increase food consumption as well as the tendency to store belly fat.[14]

- *Hair loss* Stress can trigger hair to fall out, either temporarily or permanently.[15]

- *Diabetes* People under stress often eat poorly, drink to excess, take drugs, eat junk food, or get too little sleep. All of these can alter blood sugar levels and aggravate pre-existing cases of type-2 diabetes or promote their development.[16]

- *Digestive problems* People under stress can experience nausea, vomiting, stomach pain, intestinal pain, or diarrhea. Stress hormones can cause existing digestive problems to flare. A classic example is irritable bowel syndrome.[17]

- *Loss of libido* Even in young people, stress can alter normal levels of sex hormones and this, in turn, can lead to erectile dysfunction, emotional swings, and loss of sex drive.[18]

If you experience any of these problems, a trip to the student health center may help you discover links to stress and solutions to the problems.

Stress and the Mind

Stress may be one of the single greatest contributors to mental impairment and disability and to emotional dysfunction in industrialized nations. One of the most common impairments is disrupted short-term memory, especially a person's ability to remember words as quickly as he or she could before the period of stress.[19] Animal studies show that stress hormones can actually shrink the brain's memory center (the *hippocampus*) and negatively impact verbal and other memory functions.[20] Stress can lead to mental disorders, as well. Studies have shown that environmental stressors, including divorce, marital conflict, and economic hardship can aggravate or affect the onset of mental disorders, particularly depression and anxiety (see the box Can Stress Cause Depression?).[21]

In severe cases, an individual's response to stress may develop into **post-traumatic stress disorder (PTSD)**. Traumas that can trigger PTSD include wartime experiences, rape, near-death experiences in accidents, witnessing a murder or death, being caught in a natural disaster, or a terrorist attack.

Can Stress Cause Depression?

Stress and depression have complicated interconnections based on emotional, physiological, and biochemical processes. Prolonged stress can trigger depression in susceptible people, and prior periods of depression can leave individuals more susceptible to stress.[1]

The physical links between stress and depression are strong. During the stress response, the body is flooded with cortisol and with chemicals called *cytokines.* These factors promote inflammation as part of the body's immune response. Researchers think that exposure to both kinds of chemicals can damage or kill neurons in a part of the brain called the *hippocampus* and can alter nerve transmission within the brain. One result of hippocampal damage is impaired learning and memory.[2] Another is the onset of depression symptoms in genetically susceptible individuals.[3] Research confirms that loss of hippocampal neurons is present in many who suffer depression.[4]

Realizing the important interconnections between stress and depression can help you take appropriate steps to handling one or both. Because stress and depression symptoms overlap, applying the stress-management techniques outlined in this chapter may help alleviate depression.

Physical activity is a particularly potent tool. A recent survey or more than 43,000 college students revealed that students who exercise or engage in physical activity each week have fewer feelings of depression, hopelessness, and suicidal behavior than do inactive students.[5]

If depression symptoms become severe enough to interfere with studying or other aspects of daily life, you should seek help. Potential sources for help are the student health service, the campus counseling center, a doctor or mental health professional in your community, and your local depression or suicide hotline.

Sources:
1. M. A. Ilgen and K. E. Hutchison, "A History of Major Depressive Disorder and the Response to Stress," *Journal of Affective Disorders* 86, no. 2 (2005): 143–50.
2. F. A. Scorza and others, "Neurogenesis and Depression: Etiology or New Illusion?" *Review of Brazilian Psychiatry* 27, no. 3 (2005): 249–53.
3. M. A. Ilgen and K. E. Hutchison, "A History of Major Depressive Disorder and the Response to Stress," 2005.
4. P. Price, "Stress and Depression," www.allaboutdepression.com/gen_05.html (updated June 2010).
5. L. Taliaferro and others, "Associations between Physical Activity and Reduced Rates of Hopelessness, Depression, and Suicidal Behavior among College Students," *Journal of American College Health* 57, no. 4 (2009): 427–36.

What Are the Major Sources of Stress?

College students can experience a flood of new stressors, and these can differ depending on age, sex, and year in school.[22] First-year students, for example, primarily feel academic pressure.[23] Fully 29 percent of freshman report feeling frequently overwhelmed by all they have to do.[24] Female freshmen also tend to report dieting and weight gain as stressful, while male students worry more about being underweight, relationship issues, and substance use (drugs, alcohol).[25] In addition, nontraditional and foreign students may experience other sources of stress, as described in the box International Student Stress.

Sources of Stress Can Be Internal or External

Interactions with others, expectations we and others have of ourselves, and the social and environmental conditions we live in force us to readjust constantly. Examining the causes of stress may help you identify your sources of stress and learn new ways to cope with them (Figure 9.3).

SEE IT! ONLINE
Stress at Work and Home

LIVE IT! ONLINE
Worksheet 9 Stress Tolerance Test

Change Alterations from your normal routine can cause stress. The greater the change and your necessary adjustments to it, the more stress and the greater the potential impact on your immune system.[26] Certain life events predict increased risk for stress-related illness. Knowing them can help, as you'll discover in **Lab 9.1**.

DO IT! ONLINE

Performance Demands We experience stress when we must meet higher standards or unfamiliar de-

mands. In college, competition for grades, athletic positions, club memberships, internships, graduate school acceptance, and job interviews can exert considerable pressure. We can lessen the impact of such demands by setting priorities and realistic deadlines.

Inconsistent Goals and Behaviors The negative effects of stress can be magnified when we don't match our goals with our actions. For instance, you may want good grades. But if you party and procrastinate throughout the term, your goals and behaviors are inconsistent. Behaviors that are consistent with your goals—for example, studying harder and partying less to achieve good grades—can help alleviate stress.

Overload and Burnout Time pressure, responsibilities, course work, tuition, and high expectations for yourself and those around you—coupled with a lack of support—can lead to *overload:* a state of feeling overburdened, unable to keep up, and longing for

DIVERSITY

International Student Stress

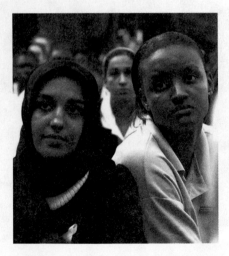

International students experience unique adjustment issues related to language barriers, cultural barriers, and a lack of social support, among other challenges. Academic stress may pose a particular problem for the more than 670,000 international students who have left support networks of family and friends in their native countries to study in the United States. Accumulating evidence suggests that seeking emotional support from others is among the most effective ways to cope with stressful and upsetting situations. Yet, many international students refrain from doing so because of cultural norms, feelings of shame, and the belief that seeking support is a sign of weakness that calls inappropriate attention to both the individual and the respective ethnic group. This reluctance, coupled with the language barriers, cultural conflicts, and other stressors, can lead international students to suffer significantly more stress-related illnesses than their American counterparts. Even if we can't solve the many problems international students encounter, there are things we can do to make one person's life (or maybe two or three persons' lives) a little less stressful: share companionship and communication and lend a helping hand. To paraphrase a popular Hindu proverb: "Help thy neighbor's boat across and thine own boat will also reach the shore."

Sources: S. Sumer, "International Students' Psychological and Sociocultural Adaptation in the United States," Georgia State University, Doctoral Dissertation, http://digitalarchive.gsu.edu/cps_diss/34 (2009); Institute of International Education, "Record Numbers of International Students in U.S. Higher Education," Press Release, http://opendoors.iienetwork.org/?p=150649 (November 2009).

Common stressors		Common stressors
Change		Traffic
Performance demands		Crowding
Inconsistent goals and behaviors		Finances
Overload and burnout		Relationships
Hassles		Racial, ethnic, or cultural isolation
		Conflict

FIGURE **9.3** Which of these stressors impact you?

escape. Overload pushes some students toward depression or substance abuse; others respond by using stress-management tools to alleviate tension before it piles up. Unrelieved overload can lead to *burnout,* a state of stress-induced physical and mental exhaustion. Teachers, nurses, and law enforcement officers, for example, experience high levels of burnout, and highly pressured professionals often use stress-management techniques to avoid reaching this point.

Hassles Petty annoyances and frustrations may seem unimportant if taken one by one: getting stuck in a long line at the bookstore, for example, or finding out that a school administrator has misplaced your paperwork. However, minor hassles can build to major stress if you perceive them negatively and let the feelings mount.[27] Regular release through stress management can counter this buildup.

Environmental Sources of Stress Environmental stress results from events occurring in the physical environment. People living in crowded urban environments tend to experience stress from things such as traffic, housing density, and a high cost of living. Meanwhile, people living in rural areas may experience different stresses such as limited employment opportunities and decreased services.

Relationships Relationships with friends, partners, family members, and co-workers can be important sources of strength and support, but they can also exert stress in our lives. These relationships can inspire and encourage us to achieve our highest goals and give us hope for the future. Staying connected can improve our mental, emotional, and physical health. Sometimes, though, relationships can diminish our self-esteem and leave us reeling from a destructive interaction. This kind of stress can diminish our wellness.

Racial, Ethnic or Cultural Isolation Those who act, speak, or dress differently sometimes face additional pressures that do not affect more "typical" students. Students perceived as different—whether due to race, ethnicity, religious affiliation, age, physical handicap, or sexual orientation—may become victims of subtle and not-so-subtle forms of bigotry, insensitivity, harassment, or hostility and this can increase the other forms of stress inherent in going to college.

Conflict Conflict occurs when we have to choose between competing motives, behaviors, or impulses, or when we must face incompatible demands, opportunities, needs, or goals. For example, what if your best friend wanted you to help her cheat on an exam, but you didn't feel right about it? College students often experience stress because their own developing set of beliefs conflicts with the values they learned from their parents.

What stresses do you face, and how are they affecting you? Lab 9.1 charts many common sources of stress for college students and others. Completing this lab will help you measure your current stress level. Reading through the next section will then supply a series of helpful stress-reduction strategies and tools for using them.

What Effective Strategies Can I Use to Manage Stress?

Most college students are able to manage their stress and do best with a low-key, multipronged approach. Figure 9.4 summarizes some of these strategies.

Internal Resources for Coping with Stress

When you perceive that your personal resources are sufficient to meet life's demands, you experience little or no stress. By contrast, when you perceive that life's demands exceed your coping resources, you are likely to feel strain and distress.

appraisal The interpretation and evaluation of information provided to the brain by the senses

psychological hardiness Personal characteristics of control, commitment, and an embrace of challenge that help individuals cope with stress

Self-Esteem and Self-Efficacy Several coping resources influence your stress **appraisal**, how you appraise the stress in your life. Two of the most important are *self-esteem* and

self-efficacy. Self-esteem is a sense of positive self-regard, or how you feel about yourself. Self-efficacy is a belief or confidence in personal skills and performance abilities. Researchers consider self-efficacy one of the most important personality traits that influence psychological and physiological stress responses.[28] Low self-esteem or low self-efficacy can lead you to feel helpless to cope with the stress in your life. Conversely, if you work to build your self-esteem and self-efficacy, you will add the benefit of less stress in your life!

Hardiness So-called "Type A" personalities are characterized as hard-driving, competitive, time-driven perfectionists. "Type B" personalities, in contrast, are more relaxed, noncompetitive, and more tolerant of others. Historically, researchers believed that people with Type A characteristics were more prone to heart attacks than their Type B counterparts.[29] Researchers today believe that personality types are more complex than previously thought—most people are not one personality type all the time, and other variables must be explored.

Psychological hardiness may negate self-imposed stress associated with Type A behavior. Psychologically hardy people are characterized by control, commitment, and an embrace of challenge.[30] People with a sense of control are able to accept responsibility for their behaviors and change those that they discover to be debilitating. People with a sense

FIGURE **9.4**   There are many effective techniques for helping you manage stress.

of commitment have good self-esteem and understand their purpose in life. People who embrace challenge see change as an opportunity for personal growth. The concept of hardiness has been studied extensively, and many researchers believe it is the foundation of an individual's ability to cope with stress and remain healthy.[31]

Exercise, Fun, and Recreational Activity

Improving your overall level of fitness may be the most helpful thing you can do to combat stress. Interestingly, research shows that exercise actually stimulates the stress response, but that a well-exercised body adapts to the *eustress* of exercise, and as a result is able to tolerate greater levels of *distress* of all kinds.[32] Compared to an unfit person, a fit individual develops a milder stress response to any given stressor.[33] Research also shows that exercise reduces both psychosocial stress and metabolic disturbances leading to belly fat, high blood pressure, high blood cholesterol, and vascular disease.[34]

Many physical activities relieve the feeling of stress and tension, while others—especially those that involve competition, high skill levels, or physical risk—may add to your stress load. Some activities are high in one value and low in the other, but many can build fitness and promote relaxation at the same time. The trick is to balance exercise, fun, and recreational activities in your free time so that you can stay fit and reduce chronic stress.

Basic Wellness Measures

Many of the habits you cultivate to improve your wellness can also fight the negative effects of stress.

Eating Well Eating nutrient-dense foods rather than fast foods and junk foods gives you more mental and physical energy, improves your immune responses, and helps you stay at a healthy weight. Undereating, overeating, or eating nutrient-poor foods can contribute to your stress levels by diminishing your overall wellness. Most claims about vitamins and supplements that reduce stress are unsupported. Vitamin and mineral supplementation beyond your daily requirements may only add to your stress—financial stress, that is!

Getting Enough Sleep Sleep is a central wellness component. As explained in the box How Does Sleep

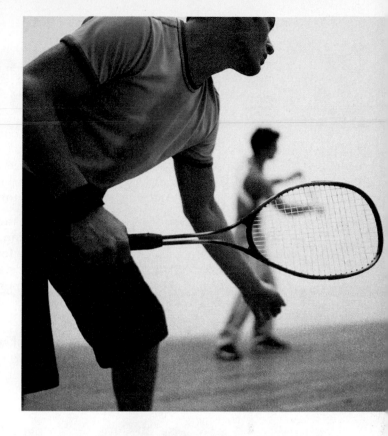

Affect My Performance and Mood?, sleep loss hinders learning, memory, academic work, and physical performance. It can also depress mood and prompt feelings of stress, anger, and sadness. *Sound* sleep is important, too. Some people find that inexpensive earplugs or eye masks from a drugstore block sleep-disturbing sound and light. Others require a quieter, darker room or more considerate roommates to solve their sleep problems.

LIVE IT! ONLINE

Worksheet 4
Sleep
Inventory

Avoiding Alcohol and Tobacco Both drinking and smoking can disrupt sleep patterns during the night. Alcohol can disrupt the length of time it takes you to fall asleep as well as the sequence and duration of your sleep states.[35] The nicotine in tobacco is highly addictive and acts as a mild stimulant. Tobacco use also impairs normal breathing and diminishes your ability to fight off colds and other infections.

Change Your Behavioral Responses

Realizing that stress is harming your fitness, wellness, relationships, or productivity is often the first step toward making positive changes. Start by assessing all aspects of a stressor, examining your typical response, determining ways to change it, and learning to cope. Often, you cannot change the stressors you face: the

How Does Sleep Affect My Performance and Mood?

Sleep experts suggest that 18- to 20-year-olds need about 8.5 to 9.25 hours of sleep per night, while adults over 21 need about 7 to 9 hours of sleep (depending on individual physiology).[1] In the 1980s, college students got an average of 7 to 7.5 hours of sleep per night. Today, however, that has slid to between 6 and 6.9 hours. In addition, the typical student sleeps less at the end of a semester than at the beginning due to the accumulation of assignments and exams.

Losing an hour or two of sleep actually does matter, even to young, active, healthy college students. Research shows that sleep loss degrades learning and memory, physical performance, and mood in both young and older adults. One piece of evidence for this is a German study that presented students with a math puzzle to work out. Most of those who "slept on it" realized a shortcut to solving the problem by morning and could accomplish the task much more quickly. Three-quarters of those who didn't "sleep on it" failed to intuit the way to a faster, simpler solution.[2] This was the first scientific proof that sleep can promote insight and problem solving.

Sleep deprivation can also increase feelings of stress, anger, anxiety, and sadness.[3] These emotional states can, in turn, make sleeping even harder. Feeling extremely stressed out and having a negative emotional response to that stress is, in fact, the best predictor that a student will have sleep problems.[4]

Poor sleep is defined as getting fewer-than-recommended hours of sleep, having irregular bedtimes and rising times, and experiencing interrupted sleep. To improve your sleep and adopt better sleep habits,

- go to bed and wake up at as regular a time as possible;
- sleep in a room that is as quiet and dark as possible;
- get regular exercise such as brisk walking or resistance training, but not too close to bedtime;[5]
- avoid caffeine in the afternoon or evening;
- avoid taking naps;
- sleep where it is cool (not cold) and ventilated (but not drafty); and
- avoid excess alcohol.

Sources:
1. National Sleep Foundation, "How Much Sleep Do We Really Need?" www.sleepfoundation.org/article/how-sleep-works/how-much-sleep-do-we-really-need (accessed October 2011).
2. U. Wagner and others, "Sleep Inspires Insight," *Nature* 427, no. 6972 (2004): 352–5.
3. B. A. Marcks, "Co-Occurrence of Insomnia and Anxiety Disorder: A Review of the Literature," *American Journal of Lifestyle Medicine* 3, no. 4 (2009): 300–9.
4. L. A. Verlander, J. O. Benedict, and D. P. Hanson, "Stress and Sleep Patterns of College Students," *Perceptual Motor Skills* 88, no. 3 (1999): 893–8.
5. M. Burman and A. King, "Exercise as Treatment to Enhance Sleep," *American Journal of Lifestyle Medicine* 4, no. 6 (2010): 500–14.

death of a loved one, the stringent requirements of your major, stacked-up course assignments, and so on. You can, however, change your reactions to them and better manage your stress.

Assess the Stressor List and evaluate the stressors in your life. Can you change the stressor itself? If not, you can still change your behavior and reactions to reduce the levels of stress you experience. For example, if you have a heavy academic workload, such as five term papers due for five different courses during the same quarter or semester, make a plan to start the papers early and space your work evenly so you can avoid panic over deadlines and all-night sessions to finish papers on time.

Change Your Response If something causes you distress—a habitually messy roommate, for example—you can (1) express your anger by yelling; (2) pick up the mess yourself but then leave a nasty note; (3) use humor to get your point across; or (4) initiate an even-tempered, matter-of-fact conversation about the problem. Before you respond, think through the most effective choice. Humor and laughter are surprisingly good ways to deescalate tense situations and to benefit your wellness generally. Laughter can boost your immune response, not to mention lightening your mood and even bringing extra oxygen into your lungs![36] A calm, rational conversation can work well, too.

Cognitive Coping Strategies Thinking things through before acting may help you avoid destructive or in-effective responses to potentially stressful events. Forethought and planning can also help you tolerate increasingly higher stress levels while limiting physical and mental wear and tear.

Prepare Before Stressful Events Preparing yourself for an event that you know will be stressful can diminish its impact. For example, practicing in front of friends may help you find and correct rough spots, and in turn, lower your levels of stress during the actual speech.

Downshift You may experience stress because you want to "have it all": a college diploma, a successful career, a family, a wide circle of friends, possessions, status in the community, and so on. But many people are **downshifting**: stepping back to a simpler life by, for example, moving from a large urban area to a smaller town, changing from a hectic high-pressure career to a low-key one, or scaling back to fewer, less-expensive possessions.

Consider some immediate and longer-term steps for simplifying your life:

- Avoid unnecessary spending.

- Choose a career that you enjoy for itself, not primarily for the salary it commands. Some lower-paying jobs are less stressful and allow more free time for relaxation.

- Clear out clutter. Having fewer unnecessary, unused items means keeping track and taking care of that much less.

Managing Your Time and Finances

The world presents us with plenty of stressors. We create some of our own through ineffective time and finance management habits. Habits are learned behaviors, and you can *unlearn* bad habits or replace them with new habits that serve you better in managing stress. Here is what to aim for.

Manage Your Time Time—or our perceived lack of it—is one of our biggest stressors. If you learn to handle demands in a more streamlined, efficient way, you can leave more time for other things, such as studying and having fun. To get a handle on time management, try working through **Lab 9.2**. The following tips can also help:

- *Use a calendar.* A calendar can help you keep track of due dates, events, commitments, and the like. Pick out a calendar that fits your life. Don't use a wall calendar if you are constantly on the go. Electronic calendars work well, especially because you can set reminders in them. Some people like the feel of paper and pen. Whatever works for you is fine, just get something you'll use.

- *Multitask only when it's truly appropriate.* Save multitasking for things that take less concentration, such as doing the laundry and paying bills.

The Multi-Tasking Myth

- *Break up big tasks.* Divide big tasks like finishing a term paper into smaller segments and then allocate a certain amount of time to each piece. If you find yourself floundering in a task, move on and come back to it when you are refreshed.

- *Clean your desk.* Periodically weed out unneeded papers and file the

downshifting Forging new values that include stepping back to a simpler life useful ones in separate folders. Promptly read, respond to, file, or toss mail into the recycle bin.

- *Accommodate your natural rhythms.* If you are a morning person, study and write papers in the morning, and take breaks when you start to slow down.

- *Avoid overcommitment.* Set your school and personal priorities and don't be afraid to say no to things you cannot or should not agree to do.

- *Avoid interruptions.* When you have a project that requires total concentration, schedule uninterrupted time. Go to a quiet room in the library or student union where no one will find you. Shut off your cell phone.

- *Remember that time is precious.* Many people learn to value their time only when they face a terminal illness. Try to value each day. Time spent not enjoying life is a tremendous waste!

Manage Your Finances Higher education can impose a huge financial burden on parents, students, and communities. In recent studies, nearly two-thirds of students indicated that they have "some" or "major" concerns regarding their ability to pay for their education. [37] The economic downturn of the past few years is pushing already financially stressed students and their families further toward the breaking point. Many students must work part- or full-time in addition to carrying heavy class loads, and some have increasing levels of credit card debt.

Here are a few tips for easing your financial stress:

- Develop a realistic budget of monthly expenses and what you really need.

- Pay bills immediately and consider online banking to avoid late fees.

- Take money management seminars and courses.

- Avoid unsolicited credit card offers.

- Take on as little new debt as possible.

Managing Your Thoughts and Emotions

Just as we can manage our time and finances, we can learn to manage how we think and react to events and to our emotions.

Manage Your Thinking Our "negative scripts" about ourselves contribute to our stress. When we see ourselves as unable to cope (that is, when we have low

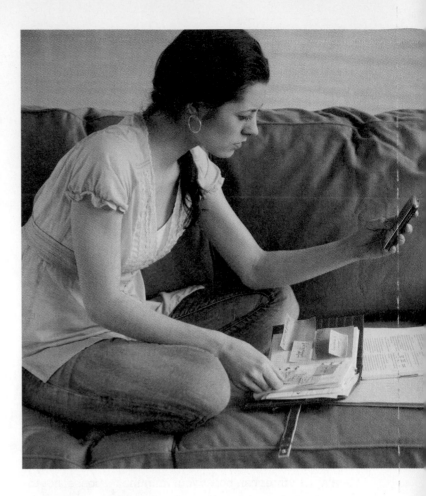

self-efficacy), we tend to handle life's problems and stresses more poorly. You can change negative scripts to more positive ones, however, and in the process reduce your stress responses. Successful stress management involves developing and practicing self-esteem skills, such as applying positive thinking and examining self-talk to reduce negative and irrational responses. Focus on your current capabilities rather than on past problems.

Here are specific actions you can take to develop better mental skills for stress management:

- *Worry constructively.* Don't waste time and energy worrying about things you can't change or events that may never happen.

- *Perceive life as changeable.* If you accept that change is a natural part of living and growing, the jolt of changes will become less stressful.

- *Consider alternatives.* Remember, there is seldom only one appropriate action. Anticipating options will help you plan for change and adjust more rapidly.

- *Moderate your expectations.* Aim high but be realistic about your circumstances and motivation.

- *Don't rush into action.* Think before you act. Tolerate mistakes by yourself and others. Rather than getting angry and stressed by mishaps, evaluate what happened, learn from them, and plan to avoid future occurrences.

- *Take things less seriously.* Try to keep the real importance of things in perspective. Ask yourself: How much will this matter in two weeks? Six months?

Manage Negative Emotions and Anger

Stress management involves learning to identify emotional reactions that are based on irrational beliefs and negative self-talk. Identifying those can allow you to deal with the belief or emotion in a healthy and appropriate way.[38]

LIVE IT! ONLINE

Worksheet 11
Anger Log

Learning how to manage anger is particularly important. Anger can be constructive if it mobilizes us to stand up for ourselves or to accomplish something others think we are incapable of. However, a habit of responding angrily when our wants or desires are thwarted can be destructive.

Hotheaded, short-fused people are at risk for health problems. Numerous studies show that anger can significantly increase the risk of heart disease. Stress hormones released during anger may constrict blood vessels in the heart or actually promote clot formation, which can trigger a heart attack.[39] Strategies for controlling and redirecting anger include practicing problem-solving techniques in place of complaining; seeking objective opinions and constructive advice from friends; anticipating situations that trigger your anger and brainstorming solutions in advance; learning to express your feelings constructively; learning to de-escalate from anger by taking deep breaths or counting to 10; and keeping a journal to observe your own reactions and progress in controlling anger.

Seeking Social Support

Making, keeping, and spending time with friends is a central stress-management tool that helps protect you against harmful stressors.[40] Social interactions are important buffers against the effects of stress: A person who is well-integrated socially is only half as likely to die from any cause at any age than is a person with few or no sources of social support.[41] This makes social connections a factor as large as being a nonsmoker versus a smoker! Social networking—through Facebook and Twitter, for example—has been an enormously popular way to stay connected. A few users do so obsessively, however, and this can become its own source of stress.[42] In addition, some recent research suggests that smoking, obesity, and other behaviors may tend to spread through networks of friends.[43] Clearly, social connectedness—pursued in moderation and with intelligent choices made toward eating, smoking, and other socially influenced behaviors—is important to wellness.

The flip side of social connectedness is social isolation, and it, too, has important health implications. Compared to students with a network of friends, isolated students experience more stress, poorer moods, and lower quality sleep.[44] Studies have found deleterious changes to the cardiovascular, immune, and nervous systems in chronically lonely people and these changes may help explain the increased risks for heart disease, infection, and depression in isolated individuals.[45] This research also suggests that a person's actual number of social contacts is less important to wellness than the subjective experience of being unpopular or lonely.[46]

While friends can be important stress reducers, people sometimes need the help of a counselor or support group. Most colleges and universities offer counseling services at no cost for short-term crises. Clergy, instructors, and dorm supervisors also may be helpful resources. Sometimes university services are unavailable and you may be concerned about confidentiality. Most communities offer low-cost counseling through mental health clinics. You may be able to find and join a stress-reduction program or stress support group through one of these professional resources. Many individual counselors and classes teach stress-reduction techniques to help you manage your stress.

relaxation breathing Inhaling deeply and rhythmically, expanding and then relaxing the abdomen; this breathing technique can help relieve tension and increase oxygen intake.

progressive muscle relaxation (PMR) A stress-management technique that identifies tension stored in the muscles and releases it, one muscle group at a time

Relaxation Techniques

Relaxation techniques tend to focus the mind and breathing while the body remains fairly stationary. Here are some of the most popular examples.

Relaxation Breathing When we're tense, we often breathe shallowly in the upper chest or even hold our breath, but this kind of breathing can increase anxiety.[47] **Relaxation breathing**—inhaling deeply and rhythmically and involving the abdominal muscles—can help relieve tension and increase oxygen levels in the blood. This, in turn, can boost energy and sharpen thinking. Relaxation breathing, also called *diaphragmatic breathing*, is easy and can be done sitting in a chair or lying down, alone or in a small group, and for a few minutes or longer. The object is to expand the lungs fully by drawing downward with the diaphragm and outward with the abdomen, then releasing fully.

Progressive Muscle Relaxation Progressive muscle relaxation (PMR) releases tension in the muscles, muscle group by muscle group. To do PMR, lie down in a quiet, comfortable place and devote 10 or 20 minutes to gradually letting go of accumulated stiffness and

TOOLS FOR **CHANGE** •

Progressive Muscle Relaxation

Progressive muscle relaxation involves systematically contracting and relaxing different muscle groups in your body. The standard pattern is to begin with the feet and work your way up your body, contracting and releasing as you go. With practice, you can quickly identify tension in your body when you are facing stressful situations and consciously release that tension to calm yourself.

Sit or lie down in a comfortable position and follow the steps below: Start with one foot. Inhale to the count of five, contracting the muscle of your foot. Hold for three seconds and notice the feeling of tension. Exhale to the count of eight, slowly releasing the muscles. Notice the feeling of tension flowing away. Repeat the same steps contracting and releasing your foot and lower leg, then your entire leg.

Follow the same sequence with your other foot and leg. Starting with one hand, follow the same sequence for both arms. Continue these isolations as you progress up your body, contracting and then relaxing your abdomen, then chest, followed by neck and shoulders, and ending with your face.

Hint: when you isolate and tense a muscle group, be sure not to contract too tightly. This can cause cramping, especially in your toes, feet, calves and neck. You many want to record the steps of PMR on a tape recorder. Some prefer to memorize the sequence of muscle groups and repeat the instructions mentally. Alternatively, ask another person to read the instructions to you out loud.

• •

tension in the affected muscles. The box Progressive Muscle Relaxation, shows you how. You can do this alone or in a group as a way to relax and refresh yourself fully. Some people also use it as a means of falling asleep.

Meditation There are dozens of forms of meditation. Most involve sitting quietly for 15 to 30 minutes and focusing on breathing. Researchers have confirmed that meditation reduces the stress response and boosts the immune response.[48] Meditation also shifts brain activity from the right prefrontal lobe, associated with unhappiness, anger, and distress, and toward the left prefrontal lobe, associated with happiness and enthusiasm. See Activate, Motivate, and Advance: A Meditation Program at the end of the chapter for guidance on beginning a meditation practice.

Biofeedback Biofeedback involves monitoring physical stress responses such as brain activity, blood pressure, muscle tension, and heart rate with a special machine and then learning to consciously alter these responses. Biofeedback is effective for several stress-related conditions, including high blood pressure, headaches, irritable bowel syndrome, and asthma.[49]

Hypnosis Hypnosis trains people to focus on one thought, object, or voice and to become unusually responsive to suggestion. A qualified hypnotherapist can implant a suggestion that directs a patient to resist habits such as smoking or overeating or to lessen phobias such as fear of snakes or air travel. The patient then learns to induce a state of selfhypnosis as a way to relax deeply and reinforce the behavioral changes.

People who exercise regularly and practice one or more of these relaxation methods—relaxation breathing, progressive muscle relaxation, meditation, biofeedback, and hypnosis—can achieve effective relief from stress symptoms.[50] Many will also see improvement in medical conditions that are worsened by stress.

Spiritual Practice

Several medical studies have discovered correlations between spirituality and wellness. Prayer, for example elicits the same relaxation response attained through other stress-management techniques: lowered

LIVE IT! ONLINE

Worksheet 7
Developing
Your Spirituality

blood pressure, heart rate, breathing and metabolism, and a more vigorous immune response.[51] Spirituality is also correlated with a reduced *perception* of stress in one's life.

Developing one's spirituality can be more than just an internal process. It can also be a social process that enhances your relationships with others. The abilities to give and take, speak and listen, and forgive and move on are integral to any process of spiritual development.

> **biofeedback** A stress-management technique that teaches you to alter automatic physiological responses such as body temperature, heart rate, or sweating.
>
> **hypnosis** A medical and psychiatric tool that trains people to focus on one thought, object, or voice and to become unusually responsive to suggestion

casestudy

CORY

"This semester was getting out of control. I was exhausted but would have trouble falling asleep, so that was a vicious cycle. I stopped working out— which I used to do twice a week but just didn't have the time for anymore. And I caught another cold at the end of October. My dad started joking that he was healthier than I was! I had to cut out something so I dropped my only elective, Spanish, even though I liked it. I used the extra time to start going back to the gym, and that actually seemed to give me back some energy. I honestly think just those two things alone helped me to get through the rest of the semester. Now, I just need to ace my MCATs ..."

THINK! What kinds of stress-related problems was Cory exhibiting? Review the section on stress-management tools. Which strategies did Cory employ?

ACT! Make a list of the stress-management strategies you use. Using that same list, put a check by the techniques that seem to be the most effective for you. How could you make the others work better?

HEAR IT! ONLINE

How Can I Create My Own Stress Management Plan?

You can use many of the fitness and wellness tools you read about in earlier chapters to help reduce your stress levels. These tools include self-assessment, drawing up a behavior change contract, and journaling. Lab 9.1 helps you assess situations that may leave you susceptible to stress. It also reveals signs of chronic stress. Using this information, target for change one or more behaviors that contribute to your increased stress.

Then, evaluate the behavior(s) you have chosen. Identify your stress-producing behavior patterns. What can you change now? What can you change in the near future? Select one stress-producing behavior pattern that you want to change. Devise an action plan and create a behavior change contract using **Lab 9.3**. As you learned earlier, your

behavior change contract should include your long-term goal for change, your short-term goals, the rewards you will give yourself for reaching these goals, potential obstacles along the way, and strategies for overcoming these obstacles.

Chart your progress in your journal. At the end of a week, evaluate how successful you were in following your plan. What helped you be successful? What obstacles to change did you encounter? What will you do differently next week? After you assess yourself, make a plan and revise it as needed. Are your short-term goals attainable? Are the rewards satisfying? Do you need to go beyond your own self-efforts and enlist the help of your peers or professionals? If you think you need professional support, start by consulting the student health service for advice and direction on finding suitable counselors, therapists, or stress-management support groups.

chapterin**review**

videos

Log on to **www.pearsonhighered.com/hopson** or MyFitnessLab to view these chapter-related videos.

Stress at Work and Home   The Multi-Tasking Myth

onlineresources

Log on to **www.pearsonhighered.com/hopson** or MyFitnessLab for access to these book-related resources, and for links to other useful websites.

 Audio case study
Audio PowerPoint lecture

 Lab 9.1 How Stressed Are You?
Lab 9.2 Managing Your Time
Lab 9.3 Your Personal Stress Management Plan

 Customizable 4-week starter and
intermediate meditation programs
Take Charge of Your Health! Worksheets:
   Worksheet 4 Sleep Inventory
   Worksheet 7 Developing Your Spirituality
   Worksheet 8 Stress Reaction
   Worksheet 9 Stress Tolerance Test
   Worksheet 11 Anger Log
Behavior Change Log Book and Wellness
Journal

Pre- and post-quizzes
Glossary flashcards

reviewquestions

1. Graduating from college and moving to a new city can create stress as well as provide an opportunity for growth. This type of stress is called
   a. strain.
   b. distress.
   c. eustress.
   d. adaptive response.

2. The physiological instinct to flee from or confront a threat is called
   a. homeostasis.
   b. the fight-or-flight response.
   c. allostasis.
   d. allostatic load.

3. *Homeostasis* describes
   a. the body's "normal" or "steady state."
   b. long-term wear-and-tear on the body.
   c. sustained stress.
   d. the exhaustion stage of the general adaptation syndrome.

4. Contemporary researchers have modified one stage of Hans Selye's general adaptation syndrome. Which one is it?
   a. The alarm stage
   b. The resistance stage
   c. The allostasis stage
   d. The exhaustion stage

5. Find the true statement:
   a. Stress reduces the risk of cardiovascular disease.
   b. Stress improves immune system function.
   c. Stress alleviates depression and anxiety.
   d. Stress reduces overall health and wellness.

6. Change, hassles, performance demands, and burn-out are all examples of
   a. psychosocial sources of stress.
   b. environmental sources of stress.
   c. internal sources of stress.
   d. homeostasis.

7. *Allostatic load* refers to
   a. changes that occur in the body to maintain homeostasis.
   b. long-term wear-and-tear on the body caused by stress.
   c. the first stage of the general adaptation syndrome.
   d. eustress.

8. Find the true statement: Effective stress management includes
   a. getting by on little sleep.
   b. reducing exercise and physical activity to allow more time for studying.
   c. eating fast food and junk food to save money and provide comfort.
   d. avoiding alcohol and tobacco.

9. *Relaxation breathing* refers to
   a. inhaling deeply and rhythmically to relieve tension and increase oxygen levels in the blood.
   b. progressive muscle relaxation.
   c. monitoring physical stress responses and then consciously working to alter those responses.
   d. biofeedback.

10. What stress-fighting technique allows people to become unusually responsive to suggestion?
    a. Meditation
    b. Massage
    c. Biofeedback
    d. Hypnosis

critical**thinking**questions

1. Compare and contrast distress and eustress. In what ways are both types of stress potentially harmful?
2. Describe the body's physiological response to stress.
3. What are some of the health risks that result from chronic stress? Summarize the main points of the general adaptation syndrome and the allostatic load model.

4. What major factors seem to influence the nature and extent of a person's susceptibility to stress? Explain how social support, self-esteem, and personality may make a person more or less susceptible.

references

1. American Psychological Association, *Stress in America 2009, Executive Summary,* www.apa.org/news/press/releases /stress-exec-summary.pdf (2009).
2. American College Health Association, *American College Health Association– National College Health Assessment II (ACHA-NCHA II) Reference Group Executive Summary Spring 2010* (Linthicum, MD: American College Health Association, 2010).
3. H. Selye, "The General-Adaptation-Syndrome" *Annual Review of Medicine* 2 (1951): 327–42.
4. D. G. Myers, *Psychology* 5th ed. (New York: Worth Publishers, 1998): 518.
5. B. McEwen and T. Seeman, "Allostatic Load and Allostasis," John D. and Catherine T. MacArthur Research Network on Socio-economic Status and Health, University of California at San Francisco (revised 2009).

6. Ibid.

7. R. Sapolsky, *Why Zebras Don't Get Ulcers: An Updated Guide to Stress, Stress-Related Diseases, and Coping* (New York: Owl Books, 2004).

8. A. Mokdal and others, "Actual Causes of Death in the United States 2000," *Journal of the American Medical Association* 291, no. 10 (2004): 1238–45.

9. S. Cohen, D. Janicki-Deverts, and G. Miller, "Psychological Stress and Cardiovascular Disease," *Journal of the American Medical Association* 298, no. 14 (2007): 1685–7.

10. F. Sparrenberger and others, "Does Psychological Stress Cause Hypertension? A Systematic Review of Observational Studies," *Journal of Human Hypertension* 23, no 1 (2009): 12–9; J. Dimsdale, "Psychological Stress and Cardiovascular Disease," *Journal of the American College of Cardiology* 51, no. 13 (2008): 1237–46.

11. S. A. Everson-Rose and T. T. Lewis, "Psychosocial Factors and Cardiovascular Diseases," *Annual Review of Public Health* 26 (2005): 469–500.

12. S. C. Segerstrom and G. E. Miller, "Psychological Stress and the Human Immune System," *Psychological Bulletin* 130, no. 4 (2004): 601–30. R. M. Lucas and others, "Mid-life Stress Is Associated with Both Up- and Down-Regulation of Markers of Humoral and Cellular Immunity," *Stress* 10, no. 4 (2007): 351–61.

13. S. C. Segerstrom and G. E. Miller, "Psychological Stress and the Human Immune System," 2004.

14. V. Vicennati and others, "Stress-Related Development of Obesity and Cortisol in Women," *Obesity* 17, no 9 (2009): 1678–83.

15. D. K. Hall-Flavin, "Stress and Hair Loss: Are They Related?" MayoClinic.com, www.mayoclinic.com/health/stress-and-hair-loss/AN01442 (2008).

16. M. Scollan-Koliopoulos, "Managing Stress Response to Control Hypertension in Type 2 Diabetes," *The Nurse Practitioner* 30, no. 2 (2005): 46–9.

17. Johns Hopkins Health Alerts, "Four Relaxation Techniques to Soothe Your Digestive Discomfort," www.johnshopkinshealthalerts.com/reports/digestive_health/2683-1.html (2008).

18. V. Bitsika, C. Sharpley, and R. Bell, "The Contribution of Anxiety and Depression to Fatigue among a Sample of Australian University Students: Suggestions for University Counselors," *Counseling Psychology Quarterly* 22, no. 2 (2009): 243–53.

19. L. Schwabe, T. Wolf, and M. Oitzl, "Memory Formation under Stress: Quantity and Quality," *Neuroscience and Biobehavioral Reviews* 34, no. 4 (2009): 584–91.

20. E. Dias-Ferreira and others, "Chronic Stress Causes Frontostriatal Reorganization and Affects Decision-Making," *Science* 325, no. 5940 (2009): 621–5.

21. D. A. Katerndahl and M. Parchman, "The Ability of the Stress Process Model to Explain Mental Health Outcomes," *Comprehensive Psychiatry* 43, no. 5 (2002): 351–60.

22. J. Burris and others, "Factors Associated with the Psychological Well-Being and Distress of University Students," *Journal of American College Health* 57, no. 5 (2009): 536–43.

23. P. Jackson and M. Finney, "Negative Life Events and Psychological Distress among Young Adults," *Social Psychology Quarterly* 65, no. 2 (2002): 186–201.

24. J. H. Pryor and others, *The American Freshman: National Norms Fall 2010* (Los Angeles: Higher Education Research Institute at UCLA, 2011): 1–4.

25. Ibid.

26. T. Holmes and R. Rahe, "The Social Readjustment Rating Scale," *Journal of Psychosomatic Research* 11 (1967): 213–8.

27. D. J. Maybery and D. Graham, "Hassles and Uplifts: Including Interpersonal Events," *Stress and Health* 17, no 2 (2001): 91–104; R. Blonna, *Coping with Stress in a Changing World,* 4th ed. (New York: McGraw-Hill, 2006).

28. A. D. Von and others, "Predictors of Health Behaviors in College Students," *Journal of Advanced Nursing* 48, no. 5 (2004): 463–74.

29. M. Friedman and R. H. Rosenman, *Type A Behavior and Your Heart* (New York: Knopf, 1974).

30. S. Kobasa, "Stressful Life Events, Personality, and Health: An Inquiry into Hardiness," *Journal of Personality and Social Psychology* 37 (1979): 1–11.

31. B. J. Crowley and others, "Psychological Hardiness and Adjustment to Life Events in Adulthood," *Journal of Adult Development* 10 (2003): 237–48.

32. A. Leal-Cerro and others, "Mechanisms Underlying the Neuroendocrine Response to Physical Exercise," *Journal of Endocrinological Investigation* 26, no. 9 (2003): 879–85.

33. U. Rimmele and others, "Trained Men Show Lower Cortisol, Heart Rate, and Psychological Responses to Psychosocial Stress Compared with Untrained Men," *Psychoneuroendocrinology* 32, no. 6 (2007): 627–35.

34. A. Tsatsoulis and S. Fountoulakis, "The Protective Role of Exercise on Stress System Dysregulation and Comorbidities," *Annals of the New York Academy of Sciences* 1083 (2006): 196–213.

35. National Institute of Alcohol Abuse and Alcoholism, "Alcohol and Sleep," *Alcohol Alert* 41, http://pubs.niaaa.nih.gov/publications/aa41.htm (1998).

36. M. Bennett and C. Lengacher, "Humor and Laughter May Influence Health IV: Humor and Immune Function," *Evidence-Based Complementary and Alternative Medicine* 6, no. 2 (2009): 159–64.

37. J. H. Pryor and others, *The American Freshman: National Norms Fall 2010,* 2011.

38. B. L. Seward, *Managing Stress: Principles and Strategies for Health and Well-Being,* 6th ed. (Sudbury, MA: Jones and Bartlett, 2009): 8.

39. L. D. Kubzansky and others, "Shared and Unique Contributions of Anger, Anxiety, and Depression to Coronary Heart Disease: A Prospective Study in the Normative Aging Study," *Annals of Behavioral Medicine* 31, no. 1 (2006): 21–9.

40. P. A. Bovier, E. Chamot, and T. V. Perneger, "Perceived Stress, Internal Resources, and Social Support as Determinants of Mental Health among Young Adults," *Quality of Life Research* 13, no. 1 (2004): 161–70; A. M. McLaughlin and others, *Determinants of Minority Mental Health and Wellness* (New York: Springer, 2009); L. Crockett and others, "Acculturative Stress, Social Support and Coping: Relations to Psychological Adjustment among Mexican American College Students," *Cultural Diversity and Ethnic Minority Psychology* 13, no. 4 (2007): 347–55; J. Ruthig and others, "Perceived Academic Control: Mediating the Effects of Optimism and Social Support on College Students' Psychological Health," *Social Psychology of Education* 12, no. 7 (2009): 233–49.

41. S. Levine, D. M. Lyons, and A. F. Schatzberg, "Psychobiological Consequences of Social Relationships," *Annals of the New York Academy of Sciences* 89, no. 7 (1999): 210–8.

42. A. Lenhart and others, "Social Media and Young Adults," Pew Internet and American Life Project, www.pewinternet.org/Reports/2010/Social-Media-And-Young-Adults.aspx (2010).

43. J. Couzin, "Friendship as a Health Factor," *Science* 323, no. 5913 (2009): 454–7.

44. J. T. Cacioppo and L. C. Hawkley, "Social Isolation and Health, with an Emphasis on Underlying Mechanisms," *Perspectives in Biology and Medicine* 46, no. 3 Suppl (2003): S39–52.

45. G. Miller, "Why Loneliness Is Hazardous to Your Health," *Science* 331, no. 6014 (2011): 138–40.

46. Ibid.

47. A. Conrad and others, "Psychophysiological Effects of Breathing Instructions for Stress Management," *Applied Psychophysiology and Biofeedback* 32, no. 2 (2007): 89–98.

48. S. Jain and others, "A Randomized Controlled Trial of Mindfulness Meditation Versus Relaxation Training: Effects on Distress, Positive States of Mind, Rumination, and Distraction," *Annals of Behavioral Medicine* 33, no. 1 (2007): 11–21; R. J. Davidson and others, "Alterations in Brain and Immune Function Produced by Mindfulness Meditation," *Psychosomatic Medicine* 65, no. 4 (2003): 564–70.

49. Mayo Clinic Staff, "Biofeedback: Using Your Mind to Improve Your Health," www.mayoclinic.com/health/biofeedback/MY01072 (January 2010).

50. Mayo Clinic Staff, "Relaxation Techniques: Try These Steps to Reduce Stress," www.mayoclinic.com/health/relaxation-technique/SR00007 (May 2011); Mayo Clinic Staff, "Exercise and Stress: Get Moving to Combat Stress," www.mayoclinic.com/print/exercise-and-stress/SR00036 (July 2010).

51. D. K. Reibel and others, "Mindfulness-Based Stress Reduction and Health-Related Quality of Life in a Heterogeneous Patient Population," *General Hospital Psychiatry* 23, no. 4 (2001): 183–92, R. Sethness and others, "Cardiac Health: Relationships among Hostility, Spirituality, and Health Risk," *Journal of Nursing Care Quality* 20, no. 1 (2005): 81–9; L. E. Carlson and others, "Mindfulness-Based Stress Reduction in Relation to Quality of Life, Mood, Symptoms of Stress and Levels of Cortisol, Dehyroepiandrosterone Sulfate (DHEAS) and Melatonin in Breast and Prostate Cancer Outpatient," *Psychoneuroendocrinology* 29, no. 4 (2004): 448–74.

LAB 9.1 • HOW STRESSED ARE YOU?

Name: _____ **Date:** _____

Instructor: _____ **Section:** _____

Purpose: To uncover your major stressors and your stress levels during the last year.

Directions: The following Life Experiences Survey lists events that can cause a buildup of chronic stress. If you did not experience a listed event, circle the zero in front of a statement. If you experienced the event but feel that it had a positive impact on your life, also mark a zero. If you experienced an event and feel it had a *negative* impact, use the scale below and circle the number 1, 2, or 3.

Life Experience Survey

3 = Extremely negative impact
2 = Moderately negative impact
1 = Somewhat negative impact
0 = No impact or a positive impact

College

0 1 2 3   Beginning a new school experience at a higher academic level

0 1 2 3   Changing to a new school at same academic level

0 1 2 3   Academic probation

0 1 2 3   Failing an important exam

0 1 2 3   Changing a major

0 1 2 3   Failing a course

0 1 2 3   Dropping a course

0 1 2 3   Joining a fraternity/sorority

0 1 2 3   Ending formal college education

0 1 2 3   Financial problems concerning college

Family

0 1 2 3   Marriage

0 1 2 3   Death of spouse

Death of a close family member

    0 1 2 3   Mother

    0 1 2 3   Father

    0 1 2 3   Brother

    0 1 2 3   Sister

    0 1 2 3   Child

    0 1 2 3   Grandmother

    0 1 2 3   Grandfather

    0 1 2 3   Other _____

0 1 2 3   Male: Wife/girlfriend's pregnancy

0 1 2 3   Female: Pregnancy

Serious illness or injury of close family member:

    0 1 2 3   Father

    0 1 2 3   Mother

    0 1 2 3   Sister

    0 1 2 3   Brother

    0 1 2 3   Grandmother

    0 1 2 3   Grandfather

    0 1 2 3   Spouse

    0 1 2 3   Child

    0 1 2 3   Other _____

0 1 2 3   Trouble with in-laws

0 1 2 3   Major change in closeness of family members (decreased or increased)

0 1 2 3   Gaining a new family member (birth, adoption, marriage of a relative)

0 1 2 3   Separation from spouse due to work, travel, school, etc.

0 1 2 3   Marital separation from mate (due to conflict)

0 1 2 3   Marital reconciliation with mate

0 1 2 3   Major change in number of arguments with spouse (a lot more, a lot fewer)

0 1 2 3   Married person: Change in a spouse's work outside the home (beginning work, loss of job, changing job, retirement, etc.)

0 1 2 3   Male: Wife/girlfriend having abortion

0 1 2 3   Female: Having an abortion

0 1 2 3   Major change in living condition of family (new home, remodeling, damage to home, loss of home)

0 1 2 3   Divorce

0 1 2 3   Son or daughter leaving home

0 1 2 3   Leaving home for first time

Fitness/Wellness Issues

0 1 2 3	Major changes in sleeping habits (much more or much less sleep)
0 1 2 3	Major change in eating habits (much more or much less food intake)
0 1 2 3	Major personal illness or injury
0 1 2 3	Sexual difficulties

Social Issues

0 1 2 3	Detention in jail or comparable institution
0 1 2 3	Minor law violation (traffic ticket, disturbing the peace, etc.)
0 1 2 3	Death of a close friend
0 1 2 3	Change of residence (moving)
0 1 2 3	Major change in church activities (increased or decreased attendance)
0 1 2 3	Major change in usual type or amount of recreation
0 1 2 3	Major change in social activities such as parties, movies, visiting (increased or decreased participation)
0 1 2 3	Serious injury or illness of close friend
0 1 2 3	Breaking up with boyfriend/girlfriend
0 1 2 3	Engagement
0 1 2 3	Reconciliation with boyfriend/girlfriend

Money Matters

0 1 2 3	Foreclosure on mortgage or loan
0 1 2 3	Major change in financial status (a lot better off, a lot worse off)
0 1 2 3	Borrowing more than $10,000 (buying a home, business, etc.)
0 1 2 3	Borrowing less than $10,000 (buying a car or TV, getting a school loan)

Work

0 1 2 3	New job
0 1 2 3	Changed work situation (different working conditions, working hours, etc.)
0 1 2 3	Trouble with employer (in danger of losing job, being suspended, demoted, etc.)
0 1 2 3	Being fired from job
0 1 2 3	Retirement from work

Additional Factors

Other experiences that have had a negative impact on your life in the past year.

_____

_____

_____

_____

RESULTS

Sum of negative scores: _____

Use the table below to find the rating of your score and write it here: _____

Life Experience Survey Scores		
Sum of Negative Score	Interpretation	Action
<6	Below-normal stress	None needed
6–9	Average stress	Consider improving your fitness and wellness
9–13	Above-average stress	Consider improving fitness and applying stress-reduction techniques
14+	Much-above-average stress	Consider improving fitness, reducing stress, and seeking counseling or group support

Source: Adapted from I.G. Sarason and others, "Assessing the Impact of Life Changes: Development of the Life Experiences Survey," *Journal of Consulting and Clinical Psychology* 46, no. 5 (1978): 932–46. Copyright 1978 by the American Psychological Association.

LAB 9.2 • MANAGING YOUR TIME

Name: _____ **Date:** _____

Instructor: _____ **Section:** _____

Purpose: Learn a concrete way to manage your time so you can accomplish the things you want to.

SECTION I: ANALYZING YOUR TIME

Every evening for a week fill out the following table, listing how much time you spent doing each activity that day.

Activity	Monday	Tuesday	Wednesday	Thursday	Friday	Saturday	Sunday	Total Hours
Getting ready								
On the road								
In class								
Working for pay								
Exercising								
Eating								
Studying								
Watching TV or videos								
Using computer (school)								
Using computer (recreational)								
Spending time with friends								
Leisure activities								
Sleeping								
Other (specify)								

At the end of the week, total the hours for each activity. Are there any activities that you would like to do more or less frequently? You can use the rest of this lab to clarify your goals and set up your calendar so that you accomplish the things that you want to accomplish.

SECTION II: CLARIFY YOUR GOALS AND CREATE YOUR TASK LIST

1. On a piece of paper or in a journal, list your goals down the left side. Goals can be anything from "go to nursing school" to "learn to play racquetball." Make the goals specific. Instead of "be more musical," come up with a concrete goal such as "learn to play guitar."

2. On the right side of the paper, break each of your goals down into specific tasks. For example, as part of the nursing school goal, you might add "make a list of possible schools" to the task list.

3. Next, prioritize the tasks by numbering them in order of importance.

SECTION III: ENTER YOUR TASKS ONTO YOUR CALENDAR

In your calendar, write the commitments you have already—classes, job, exercise, rehearsals, and so on. Be sure to look at the schedule you filled out in section one. Now is your chance to think about what activities you want to continue and which you would like to curb.

When you have all of your commitments written in, you'll be able to see where your free time is. Now review your task list from section two above and choose the most important tasks to put in your free time. Make sure these tasks are things that are really important to you to accomplish.

SECTION IV: MAKE IT HAPPEN

Go over your schedule at the start of each day. This gives you a chance to prepare for the day and remember things that you need to take with you. At the end of the day, cross off tasks you were able to accomplish and re-arrange (or delete) tasks that you didn't do.

SECTION IV: REFLECTION AND EVALUATION

1. Describe any times you found yourself procrastinating. What do you think caused that? Were you bored? Were you overwhelmed? What specific thing could you do next time to get back on track quicker? For example, if you were overwhelmed, is there an advisor you could talk to who could help you prioritize?

_____

_____

2. Did you check your planner each morning, writing in tasks, checking them off, doing weekly planning? If not, what got in the way? What could you do differently next time?

_____

_____

3. Did you find other people encroaching on your time? What happened? How could you handle that differently next time?

_____

_____

4. Review your goals and tasks for the next week, adjust the list to reflect things you've accomplished or any other changes, and then block off time on your calendar for the most important things. Remember that time management is an ongoing exercise. Spend at least 20 minutes at the start of your week planning for the upcoming week, then stay focused on the things you want to accomplish!

Name: _____ Date: _____

Instructor: _____ Section: _____

Purpose: To develop a stress-management plan that targets the key sources of stress in your life.

SECTION I: EXAMINE YOUR BEHAVIOR AND ATTITUDES

1. Enter your results from Lab 9.1 here:

Score: _____ Interpretation: _____

Action: _____

2. Do you feel that stress is a problem in your life right now? ☐ Yes ☐ No

If you scored above average in Lab 9.1, indicating relatively high exposure to stressors and fairly high stress levels, and yet you don't see stress as an issue to address, consider your readiness for change.

SECTION II: IDENTIFY MAJOR SOURCES OF STRESS

After reviewing your entries in the Life Experiences Survey in Lab 9.1, describe your main sources of stress, grouping them into the following categories:

College

_____

_____

Family

_____

_____

Fitness/Wellness Issues

_____

_____

Social Issues

_____

_____

_____

_____

Time-Management Issues

_____

_____

SECTION III: SET REALISTIC GOALS

Use this chart to rank your top five stressors from Section II, in order of urgency. Note ways to modify or eliminate each stressor. Note stress-reduction techniques that you can apply when the stressor arises.

	Stressors	Can I Modify or Eliminate the Stressor? Y/N	Can I Reduce Stress Symptoms? Y/N
Most urgent	1.		
⇓	2.		
⇓	3.		
⇓	4.		
Least urgent	5.		

SECTION IV: DEVISE A STRATEGY AND AN ACTION PLAN

Use this section to target the most urgent source of stress in your life first, and then address additional stressors as you feel ready to work on them.

1. Stressor: _____

2. Is it possible that I will need help from others?   ☐ Y   ☐ N

If yes, ask yourself the following:

What professional resources are available where I live, work, or go to school? _____

_____

_____

How can I get my friends or family involved? _____

_____

3. List general strategies for modifying or eliminating environmental stressors that apply to more than one of your most urgent examples: _____

_____

4. What stress-management techniques can I use to relieve my own ongoing or recurrent symptoms of stress? (Consider relaxation breathing, progressive muscle relaxation, visual imagery, meditation, yoga, improved fitness, improved diet, better time-management skills, and enhanced spiritual connectedness.)

_____

_____

5. How can I plan ahead to avoid this stressor in the future?

_____

_____

6. How will I reward myself for sticking to my plan? _____

_____

SECTION V: CREATE A BEHAVIOR CHANGE CONTRACT

Use the information from Part IV to develop a behavior change contract that targets the stressor(s) you selected. A basic behavior change contract is included at the front of this book.

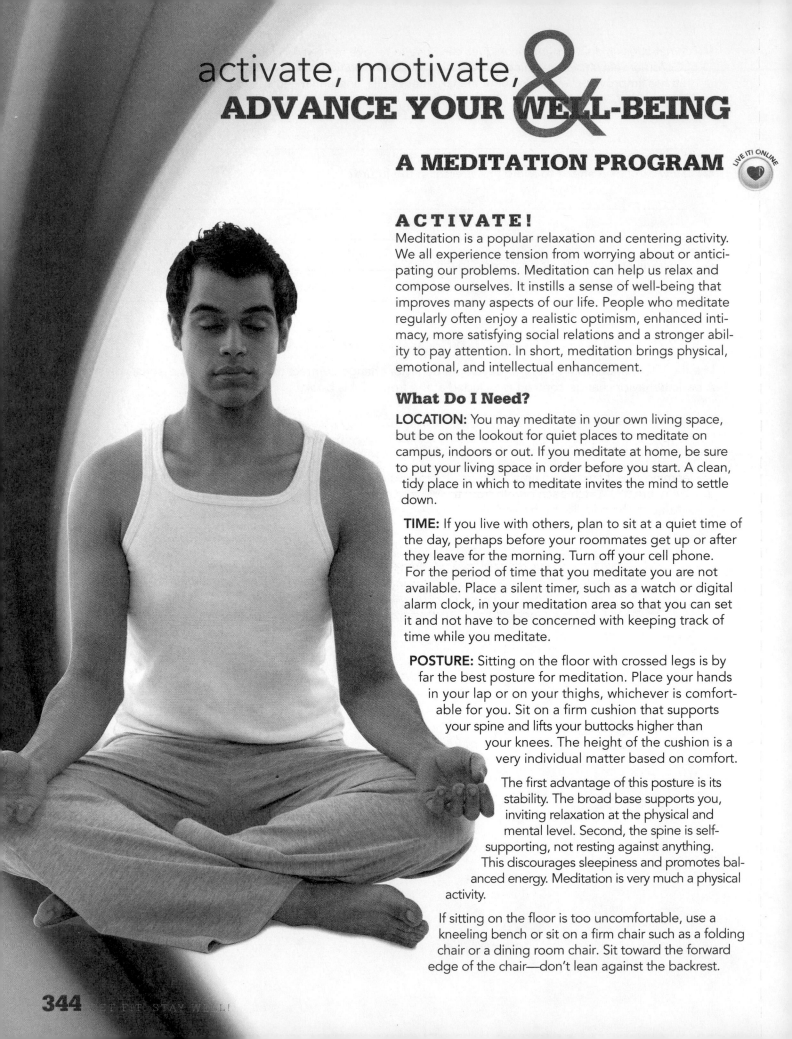

activate, motivate, & ADVANCE YOUR WELL-BEING

A MEDITATION PROGRAM

LIVE IT! ONLINE

ACTIVATE!

Meditation is a popular relaxation and centering activity. We all experience tension from worrying about or anticipating our problems. Meditation can help us relax and compose ourselves. It instills a sense of well-being that improves many aspects of our life. People who meditate regularly often enjoy a realistic optimism, enhanced intimacy, more satisfying social relations and a stronger ability to pay attention. In short, meditation brings physical, emotional, and intellectual enhancement.

What Do I Need?

LOCATION: You may meditate in your own living space, but be on the lookout for quiet places to meditate on campus, indoors or out. If you meditate at home, be sure to put your living space in order before you start. A clean, tidy place in which to meditate invites the mind to settle down.

TIME: If you live with others, plan to sit at a quiet time of the day, perhaps before your roommates get up or after they leave for the morning. Turn off your cell phone. For the period of time that you meditate you are not available. Place a silent timer, such as a watch or digital alarm clock, in your meditation area so that you can set it and not have to be concerned with keeping track of time while you meditate.

POSTURE: Sitting on the floor with crossed legs is by far the best posture for meditation. Place your hands in your lap or on your thighs, whichever is comfortable for you. Sit on a firm cushion that supports your spine and lifts your buttocks higher than your knees. The height of the cushion is a very individual matter based on comfort.

The first advantage of this posture is its stability. The broad base supports you, inviting relaxation at the physical and mental level. Second, the spine is self-supporting, not resting against anything. This discourages sleepiness and promotes balanced energy. Meditation is very much a physical activity.

If sitting on the floor is too uncomfortable, use a kneeling bench or sit on a firm chair such as a folding chair or a dining room chair. Sit toward the forward edge of the chair—don't lean against the backrest.

CLOTHING: Loose-fitting pants allow the abdomen to relax and they give room for the thighs to rotate out. Bare feet are most comfortable for sitting cross-legged. It's a good idea to wear a long-sleeved shirt for warmth.

How Do I Start?

BEGIN BY FOCUSING YOUR ATTENTION ON YOUR BREATH: Close your eyes and draw your attention to the area of your abdomen where you find the sensations of breathing most obvious; Follow the sequence of sensations occurring as you inhale and exhale. As you mindfully observe the rising and falling of the abdomen, make soft mental notes, "rising" and "falling." Noticing the breath is the primary activity of meditation, and it helps to sharpen and strengthen your attention.

Don't exaggerate the breath, let it be natural. Don't use your imagination to create an image of the breath, just attend to the sensations that are actually occurring.

You may find that your mind wanders off. Gently reapply your attention to your breath. Your mind may wander, and you cannot control it with your will power. Relax! Make a mental note, "wandering, wandering," and aim your focus on the breath again. Already you are learning about stress and how to let go. Try to notice every breath. Watch each breath from the beginning, through the middle, to the end. As a beginner you won't be able to be present with every breath, but you must try. To be patient about this wandering, appreciate how passive your attention is generally. Your attention is drawn to stimulating things and is held there by the excitement. Think about the opening moments of a movie. Does it excite your interest? Must you make a special effort to stay with it, or are you swept along?

By contrast, in meditation you focus inward, on your breath. To avoid boredom, sleepiness, and wandering thoughts you attend to your breath. Through noticing the breath and the sensations of the rising and falling of the abdomen—stretching, tightness, swelling; and softness, cascading, and deflation—you will feel stress leave you.

As you become more skilled, your attention will become sustained and steadier for longer periods of time. Gradually your mind will settle down and your body will relax. This composure of mind and body is energizing, bright, and pleasant.

FOCUSING ATTENTION ON THE FELT SENSE OF DISCOMFORT: Physical pain or mental pain can be difficult for the body and mind. In trying to push them away, you may experience tension and stress. Try to turn toward what you have been avoiding. The rewards will be immediate.

When physical pain or mental displeasure arises for you, track and scrutinize the sensation, applying a soft mental label "pain" or "disliking" three or so times. As best you can, track the changing sensations of pressure, hardness, and heat, for example. The fear of pain will start to lose its grip as you see that pain is a collection of intense sensations.

When you are disturbed by thinking about someone you dislike, try saying this mantra: "If I have hurt, harmed, or offended anyone knowingly or unknowingly, may I be forgiven." Repeat that several times and then continue with this: "And anyone who may have hurt, harmed, or offended me knowingly or unknowingly, I freely forgive them."

When the strength of attention on the discomfort weakens, turn back to the breath to make a fresh start, setting aside the negativity. Your composure will grow as you focus on the breath.

ENDING THE SESSION: When it is time to stop meditating, move slowly. Take a little time to stretch and rest, write in your journal, and transition from quiet and stillness into activity. Wait for 20 minutes or so before making phone calls, texting, or getting into conversations.

Four-Week Beginning Meditation Program

After you sit, take a few minutes to record notes. Write down what you observed of the breath. The purpose of this exercise is to enhance your ability to pay attention to the breath as it is, in the same spirit as if you were an artist who kept a sketchbook in which to record things seen during the day.

PROGRAM A **GOAL:** Sit for 15 minutes every other day for four weeks.

	Mon	Tue	Wed	Thurs	Fri	Sat	Sun
Week 1	15 min		15 min		15 min		15 min
Week 2		15 min		15 min		15 min	
Week 3	15 min		15 min		15 min		15 min
Week 4		15 min		15 min		15 min	

MOTIVATE!

Create a journal—or use the log on the companion website—to keep track of your meditation sessions and become aware of the changing quality of your meditation experiences. Here are some other things to bear in mind and potential motivators to consider as you progress in your meditation practice:

ACCEPT THE CHALLENGE: Meditation can bring the benefits of centeredness, relaxation, and brightness of mind. Learning to meditate is a lifelong endeavor. To sit still, watch the breath, focus attention and calm down sounds simple, but it's a challenge! To do it, one must meet and overcome doubt, boredom, desire, irritability, and restlessness in turn.

FACE DISTRACTIONS: When you find yourself stopped by doubt, remember that being able to meet life's challenges with a calm mind is a valuable thing—worth working for. If you keep wanting to get up and eat something or check for text messages, then observe each mental interruption, acknowledge it, and let it go.

ENJOY THE FREEDOM: It is usually a great relief to detach from discomfort and from taking things personally. It is uplifting to be able to relax in the face of annoyances that previously would have provoked resistance and retaliation. When you truly attend to displeasure, annoyances don't dominate or push you around as they used to. Introspection gives rise to insight and inner freedom.

JOIN A GROUP: Beginners can find it motivating to join a meditation class with a teacher. You may be able to find such a meditation class through a yoga center, through your fitness instructor, or in a local alternative newspaper. If you sit with a group you will enjoy the inspiration and support of the group energy and can begin to feel confident about the benefits of daily practice. If you can't find an established group, you may form your own group of people with similar goals. In a quiet setting, you may want to read a book together, selecting an interesting passage to precede the sitting, or listen to a recorded talk from the Internet before you sit.

ATTEND A RETREAT: In addition to a weekly sitting group, you may want to deepen your learning by going on a silent retreat. Retreats may be for a weekend or for as long as three months! Some retreats are specifically for young people.

ADVANCE!

Meditation is a lifelong affair. When you learn how to meditate you learn how to be attentive and reflective all the time. You will want to sit every day. People often find that 45 minutes to an hour daily is enough to see real effects in personality, friendships, and ability to concentrate on work.

PROGRAM B

 LIVE IT! ONLINE

GOAL: Sit for 20 minutes five days a week, working up to sitting daily for a minimum of 20 minutes.

	Mon	Tue	Wed	Thurs	Fri	Sat	Sun
Week 1	20 min	20 min	20 min	20 min	20 min		
Week 2	20 min	20 min	20 min	20 min	20 min		
Week 3	20 min	20 min	20 min	20 min	20 min	20 min	
Week 4	20 min	20 min	20 min	20 min	20 min	20 min	20 min

10 Reducing Your Risk of Cardiovascular Disease

Learning Outcomes

1. Define cardiovascular disease (CVD).

 Audio case study and audio PowerPoint lecture

2. Explain why a college student should be concerned about CVD.

3. List the human and economic impacts of CVD.

 Heart Disease in America

4. Explain how CVD affects the heart and blood vessels, and the symptoms it produces.

5. Describe various forms of CVD, including hypertension, atherosclerosis, stroke, heart disease, and others.

6. Outline the main risk factors for CVD, including those you can and cannot control. Lab 10.1 Understand Your CVD Risk

 Tips to Raise Good Cholesterol

7. Create a plan and apply behavior-change skills to lower your own risk of CVD. Take Charge of Your Health worksheets and Behavior Change Logs for assessing your CVD risk and creating a change plan

Pre- and post-quizzes and glossary flashcards

casestudy

DARYL

"Hi, I'm Daryl. I'm a junior, majoring in education. I'm also a jazz pianist and I play at clubs around town about three times a week. I love jazz, and the gigs help me pay my college tuition.

"I think I'm pretty healthy—I've never been hospitalized for anything in my life—but I do have a family history of heart disease. Both of my grandfathers died from heart attacks when they were in their 40s. My dad died of a stroke when I was 10, and my mom is currently getting treatment for high blood pressure and high cholesterol. I know I'm still young, but given the family history, I'm worried. Are there things I can be doing to protect myself? And how can I help my mom?"

• •

Cardiovascular disease (CVD) is the term commonly used to describe diseases of the heart and the blood vessels brought on by a build-up of fatty, waxy accumulations that restrict or block blood flow. CVD can bring on potentially devastating consequences such as a heart attack and stroke, which are the number one and number three leading causes of death in America (cancer being number two).[1] You may think that cardiovascular problems strike only older people but in fact, 9 to 15 percent of women and men under age 40 have some form of CVD.[2] The prevalence rises to about 40 percent in middle-aged adults of both sexes and then climbs sharply after age 60, involving about three-quarters or more of older Americans.[3] Among Americans of all age groups, approximately one out of every three has some form of cardiovascular disease.[4]

cardiovascular disease (CVD)
A disease of the heart and/or blood vessels

Why Should I Worry about Cardiovascular Disease?

As a college student, your most pressing concerns are probably things like getting good grades, paying tuition, and landing a job. Cardiovascular disease could be the furthest thing from your mind. However, it is not too early to start learning about CVD. For many people, the earliest manifestations of heart and blood vessel diseases take root during childhood and early adulthood.[5] While genetic predisposition plays an important role, lifestyle choices that you make now—such as whether or not to smoke, how often to exercise, your stress level, and what you eat—can also greatly influence your risk for developing cardiovascular disease later.

LIVE IT! ONLINE
Worksheet 39
Healthy Heart
I.Q.

Cardiovascular Disease Is America's Biggest Killer

Cardiovascular disease and stroke kill about 30 percent of all those who die in the United States each year—more than any other single cause of death in America.[6] In fact, cardiovascular disease has been the leading cause of death in the U.S. every year since 1900, except in 1918, when pandemic flu killed more Americans. If we completely eliminated CVD in the United States, experts estimate our average life expectancy would rise by almost 7 years.[7] Together, heart disease and strokes kill more Americans each year—both men and women and people of various races—than cancer or any other cause (Table 10.1; also, see the box Men, Women, and Cardiovascular Disease).

SEE IT! ONLINE
Heart Disease
in America

Figure 10.1 shows the prevalence of CVD throughout the country. Cardiovascular disease costs Americans an estimated $475.3 billion each year, a figure that includes the costs of actual care (physicians, hospitals, nursing homes, and medications) as well as lost productivity.[8] By 2030, the prevalence of cardiovascular disease is expected to increase 9.9 percent, with the prevalence of heart failure and stroke increasing approximately 25 percent, and annual direct costs are expected to increase to $818 billion, with another $276 billion in lost productivity.[9]

Cardiovascular disease is a global problem, and CVD is the number one cause of death globally.

HEAR IT! ONLINE

TABLE 10.1 Five Leading Causes of Death in the U.S.	
Cause	Number of deaths
Heart disease and Stroke	727,210
Cancer	568,668
Chronic lower respiratory diseases	137,082
Accidents (unintentional injuries)	117,176
Alzheimer's disease	78,889

Source: K. D. Kochanek, "Deaths: Preliminary Data for 2009," *National Vital Statistics Reports* 59, no. 4 (Hyattsville, MD: National Center for Health Statistics, 2011).

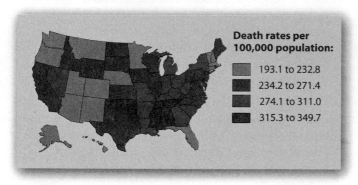

Death rates per 100,000 population:

- 193.1 to 232.8
- 234.2 to 271.4
- 274.1 to 311.0
- 315.3 to 349.7

FIGURE **10.1** Cardiovascular disease age-adjusted death rates by state.

Reprinted with permission from CIRCULATION 2011; 123:e18-e209. © 2010, American Heart Association, Inc.

Of an estimated 17.3 million global deaths from CVD in 2008, about 7.3 million were due to coronary heart disease and 6.2 million were due to stroke.[10] The World Health Organization predicts that by 2030, CVD will still be the single leading cause of death and will claim almost 23.6 million lives each year, mainly from heart disease and stroke.[11]

Among developed nations, eastern European countries such as Russia, Bulgaria, and Romania have the highest incidence of deaths attributed to CVD, with over 500 deaths per 100,000 population per year.[12] France, Japan, Switzerland, Spain, and Italy are at the bottom of the list, with about 200 deaths or fewer per 100,000 population. The United States is in the middle—along with countries such as England, Denmark, New Zealand, and Germany—with 300 to 400 deaths per 100,000 population per year, depending on demographic groups within the populations.[13]

Cardiovascular Disease Can Greatly Decrease Your Quality of Life

The potential of cardiovascular disease to cause death is obviously its most serious consequence, but even when it is not fatal, it can seriously impact daily life. Heart attack and stroke survivors may lose their ability to walk, talk, read, exercise, or carry out other daily activities normally. Cardiovascular disease can cause chest pain, shortness of breath, and damage to internal organs. It can also require expensive drugs, which have their own negative side effects.

Cardiovascular Disease Can Begin Early in Life

Childhood and early adolescence are often the time when people first start experiencing the risk factors for cardiovascular disease—poor diet, lack of exercise, BMI above 25, and smoking. These, in turn, can trigger physical processes that initiate the start of cardiovascular disease itself surprisingly early in life. In a classic study of blood vessel tissue from 3,000 young people between the ages of 15 and 34 who had died of accidents, homicides, or suicides, researchers found glistening streaks of fat and fatty, waxy buildup in some of the vessel specimens— deposits that marked the unmistakable beginnings of cardiovascular disease. The researchers found early signs of CVD in 2 percent of males aged 15 to 19. They also observed advanced markers of CVD in 20 percent of 30- to 34-year-old males, and 8 percent of females in the same age group. In examining the individual health records of those young people with blood vessel deposits, the researchers found a higher incidence of poor diet, lack of exercise, high BMI, and smoking than in healthier young people lacking those deposits.[15] These same habits continue to contribute to cardiovascular disease in middle-aged and older adults. More recent studies reflect the result of those early risk factors and blood vessel deposits: A 2011 CDC study revealed that stroke-related hospitalizations rose dramatically in 15- to 44-year-olds between the years 1994 and 2007.[16] Among 15- to 34-year-old men, they found a 51 percent jump in stroke hospitalizations, and among boys and girls aged 5 to 14, a 30 percent rise. The actual numbers of young people who suffer strokes are small but the trend is clear; CVD prevention must begin in childhood.

Men, Women, and Cardiovascular Disease

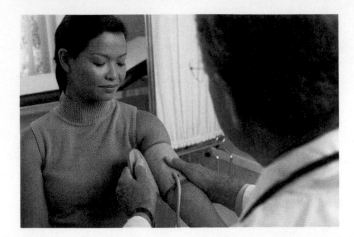

Many people are aware that cardiovascular disease is the leading cause of death in men in the United States, claiming 388,049 male victims in 2007.[1] Few realize, however, that cardiovascular disease is the leading cause of death in American women as well—and in fact kills more women than men each year; in 2007, CVD claimed 418,107 female victims. This figure is higher than the number of female lives lost in 2007 due to cancer, Alzheimer's, diabetes, and accidents *combined*.

Even physicians can harbor misconceptions about women and cardiovascular disease. In one study, fewer than one doctor in five knew that CVD kills more women than men annually.[2] Another study has shown that doctors are more likely to screen male patients for heart disease and make recommendations for intervention than they are to screen or treat female patients for the same.[3]

Researchers have also found significant differences in the ways men and women tend to express patterns and symptoms of cardiovascular disease. For example:

- Men tend to develop heart disease 10 to 15 years earlier than women. Women rarely have heart attacks before menopause (early 50s); they show rates of CVD two or three times higher after menopause than before.

- While having a heart attack, men tend to experience the classic "squeezing" sensation in the chest, pain in the chest or arm, and/or shortness of breath. Women, however, are less likely to feel these symptoms. Instead, they are more likely to experience shortness of breath, weakness or fatigue, a cold sweat, or dizziness. If they feel any localized pressure, it tends to be between the shoulder blades rather than in the chest or arm. Women are also more likely than men to have early warning symptoms up to one month before, including unusual fatigue, sleep disturbances, shortness of breath, indigestion, and anxiety.[4]

- Looking at cardiovascular disease as a whole, men are more likely to have heart attacks, while women with CVD are more likely to have strokes. This is perhaps based on the smaller size of blood vessels throughout the body, including the brain.[5]

- Doctors have long prescribed daily aspirin to both sexes as a way to prevent heart attacks. Recent studies, however, have shown that aspirin seems to prevent some heart attack deaths in men and some stroke deaths in women but does not seem to prevent stroke deaths in men or heart attack deaths in women.[6]

Sources:
1. J. Xu and others, "Deaths: Final Data for 2007," *National Vital Statistics Reports* 58, no. 19 (Hyattsville, MD: National Center for Health Statistics, 2010).
2. L. Mosca and others, "National Study of Physician Awareness and Adherence to Cardiovascular Disease Prevention Guidelines," *Circulation* 111, no. 4 (2005): 499–510.
3. J. H. Mieres, "Review of the American Heart Association's Guidelines for Cardiovascular Disease Prevention in Women," *Heart* 92, Suppl 3 (2006): iii10–3.
4. J. C. McSweeney and others, "Women's Early Warning Symptoms of Acute Myocardial Infarction," *Circulation* 108 (2003): 2619–23.
5. T. Kurth and others, "Healthy Lifestyle and the Risk of Stroke in Women," *Archives of Internal Medicine* 166, no. 13 (2006): 1403–9.
6. J. S. Berger and others, "Aspirin for the Primary Prevention of Cardiovascular Events in Women and Men: A Sex-Specific Meta-analysis of Randomized Controlled Trials," *Journal of the American Medical Association* 295, no. 3 (2006): 306–13.

How Does Cardiovascular Disease Affect the Body?

Learning about how cardiovascular disease affects your body is useful for understanding why it causes the symptoms it does and what you can do to keep your cardiovascular system healthy.

Cardiovascular Disease Affects the Heart and Blood Vessels

Your body contains trillions of living cells, all needing a continuous supply of oxygen and energy compounds. The cardiovascular system—the heart and blood vessels—does the critical work of delivering that oxygen and energy *to* your cells. It also removes carbon dioxide and other wastes *from* your cells. (To review the anatomy of the cardiovascular, or circulatory, system, see Chapter 3.)

In a healthy 10-year-old, the heart is almost adult size. The blood vessel walls are smooth inside and out. The walls of the arteries are strong and elastic, while the walls of the veins are thinner and more fixed in diameter. Blood can flow freely down the long narrow opening in the middle of each vessel. The ventricles fill smoothly and forcibly push blood out. Tight-closing valves help prevent blood from flowing backward. The circulating blood reaches all the distant capillary beds in the brain, limbs, kidneys, skin, and other organs, then returns quickly through the venous system.

Atherosclerosis Starting at age 10 or even earlier, abnormal accumulations inside the blood vessels can begin to restrict blood flow. The process of accumulation and restriction in blood vessels is known as **atherosclerosis** (from the Greek words "athero," meaning gruel, and "sclerosis," meaning hardness.) Atherosclerosis is a major factor in many forms of cardiovascular disease. Both lifestyle and genetic factors can cause deposits of fatty, waxy, yellowish, sludgelike debris called *atheromas* to accumulate inside arteries and smaller arterioles. Other substances such as calcium salts, cholesterol, cellular waste, blood clotting proteins, and white blood cells can accumulate around the atheromas, enlarging and solidifying the yellowish deposits into hardened blockages called **plaques**. These plaques, in turn, tend to bulge inward and cause a narrowing of the vessels' inner channels. This narrowing is called **arterial stenosis**. Plaques can eventually grow large enough to block blood passage through the vessel (see Figure 10.2) or even cause the vessel to rupture. The buildup process can take decades, but atherosclerosis can start in childhood, especially in the overweight and obese.[17]

Arteries with plaques that cause a narrowed channel or inward-bulging side walls transport less blood and are stiffer and less flexible. Just as the pressure builds up in a hose if you prevent normal water flow with your thumb, channel narrowing and plaque buildup can increase pressure within the blood vessels. Unhealthy lifestyle characteristics including smoking, chronic stress, inactivity, high alcohol consumption, high blood sugar, high blood pressure, obesity, and unfavorable levels of certain fats and cholesterol in the blood can all increase the speed and severity of atherosclerosis and, in turn, contribute to CVD.[18] Atherosclerotic cardiovascular disease is America's leading cause of death and disability.[19]

In recent years, medical researchers have studied the role of *inflammation* in atherosclerosis. Inflammation is an immune response that causes redness and swelling in response to injury. Researchers think that LDL (low-density lipoprotein) cholesterol, cigarette smoking, hypertension, diabetes mellitus, and disease-causing bacteria may all promote inflammation. The most likely disease-causing bacteria are *Chlamydia pneumoniae* (a common cause of respiratory infections), *Helicobacter pylori* (which causes ulcers), herpes simplex virus (to which the majority of Americans are exposed by the age of 5), and cytomegalovirus (another herpes virus transmitted through body fluids and infecting most Americans before the age of 40).

During an inflammatory reaction, researchers can often detect high levels of two or more substances. One is a set of proteins called *C-reactive proteins* (CRPs), the other is an amino acid called *homocysteine*. These substances may inflame the inner linings of arteries and promote plaque deposits and blood-clot formation. At the very least, their presence is an indicator of inflammation. In the near future, physicians may be able to order sensitive tests that detect CRPs and homocysteine as markers of atherosclerosis.[20] Lifestyle changes such as regular exercise, weight management, smoking

atherosclerosis Hardening or stiffening of the arteries as plaque accumulates, often at injury sites, in the inner linings of arteries

plaques A pinpoint area of fatty, waxy debris that accumulates at a site along the inner wall of an artery or arteriole

arterial stenosis A narrowing of the inner channel of arteries and smaller arterioles due to the buildup of a sludge-like layer of fatty, waxy debris

Normal blood flow

Restricted blood flow

Atherosclerotic plaque

(a) Healthy artery   **(b)** Narrowed artery

FIGURE **10.2**   (a) Cross-section of a healthy artery, allowing normal blood flow. (b) Cross-section of an artery with plaque buildup narrowing the channel and restricting blood flow.

cessation, moderation of alcohol intake, and eating less saturated fat and cholesterol appear to reduce inflammation and its markers in the blood.

Cardiovascular Disease Takes Many Forms

Table 10.2 identifies the most common forms of cardiovascular disease and their prevalence in American adults. Let's look at each of these forms of CVD in more detail.

Hypertension Hypertension, or sustained high blood pressure, is the most common form of cardiovascular disease. It is also considered a risk factor for other forms of CVD. About 30 percent of all Americans have hypertension.[21] Because it has no initial symptoms,[22] many are unaware they have the condition, causing experts to refer to it as a "silent killer." Hypertension causes blood vessel damage and promotes plaque development.[23] As mentioned earlier, plaque deposits and vessel-channel narrowing can in turn increase resistance to blood flow throughout the circulatory system and can cause blood pressure to rise further, creating a damaging vicious cycle. In addition to leading to other forms of CVD, hypertension can cause your thinking to slow down or make you more susceptible to dementia later in life.[24] You may think of high blood pressure as an older person's disease, but it can begin in your college years and is common by middle age.[25] The condition can result from consuming too much sodium in the diet, leading to water retention and increased blood volume. Other causes of hypertension include kidney or heart abnormalities, aging, inherited tendencies, obesity, sleep apnea, stress, or certain kinds of tumors. Could hypertension impact you? See the box College Students and Hypertension to find out more.

A blood pressure device can help diagnose hypertension. Such devices measure your blood pressure in two parts, expressed as a fraction—for example, 120/80. Both values are measured in millimeters of mercury (mm Hg). The first number refers to **systolic pressure**, or the pressure being applied to the walls of the arteries when the heart contracts, pumping blood to the rest of the body. The second value is **diastolic pressure**, or the pressure applied to the walls of the arteries during the heart's relaxation phase. During this phase, blood is reentering the heart's chambers, preparing for the next heartbeat.

Normal blood pressure varies, depending on an individual's weight, age, physical condition, gender, and ethnic background. Systolic blood pressure tends to increase with age, while diastolic blood pressure tends to increase until age 55, and then decline. Generally, men have a greater risk for high

hypertension Sustained blood pressure over 130/85 mm Hg

systolic pressure The pressure applied to the walls of the arteries when the heart contracts

diastolic pressure The pressure applied to the walls of the arteries during the heart's relaxation phase

TABLE 10.2 Major Types of Cardiovascular Disease and Prevalence of Each	
Type of Cardiovascular Disease	Prevalence in the United States
Hypertension	76.4 million
Coronary heart disease (including heart attack)	16.3 million
Angina pectoris	9.0 million
Arrhythmia	2.2 million
Congestive heart failure	5.7 million
Congenital cardiovascular defects	Eight defects per 1,000 live births
Stroke	7.0 million; 795,000 new or recurrent cases of stroke each year

Data from American Heart Association *Heart Disease and Stroke Statistics 2011 Update* (2011).

DIVERSITY

College Students and Hypertension

Our discussion of increased hospitalizations for stroke among young people is part of a bigger trend: increased hypertension in people from 20 to 44. A revealing study of 800 students at the University of New Hampshire, for example, showed that one-third were overweight or obese and that fully 60 percent of male students had high blood pressure.[1] Other reports have shown that more than four million young adults (about 4 percent) are now taking anti-cholesterol medications, while 8.5 million (8 percent) are now taking medications to combat high blood pressure (hypertension).[2]

As with the general U.S. adult population, college students of both sexes are at risk of hypertension based on the prevalence of obesity, poor diet, and sedentary lifestyles in our culture. But young men, particularly young African American men, seem to be at highest risk.[3] This may be partly because men under age 35 are more likely to ignore early symptoms and delay return visits to doctors after a preliminary discussion about their high blood pressure. Depression and high alcohol consumption can also increase the risk for hypertension, and both are common among college students of both sexes.[4]

Hypertension can have devastating long-term effects on nearly every organ of the body. Among the many health problems that they may encounter, men with prehypertension and hypertension are nearly three times as likely to experience erectile dysfunction as men without these cardiac problems. Reducing sodium consumption, losing weight, and exercising, among other measures, can make a huge difference in risk reduction and help you avoid the need for medical intervention.

Sources:
1. University of New Hampshire, "College Students Face Obesity, High Blood Pressure, Metabolic Syndrome," *ScienceDaily*, www.sciencedaily.com /releases/2007/06/070614113310.htm (June 18, 2007).
2. J. T. Flynn, "Pediatric Hypertension Update," *Current Opinion in Nephrology and Hypertension* 19, no. 3 (2010): 292–7; *Washington Times*, "Heart Patients Getting Younger," www.washingtontimes.com/news/2007/oct /30/heart-patients-getting-younger (October 30, 2007).
3. B. Rosner, "Blood Pressure Differences by Ethnic Group among United States Children and Adolescents," *Hypertension* 54, no. 3 (2009): 502–8; D. T. Lackland, "High Blood Pressure: A Lifetime Issue," *Hypertension* 54, no. 3 (2009): 457–8.
4. S. B. Patten and others, "Major Depression as a Risk Factor for High Blood Pressure: Epidemiologic Evidence from a National Longitudinal Study," *Psychosomatic Medicine* 71, no. 3 (2009): 273–9.

blood pressure than women until age 55; at that point, the risks become about equal. After age 75, women are more likely to have high blood pressure than men.[26]

For a healthy adult, normal systolic blood pressure is less than 120, and normal diastolic blood pressure is less than 80.[27] A physician may diagnose *prehypertension* or the potential beginnings of hypertension when systolic pressure is between 120 and 139 and diastolic pressure is between 80 and 89. *High blood pressure* (HBP) is usually diagnosed when systolic pressure is 140 or above and diastolic pressure is 90 or above (although the latter reading may not necessarily be elevated). When only systolic pressure is high, the condition is known as *isolated systolic hypertension* (ISH), the most common form of high blood pressure in older Americans. If your blood pressure exceeds 140/90, you need to work with your physician to lower it through diet, exercise, stress reduction, and prescription drugs. Table 10.3 presents a summary of blood pressure values.

If you are diagnosed with high blood pressure in college, you can do something about it. Lifestyle modifications are helpful in reducing or preventing hypertension in early adulthood. These include losing weight, exercising, reducing stress, and reducing dietary salt and sugar (see the box Do Salt and Sugar Increase My Risk of Cardiovascular Disease?).[28]

TABLE 10.3 Blood Pressure Readings

Classification	Systolic Reading (mm Hg)	Diastolic Reading (mm Hg)
Normal	Less than 120	Less than 80
Prehypertension	120–139	80–89
Hypertension		
Stage 1	140–159	90–99
Stage 2	160 or higher	100 or higher

Note: If systolic and diastolic readings fall into different categories, treatment is determined by the highest category. Readings are based on the average of two or more properly measured, seated readings on each of two or more health care provider visits.

Source: National Heart, Lung, and Blood Institute, *Seventh Report of the Joint National Committee on Prevention, Detection, Evaluation, and Treatment of High Blood Pressure* (NIH Publication No. 03-5233) (Bethesda, MD: National Institutes of Health, May 2003).

Coronary Heart Disease When atherosclerosis occurs in the heart's main blood vessels, it is called **coronary artery disease (CAD)** or **coronary heart disease (CHD)**. When it occurs in the feet, ankles, calves, hands, or forearms, it is called *peripheral artery disease*. Of all the types of cardiovascular disease, CHD is the greatest killer. Each year, an estimated 1.25 million Americans will suffer a *coronary attack* or heart attack: 785,000 will have their first heart attack and 470,000 will have a recurrent attack.[29] The American Heart Association calculates that approximately every *minute*, somewhere in the U.S., someone dies of a first or subsequent heart.

A heart attack, also called a **myocardial infarction (MI)**, occurs when an area of the heart suffers permanent damage after its normal blood supply has been blocked. The blockage can be caused by a blood clot in a coronary artery or by atherosclerotic narrowing. When blood flow slows dramatically or stops, the surrounding tissue is deprived of oxygen. If the blockage is extremely minor, an otherwise healthy heart will adapt over time as small blood vessels reroute needed blood through other areas.

When heart blockage is more severe, a person can experience the symptoms of a heart attack and will require life-saving support. The box In the Event of a Heart Attack, Stroke, or Cardiac Arrest (on page 357) describes how you should respond if you recognize such symptoms in someone else or yourself.

Angina Pectoris Atherosclerosis and other circulatory impairments may reduce the heart's blood and oxygen supply and cause a condition called **ischemia**. People with ischemia often suffer from varying degrees of chest pain, also called **angina pectoris**. The American Heart Association estimates that more than nine million Americans suffer from angina.[30] Many people experience short episodes of angina whenever they exert themselves physically. Symptoms may range from slight indigestion to a feeling that the heart is being crushed. Generally, the more serious the oxygen deprivation, the more severe the pain.

Doctors currently use several methods of treating angina. In mild cases, they prescribe rest. To treat more serious chest pain, they may recommend nitroglycerin tablets to relax veins and lessen the heart's workload. Calcium channel blockers can also relieve angina caused by spasms of the coronary arteries. Drugs called *beta blockers* can control potential overactivity of the heart muscle.[31]

Arrhythmias An **arrhythmia**, or irregular heartbeat, is relatively common: More than 2.2 million Americans experience it each year.[32] The disturbance of heartbeat rhythm can take several forms: a racing heart in the absence of exercise or anxiety (called *tachycardia*); an abnormally slow heartbeat (called *bradycardia*); or a sporadic, quivering pattern called *fibrillation*. **Fibrillation** renders the heart extremely inefficient at pumping blood

coronary artery disease (CAD) or **coronary heart disease (CHD)** Atherosclerosis (the buildup of plaque deposits) in the main arteries that supply oxygen and other materials to the heart muscle.

myocardial infarction (MI) Medical term for a heart attack; involves permanent damage to an area of the heart muscle brought on by a cessation of normal blood supply

ischemia A damaging reduction in the blood (and therefore the oxygen supply) to a region of the heart, brain, or other organ

angina pectoris Chest pain due to ischemia, or reduction in blood flow to the heart muscle and surrounding tissues

arrhythmia Irregular heartbeat; can involve abnormally fast or slow heartbeat or the disorganized, sporadic beat of fibrillation

fibrillation A sporadic, quivering heartbeat pattern that results in inefficient pumping of blood

Do Salt and Sugar Increase My Risk of Cardiovascular Disease?

The average American adult consumes 3,466 mg of sodium per day in salt (NaCl)[1]—more than twice the USDA-recommended level of 1500 mg for those over 50, African Americans, and those who have high blood pressure. The 2010 Federal Dietary Guidelines recommend that all other adults consume below 2300 mg per day (the American Heart Association recommends a more conservative limit of 1500 mg per day for adults and children of all ages). These health organizations advocate limiting salt because excess sodium induces fluid retention. This, in turn, elevates blood pressure and contributes to hypertension and CVD. To get below 2300 mg, most adults would have to cut overall salt consumption by about half a teaspoon.

Most of the salt in our national diet comes from foods high in processed grains (such as pizza and cookies) and from meats, poultry, and lunch meats.[2] Researchers estimate that a population-wide average drop in dietary salt by 1200 mg/day would annually cut new cases of cardiovascular disease by 60,000 to 120,000 and prevent 32,000 to 66,000 new strokes, 54,000 to 99,000 new heart attacks, and 44,000 to 92,000 deaths. They also projected this trend would save $10 to $24 billion in annual health care costs.[3] Some medical researchers have criticized a few of the team's assumptions and thus disagree with their specific figures.[4] However, few, if any, disagree with the major premise that dietary salt causes hypertension and cutting consumption would help improve and prevent CVD.

What about sugar? The average American consumes more than 150 pounds of caloric sweeteners (sugar, corn syrup, brown sugar, honey, agave syrup, concentrated fruit juice, and so on) each year. That's almost three pounds per week![5] Most of this extra sugar comes from sweetened sodas, sports drinks, energy drinks, coffee drinks, and tea drinks. Like salt, sugar takes a toll on our cardiovascular health by increasing weight gain and by raising both glucose and triglyceride levels in the blood. Consuming an extra 2.6 ounces per day of corn syrup (the amount in two or three sweetened drinks) doubles a person's risk for high systolic blood pressure.[6] In one large study, women who consumed two sweetened drinks per day had a 20 percent greater risk of heart disease over those who drank sugary drinks only about once per month.[7] In another large study, drinking one sugary drink per day increased the risk of metabolic syndrome by 44 percent.[8] Dietary sugar, in other words, increases the risks of CVD, just as salt does.

Sources:

1. Centers for Disease Control and Prevention, "CDC Survey Find Nine in Ten U.S. Adults Consume Too Much Sodium," Press Release www.cdc.gov/media/pressrel/2010/r100624.htm (2010).
2. Ibid.
3. K. Bibbins-Domingo and others, "Projected Effect of Dietary Salt Reductions on Future Cardiovascular Disease," The New England Journal of Medicine 362, no. 7 (2010): 590–9.
4. P. Belluck, "Big Benefits Are Seen from Eating Less Salt," New York Times, www.nytimes.com/2010/01/21/health/nutrition/21salt.html (January 20, 2010).
5. USDA, "Chapter 2: Profiling Food Consumption in America," Agricultural Fact Book 2001–2002, www.usda.gov/factbook/chapter2.htm (2002).
6. D. I. Jalal and others, "Increased Fructose Associates with Elevated Blood Pressure," Journal of the American Society of Nephrology 21, no. 9 (2010): 1543–9.
7. T. T. Fung and others, "Sweetened Beverage Consumption and Risk of Coronary Heart Disease in Women," American Journal of Clinical Nutrition 89, no. 4 (2009): 1037–42.
8. R. Dhingra and others, "Soft Drink Consumption and Risk of Developing Cardiometabolic Risk Factors and the Metabolic Syndrome in Middle-Aged Adults in the Community," Circulation 116, no. 5 (2007): 480–8.

through the vessels. If a fibrillation incident or series of incidents go untreated, the condition may be fatal. Even without cardiovascular disease, you may feel heart arrhythmias from drinking too much caffeine or from the nicotine in tobacco. Mild cases like this are seldom life-threatening. If you develop a severe case due to disease, you may require drug therapy or a pacemaker.

Congestive Heart Failure More than five million Americans suffer from **congestive heart failure (CHF)** each year.[33] Causes include past heart attack, high blood pressure, heart valve defects or damage, birth defects, or damage to the heart from infection or inherited disease. In CHF, the heart muscle is damaged or overworked, the pumping chambers are often taxed to the limit, and the heart lacks the strength to keep blood circulating normally through the body. Heart muscle damage can result from viral or bacterial pneumonia, heart attack, other cardiovascular problems, or even treatments for cancer. The weakened heart pumps less blood out through the arteries. As a result, the "return" blood can't flow back through the veins to the heart in normal amounts. As the blood begins to back up, it causes congestion in body tissues. Blood pooling enlarges the heart, making it even less efficient, and fluid accumulates in the legs, ankles, or lungs, where it can cause swelling or difficulty in breathing.

Congestive heart failure can be fatal if untreated, but most cases respond well to drug treatment. Diuretics (water pills) increase urination and reduce fluid accumulation, drugs such as digitalis increase the heart's pumping action, and vasodilators expand blood vessels so blood can flow through more easily and reduce the heart's workload.

Congenital Heart Disease Congenital heart disease, meaning heart disease present at birth, affects nine out of every 1,000 live births.[34] A baby may be born with a slight *heart murmur,* an audible sound based on an irregular heart valve that allows turbulent blood flow through the heart. Some children outgrow such heart murmurs and have no further problems. Others, however, can have more serious

congenital irregularities with heart anatomy or function that require surgical repair. Causes may include hereditary factors, a mother's case of rubella or certain other infections during pregnancy, or the mother's use of alcohol or drugs during fetal development. Advances in treatment continually improve the prospects for children with congenital heart defects.

Stroke The American Heart Association's most recent statistics show that approximately seven million Americans alive today have suffered a stroke at some point in their lives. Each year more than 795,000 people experience a new or recurrent stroke, and 136,000 of them die, making stroke the third leading cause of death after heart disease and cancer.[35] In recent years, the incidence of stroke has been rising in adults aged 15 to 44.

We saw that a heart attack can occur when a blocked vessel prevents a region of the heart from getting enough oxygenated blood. In a similar way, a **stroke** is a sudden loss of function in a region of the brain caused by blockage in or rupture of a blood vessel, leading to oxygen deprivation and cell damage or death. *Ischemic* strokes are the result of a plaque-blocked vessel or a floating blood clot that lodges in a vessel and cuts off blood supply to a brain region. *Hemorrhagic* strokes occur when a blood vessel bursts, spilling oxygenated blood rather than transporting it to a distal brain region, allowing that unsupplied area to become damaged through oxygen deprivation. Family history, advancing age, atherosclerosis, heart disease, congestive heart failure, hypertension, smoking, diabetes, inactivity, overweight, heavy drinking, stimulant drug use, and other factors can all contribute to triggering strokes.[36]

Some strokes are mild and cause only temporary dizziness or slight weakness or numbness. If an affected area is large or in a crucial part of the brain, stroke may cause speech impairments, memory problems, loss of motor control, or death. About 1 in 10 major strokes is preceded days, weeks, or months earlier by *transient ischemic attacks (TIAs),* brief interruptions of the blood supply to the brain that cause only temporary dizziness, weakness, paralysis, numbness, or other symptoms.[37] Deaths due to strokes have decreased in recent years thanks to better diagnosis, better surgical options, new clot-busting drugs that can be injected immediately after a stroke has occurred, and better aftercare for stroke patients. Campaigns to teach awareness and avoidance of risk factors could prevent up to half of annual strokes if people followed them carefully.

congestive heart failure (CHF) A cardiovascular disease in which the heart muscle is damaged or overworked, and the heart lacks the strength to keep blood circulating normally through the body

congenital heart disease Heart disease present at birth

stroke A sudden loss of function in a region of the brain caused by blockage in or rupture of a blood vessel, leading to oxygen deprivation, cell damage, or death

In the Event of a Heart Attack, Stroke, or Cardiac Arrest

Knowing what to do in a cardiovascular emergency could save a friend's life—or your own.

Warning Signs of a Heart Attack

- Uncomfortable pressure, fullness, squeezing, or pain in the center of the chest (more likely in men) or between the shoulder blades (more likely in women), lasting two minutes or longer

- Jaw pain and/or shortness of breath

- Pain spreading to the shoulders, neck, or arms

- Dizziness, fatigue, fainting, sweating, and/or nausea

Not all of these warning signs occur in every heart attack. For instance, a woman's heart attack may show up as shortness of breath, fatigue, and jaw or shoulder blade pain or pressure, stretched out over hours rather than minutes. If any of these symptoms appear, don't wait. Get help immediately!

Warning Signs of a Stroke

- Sudden numbness or weakness, especially on one side of the body, affecting face, arm, and/or leg

- Sudden mental confusion, especially trouble speaking or understanding words

- Sudden vision problems in one or both eyes

- Sudden dizziness, loss of balance, lack of coordination, or trouble walking

- Sudden severe headache without apparent cause

Warning Signs of a Cardiac Arrest

- Sudden loss of responsiveness (won't respond if tapped on either shoulder)

- Cessation of normal breathing (tilt head up; check for breathing for 5 seconds)

Know What to Do before an Emergency Strikes

- Find out which hospitals in your area have 24-hour emergency cardiac care.

- Determine (in advance) the hospital or medical facility that is nearest your home and office and tell your family and friends to call this facility in an emergency.

- Keep a list of emergency rescue service numbers next to your telephone and in your pocket, wallet, or purse. Remember 911 if you don't have time to call emergency rescue numbers.

- If you have chest or jaw discomfort that lasts more than two minutes, call the emergency rescue service or 911. Do not drive yourself to the hospital unless there is no other alternative.

Be a Lifesaver during a Crisis

- If you are with someone who is showing signs of a heart attack or stroke and the warning signs last for two minutes or longer, act immediately.

- Expect a denial. It is normal for a person with chest discomfort to deny the possibility of anything as serious as a heart attack. Don't take no for an answer. Insist on taking prompt action.

- Call 911 or an emergency rescue service, or get to the nearest hospital emergency room that offers 24-hour emergency cardiac care.

- If you are with someone in cardiac arrest and if you are properly trained, give chest compressions and mouth-to-mouth breathing. Continual chest compressions appear to be more important for adult heart attack victims; combined compressions and breathing (CPR or cardiopulmonary resuscitation) seem to be more important for children having a heart, stroke, or breathing-related emergency. Get instructions on which to use from a 911 operator, emergency medical technician, or other rescue personnel if possible.

- An automated external defibrillator (AED) may save a person during cardiac arrest. These devices are increasingly common in public places—workplaces, restaurants, health clubs, sports stadiums, schools, shopping centers, airports, hotels, and so on. Try to cultivate the habit of noticing their location in case of emergency.

Source: Adapted from American Heart Association, "Heart Attack, Stroke, and Cardiac Arrest Warning Signs," www.americanheart.org, March 18, 2011.

What Are the Main Risk Factors for Cardiovascular Disease?

The prevalence of cardiovascular disease is an unfortunate reality. However, we can modify many of our individual risk factors. By identifying your risks and understanding which are controllable, (see **Lab 10.1**), you can learn to modify risk-promoting behaviors and lower your chances of developing CVD.

Risks You Can Control

Experts have identified at least 10 significant risk factors for CVD: tobacco use, hypertension, high blood fats, obesity/overweight, physical inactivity, type 2 diabetes, metabolic syndrome, heavy alcohol consumption, poor diet, and uncontrolled stress. Since lifestyle choices underlie many of these risk factors, changes to daily habits can often reduce the chances of developing cardiovascular disease. Many people have multiple risk factors for CVD; the more risk factors they have, the greater their chances of experiencing a heart attack, stroke, angina, atherosclerosis, and other specific forms of CVD.[38] Let's look at each of these risk factors more closely.

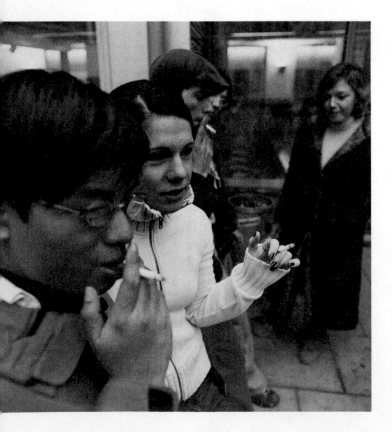

Tobacco Use In 1964, the Surgeon General of the United States asserted that smoking was the greatest risk factor for heart disease. Today, more than 20 percent of deaths from CVD are directly related to smoking. The risk for cardiovascular disease is 70 percent greater for smokers than for nonsmokers. Smokers who have a heart attack are more likely to die suddenly (within one hour) than are nonsmokers.[39] Evidence also indicates that an estimated 46,000 *non*smokers die from cardiovascular disease each year as a result of chronic exposure to environmental tobacco smoke.[40]

How does tobacco use damage the cardiovascular system? Researchers have several plausible explanations. One is that the nicotine in all forms of tobacco (cigarettes, cigars, chewing tobacco, etc.) increases heart rate, heart output, blood pressure, and oxygen use by the heart muscle. Another is that cigarette smoke is filled with carbon monoxide, which displaces oxygen in heart tissue and requires a smoker's heart to work harder to obtain enough oxygen. Chemicals in smoke can cause injuries to arteries that lead to both plaque formation and inflammation. Finally, smokers have a higher level of a natural blood-clotting factor, and these increased levels may contribute to the blood clots that trigger heart attacks and strokes.[41]

Hypertension We have seen that hypertension can damage artery walls and lead to atherosclerosis. It can also weaken artery walls and lead to an *aneurysm,* an abnormal, blood-filled bulge in a blood vessel that has the potential to rupture. Hypertension can damage coronary arteries, enlarge the heart, or weaken the heart muscle. By affecting blood vessels in the brain, hypertension can cause strokes and TIAs, promote dementia, and impair cognitive functioning. By damaging delicate blood vessels in the kidneys and eyes, hypertension can lead to kidney damage or failure and to impaired vision or vision loss. In addition, hypertension can reduce sexual function, disrupt sleep, and magnify the bone loss of osteoporosis.[42] Reducing dietary sodium, blood fats, and excess weight can help lower blood pressure, as can managing stress and taking certain prescription drugs.

High Levels of Fats in Your Blood *Hyperlipidemia*—or high levels of cholesterol, triglycerides, and other fats in the blood—is correlated with increased risk of several cardiovascular diseases. According to a recent report, more than 50 percent of American men aged 65 and older and 40 percent of Amercian women aged 65 or older are on some type of anti-hyperlipidemia prescription drug, including such medications as the "statins"

(Lipitor, Crestor, Zocor) and others drugs designed to reduce blood fats.[43] Unfortunately, many of these medications carry significant risks of their own. Additionally, many people use these medications as "crutches" and continue to eat high fat-foods, assuming that the medications will keep any risks from CVD at bay.

Diets high in saturated fats and/or *trans* fats can raise blood cholesterol levels and contribute to atherosclerosis. They can also switch on the body's blood-clotting system, making the blood thicker and stickier. All of these blood changes increase the risk of heart attack or stroke.

Increases in blood cholesterol can also contribute to hardening of the arteries, or atherosclerosis, with its long-term effects on CVD. Table 10.4 shows recommended levels for blood cholesterol. People with several risk factors for CVD should follow the most stringent range of the guidelines.

Total cholesterol levels are just one measure of cardiovascular disease risks. Another is the ratio of "bad" to "good" cholesterol. Low-density lipoprotein (LDL), often referred to as "bad" cholesterol, is believed

SEE IT! ONLINE

Tips to Raise Good Cholesterol

to contribute to plaque buildup on artery walls. High-density lipoprotein (HDL), or "good" cholesterol, appears to remove plaque from artery walls, thus serving as a protector. In theory, if LDL levels get too high relative to HDL levels, plaque will tend to accumulate inside arteries and lead to cardiovascular problems. The LDL/HDL ratio can increase because of too much saturated fat in the diet, lack of exercise, high stress levels, or genetic predisposition.

It can be useful to obtain an accurate assessment of your total cholesterol and LDL and HDL levels. This analysis requires a fasting blood test (no eating or drinking for 12 hours prior to the test) administered by a reputable health provider. You can compare your numbers to Table 10.4 and discuss their significance with your physician.

A second type of blood fat called *triglycerides* also appears to promote atherosclerosis. As people get older, heavier, or both, their triglyceride and cholesterol levels tend to rise. No one has yet proved that high triglyceride levels cause atherosclerosis and thus underlie CVD. However, these blood fats may contribute to faster plaque development.

Overweight and Obesity Being overweight or obese can strain the heart, forcing it to push blood through "extra" miles of capillaries that supply each pound of fat. A heart that must continuously move blood through an overabundance of vessels has to work harder and may become weakened or damaged. The same high-fat, high-sugar, and high-calorie diets that lead to overweight and obesity can also contribute to plaque formation.

Overweight people are more likely to develop heart disease and stroke even if they have no other CVD risk factors.[44] Losing even 5 to 10 pounds can make a significant difference to CVD risk.[45] This is especially true for people who tend to store fat around the upper body and waist (an "apple" shape) as opposed to those who tend to store fat around the hips and thighs (a "pear" shape.)

Physical Inactivity A sedentary lifestyle is one of the most significant risk factors for CVD. Elevating the heart rate and blood flow through moderate to vigorous activity benefits the heart muscle and helps prevent plaque deposits on artery walls. Conversely, inactivity decreases the efficiency of the heart muscle and allows plaque buildup to occur more easily. Even modest levels of low-intensity physical activity—walking, gardening, housework, dancing—are beneficial if done regularly and over the long term. Despite the clear

TABLE 10.4 LDL, Total, and HDL Cholesterol and Triglycerides (mg/dL) Levels for Adults	
LDL Cholesterol	
Less than 100	Optimal
100–129	Near optimal/above optimal
130–159	Borderline high
160–189	High
190 or higher	Very high
Total Cholesterol	
Less than 200	Desirable
200–239	Borderline high
240 or higher	High
HDL Cholesterol	
Less than 40	Low
60 or higher	Desirable
Triglycerides	
Less than 150	Normal
150–199	Borderline high
200–499	High
500 or higher	Very high

Source: National Heart, Lung, And Blood Institute, "Detection, Evaluation, and Treatment of High Blood Cholesterol in Adults" (NIH Publication No. 02-5215), 2002.

benefits of regular exercise, only 34.4 percent of Americans over age 18 engage in any regular physical activity.[46]

Diabetes Mellitus Chronic diseases are interrelated: people who have one tend to have others. This connection is especially clear when it comes to diabetes and cardiovascular disease. Having diabetes significantly increases one's risk for CVD even if blood sugar levels are well controlled. When they're uncontrolled, the risks are even higher. People with diabetes have death rates from CVD that are 2–4 times higher than those of people without diabetes.[47] Some experts estimate that as many as 50 percent of people with diabetes eventually die of CVD.[48] In fact, the risk is so great, many physicians consider someone with pre-diabetes or with the early stages of diabetes to have the same risks as someone who has already had their first heart attack. Diabetics also tend to have elevated blood fat levels, increased atherosclerosis, and a tendency toward deterioration of small blood vessels, particularly in the eyes and extremities.

Metabolic Syndrome Metabolic syndrome refers to a cluster of obesity-related risk factors associated with CVD and type 2 diabetes.[49] People with metabolic syndrome have several characteristics in common (see Figure 10.3):

metabolic syndrome A group of metabolic conditions occurring together that increase a person's risk of heart disease, stroke, and diabetes

- Abdominal obesity, meaning a large waistline (more than 40 inches in men or 35 inches in women).

- Elevated levels of triglycerides in the blood (more than 150 mg/dL).

- Low levels of "good cholesterol" (HDLs below 40 mg/dL in men or 50 mg/dL in women)

- High blood pressure (greater than 130/85 mm Hg)

- High levels of the sugar glucose in the blood (more than 100 mg/dL after fasting)

- High levels of C-reactive protein (more than 10 mg/L), indicating inflammation

The National Heart, Lung, and Blood Institute estimates that 47 million American adults—fully one quarter of our adult population—have metabolic syndrome.[50] By definition, they have multiple risk factors for CVD, and thus their overall risk of developing cardiovascular illness is high.

The prevalence of metabolic syndrome in adolescents and young adults is causing concern among many health professionals. A recent study of nearly 2,000 teenagers revealed that one-third of overweight or obese teens had metabolic syndrome, as did 10 percent of all the adolescents tested.[51] Nutrition—specifically low intake of fruits and vegetables and high intake of sweetened beverages—can play an important role in this early onset.[52]

Studies of college students have found similar rates of metabolic syndrome, with both low levels of fitness and overweight status correlating with higher risk for metabolic syndrome.[53] As with adolescents, only 10 percent of college students in one study had several of the measurable parameters that define metabolic syndrome; however, 43 percent had at least one of the indicators.[54] The message here is clear: Being young does not make you immune to metabolic syndrome and its multiple risk factors for cardiovascular disease.

ELEVATED BLOOD TRIGLYCERIDES
- Greater than or equal to 150 mg/dL

REDUCED BLOOD HDL CHOLESTEROL
- *Men:* Less than 40 mg/dL
- *Women:* Less than 50 mg/dL

ELEVATED FASTING BLOOD GLUCOSE
- Greater than or equal to 100 mg/dL

ELEVATED BLOOD PRESSURE
- *Systolic* blood pressure greater than or equal to 130 mm Hg
- *Diastolic* blood pressure greater than or equal to 85 mm Hg

INCREASED WAIST CIRCUMFERENCE
- *Men:* Greater than or equal to 40 inches
- *Women:* Greater than or equal to 35 inches

FIGURE **10.3** Risk factors associated with metabolic syndrome.

Other Controllable Factors Stress can act as a risk factor for CVD. Your body's stress response can cause blood pressure to rise and can trigger blood-clotting and heart rhythm abnormalities.[55] Stress can also foster habits that promote CVD, such as overeating or smoking.

Poor nutrition also increases CVD risk. Too much saturated fat, salt, and refined carbohydrates and too little fiber and too few fruits and vegetables all heighten risk, while improved nutrition lowers risk.

Although some studies have suggested that *moderate* amounts of alcohol may help lower the risk of cardiovascular disease, excessive alcohol consumption can raise blood triglycerides, trigger arrhythmias, raise blood pressure, promote obesity, and contribute to heart failure and strokes. Stimulant drugs, such as amphetamines or cocaine, can also trigger strokes—even in young people.[56]

Risks You Cannot Control

Unfortunately, there are risk factors for cardiovascular disease that you cannot control, including the following:

Heredity A family history of cardiovascular disease—that is, CVD in several generations of an extended family—appears to increase risk significantly. Researchers are unsure whether the increase is due to genetics, to the environment in which you were raised (including diet, exercise, and stress levels), or both.

Age Seventy-five percent of all heart attacks occur in people over age 65. The risk for CVD increases with age for both sexes.[57]

Gender Men are at greater risk for CVD until about age 60.[58] Women under 35 have a fairly low risk unless they have high blood pressure, kidney problems, or diabetes. Being a smoker while using oral contraceptives also increases a woman's risk. Hormonal factors appear to protect women before menopause; after menopause or after estrogen levels decline due to hysterectomy or ovary disease, a woman's LDL levels tend to rise and with them, the chances of developing cardiovascular disease.[59]

Race Members of certain racial/ethnic groups may face increased cardiovascular disease risk (see Figure 10.4).[60] African Americans have the highest rates of cardiovascular disease, followed by Caucasian Americans and Mexican Americans. Rates for Asian Americans are below 25 percent.[61]

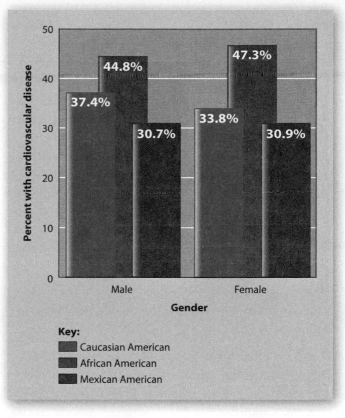

FIGURE 10.4 Cardiovascular disease affects a disproportionate percentage of African Americans.

Data from American Heart Association, *Heart Disease and Stroke Statistics 2010 Update-at-a-Glance*. Comparable data on Hispanic American and Asian American populations were not available in this report.

casestudy

DARYL

"I took my mom in for a check-up the other day. The good news is that her blood pressure and cholesterol have both come down since her last visit. While I was sitting in the waiting room, though, I read a brochure about risk factors for heart disease. I knew genetics was a factor, but I was surprised at how many other risk factors I had: not being very active (unless you count playing the piano!), breathing in other people's smoke at jazz clubs, too much fast food, and stress."

THINK! What else could Daryl do to assess his risk for cardiovascular disease? What risk factors for cardiovascular disease do you have?

ACT! Sort your risk factors by "controllable" and "non-controllable." For each controllable risk factor, list ways you could change your lifestyle to reduce your vulnerability.

How Can I Avoid Cardiovascular Disease?

Worksheet 38 Cardiovascular Risk Assessment

People often wait until they get a scary medical diagnosis before changing their habits. If you have risk factors for cardiovascular disease, the earlier you confront them, the better your chances of avoiding CVD later. Identifying the controllable risk factors for cardiovascular disease in your life, and making simple changes to reduce them, will give you a head start toward protecting your cardiovascular health throughout adulthood!

Lower Your Controllable Risks

Here are specific behavioral tips for avoiding cardiovascular disease by reducing the risk factors you can control.

Don't Use Tobacco According to the American Heart Association, smoking is the greatest preventable cause of disease and death. Even light smoking—just two cigarettes per day—increases your CVD risk. When people stop smoking, regardless of how long or how much they have smoked, their risk of heart disease declines rapidly. Three years after quitting, the risk of death from heart disease and stroke for people who smoked a pack a day or less is almost the same as for people who never smoked. Women appear to recover lung function more fully than men.[62] Since secondhand smoke is a potent risk factor, avoid smoky places when possible. Avoid all forms of tobacco, since nicotine increases blood pressure, heart rate, blood clotting, and plaque buildup.

Eat Well There are numerous ways you can promote cardiovascular health through better nutrition. The American Heart Association recommends the following:[63]

- Aim to use up at least as many calories as you consume.

- Eat a wide variety of foods from all the basic food groups.

- Aim to have a diet that consists of mainly nutrient-rich foods such as vegetables, fruits, and whole-grain products. Fruits and vegetables are high in vitamins, minerals, and fiber, and are low in calories. Meanwhile, the fiber in unrefined whole-grain foods can help lower cholesterol and help you feel full (which can help with weight management).

- Eat fish at least twice a week. The omega-3 fatty acids in fish such as salmon and trout may help lower the risk of death from coronary artery disease.

- Consume lean meats without skin, and cook them without added saturated and *trans* fat. Or substitute beans and legumes as a protein source instead of meats.

- Avoid high-fat dairy products, and instead consume fat-free, 1 percent fat, or low-fat dairy products.

- Reduce your consumption of foods containing partially hydrogenated vegetable oils to lower the amount of *trans* fat in your diet.

- Cut back on foods high in dietary cholesterol. Aim to eat less than 300 milligrams of cholesterol each day.

- Cut back on beverages and foods with added sugars.

- Reduce your intake of sodium to 1,500 milligrams or less per day.

- Drink alcohol in moderation.

- Be aware of portion sizes, especially while dining out.

If you have (or are at risk of developing) hypertension, your physician may suggest that you adopt the DASH (Dietary Approaches to Stop Hypertension) diet. Following this diet can help lessen your risk of hypertension and other forms of cardiovascular disease. The box on the DASH Diet discusses the diet's specific recommendations.

Exercise Regularly Regular cardiovascular exercise strengthens the heart muscles and helps keep the blood vessels resilient. Performing 30 to 60 minutes or more of moderate activity most days of the week will help prevent cardiovascular disease, especially if you reach your target heart rate. Strength training and flexibility are also important components of your exercise plan for cardiovascular wellness, helping you to maintain muscle mass, speed metabolism, control weight, and prevent injury.

Manage Your Stress The physiological stress response raises blood pressure, speeds the heart rate, and floods the bloodstream with glucose. All of these, in turn, can promote cardiovascular disease by damaging the blood vessels and directly contributing to atherosclerosis, and by weakening the heart through electrical and hormonal overstimulation. Learning specific techniques for stress reduction, relaxation, and anger management can give you important tools for lowering your risk of cardiovascular disease.

Control Diabetes Because elevated sugar levels in the blood greatly increase the risk for heart disease, stroke, and artery disease, people with diabetes are at tremendous risk. The very factors that contribute to the development of diabetes (obesity, hypertension, elevated blood cholesterol and triglycerides, inactivity) are additional risks for CVD. Careful diet, increased exercise, and medication help most diabetics control their condition and lower their CVD risk.

Avoid Alcohol and Drug Abuse If you drink, keep your consumption below one drink per day for women and two per day for men. Greater consumption raises blood sugar and triglyceride levels. Avoid recreational drugs, especially stimulants.

TOOLS FOR **CHANGE** ●

The DASH Diet

The DASH (Dietary Approaches to Stop Hypertension) diet is a set of nutritional guidelines designed to reduce blood pressure. Recommended by the National Heart, Lung, and Blood Institute and the American Heart Association, it is characterized by the following:

- Reduced consumption of saturated fat, total fat, red meats, sodium, sweets, added sugars, and sugar-containing beverages

- Increased consumption of fruits, vegetables, fat-free or low-fat dairy products, whole-grain foods, fish, poultry, and nuts

- Special care to consume recommended levels of potassium, magnesium, calcium, protein, and fiber

You can find the entire DASH eating plan—including nutrient goals and serving recommendations at different calorie levels for various food groups—online at www.nhlbi.nih.gov/health/public/heart/hbp/dash/new_dash.pdf.

In addition to these guidelines, the DASH diet provides tips for reducing sodium—often hidden in processed foods—that can benefit virtually everyone:

- Buy the low- or reduced-sodium versions of soups, condiments, crackers, and other packaged foods. Read labels carefully and watch for sodium in such items as breakfast cereals and salad dressings.

- Choose fresh or frozen vegetables. If buying canned, look for no-sodium or low-sodium versions.

- Watch out for canned, smoked, cured, or processed meats and brined foods such as pickles and olives, which are usually very high in sodium. Rinse when practical to wash away some of the salt.

- Some processed foods have so much sodium you may simply have to avoid them; examples include packaged cake and sauce mixes, pizzas, and frozen dinners.

Source: U.S. Department of Health and Human Services, National Institutes of Health, National Heart, Lung, and Blood Institute, *DASH Eating Plan: Lower Your Blood Pressure* (NIH Publication #06-4082, Revised April, 2006).

● ●

chapterin**review**

videos

Log on to **www.pearsonhighered.com/hopson** or MyFitnessLab to view these chapter-related videos.

Heart Disease in America   Tips to Raise Good Cholesterol

onlineresources

Log on to **www.pearsonhighered.com/hopson** or MyFitnessLab for access to these book-related resources, and for links to other useful websites.

 Audio case study
Audio PowerPoint lecture

 Lab 10.1 Understand Your CVD Risk

 Take Charge of Your Health! Worksheets:
    Worksheet 38 Cardiovascular Risk
        Assessment
    Worksheet 39 Healthy Heart I.Q.
Behavior Change Log Book and Wellness
Journal

 Pre- and post-quizzes
Glossary flashcards

reviewquestions

1. Cardiovascular disease and stroke are responsible for about _____ of deaths in the United States each year.
   a. one-half
   b. one-tenth
   c. one-sixth
   d. one-third

2. In annual medical care costs and lost productivity, CVD collectively costs Americans
   a. about $475,000.
   b. about $47.5 million.
   c. about $475 million.
   d. about $475 billion.

3. Which of the following is an example of cardiovascular disease (CVD)?
   a. Diabetes
   b. Low blood pressure
   c. Coronary heart disease
   d. Systolic pressure

4. Which of the following accurately describes *hypertension*?
   a. Sustained high blood pressure
   b. A thickening or hardening of the arteries
   c. Heart blockage
   d. Irregular heartbeat

5. Which of the following is characteristic of cardiovascular disease?
   a. Joint pain
   b. Feeling energized
   c. Having no symptoms at all
   d. Dry skin

6. When atherosclerosis occurs in the heart's main blood vessels, it is called
   a. peripheral artery disease.
   b. coronary artery disease.
   c. inflammation.
   d. homocysteine.

7. Which of the following is a significant risk factor for CVD?
   a. Regular exercise
   b. Managed stress
   c. Underweight
   d. Tobacco use

8. A person with metabolic syndrome is likely to have which one of the following?
   a. Abdominal obesity or a large waistline
   b. Depressed levels of triglycerides in the blood
   c. High levels of "good" cholesterol (HDLs)
   d. Hypoglycemia or low blood sugar

9. Which of the following statements is true?
   a. The earliest manifestations of cardiovascular disease often take root during childhood.
   b. Only seniors need to worry about cardiovascular disease.
   c. Heavy alcohol consumption is unrelated to your risks for developing cardiovascular disease.
   d. People who are skinny are protected against cardiovascular disease.

10. Low-density lipoprotein (LDL) is often referred to as
    a. "good" cholesterol.
    b. "bad" cholesterol.
    c. diabetes mellitus.
    d. metabolic syndrome.

critical**thinking**questions

1. List six different forms of CVD. Compare and contrast their risk factors, symptoms, and prevention.
2. Describe the atherosclerosis process and explain the medical term "atherosclerotic cardiovascular disease."
3. Discuss the evidence that people in your age group are at risk for developing CVD.
4. Discuss specific ways that exercise and dietary changes can help prevent CVD.

references

1. National Center for Health Statistics (NCHS), "FastStats: Leading Causes of Death," www.cdc.gov/nchs/fastats/lcod .htm (updated September 2011).
2. American Heart Association, "Heart Disease and Stroke Statistics 2011 Update: A Report from the American Heart Association," *Circulation* 123, no. 4 (2011): e18–209.
3. Ibid.
4. Ibid.
5. L. L. Hayman, "Starting Young: Promoting a Healthy Lifestyle with Children," *Journal of Cardiovascular Nursing* 25, no. 3 (2010): 228–32; American Heart Association, "Heart Disease and Stroke Statistics 2011 Update," 2011.
6. J. Xu and others, "Deaths: Final Data for 2007," *National Vital Statistics Reports* 58, no. 19 (Hyattsville, MD: National Center for Health Statistics, 2011); M. Heron, "Deaths: Leading Causes for 2006," *National Vital Statistics Reports* 58, no. 14 (Hyattsville, MD: National Center for Health Statistics, 2010); K. D. Kochank and others, "Deaths: Preliminary Data for 2009," *National Vital Statistics Reports* 59, no. 4 (Hyattsville, MD: National Center for Health Statistics, 2011).
7. American Heart Association, "American Heart Association Scientific Statement: Combined Behavioral Interventions Best Way to Reduce Heart Disease Risk," http://newsroom.heart.org/pr/aha/1073 .aspx (July 12, 2010).
8. American Heart Association, "Cardiovascular Disease Cost," www.americanheart .org/presenter.jhtml?identifier=4475 (2011).
9. P. A. Heidenreich and others, "Forecasting the Future of Cardiovascular Disease in the United States: A Policy Statement from the American Heart Association," *Circulation* 123, no. 8 (2011): 933–44.
10. World Health Organization, "Cardiovascular Diseases (CVDs)," Fact sheet no. 317, www.who.int/mediacentre/factsheets /fs317/en/index.html (September 2011).
11. Ibid.

12. World Health Organization, "Cardiovascular Disease: Prevention and Control," Global Strategy on Diet, Physical Activity, and Health, www.who.int/dietphysicalactivity /publications/facts/cvd/en/index.htm (accessed August 2007).
13. World Health Organization, "Cardiovascular Diseases (CVDs)," 2011.
14. H. C. McGill and others, "Origin of Atherosclerosis in Childhood and Adolescence," *American Journal of Clinical Nutrition* 72, no. 5 (2000): 1307S–15S.
15. H. C. McGill and others, "Association of Coronary Heart Disease Risk Factors with Microscopic Qualities of Coronary Atherosclerosis in Youth," *Circulation* 102, no. 4 (2000): 374–9.
16. T. Parker-Pope, "Stroke Rising among Young People," *New York Times* http: //well.blogs.nytimes.com/2011/02/10 /stroke-rising-among-young-people (February 10, 2011).
17. P. Franks and others, "Childhood Obesity, Other Cardiovascular Risks, and Premature Death," *New England Journal of Medicine* 362, no. 6 (2010): 485–93; D. H. Whincup and J. E. Deanfield, "Childhood Obesity and Cardiovascular Disease: The Challenge Ahead," *Nature Clinical Practice Cardiovascular Medicine* 2, no. 9 (2005): 432–3; R. E. Kavey and others, "American Heart Association Guidelines for Primary Prevention of Atherosclerotic Cardiovascular Disease Beginning in Childhood," *Circulation* 107, no. 11 (2003): 1562–6.
18. A. G. Mainous III and others, "Life Stress and Atherosclerosis: A Pathway through Unhealthy Lifestyle," *International Journal of Psychiatry in Medicine* 40, no. 2 (2010): 147–61; Mayo Clinic Staff, "Arteriosclerosis /Atherosclerosis: Causes," www.mayoclinic .com/health/arteriosclerosisatherosclerosis /DS00525 (June 2010).
19. R. E. Kavey, "American Heart Association Guidelines for Primary Prevention of Atherosclerotic Cardiovascular Disease," 2003.
20. "Inflammation, Heart Disease, and Stroke: The Role of C-Reactive Protein," American

Heart Association, www.americanheart .org/presenter.jhtml?identifier=4648 (March 2011).
21. B. M. Egan, Y. Zhao, and R. N. Axon, "US Trends in Prevalence, Awareness, Treatment, and Control of Hypertension, 1988–2008," *Journal of the American Medical Association* 303, no. 20 (2010): 2043–50.
22. Mayo Clinic Staff, "High Blood Pressure (Hypertension)," www.mayoclinic.com /health/high-blood-pressure/DS00100 (March 2011).
23. S. I. Sharp and others, "Hypertension Is a Potential Risk Factor for Vascular Dementia: Systematic Review," *International Journal of Geriatric Psychiatry* 26, no. 7 (2011): 661–9; F. D. Testai and P. B. Gorelick, "Vascular Cognitive Impairment and Alzheimer's Disease: Are These Disorders Linked to Hypertension and other Cardiovascular Risk Factors?" in V. Aiyagari and P. B. Gorelick (eds.) *Hypertension and Stroke: Pathophysiology and Management* (New York: Humana Press, 2011): 195–210.
24. Ibid.
25. C. L. Williams and B. A. Strobino, "Childhood Diet, Overweight, and CVD Risk Factors: The Healthy Start Project," *Preventive Cardiology* 11, no. 1 (2008): 11–20; P. K. Elias and others, "Blood Pressure-Related Cognitive Decline: Does Age Make a Difference?" *Hypertension* 44, no. 5 (2004): 631–6.
26. American Heart Association, "About High Blood Pressure," www.heart.org /HEARTORG/Conditions/HighBlood Pressure/AboutHighBloodPressure /About-High-Blood-Pressure_UCM_002050 _Article.jsp (updated June 2011).
27. Ibid.
28. J. Flynn, "Hypertension in the Young: Epidemiology, Sequelae, and Therapy," *Nephrology, Dialysis, Transplantation* 24, no. 2 (2009): 370–75.
29. American Heart Association, "Heart Disease and Stroke Statistics 2011 Update," 2011.
30. Ibid.

31. Mayo Clinic Staff, "Angina," www .mayoclinic.com/health/angina/DS00994 (June 2011).

32. American Heart Association, "About Arrhythmia," www.heart.org/HEARTORG /Conditions/Arrhythmia/AboutArrhythmia /About-Arrhythmia_UCM_002010_Article .jsp (updated June 2011).

33. American Heart Association, "About Heart Failure," www.heart.org/HEARTORG /Conditions/HeartFailure/AboutHeartFailure /About-Heart-Failure_UCM_002044_Article .jsp (updated September 2011).

34. American Heart Association, "About Congenital Heart Defects," www.heart.org /HEARTORG/Conditions/Congenital HeartDefects/AboutCongenitalHeart Defects/About-Congenital-Heart-Defects _UCM_001217_Article.jsp (updated January 2011).

35. American Heart Association, "Heart Disease and Stroke Statistics 2011 Update," 2011.

36. Mayo Clinic Staff, "Stroke: Risk Factors," www.mayoclinic.com/health/stroke /DS00150 (July 2011).

37. Mayo Clinic Staff, "Transient Ischemic Attack (TIA)," www.mayoclinic.com /health/transient-ischemic-attack/DS00220 (March 2011).

38. National Heart, Lung, and Blood Institute, "What Are Coronary Heart Disease Risk Factors?" www.nhlbi.nih.gov/health/dci /Diseases/hd/hd_prevention.html (February 2011).

39. U.S. Department of Health and Human Services, *The Health Consequences of Smoking: A Report of the Surgeon General* (Atlanta: U.S. Department of Health and Human Services, Centers for Disease Control and Prevention, National Center for Chronic Disease Prevention and Health Promotion, Office on Smoking and Health, 2004), available at www.surgeongeneral .gov/library/smokingconsequences/index .html.

40. American Cancer Society, "Secondhand Smoke," www.cancer.org/cancer/cancer causes/tobaccocancer/secondhand-smoke (revised June 2011).

41. American Heart Association, "Why Quit Smoking?" www.heart.org/HEARTORG /GettingHealthy/QuitSmoking /QuittingSmoking/Why-Quit-Smoking _UCM_307847_Article.jsp (updated August 2011); V. F. Tapson, "The Role of Smoking in Coagulation and Thromboembolism in Chronic Obstructive Pulmonary Disease," *Proceedings of the American Thoracic Society* 2, no. 1 (2005): 71–7.

42. Mayo Clinic Staff, "High Blood Pressure Dangers: Hypertension's Effects on Your Body," www.mayoclinic.com/health /high-blood-pressure/HI00062 (January 2011).

43. National Center for Health Statistics, *Health, United States, 2010: With Special Feature on Death and Dying* (Hyattsville, MD: U.S. Department of Health and Human Services, 2011) Table 95.

44. American Heart Association, "Heart Disease and Stroke Statistics 2011 Update," 2011.

45. Mayo Clinic Staff, "Top 5 Lifestyle Changes to Reduce Cholesterol," www.mayoclinic .com/health/reduce-cholesterol/CL00012 (May 2010).

46. National Center for Health Statistics, "National Health Interview Survey, 1997–2010, Leisure-Time Physical Activity," www.cdc.gov/nchs/data/nhis/earlyrelease /201106_07.pdf (June 2011).

47. American Diabetes Association, "Diabetes Statistics: 2011 National Diabetes Fact Sheet," www.diabetes.org/diabetes-basics/diabetes-statistics (January 2011).

48. World Heart Federation, "Diabetes and Cardiovascular Disease," www.world-heart-federation.org/press/fact-sheets /diabetes-and-cvd (January 2011).

49. American Heart Association, "Heart Disease and Stroke Statistics 2011 Update," 2011.

50. National Heart, Lung, and Blood Institute, "What Is Metabolic Syndrome?" www .nhlbi.nih.gov/health/dci/Diseases/ms /ms_whatis.html (April 2011).

51. S. D. de Ferranti and others, "Prevalence of the Metabolic Syndrome in American Adolescents: Findings from the Third National Health and Nutrition Examination Survey," *Circulation* 110, no. 16 (2004): 2494–7.

52. American Diabetes Association, "Metabolic Syndrome Risk Factors in Young Adults," *DOC NEWS* 2, no. 1 (2005): 23.

53. J. Schilter and L. Dalleck, "Fitness and Fatness: Indicators of Metabolic Syndrome and Cardiovascular Disease Risk Factors in College Students?" *Journal of Exercise Physiology* 13, no. 4 (2010): 29–39.

54. T. L. Keown, C. B. Smith, and M. S. Harris, "Metabolic Syndrome among College Students," *The Journal for Nurse Practitioners* 5, no. 10 (2009): 754–9.

55. M. Esler and others, "Chronic Mental Stress Is a Cause of Essential Hypertension: Presence of Biological Markers of Stress," *Clinical and Experimental Pharmacology and Physiology* 35, no. 4 (2008): 498–502; A. Flaa and others, "Sympathoadrenal Stress Reactivity Is a Predictor of Future Blood Pressure: An 18-Year Follow-Up Study," *Hypertension* 52, no. 2 (2008): 336–41; T. Chandola et al., "Work Stress and Coronary Heart Disease: What Are the Mechanisms?" *European Heart Journal* 29, no. 5 (2008): 640–8.

56. A. N. Westover, S. McBride, and R. W. Haley, "Stroke in Young Adults Who Abuse Amphetamines or Cocaine," *Archives of General Psychiatry* 64 (2007): 495–502.

57. American Heart Association, "Heart Disease and Stroke Statistics 2011 Update," 2011.

58. Ibid.

59. National Heart, Lung, and Blood Institute, National Cholesterol Education Program, "High Blood Cholesterol: What You Need to Know," NIH Publication No. 05-3290, www.nhlbi.nih.gov/health /public/heart/chol/wyntk.htm (revised June 2005).

60. American Heart Association, "Heart Disease and Stroke Statistics 2011 Update," 2011.

61. Ibid.

62. Centers for Disease Control and Prevention, "Tobacco Use: Targeting the Nation's Leading Killer—At A Glance 2011," www .cdc.gov/chronicdisease/resources /publications/AAG/osh.htm (updated February 2011).

63. American Heart Association, "American Heart Association Supports New USDA /HHS Dietary Guidelines and Encourages Adherence: AHA Also Expresses Disappointment That Sodium, Saturated Fat Guidance Is Weak." Press Release http://newsroom.heart.org/pr/aha/1243 .aspx (January 2011).

LAB 10.1 • UNDERSTAND YOUR CVD RISK

Name: _____ Date: _____

Instructor: _____ Section: _____

Purpose: To engage students in critical thinking about their own risk factors for CVD.

Directions: Complete each of the following questions about CVD risk and total your points in each section—the higher the score, the greater your risk. If you answered "don't know" for any question, talk to your parents or other family members as soon as possible to find out whether you have any unknown risks.

SECTION I: ASSESS YOUR FAMILY RISK FOR CVD

	Yes	No	Don't Know
1. Do any of your primary relatives (mother, father, grandparents, siblings) have a history of heart disease or stroke?	1	0	
2. Do any of your primary relatives (mother, father, grandparents, siblings) have diabetes?	1	0	
3. Do any of your primary relatives (mother, father, grandparents, siblings) have high blood pressure?	1	0	
4. Do any of your primary relatives (mother, father, grandparents, siblings) have a history of high cholesterol?	1	0	
5. During the time you lived at home, did your family consume red meat and high-fat dairy products several times per week?	1	0	
Total for Section I = _____			

SECTION II: ASSESS YOUR LIFESTYLE RISK FOR CVD

	Yes	No	Don't Know
1. Do you have high blood pressure?	1	0	
2. Is your total cholesterol level higher than recommended? (See Table 10.4)	1	0	
3. Have you been diagnosed as pre-diabetic or diabetic?	1	0	
4. Do you smoke three or more cigarettes per day?	1	0	
5. Would you describe your life as being highly stressful?	1	0	
Total for Section II = _____			

SECTION III: ASSESS YOUR ADDITIONAL RISKS FOR CVD

1. How would you best describe your current BMI?	
<18.5 (1 point)	25–29.9 (1 point)
18.5–24.9 (0 point)	≥30 (2 points)

2. How would you describe your level of exercise?

Moderate activity for 30 to 60 minutes on fewer than 3 days per week, plus fewer than three cardio workouts per week and fewer than two strength-training workouts per week	1 point
Moderate activity for 30 to 60 minutes most days of the week, plus three cardio workouts and two strength-training workouts per week	0 points
Moderate activity for 60 minutes or more most days of the week, plus more than three cardio workouts and two strength-training workouts per week	0 points

3. How would you describe your dietary behaviors?

I eat more than the recommended number of calories each day.	1 point
I eat about the recommended number of calories/day for my age, BMI, and activity level.	0 points
I eat fewer than the recommended number of calories each day.	0 points

4. Which of the following best describes your typical dietary behavior?

I eat several servings of red meat per week and consume saturated fat from other meats and high-fat dairy products most days.	1 point
I eat from the major food groups, trying hard to get the recommended fruits and vegetables.	0 points
Whenever possible, I try to substitute olive oil or canola oil for other forms of dietary fat.	0 points

Total for Section III = _____

Scoring: Look at each section. If your total score for that section is 0, your CVD risk is minimal. Keep up the good work! If your score is between 1 and 3, your risk is moderate and you should initiate some change to lower it. If you score a 4 or 5, you should make substantial changes in those factors that you can control. Your behavior change plan for the chapter will help, and you can get additional advice from your instructor.

SECTION IV: REFLECTION

1. What are your risk factors for CVD? Identify any behaviors that put you at risk for CVD. What can you change right now? What can you change in the future to reduce your risk?

_____

_____

2. Which risk factors for CVD are outside of your control? What can you do to reduce your risk of CVD, even though you have some uncontrollable risk factors?

_____

_____

11

Reducing Your Risk of Diabetes and Other Chronic Diseases

Learning Outcomes

1. Define *chronic disease*.

2. Explain why Americans should be concerned about chronic disease now and in the future.

  Audio case study and audio Power-Point lecture

3. Describe *type 2 diabetes*, America's fastest-growing chronic disease.

 Lab 11.1 Are You at Risk for Diabetes?

  Will Diabetes Cases Double in 25 Years?

Diabetes Plagues West Virginia County

4. Explain *chronic lung disease* and why it is far more common than lung cancer.

5. Define *osteoporosis* and explain how it heightens the risk for brittle and broken bones.

6. Provide details on *arthritis* and how it limits activity for 16 million Americans.

  Understanding Over-the-Counter Painkillers

7. Identify the common and specific risk factors for these major chronic diseases.

8. Identify ways to lower your own risk of developing a chronic disease.

 Take Charge of Your Health worksheets and Behavior Change Logs for assessing your chronic disease risk and creating a change plan

Pre- and post-quizzes and glossary flashcards

casestudy

GRACE

"I'm Grace. I'm a nursing student and just found out that my blood sugar level is high enough to put me in the category for pre-diabetes. In class, I learned about patients with diabetes and other common diseases like emphysema, osteoporosis, and arthritis. Now it looks like I'm going to be a patient myself. Are some people more likely to develop diabetes than others? What can I do to keep my condition from getting any worse?"

HEAR IT! ONLINE

• •

Y ou probably have a friend or family member with a **chronic disease**: a disease that tends to develop gradually and persist for months or years, often causing pain and disability. Generally, vaccines do not prevent chronic diseases and treatments do not provide a cure. However, lifestyle changes can often delay the onset of symptoms and medications and treatments can relieve them. Common chronic diseases include cardiovascular disease (Chapter 10), cancer (Chapter 12), and the main topics of this chapter: diabetes, chronic lung diseases, osteoporosis, and arthritis. Chronic *conditions* are

> **chronic disease** A medical condition that persists for a long period of time

usually less severe medical issues and include allergies, back pain, migraine headaches, and irritable bowel syndrome.

Your chance of developing chronic diseases and conditions increases as you get older. College students are not immune, however, as Figure 11.1 shows. The roots of many long-term diseases lie in poor health behaviors developed during childhood and in early adulthood. Three behaviors—smoking, eating poorly, and not exercising—are the underlying causes of over 35 percent of all chronic disease deaths in the United States today.[1] Learning about chronic disease now can inspire you to establish lifelong exercise, nutrition, and health care habits that may help you prevent or delay illness later in life.

Having one chronic disease can increase your susceptibility to developing other chronic diseases.[2] For example, having arthritis or osteoporosis makes exercise more difficult, which in turn may result in weight gain and exacerbate cardiovascular disease. And in people with diabetes, uncontrolled high levels of blood glucose can increase the risk of CVD and kidney disease, among others. By making plans for behavior change in the earlier chapters of this textbook, you have already built a good foundation for lowering your risks of developing chronic disease. Take a look at the box Tips to Reduce Your Risk of Chronic Disease for suggestions of other

FIGURE **11.1** Proportion of College Students Diagnosed with or Treated for Chronic Conditions in the Past 12 Months.

Data are from American College Health Association, *American College Health Association—National College Health Assessment II (ACHA-NCHA II): Reference Group Data Report Fall 2010* (Baltimore: American College Health Association, 2010).

Tips to Reduce Your Risk of Chronic Disease

The major risk factors for diabetes, chronic lung diseases, osteoporosis, and arthritis include obesity, inactivity, poor diet, and smoking. Fortunately, the same behavioral choices that increase overall wellness can also help you avoid chronic disease.

- Exercise daily
- Eat more fruits, vegetables, beans, nuts, whole grains, and heart-healthy fats
- Limit salt and sugar in your diet
- Maintain your recommended BMI

- Manage stress
- Avoid tobacco as well as drug and alcohol abuse
- Get enough sleep.

Sleep aids in immune function and increased ability to ward off infection. Sleep deprivation can increase risks for diabetes, hypertension, stress-related muscle aches and pains, and a host of other problems.[1]

Sources:
1. K. Knutson and others, "The Metabolic Consequences of Sleep Deprivation." *Sleep Medicine Review* 11, no. 2 (2007): 163–78; L. Rafalson and others, "Short Sleep Duration Is Associated with the Development of Impaired Fasting Glucose: The Western New York Health Study," *Annals of Epidemiology* 20, no. 12 (2010): 883–9.

---

behaviors you might need to change to avoid chronic disease. In the next sections, we take a closer look at four common chronic diseases: diabetes, chronic lung disease, osteoporosis, and arthritis.

What Is Diabetes?

SEE IT! ONLINE

Will Diabetes Cases Double in 25 Years?

Diabetes mellitus is the fastest-growing chronic disease in America.[3] Today, diabetes affects 25.8 million Americans. By 2050, those numbers could more than double, with one-third of all Americans born after 2000 developing diabetes in their lifetimes.[4] Diabetes seems to be increasing more dramatically among younger adults than among older Americans. One study by the Centers for Disease Control and Prevention (CDC) showed a rise in cases of almost 70 percent among those in their thirties.[5]

SEE IT! ONLINE

Diabetes Plagues West Virginia County

Diabetes Is the Inability to Properly Produce or Use Insulin

In healthy people, the pancreas secretes *insulin,* a hormone that is needed to convert sugar, starches, and other food into energy needed for life. **Type 1 diabetes** is an **autoimmune disease** in which the body's immune system creates antibodies that destroy the pancreas's ability to make insulin. The disease has a strong genetic basis and usually develops during childhood or adolescence.

Type 1 diabetes represents 5 percent of all cases of diabetes mellitus.[6] People with type 1 diabetes depend on insulin injections or infusions and must pay careful attention to diet, exercise, and stress levels to control their blood glucose.

In people with **pre-diabetes**, blood glucose levels are higher than normal but not high enough to be classified as diabetes.[7] An estimated 57 million Americans age 20 or older have pre-diabetes.[8] If you're like Grace from our case study, you can probably halt or slow the progression of your pre-diabetes or type 2 diabetes by losing weight and exercising more.[9]

In **type 2 diabetes**, the pancreas may produce too little insulin, or it may secrete sufficient insulin but the body's cells are

diabetes mellitus A disorder characterized by inadequate secretion or utilization of insulin, excessive urine production, excessive amounts of sugar in the blood and urine, and thirst, hunger, and weight loss

type 1 diabetes An autoimmune disease that destroys the insulin-producing cells of the pancreas, compromising the body's ability to make insulin and to properly regulate blood sugar

autoimmune disease A disorder in which the body's immune system creates antibodies that attack the person's own living cells

pre-diabetes A condition marked by blood glucose levels that are higher than normal but not yet diabetic

type 2 diabetes A disease linked to obesity and inactivity in which the body loses its ability to respond to insulin and cannot properly regulate blood sugar unable to use the hormone properly to convert glucose into cellular energy (Figure 11.2). This results in elevated glucose levels in the blood and urine, a condition known as *hyperglycemia*. Over time, high blood glucose levels can result in blindness, nerve damage, and significant circulatory system damage. In adults, type 2 diabetes represents 90 to 95 percent of all cases of diabetes mellitus.[10] It is most common in older Americans; one in four adults over age 65 has the disease.[11] Physicians used to refer to type 2 diabetes as *adult-onset diabetes*; now, however, they are diagnosing it in younger adults and even in children and teens. In the United States prior to the year 2000,

only 1 to 2 percent of patients below age 18 diagnosed with diabetes had type 2. But recent reports indicate that as many as 33 percent of Americans born after the year 2000 could one day develop type 2 diabetes.[12] The disease has a weak genetic basis and is linked to obesity and inactivity, so people are often able to control their diabetes through weight loss, increased activity, improved diet, and sometimes medications.

A third form of diabetes, *gestational diabetes,* can develop in women during pregnancy. The condition usually disappears after childbirth but can leave the woman at greater risk of developing type 2 diabetes.[13] Gaining

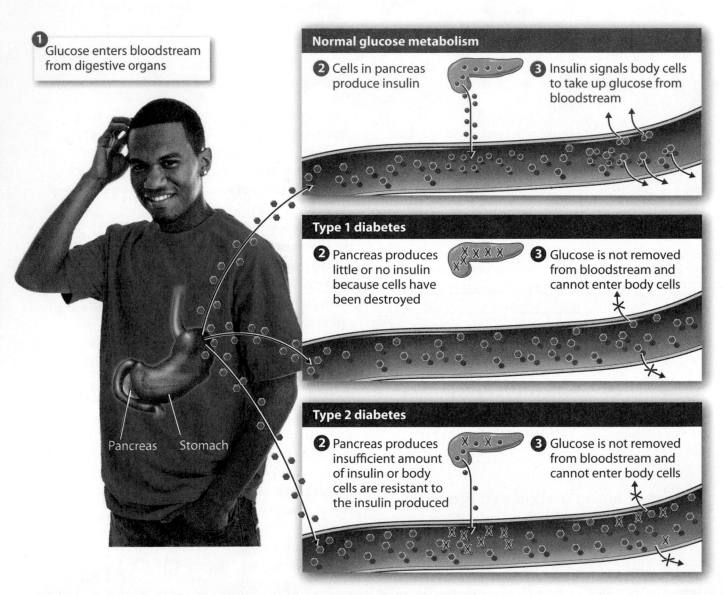

FIGURE **11.2**   In type 1 diabetes, the pancreas produces too little insulin. In type 2 diabetes, either the pancreas doesn't produce enough insulin or the body cells have developed resistance to insulin so they cannot properly respond to it. Both diseases result in body cells lacking energy because they cannot take up glucose from the bloodstream. Glucose accumulates in the blood causing high blood sugar levels that can lead to damage of nerves, kidneys, eyes, and blood vessels.

weight between pregnancies also increases the risk of type 2 diabetes.

Common symptoms of diabetes include excessive thirst and frequent urination. Physicians confirm a diagnosis of diabetes by measuring the levels of glucose in blood or urine.

You Can Lower Your Risk of Developing Diabetes

You may have an elevated risk for type 1 diabetes if you have a family history of diabetes or of autoimmune diseases.[14] Your risks for developing type 2 diabetes increase with the following factors:

- Age between 35 and 64

- High BMI (30 or above)

- Physical inactivity

- Poor diet

- A family history of type 2 diabetes

- Gestational diabetes during pregnancy

- Ethnic status (Native Americans, African Americans, or Hispanic Americans are twice as likely as Caucasian or Asian Americans to develop type 2 diabetes)

- A diagnosis of pre-diabetes

If you have several risk factors for diabetes, consult a physician and get your blood sugar tested. Early diagnosis of pre-diabetes or diabetes can allow earlier and better control of blood sugar and can help reduce blood vessel and nerve damage. If you are diagnosed with diabetes or pre-diabetes, closely follow your doctor's recommendations for diet, exercise, and drug treatments. While you cannot control your genetics, you can make lifestyle choices that can significantly lower your risk of developing type 2 diabetes.[15]

Eat a Healthy Diet You can lower your risk of type 2 diabetes by eating five to nine servings of fruits and vegetables and several servings of whole-grain foods each day.[16] Choose proteins and dairy products low in saturated fat and consume heart-healthy mono- and polyunsaturated oils.[17] Avoid refined carbohydrates and sugars: white bread, white potatoes, white rice, sweets (candy, cookies, desserts, and so on), sodas, and sweetened juices.[18] Surges in blood sugar followed by spikes in

insulin production can stimulate appetite and reduce your cells' sensitivity to insulin.[19] Proper combinations of protein, fiber, and carbohydrates/sugars (in reasonable portions) can control blood sugar levels throughout the day. For example, drink orange juice and eat some protein and fiber to help control blood glucose and to feel full longer.

Exercise Regularly Consistent physical activity plus a healthy diet can cut your risk of developing type 2 diabetes by nearly 60 percent.[20] Exercise builds muscle tissue, which is more sensitive to insulin and uses it more efficiently that other tissue. Thus exercise can help you prevent impaired glucose tolerance and maintain better blood glucose. Conversely, inactivity can increase your risks.[21] Researchers have estimated that 43 percent of new cases of type 2 diabetes could be prevented if adults viewed less than 10 hours of television per week and did the equivalent of 30 minutes or more of brisk walking each day.[22] The box Does Exercise Reduce the Risk for Chronic Diseases? covers the role of exercise in preventing all forms of chronic disease.

case study

GRACE

"The doctor told me that several things put me at high risk of becoming diabetic: lack of exercise, a high BMI, being Hispanic, and my family medical history—my aunt has diabetes. He also said that pre-diabetes is pretty common and that to keep it from getting worse, I should lose weight and start exercising. I'll admit it—I hate to sweat, and I know I don't always eat the healthiest foods! But if that is what it takes to keep from getting diabetes, I'm willing to give it a try."

THINK! What are the risk factors for type 2 diabetes? Do any of these risk factors apply to you?

ACT! Make a list of your personal risk factors for type 2 diabetes. List two to three simple things you could do to start addressing the easiest one.

Does Exercise Reduce the Risk for Chronic Diseases?

Compared to our predecessors in the first half of the twentieth century and before, we live longer lives and are safer, more amply fed, better housed, and better rested. Health-wise, too much so: Researchers have documented a downhill trend from activity to inactivity, and the price we are now paying for this unprecedented leisure is a dramatic rise in chronic illness.[1] We can change this trend, though; it just requires a little work. Where our predecessors had their exercise built into their day—chopping wood, gathering food, bringing water from a well—we may have be a little more creative to make exercise a part of our routines.

The National Institute of Diabetes and Digestive and Kidney Diseases (NIDDK) reports that losing weight and increasing physical activity over a three-year period reduced the development of type 2 diabetes by 58 percent in those with high risk for the disease. In those with pre-diabetes, such lifestyle changes helped prevent or delayed the onset of disease and was more cost-effective than medications.[2] An ideal program would include better nutrition and appropriate calorie-intake plus 150 minutes per week of moderate or vigorous aerobic exercise and resistance training.[3]

For people with chronic lung disease, regular physical activity (particularly aerobic exercise) can improve circulation and oxygen use by tissues, strengthen the heart, and build lung capacity.[4] The best prevention remains avoiding smoking.

To prevent osteoporosis, the National Osteoporosis Foundation recommends this as the best approach: Starting early in life, get enough calcium and vitamin D as well as regular weight-bearing and strengthening exercise such as running, field or court sports, and resistance training.[5] A recent review of animal and human studies on resistance exercise showed that bone responds to resistance training with slowed loss of mass and often increased mineral density.[6]

Finally, arthritis, too, responds to increased physical activity. The Centers for Disease Control and Prevention (CDC) reports that among adults with arthritis, 44 percent had no leisure-time activity, while 36 percent of adults without arthritis took no exercise.[7] The CDC also reports that people with arthritic knees can reduce their disability by 47 percent by engaging in physical activity (swimming is often recommended as easier on sore joints) at least three times per week.[8]

Clearly, increased exercise is a good way to prevent chronic disease and to help alleviate it!

Sources:

1. G. Heath, "Physical Activity Transitions and Chronic Disease," *American Journal of Lifestyle Medicine* 3, no. 1 (2009): 27S–31S.

2. National Diabetes Information Clearinghouse, National Institute of Diabetes and Digestive and Kidney Diseases (NIDDK), *National Diabetes Statistics, 2011* (Bethesda, MD: National Institutes of Health, 2011) NIH Publication no. 11–3892.

3. M. B. Weber and others, "Lifestyle Interventions and the Prevention and Treatment of Type 2 Diabetes," *American Journal of Lifestyle Medicine* 4, no. 6 (2010): 468–80.

4. "COPD Exercise and Activity Guidelines," Cleveland Clinic, http://my.clevelandclinic.org/disorders/chronic_obstructive_pulmonary_disease_copd/hic_copd_exercise_and_activity_guidelines.aspx (2011).

5. National Osteoporosis Foundation, "Fast Facts," www.nof.org/node/40 (2011).

6. S. Going and M. Laudermilk, "Osteoporosis and Strength Training," *American Journal of Lifestyle Medicine* 3, no. 4 (2009): 310–9.

7. Centers for Disease Control and Prevention, "Arthritis-Related Statistics," www.cdc.gov/arthritis/data_statistics/arthritis_related_stats.htm (updated October 2010).

8. Ibid.

What Is Lung Disease?

Lung disease is the fourth leading cause of death in the United States, after heart disease, cancer, and stroke. In 2009, lung disease was responsible for one death in six, or more than 400,000 people. Today, more than 35 million Americans are living with chronic lung diseases such as asthma, emphysema, and bronchitis.[23]

Asthma Has a Wide Range of Triggers

LIVE IT! ONLINE

Worksheet 43
Check Your
Asthma I.Q.

Asthma is a chronic disease in which the lungs' airways swell, restricting airflow. Increased mucous makes breathing more difficult and tiny airways often react with spasms that lead to wheezing, coughing bouts, and shortness of breath (Figure 11.3). Air restriction can be so severe that an individual loses consciousness and can even die during a prolonged asthma attack. Controlling asthma requires medical care as well as avoiding or responding to triggers, such as smoke, dust mites, air pollution, cockroaches, pets, mold, flu, strenuous exercise, and in some cases, stress and strong emotional responses.

If you have asthma, learn to anticipate and avoid its triggers. Carry asthma inhalers and other medications and use them as prescribed by your physician to prevent serious asthma-related problems.

COPD

Chronic obstructive pulmonary disease (COPD) affects about 12 million Americans—25 times more people than lung cancer.[24] COPD is the fourth leading cause of death in America.[25] Chronic obstructive pulmonary disease refers to two lung diseases that disrupt airflow and cause breathing problems: **emphysema** and **chronic bronchitis**.

Emphysema Emphysema begins when toxic substances such as tobacco smoke damage the millions of tiny air sacs (called *alveoli*) in the lungs. As alveoli are destroyed, emphysema patients find it more and more difficult to exhale. Their chest cavities can gradually begin to expand, producing a characteristic "barrel-shaped" chest. They may become winded by limited exertion and feel as though they are suffocating. Over time, the condition taxes the heart and can lead to hospitalization or death.

Chronic Bronchitis In **chronic bronchitis**, cigarette smoke, air pollution, mold, infectious agents, or other irritants cause the bronchial tubes to become inflamed. Symptoms of chronic bronchitis include chronic cough, increased mucus, frequent clearing of the throat, and shortness of breath

asthma A condition in which air passages to and within the lungs "overreact" to smoke, allergens, or other triggers

chronic obstructive pulmonary disease (COPD) Progressive lung disease that causes breathing difficulties; includes emphysema and chronic bronchitis

emphysema A type of COPD involving damage to the air sacs (alveoli) in the lungs

chronic bronchitis A type of COPD characterized by inflammation of the main air passages (bronchi) in the lungs

❶ Air enters the respiratory system from the nose and mouth and travels through the bronchial tubes.

❷ In a nonasthmatic person, the muscles around the bronchial tubes are relaxed and the tissue thin, allowing for easy airflow.

❸ In an asthmatic person, the muscles of the bronchial tubes tighten and thicken, and the air passages become inflamed and mucus-filled, making it difficult for air to flow.

FIGURE **11.3** Asthma is an inflammation of the airways within the lungs.

that tend to persist and reoccur. Continued exposure to the irritants can cause scarring in the bronchial tubes that leads to a chronically thicker mucus layer. A person with chronic bronchitis is more susceptible to pneumonia, cardiovascular diseases, and other medical conditions.[26]

You Can Reduce Your Risk of Developing COPD

In 85 to 90 percent of emphysema and chronic bronchitis cases, smoking is the primary risk factor.[27] So, don't smoke or spend time in smoky areas! Some chronic bronchitis and emphysema cases, however, can be attributed to poor urban air quality or to home and workplace air pollution, including frequent fireplace use or industrial exposures. Changing your habits or your home/work environments may be necessary to reduce your risks.

Respiratory infections can trigger some COPD cases and make existing cases worse. People with COPD or COPD risk factors should try to avoid colds and flu by getting flu shots, by observing general wellness behaviors, by washing hands regularly—particularly after being around crowds in confined spaces—and by keeping hands away from the mouth, nose, and eyes. People who are short of breath and feel as though they are suffocating are often reluctant to exert themselves by exercising. This reluctance, however, can lead to progressive physical deterioration and even disability.[28] Started slowly and built up gradually under medical supervision, exercise programs can give COPD patients more physical capacity and less fatigue and breathlessness. For people with risk factors for COPD but no current breathing problems, exercise is essential for maintaining lung function.[29]

What Is Osteoporosis?

Do you have a grandmother who looks a bit stooped forward or hunched around the shoulders, or perhaps has broken a bone during a fall? These symptoms describe a common condition of older Americans: **osteoporosis**. Fifty-five percent of all Americans over 50 have osteoporosis or early signs of it: 10 million people have the full-blown disease and another 34 million have *osteopenia* (diminished bone mass; also called low bone density), putting them at heightened risk for the disease.[30]

osteoporosis A chronic degenerative bone disease characterized by diminished bone mass and porous, brittle bones

Osteoporosis Is Characterized by Thinning, Brittle Bones

Osteoporosis literally means "porous bone," and indeed, in this chronic degenerative bone disease, the bones become full of holes, brittle, and susceptible to breaking (see Figure 11.4). The thinning can be so extreme that a simple cough, sneeze, or bend can cause a bone to break. Osteoporosis develops over a period of years, beginning with diminished bone mass that is often rooted in the eating, smoking, drinking, and exercise habits of youth. Race, age, frame size, family history, and other factors can increase your risk. In general, women are more susceptible than men but the incidence of osteoporosis is rising in males. Because most of your bone mass accumulates before adulthood, building strong bones during childhood and adolescence can help prevent osteoporosis later in life.[31]

Your body builds bone tissue in response to the physical demands you place on it. Weight-bearing

(a) Normal bone

(b) Osteoporotic bone

FIGURE **11.4** Osteoporosis causes bones to become more porous.

exercise (during which you bear your body weight on your legs) and resistance exercise (such as weight lifting) are both conducive to building bone tissue. The body also stores excess calcium and phosphates in bone tissue and draws upon them when these minerals are needed elsewhere. Physical inactivity signals a diminished need for fortified bones, leading the body to release more minerals and resulting in decreased reserves.[32] In postmenopausal women, declining levels of certain hormones also cause the body to retain fewer minerals in bone tissue, making bones more vulnerable to osteoporosis.

A simple, noninvasive procedure called a *bone mineral density test* can evaluate your bone mass. Bone-density testing is important for people in high-risk groups for osteoporosis, because the disease is essentially symptom free.

You Can Reduce Your Risk for Developing Osteoporosis

You are at greater risk of osteoporosis if you are female, if you are thin or have a small frame, if you are over 50 (Figure 11.5), if you have broken a bone over age 50, or if you have a low bone mass reading. Beyond these factors, there are four groups of risk factors for osteoporosis: genetic, hormonal, nutritional, and lifestyle choices. Your wellness choices can lessen many of the individual risk factors within each group.

- *Genetic factors.* Having a close relative who has been diagnosed with osteoporosis or has suffered a fracture after age 50 increases your risk. You can't change these factors, but they can alert you to osteoporosis risk and inspire greater effort toward prevention.

- *Hormonal factors.* Diminishing estrogen levels in women—and to a lesser extent, testosterone in men—can lead to bone "dismantling," calcium release, osteopenia, or full-fledged osteoporosis. Women are particularly at risk and can lose up to 20 percent of bone mass in the first five to seven years after menopause.[33] Also at risk are women whose menstrual periods stop prematurely due to heavy exercise, extreme dieting, or illness.

- *Nutritional factors.* We all need calcium in our daily diet to build strong bones. We also need vitamin D so that the body can transport calcium out of the digestive tract and deliver it to bone-building cells. Getting enough calcium (1,300 mg/day during adolescence; 1,000 mg/day from ages 19 to 50; and 1,200 mg/day after age 50) and enough vitamin D (400 to 800 IU/day) is important to stave off osteoporosis.[34] In other words, build the best skeletal support you can now, and continue those good habits throughout life!

- *Lifestyle choices.* Your daily habits can increase or decrease osteoporosis risk. Try to get enough calcium and vitamin D each day. Make regular weight-bearing exercise and resistance exercise part of your fitness routine. Avoid smoking and drinking. Both can reduce your body's ability to retain calcium. If you have risk factors for osteoporosis, get a bone-density test. Avoid caffeine, carbonated sodas, and too much salt.

What Is Arthritis?

Arthritis is acute or chronic inflammation of a joint that can cause stiffness, aching, swelling, or permanent deformation and dysfunction. About one in five American adults or 46 to 50 million people have some form of the one hundred diseases and conditions that fall under the category of arthritis.[35] It limits daily activity such as walking, dressing, and bathing for seven million Americans, making it the leading cause of disability in the United States.[36]

The most common types of arthritis

> **arthritis** Inflammation of joints, typically accompanied by pain, swelling, and stiffness

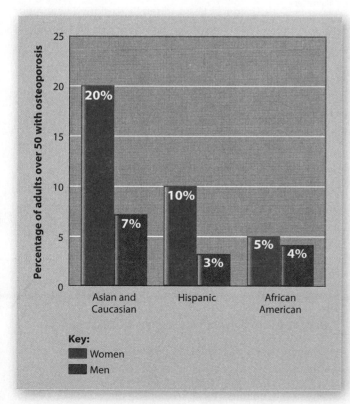

FIGURE **11.5** Osteoporosis is most prevalent among Asian and Caucasian females over age 50.

Source: National Osteoporosis Foundation, "Fast Facts," www.nof.org/node/40 (2011).

bone can start grinding against bone, causing pain and sometimes creating detached bone, cartilage fragments, or little projections called *bone spurs*. Extra joint fluid builds up, acting like a buffer but also enlarging the joint in a way that restricts movement. Osteoarthritis usually affects the hips, knees, toes, fingers, or joints in the spine (Figure 11.6).

Rheumatoid Arthritis

Rheumatoid arthritis is a chronic inflammation of the joints that tends to appear between ages 25 and 40 and affects about 1.5 million Americans.[38] The body's immune system triggers an attack on one or more joints, with white blood cells crowding into the tight areas and releasing chemicals that increase blood flow. The influx usually causes redness, warmth, fluid buildup, and swelling. This inflammation, in turn, irritates the joint, wears down the cartilage, and eventually leads to bone-on-bone grinding. Hands with painfully misshapen knuckles are characteristic of rheumatoid arthritis, although the condition can affect knees and other joints as well.

Understanding Over-the-Counter Painkillers

Swelling, pain, and stiffness in a joint are all symptoms of arthritis; redness and warmth to the touch can distinguish rheumatoid arthritis from osteoarthritis. Pain-relieving medications and physical therapy have been found to help ease some of the pain and dysfunction of arthritis. In large, carefully designed scientific trials, supplements such as glucosamine and chondroitin appear to be no more effective than placebos.[39]

You Can Reduce Your Risks of Developing Arthritis

Your likelihood of developing rheumatoid arthritis is only one-tenth as great as your chances of developing osteoarthritis, and the risk factors are quite different for the two conditions. Because rheumatoid arthritis is a genetically determined autoimmune disease, your risk for it rises if you or a close relative have had asthma, lupus, or type 1 diabetes. The risk factors for osteoarthritis include:

- Advanced age

- Genetics

- Injuries (a single accident, or repeated stress)

- Obesity (extra weight adds pressure on weight-bearing joints and may cause premature wear and tear)

- Physical weakness (weak muscles, inactivity, or certain diseases can atrophy the muscles that surround and normally protect joints)

FIGURE **11.6** Stiff, aching joints are characteristic of both osteoarthritis and rheumatoid arthritis.

are *osteoarthritis*, caused by long-term wear and tear of cartilage, and *rheumatoid arthritis*, caused by autoimmune activity.[37]

Osteoarthritis

In a joint, two bones are attached by tendons and ligaments, allowing one or both bones to move relative to the other. A layer of *cartilage* (connective tissue) separates the bones, allowing smooth movement. **Osteoarthritis** is a slow, progressive joint disease that involves a breakdown of cartilage due to injury, repetitive use, joint deformity, the physical strain of obesity, muscle weakness, and other causes. After years of wear and tear,

osteoarthritis A type of arthritis characterized by stiffness, aching, swelling, or permanent deformation and dysfunction of a joint, caused primarily by wear and tear

rheumatoid arthritis A type of arthritis characterized by chronic inflammation, swelling, and pain in a joint brought about by an autoimmune attack

- Hormone deficiency (especially in women after menopause)
- Vitamin deficiency (vitamin D promotes healthy cartilage)

A good strategy is to avoid hard-hitting activities such as football, or to at least alternate such activities with less percussive sports—especially if joint problems start to appear. The kinds of repetitive motions that go into practicing and excelling at nearly any sport will eventually cause joint wear and tear. High-level and competitive sports performance is a choice people make for many reasons—including benefit to fitness and wellness—despite the inevitable costs. Good athletes, trainers, and coaches keep athletes' future joint problems in mind, including switching to milder forms of activity when the prospect of joint damage and future disability starts to emerge.

Finally, to avoid deficiencies, be sure to get the proper amount of vitamin D and to consult a doctor about potential hormonal deficiencies.

casestudy

GRACE

"I have a cousin, Bart, who plays college football. He's been playing since junior high school, and his apartment is full of trophies. But his neck, back, and knees are already starting to bother him. In fact, he has to use ice and aspirin to get the swelling down in his joints after most of the practices and games. He's heard that college and professional athletes can wind up with arthritis later on, and he wants to keep that from happening. But football is Bart's life and if he could get into the pros he'd be ecstatic."

THINK! What steps could an athlete like Bart take to prevent arthritis? What steps could you take to reduce your risk?

ACT! Make a list of your risk factors for arthritis. List 2–3 simple things you could do to start addressing the easiest one.

chapterin**review**

videos

Log on to **www.pearsonhighered.com/hopson** or MyFitnessLab to view these chapter-related videos.

Will Diabetes Cases Double in 25 Years?

Diabetes Plagues West Virginia County

Understanding Over-the-Counter Painkillers

onlineresources

Log on to **www.pearsonhighered.com/hopson** or MyFitnessLab for access to these book-related resources, and for links to other useful websites.

Audio case study
Audio PowerPoint lecture

Take Charge of Your Health! Worksheets:
Worksheet 43 Check Your Asthma I.Q.
Behavior Change Log Book and
Wellness Journal

Lab 11.1 Are You at Risk for Diabetes?

Pre- and post-quizzes
Glossary flashcards

reviewquestions

1. Which one of the following is true about chronic diseases?
   a. In the United States, chronic diseases cause 7 percent of deaths and kill 170,000 Americans per year.
   b. Chronic diseases are mainly a problem in the developing world.
   c. Getting one chronic disease usually gives you immunity from other chronic diseases.
   • d. Smoking, poor diet, and physical inactivity are the underlying causes of more than 30 percent of chronic disease deaths in the U.S.
2. Which one of these statements is true about chronic diseases?
   a. They tend to come on suddenly.
   b. They usually last for short periods and often resolve without treatment.
   c. Pharmaceutical companies have developed many effective vaccines for preventing chronic diseases.
   • d. They have multiple causes.
3. Which one of the following can help you reduce your risk of type 2 diabetes and cardiovascular disease?
   a. Eating one serving of fruits and vegetables per day
   b. Eating more foods that contain saturated fat
   • c. Maintaining a BMI above 25
   d. Avoiding drug and alcohol abuse
4. Which one of the following statements is true about type 2 diabetes?
   • a. It is the fastest growing chronic disease in America.
   b. It has a strong genetic basis and usually develops during childhood.
   c. Body cells can still use insulin properly, but the pancreas usually stops making insulin.
   d. Exercise is unimportant in its prevention and management.
5. The biggest risk factor for chronic obstructive pulmonary disease is
   a. allergies.
   b. genetics.
   • c. smoking.
   d. physical inactivity.
6. Which one of the following statements about COPD is correct?
   a. A smoker's chances are far higher of developing lung cancer than COPD.
   b. A smoker's chances are far higher of dying from lung cancer than COPD.
   c. You can develop emphysema or chronic bronchitis but avoid COPD.
   • d. Ephysema destroys alveoli and lung capacity.
7. Which of the following is a risk factor for developing osteoporosis?
   a. Regular weight-bearing exercise
   • b. Being thin or having a small frame
   c. Getting excess calcium in the diet
   d. Having high levels of estrogen hormones
8. Diminished bone mass usually has its roots in behaviors established during
   • a. childhood or young adulthood.
   b. menopause.
   c. middle age.
   d. old age.
9. Which of the following statements is true about osteoporosis?
   a. Women have to worry about it, but men don't.
   b. Getting enough protein in the diet can help prevent osteoporosis.
   c. Females needn't worry about osteoporosis until after menopause.
   • d. More than half of all Americans over 50 have osteoporosis or osteopenia.
10. Which one of these will increase your risk of osteoarthritis?
    a. Maintaining a healthy BMI
    b. Regular weight-bearing exercise
    c. Regular resistance exercise
    • d. Playing competitive football

critical**thinking**questions

1. Give an example of two chronic diseases that are interrelated. Explain how they are interrelated.

2. Identify five behaviors that can help you avoid chronic diseases, and explain why these behaviors can lower your risks.

references

1. Centers for Disease Control and Prevention, "Chronic Diseases and Health Promotion," www.cdc.gov/chronicdisease/overview/index.htm (updated July 2010).

2. R. M. Merrill, *Introduction to Epidemiology* (Jones and Bartlett: Sudbury MA, 2011): 274.

3. Centers for Disease Control and Prevention (CDC), "Diabetes Successes and Opportunities for Population-Based Prevention and Control: At A Glance 2011," www.cdc.gov/chronicdisease/resources/publications/AAG/ddt.htm (updated August 2011).

4. Ibid.

5. Centers for Disease Control and Prevention, "Diabetes Data & Trends," http://apps.nccd.cdc.gov/ddtstrs (2008).

6. CDC, "Diabetes Successes and Opportunities for Population-Based Prevention and Control," 2011.

7. American Diabetes Association, "Diabetes Basics: Pre-Diabetes FAQs" www.diabetes.org/diabetes-basics/prevention/prediabetes/pre-diabetes-faqs.html (accessed October 2011).

8. National Diabetes Information Clearinghouse, National Institute of Diabetes and Digestive and Kidney Diseases (NIDDK), *National Diabetes Statistics, 2011* (Bethesda, MD: National Institutes of Health, 2011) NIH Publication no. 11–3892.

9. Ibid.

10. Ibid.

11. Ibid.

12. H. Rodbard, "Diabetes Screening, Diagnosis, and Therapy in Pediatric Patients with Type 2 Diabetes," *Medscape Journal of Medicine* 10, no. 8 (2008): 184.

13. CDC, "Diabetes Successes and Opportunities for Population-Based Prevention and Control," 2011.

14. Ibid.

15. National Diabetes Education Program, *Small Steps. Big Rewards. Your GAME PLAN to Prevent Type 2 Diabetes: Information for Patients* (Bethesda, MD: National Institutes of Health, 2006) NIH Publication no. 06-5334.

16. J. de Munter and others, "Whole Grain, Bran, and Germ Intake and Risk of Type 2 Diabetes: A Prospective Cohort Study and Systematic Review," *PLoS Medicine* 4, no.8 (2007): e261; J. Anderson and others, "Health Benefits of Dietary Fiber," *Nutrition Reviews* 67, no. 4 (2009): 188–205; B. Hopping and others, "Dietary Fiber, Magnesium, and Glycemic Load Alter Risk of Type 2 Diabetes in a Multiethnic Cohort in Hawaii," *Journal of Nutrition* 140, no. 1 (2010): 68–74.

17. M. Lankinen and others, "Fatty Fish Intake Decreases Lipids Related to Inflammation and Insulin Signaling—A Lipidomics Approach," *PLoS One* 4, no. 4 (2009): e5258.

18. Linus Pauling Institute, "Glycemic Index and Glycemic Load," http://lpi.oregonstate.edu/infocenter/foods/grains/gigl.html (updated April 2010).

19. CDC, "Diabetes Successes and Opportunities for Population-Based Prevention and Control," 2011.

20. Ibid.

21. Ibid; F. B. Hu and others, "Television Watching and Other Sedentary Behaviors in Relation to Risk of Obesity and Type-2 Diabetes Mellitus in Women," *Journal of the American Medical Association* 289, no. 14 (2003): 1785–91.

22. Ibid.

23. American Lung Association, "Lung Disease," www.lungusa.org/lung-disease (2010).

24. National Heart, Lung, and Blood Institute, Diseases and Conditions Index, "What Is COPD?" www.nhlbi.nih.gov/health/dci/Diseases/Copd/Copd_WhatIs.html (June 2010).

25. Ibid.

26. American Lung Association, "Chronic Obstructive Pulmonary Disease (COPD) Fact Sheet," www.lungusa.org/lung-disease/copd/resources/facts-figures/COPD-Fact-Sheet.html (February 2011).

27. Ibid.

28. R. H. Dressendorfer and others, American College of Sports Medicine, "ACSM Current Comment: Exercise for Persons with COPD," October 2002.

29. Ibid.

30. National Osteoporosis Foundation, "Fast Facts," www.nof.org/node/40 (2011).

31. CDC, "Calcium and Bone Health," www.cdc.gov/nutrition/everyone/basics/vitamins/calcium.html (2011); National Osteoporosis Foundation, "Fast Facts," 2011.

32. John Postlethwait and Janet L. Hopson, *Explore Life* (Pacific Grove, CA: Brooks/Cole Publishing Company, 2003): 516–7.

33. Ibid.

34. Office of Dietary Supplements, National Institutes of Health, "Dietary Supplement Fact Sheet: Calcium," http://ods.od.nih.gov/factsheets/calcium/ (reviewed August 2011).

35. Arthritis Foundation, "Arthritis Facts," www.arthritis.org/facts.php (2011).

36. Ibid.

37. Arthritis Foundation, Disease Center, "What Is Osteoarthritis?" www.arthritis.org/what-is-osteoarthritis.php (2011); Arthritis Foundation, Disease Center, "What Is Rheumatoid Arthritis?" www.arthritis.org/types-what-is-rheumatoid-arthritis.php (2011).

38. CDC, "Rheumatoid Arthritis," www.cdc.gov/arthritis/basics/rheumatoid.htm (updated September 2011).

39. A.D. Sawitzke, "Clinical Efficacy and Safety of Glucosamine, Chondroitin Sulphate, Their Combination, Celecoxib or Placebo Taken to Treat Osteoarthritis of the Knee: 2-Year Results from GAIT," *Annals of the Rheumatic Diseases* 69, no. 8 (2010): 1459–64.

LAB 11.1 • ARE YOU AT RISK FOR DIABETES?

Name: _____ Date: _____

Instructor: _____ Section: _____

Purpose: To assess your personal risk factors for developing diabetes.

Directions: Answer the questions below.

	Yes	No
1. Do you have a history of diabetes in your family?	☐ Yes	☐ No
2. Do any of your primary relatives (mother, father, sister, brother, or grandparents) have diabetes?	☐ Yes	☐ No
3. Are you overweight (BMI above 25) or obese (BMI above 30)?	☐ Yes	☐ No
4. Are you typically sedentary (seldom, if ever, engage in vigorous aerobic exercise)?	☐ Yes	☐ No
5. Have you noticed an increase in your craving for water or other beverages (not related to physical activity or summer heat)?	☐ Yes	☐ No
6. Have you noticed that you have to urinate more frequently than you used to during a typical day?	☐ Yes	☐ No
7. Have you noticed any tingling or numbness in your hands and feet, which might indicate circulatory problems?	☐ Yes	☐ No
8. Do you often feel a gnawing hunger during the day, even though you usually eat regular meals?	☐ Yes	☐ No
9. Have you noticed that you are losing weight without conscious dieting and/or increase in exercise?	☐ Yes	☐ No
10. Are you often so tired that you find it difficult to stay awake to study, watch television, or engage in other activities?	☐ Yes	☐ No
11. Have you noticed that you have skin irritations more frequently and that minor infections don't heal as quickly as they used to?	☐ Yes	☐ No
12. Have you noticed any unusual changes in your vision (blurring, difficulty in focusing, etc.)?	☐ Yes	☐ No
13. Have you noticed unusual pain or swelling in your joints?	☐ Yes	☐ No
14. Do you often feel weak or nauseated if you wait too long to eat a meal?	☐ Yes	☐ No
15. If you are a woman, have you had several vaginal (yeast) infections during the past year?	☐ Yes	☐ No

If you answer yes to three of more of these questions, consider seeking medical advice. Talk to health professionals at your student health center or make an appointment with your family physician.

12

Reducing Your Risk of Cancer

Learning Outcomes

1. Define cancer and explain how it develops and spreads.

 HEAR IT! ONLINE Audio case study and audio Power-Point lecture

2. Discuss the causes of cancer.

3. List seven major types of cancer and the risk factors for each.

 SEE IT! ONLINE Tanning Beds Mammogram Controversy

4. Describe the factors that affect an individual's risk of developing cancer, including lifestyle choices, biological factors, and environmental exposures.

 SEE IT! ONLINE Alcohol and Cancer

5. Identify your own risk factors and make choices to reduce those risks.

 DO IT! ONLINE Lab 12.1 Assess Your Personal Risk of Cancer

Lab 12.2 Plan for Cancer Prevention

6. Discuss approaches to cancer treatment and recovery.

 SEE IT! ONLINE Treating Cancer with Bone Drugs

Possible Melanoma Treatment

 LIVE IT! ONLINE Take Charge of Your Health worksheets and Behavior Change Logs for assessing your cancer risk and creating a change plan

Pre- and post-quizzes and glossary flashcards REVIEW IT! ONLINE

385

casestudy

TIM

"I'm Tim. I'm in my second year of community college in Arizona and I work part-time in the pro shop at the local golf course. I'm a recreation major; between my classes, labs, and job, I spend half of my time outside. I really like being outdoors, and I like having a tan. I know that I should use sunscreen, but I just get lazy about it. Anyway, skin cancer is mainly a problem for very light-skinned people, right?"

Cancer is second only to cardiovascular disease as a cause of death in the United States; in 2011, cancer killed an estimated 572,000 Americans.[1] Nearly half of all American males and one-third of all American females will develop cancer at some point during their lives.[2] Lifestyle choices have a dramatic impact on cancer risk: Scientific evidence suggests that tobacco use causes 30 percent of cancer deaths, while another one-third of the deaths are related to overweight or obesity, physical inactivity, and poor nutrition.[3] Overexposure to the sun's harmful rays and exposure to certain viruses and other infectious agents can also contribute to skin cancer and cancers at various other sites.[4] Understanding the relationships between cancer and lifestyle choices can help you identify unhealthy behaviors to change in order to reduce your risk of developing these potentially deadly diseases.

cancer The name given to a large group of diseases characterized by the uncontrolled growth and spread of abnormal cells

tumor A clumping of cells that grows more rapidly than surrounding tissue

benign Harmless; refers to a noncancerous tumor

malignant Very dangerous or harmful; refers to a cancerous tumor

metastasis Process by which cancer spreads from one area to different areas of the body

What Is Cancer?

Cancer is the name given to a large group of diseases characterized by the uncontrolled growth and spread of abnormal cells.

Cancer Is the Unchecked Growth of Abnormal Cells

Living cells contain biochemical instructions called DNA that control the cell's growth, division, and daily functions. Sometimes a segment of a DNA molecule inside a cell becomes damaged. This may cause a *mutation* or a change in the genetic instructions that can override the cell's normal cycle of growing and dividing. The offspring of that mutated cell can form a **tumor**—a mass of cells that serves no physiological function and that may grow and spread into other areas.

Most tumors are **benign** (noncancerous)—they are generally harmless unless their growth obstructs or crowds out normal tissue. A benign tumor is usually enclosed in a capsule of collagen that prevents it from spreading to other areas of the body (Figure 12.1).

Cancerous tumors may stay localized; these are called *in situ* carcinomas. Lacking a capsule, *in situ* carcinomas can grow in place and disrupt neighboring tissues. Or they can further mutate into malignant tumors. **Malignant** tumors invade surrounding tissue. *Metastases,* or clusters of malignant cells, can break off of them and migrate to other parts of the body through the bloodstream in the process of **metastasis** (Figure 12.2). Once lodged in new places, metastases can disrupt normal cell functioning and lead to more mutations. As the invaded, now mutated cells divide

FIGURE **12.1** A mutation in the genetic material of a skin cell triggers abnormal cell division, resulting in a benign tumor. A capsule of normal cells keeps the tumor localized.

Genetically altered skin cell · Basement membrane · Abnormal new growth · Benign tumor

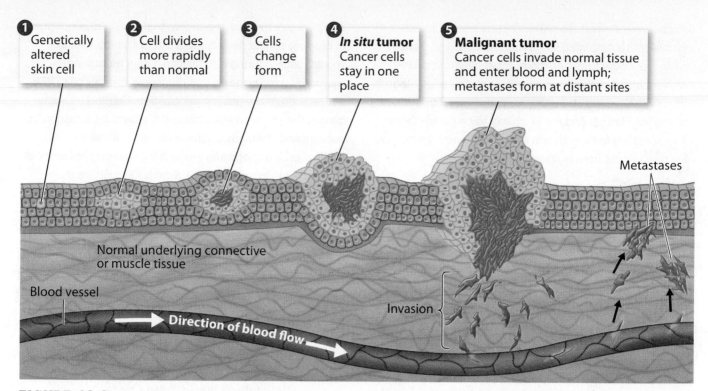

FIGURE 12.2 A mutation in the DNA of a skin cell triggers abnormal cell division and changes cell formation, resulting in a cancerous tumor. *In situ* cancer remains localized; malignant cancer spreads to neighboring tissues and can metastasize to other parts of the body.

and metastasize further, the cancer spreads. A **biopsy** (a surgical retrieval of cells, followed by microscopic or biochemical examination of their characteristics) can usually determine whether a given tumor is benign or malignant.

To grow much beyond the size of the tip of a ballpoint pen, a tumor must have its own blood supply.[5] In a process called **angiogenesis**, malignant cells give off growth factors that induce new blood capillaries to grow toward the tumor. The new capillaries supply the tumor cells with oxygen and nutrients and carry off wastes, allowing the tumor to grow much faster and larger. Some cancer treatments prevent the growth of new blood vessels and thus the growth of the tumor as well.[6]

Cancers Are Assigned Classes and Stages

There are four different classes of cancerous tumors:

- **Carcinomas** are solid tumors that occur in epithelial tissue (the tissues covering body surfaces and lining most body cavities). Carcinomas are the most common class of tumors and include those of the breast, lung, intestines, skin, and mouth.

- **Sarcomas** are solid tumors that occur in middle layers of tissue—for example, in bones, muscles, and other connective tissue. Less common than carcinomas, sarcomas generally grow faster and become dangerous more quickly.

- **Lymphomas** are malignant cells that develop in the lymph nodes, lymph vessels, or related infection-fighting organs of the body. They generally fall into one of two categories: *non-Hodgkin's* lymphoma or *Hodgkin's* lymphoma.

- **Leukemias** are nonsolid cancers characterized by an increased number of white blood cells in blood-forming parts of the body, particularly the bone marrow and spleen.

A doctor who specializes in cancer treatment (called an **oncologist**)

biopsy Surgical retrieval of cells and microscopic examination of tissue to determine if a cancer is present

angiogenesis Process in which malignant cells induce new blood capillaries to grow toward the tumor

carcinomas Solid tumors that occur in epithelial tissues (the tissues covering body surfaces and lining most body cavities)

sarcomas Solid tumors that occur in middle layers of tissue (for example, in bones, muscles, and connective tissue)

lymphomas Tumors that develop in lymph nodes, lymph vessels, or related infection-fighting regions of the body

leukemias Nonsolid cancers characterized by an increase in the number of white blood cells, particularly the bone marrow and spleen

oncologist A doctor who specializes in cancer detection and treatment determines the class of a patient's tumor and rates its seriousness, assigning a stage number from 1 to 4 based on the size of the tumor(s), the number of lymph nodes involved, and the degree of spread (or metastasis). Stage 1 tumors are localized and often curable. Stage 2 to 4 cancers have spread farther and are less likely to be cured. Table 12.1 shows the most common cancer sites and the number of annual deaths from each type.

What Causes Cancer?

Most research supports the idea that cancer is caused by both *external* factors, such as chemicals, radiation, viruses, and lifestyle, and *internal* factors, like hormones, immune conditions, and inherited mutations.[7]

carcinogens Cancer-causing agents

oncogenes Suspected cancer-causing genes

These factors may act separately, together, or in sequence to promote cancer development. Some mutations arise spontaneously during cell division. Other mutations are caused by **carcinogens** that damage a normal cell's DNA and reprogram the genetic information. Common carcinogens in the environment include the ultraviolet radiation in sunlight and the tar in cigarette smoke.[8] Cancer may also be caused by **oncogenes**—genes that researchers suspect play a role in uncontrolled cell growth. Oncogenes may initially be dormant but become activated by age, stress, viral infection, radiation, or exposure to other carcinogens, transforming healthy cells into cancerous ones. Women, for example, who inherit a mutation of oncogenes are significantly more likely to develop breast cancer.[9]

Most experts agree that many cancers are preventable through modifying environmental factors and avoiding risk-related behaviors. For example, at

TABLE 12.1 Leading Sites of New Cancer Cases and Deaths, 2011 Estimates			
Estimated New Cases of Cancer		**Estimated Deaths from Cancer**	
Site	Incidence (% of all cases)	Site	Mortality (% of all deaths)
Male			
Prostate	240,890 (29%)	Lung & bronchus	85,600 (28%)
Lung & bronchus	115,060 (14%)	Prostate	33,720 (11%)
Colon & rectum	71,850 (9%)	Colon & rectum	25,250 (8%)
Urinary bladder	52,020 (6%)	Pancreas	19,360 (6%)
Melanoma of the skin	40,010 (5%)	Liver & intrahepatic bile duct	13,260 (4%)
Kidney & renal pelvis	37,120 (5%)	Leukemia	12,740 (4%)
Non-Hodgkin lymphoma	36,060 (4%)	Esophagus	11,910 (4%)
Oral cavity & pharynx	27,710 (3%)	Urinary bladder	10,670 (4%)
Leukemia	25,320 (3%)	Non-Hodgkin lymphoma	9,750 (3%)
Pancreas	22,050 (3%)	Kidney & renal pelvis	8,270 (3%)
All Sites	822,300 (100%)	All Sites	300,430 (100%)
Female			
Breast	230,480 (30%)	Lung & bronchus	71,340 (26%)
Lung & bronchus	106,070 (14%)	Breast	39,520 (15%)
Colon & rectum	69,360 (9%)	Colon & rectum	24,130 (9%)
Uterine corpus	46,470 (6%)	Pancreas	18,300 (7%)
Thyroid	36,550 (5%)	Ovary	15,460 (6%)
Non-Hodgkin lymphoma	30,300 (4%)	Non-Hodgkin lymphoma	9,570 (4%)
Melanoma of the skin	30,220 (4%)	Leukemia	9,040 (3%)
Kidney & renal pelvis	23,800 (3%)	Uterine corpus	8,120 (3%)
Ovary	21,990 (3%)	Liver & intrahepatic bile duct	6,330 (2%)
Pancreas	21,980 (3%)	Brain & other nervous system	5,670 (2%)
All Sites	774,370 (100%)	All Sites	271,520 (100%)

Data from: The American Cancer Society, *Cancer Facts and Figures* 2011 (Atlanta: American Cancer Society, 2011).

casestudy

TIM

"One of my good friends, Kevin, was recently diagnosed with skin cancer. He's a surfer and a life-guard, and I've never seen him without a tan. Fortunately, they caught it early and he's going to be OK. Ever since his diagnosis, he's been lecturing me about wearing sunscreen and about how I should learn from his mistakes. The other day, I counted up the number of hours I spend in the sun—it's at least ten hours each week."

THINK! Count the number of hours per week you spend in the sun. Do you wear protective clothing and sunscreen with a SPF of at least 15 ?

ACT! Write down two things you could do differently to protect your skin.

HEAR IT! ONLINE

· ·

least 30 percent of all cancer deaths and 87 percent of lung cancer deaths are attributable to smoking.[10]

What Are the Most Common Types of Cancers?

There are many different types of cancers. This section surveys the most common types.

Skin Cancer Is the Most Common

More than 3.5 million cases of skin cancer are diagnosed in the United States each year.[11] Most skin cancer cases are *basal cell carcinoma* or *squamous cell carcinoma* and are highly curable. **Malignant melanoma** accounts for only about 5 percent of skin cancer cases, but causes

most of the deaths from skin cancer each year. Once melanoma has spread, it is extremely difficult to treat. Malignant melanoma has become the most frequent cancer in Caucasian women aged 25 to 29; in women aged 30 to 34, it is second only to breast cancer.[12]

> **malignant melanoma** An invasive cancer of the pigment-producing cells of the skin

The risk of skin cancer is greatest for people with light skin; with blond, red, or light brown hair; and with blue, green, or gray eyes. A Caucasian's risk of melanoma is ten times higher than an African American's. risk.[13] You are also at risk if you burn easily, peel readily, and spend lots of time outdoors. High-altitude exposure, having a relative who has been treated for skin cancer, and inadequate use of sunscreen (e.g., using an SPF below 15 or failing to reapply every two hours) can further increase your risk.

Many people do not know what to look for when examining themselves for skin cancer. Basal and squamous cell carcinomas show up most commonly on the face, ears, neck, arms, hands, and legs as warty bumps, colored spots, or scaly patches (see Figure 12.3a, b). Many skin cancers begin in less obvious places, such as between the toes, near the genitals or anus, or on the scalp. Surgery may be necessary to remove the growths, but they are seldom life-threatening. By contrast, melanoma starts as a normal-looking mole but quickly develops abnormal characteristics (Figure 12.3c). Remember the simple "ABCD" guidelines to help you detect the warning signs of melanoma:

- **A**symmetry: One half of the mole does not match the other half.

- **B**order irregularity: The edges of the mole are uneven, notched, or scalloped.

- **C**olor: Pigmentation is not uniform. Melanoma may vary in color from tan to deeper brown, reddish black, black, or deep bluish black.

(a) Basal cell carcinoma

(b) Squamous cell carcinoma

(c) Malignant melanoma

FIGURE **12.3** The three main types of skin cancers: (a) Basal cell carcinoma starts as a small bump, then develops a central crater that crusts and bleeds. (b) Squamous cell carcinoma is often a small nodule surrounded by inflamed tissue. (c) Malignant melanoma is usually irregular in shape, darkly pigmented, and larger than pea size.

Can Having a Tan Protect Me from Skin Cancer?

Can a person's tanned skin, being darker than its natural color, offer protection from the sun's damaging UV rays? No, according to the American Cancer Society. Tanned skin (whether darkened by direct sunlight or from the light in a tanning booth) can only provide about the equivalent of SPF 4 sunscreen—much too weak to be considered protective.[1]

The idea that tanning is protective has at least three inherent fallacies. First, tanned skin is already injured skin that has sustained UV-induced damage to the genetic material and cell structures in the deep dermal layers below the dry epidermal surface. Over time, UV damage can trigger skin cancers to develop.

Second, an SPF of at least 15 is needed to protect light-colored skin for three to four hours and must be reapplied every two hours to compensate for sweating and rubbing off. An SPF of 30 or higher is twice as long-lasting. People with naturally dark skin tones have a lower risk of skin cancer and this persuades many to skip sun-protection.[2] Nevertheless, they *can* develop basal and squamous cell carcinomas and melanomas.[3]

Third, a "base tan" can put you at increased risk of sun damage by conferring a false sense of security. Tan people are likely to stay out in the sun longer than untanned people—often without sunscreen. Therefore, they tend to sustain increased sun damage.

The best protection against skin cancer is to protect your skin from sun damage by wearing sunscreens, long sleeves, hats, and sunglasses and limiting UV exposure, especially between 10:00 a.m. and 4:00 p.m. Finally, stay away from indoor tanning beds. The International Agency for Research on Cancer (part of the World Health Organization) in 2009 classified tanning beds as official human carcinogens! The U.S. Food and Drug Administration is now considering doing the same.[4]

Sources:
1. American Cancer Society, "What's Your Sun-Safety IQ?" www.cancer.org/healthy/toolsandcalculators/quizzes/app/sun-safety-quiz (2011).
2. L.C. Pichon and others, "Sun-Protection Behaviors among African Americans," *American Journal of Preventative Medicine* 38, no. 3 (2010): 288–95.
3. R. C. Rabin, "For Some, Delays in Skin Cancer Diagnosis," *New York Times*, December 29, 2009.
4. R. C. Rabin, "Hazards: Indoor Tanning Is Linked to Skin Cancer," *New York Times*, June 1, 2010.

- **D**iameter: The diameter of the mole is greater than 6 millimeters (about the size of a pea).

If you notice any of these symptoms, or if there is a rapid change in the size or color of a mole, skin tag, or area of the skin, consult a physician promptly.

Contrary to what some may believe, a "base tan" does *not* protect you from skin cancer, as explained in the box Can Having a Tan Protect Me from Cancer?

Tanning Beds

Lung Cancer Is the Leading Killer

Lung cancer kills more men and women than any other cancer.[14] Although more women develop breast cancer each year, more die from lung cancer. The good news is that smoking rates have declined over the past 30 years, and with them, lung cancer rates in men (Figure 12.4).[15] Lung cancer rates have also leveled off in women, after rising for many decades. Most lung cancer patients are smokers or former smokers, but people who have only experienced secondhand smoke or no exposure to smoking may develop the disease.[16]

Warning signs of lung cancer include pain, shortness of breath, persistent wheezing or hoarseness, repeated bouts of pneumonia or bronchitis, a cough that won't go away (or gets worse), weight loss, loss of appetite, coughing up blood, or fever. Treatments for lung cancer include surgery, radiation, or chemotherapy. Despite medical advances, only 16 percent of all lung cancer patients survive for five or more years after diagnosis.[17]

Breast Cancer Strikes Mainly Women

Breast cancer is the second leading cause of cancer death in American women, but it can also occur in men. Earlier diagnosis and better treatments are helping cut the death rate, especially in women under 50. Risk factors associated with breast cancer include a prior history of breast cancer, a primary relative with breast cancer, unusual cell growths in the breast confirmed by biopsy, obesity after menopause, never having children or having a first child after age 30, consuming two or more drinks of alcohol per day, higher education and socioeconomic status, and hormone replacement therapy after menopause. Other possible risk factors include a high-fat diet, genetic predisposition due to oncogenes *BRCA1* and *BRCA2*, exposure to pesticides and other chemicals, weight gain, and physical inactivity. The box Do Birth Control Pills Increase Cancer Risk? presents the conflicting research studies on oral contraceptives and cancer risk.

Regular breast self-examinations and medical check-ups (including *mammography*—breast X rays) can detect cancer early, at its most treatable stage. The box Breast Awareness and Self-Exam walks you through performing breast self-exams. The American Cancer Society recommends that women begin monthly breast self-examinations at age 20 with a clinical breast exam at least every three years, and yearly clinical breast exams and mammograms beginning at age 40.[18] The U.S. Preventive Services Task Force recommends mammograms every two years for women over 50 to minimize radiation exposure.[19] Keep in mind that most breast lumps are harmless cysts or fibrous tissue. A physician may investigate a lump with a biopsy, an ultrasound, or

Mammogram Controversy

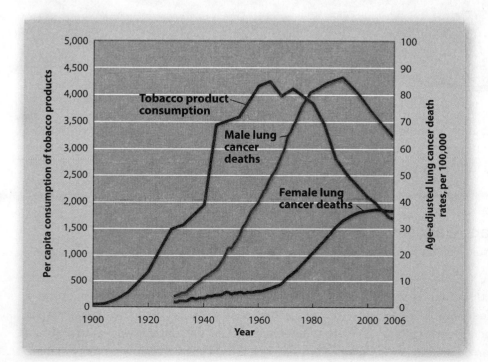

FIGURE **12.4** For decades, lung cancer was by far the biggest cancer killer of American men, but incidence has fallen along with smoking rates. Lung cancer deaths for women have also begun to plateau.

Data from: Death Rates: U.S. Mortality Files, National Center for Health Statistics, Centers for Disease Control and Prevention, 2010; Cigarette Consumption: U.S. Department of Agriculture, 1900–2006.

Do Birth Control Pills Increase Cancer Risk?

The question of whether using oral contraceptives increases the risk of cancer in women remains controversial. In 1996, a large, widely publicized study concluded that women who took birth control pills had a slightly increased risk of developing breast cancer both while they were taking the pills and for 10 years after stopping use.[1] A 2002 study published in the *New England Journal of Medicine*, however, found no increased breast cancer risk among women who took birth control pills—regardless of how long they took the pills and what type of pills they took.[2] Another large study sponsored by the National Cancer Institute looked at thousands of women diagnosed with breast cancer.[3] Women between ages 20 and 34 who had used birth control pills within five years of their diagnosis had the highest additional risk, although the elevated risk itself was small. To complicate matters, several studies, including a major study published in 2008, concluded that oral contraceptives *lower* a woman's risk for ovarian cancer.[4] Additional health questions about oral hormones remain in dispute, including whether or not they increase the risk of strokes or other cardiovascular diseases, especially when used after menopause. The decision to take oral contraceptives and hormones is a personal one. Women should consult their doctors and weigh the risks and benefits for themselves.

Sources:
1. Collaborative Group on Hormonal Factors in Breast Cancer, "Breast Cancer and Hormonal Contraceptives: Collaborative Reanalysis of Individual Data on 53,297 Women with Breast Cancer and 100,239 Women without Breast Cancer from 54 Epidemiological Studies," *Lancet* 347, no. 9017 (1996): 1713–27.
2. P. A. Marchbanks and others, "Oral Contraceptives and the Risk of Breast Cancer," *New England Journal of Medicine* 346, no. 26 (2002): 2025–32.
3. M. D. Althuis and others, "Breast Cancers among Very Young Premenopausal Women (United States)," *Cancer Causes and Control* 14, no. 2 (2003): 151–60.
4. Collaborative Group on Epidemiological Studies of Ovarian Cancer, "Ovarian Cancer and Oral Contraceptives: Collaborative Reanalysis of Data from 45 Epidemiological Studies Including 23,257 Women with Ovarian Cancer and 87,303 Controls," *Lancet* 371, no. 9609 (2008): 303–14.

a noninvasive technique that measures the elasticity of a mass with pressure waves. If invasive cancer is discovered, treatments include surgery, radiation, and chemotherapy.

Female Reproductive Tract Cancers

Cancers of the female reproductive tract include ovarian, uterine, and cervical cancer.

Ovarian Cancer Among reproductive tract cancers in women, ovarian cancer is the deadliest. It is also the fifth leading cause of cancer death among American women.[20] Because ovarian cancer has few overt signs (symptoms include feeling bloated, a constant feeling of fullness, changes in bowel or bladder activity, and pain in the pelvis, abdomen, or back), it often progresses to an advanced stage before it's discovered.[21]

A woman's risk of ovarian cancer increases if she has a prior history of (or has a close relative with) breast, colon, or ovarian cancer. The risk also increases if a woman is over 50 and has had few or no children. Other suspected risk factors are the use of fertility drugs before menopause and the use of hormone replacement drugs after menopause. Factors that appear to *lower* risk include eating a low-fat diet, consuming plenty of fruits

Breast Awareness and Self Exam

Women should know how their breasts normally look and feel and report any new breast changes to a health professional as soon as these changes are noted. The best time for a woman to examine her breasts is when the breasts are not tender or swollen. The American Cancer Society recommends the use of mammography and clinical breast exam in addition to self-examination.

How to Examine Your Breasts

- Lie down and place your right arm behind your head. In this position, breast tissue spreads evenly over the chest wall and is as thin as possible.

- Use the finger pads of the three middle fingers on your left hand to feel for lumps in the right breast. Use overlapping, dime-sized circular motions of the finger pads to feel the tissue.

- Use three different levels of pressure to feel all the breast tissue. If you're not sure

how hard to press, talk with your doctor or nurse. Use each pressure level to feel the breast tissue before moving on to the next spot.

- Move around the breast in an up-and-down pattern starting at an imaginary line drawn straight down your side from the underarm and moving across the breast to the middle of the chest bone.

- Repeat the exam on your left breast, using the finger pads of the right hand.

- While standing in front of a mirror with your hands pressing firmly down on your hips, look at your breasts for any changes of size, shape, contour, or dimpling and redness or scaliness of the nipple or breast skin.

- Examine each underarm while sitting up or standing and with your arm only slightly raised so you can easily feel in this area.

Source: American Cancer Society, "Can Breast Cancer Be Found Early?" Revised September 2010, www.cancer.org/Cancer/BreastCancer/DetailedGuide/breast-cancer-detection. Reprinted by the permission of the American Cancer Society, Inc., from www.cancer.org. All rights reserved.

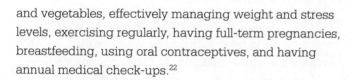

and vegetables, effectively managing weight and stress levels, exercising regularly, having full-term pregnancies, breastfeeding, using oral contraceptives, and having annual medical check-ups.[22]

Uterine and Cervical Cancer Most uterine cancers develop in the body of the uterus, usually in the endometrium (lining). The rest develop in the cervix, at the base of the uterus.

Risk factors for uterine (endometrial) cancer include increasing age, race (Caucasian women are at higher risk), endometrial tissue buildup due to hormone imbalances, estrogen replacement therapy, overweight or obesity, diabetes and high blood pressure, a history of other cancers, having few or no children, and menopause late in life.[23] Early symptoms of uterine cancer may include bleeding outside the normal menstrual period or after menopause, or persistent unusual vaginal discharge.

The main cause of cervical cancer is infection by the human papillomavirus (HPV).[24] Activities that increase the risk of acquiring HPV infection, such as early age at first intercourse and multiple sex partners, also increase the risk of cervical cancer, as do smoking and infection by the herpes virus.[25] The **Pap smear** is very effective for detecting early stage cervical cancer and has helped reduce the incidence of dangerous later-stage cancers. There are also new vaccines for females aged 9 to 26 that protect against HPV, which can in turn decrease the risk of developing cervical cancer.[26]

Screening for cervical cancer should begin 3 years after a woman begins having vaginal

Pap smear A procedure in which cells taken from the cervical region are examined for abnormal cellular activity

Testicular Self-Exam

Most testicular cancers can be found at an early stage. The American Cancer Society (ACS) advises men to be aware of testicular cancer and to see a doctor right away if they find a lump in a testicle. If you have certain risk factors that increase your chance of developing testicular cancer (e.g., an undescended testicle, previous germ cell tumor in one testicle, or a family history), you should talk to your doctor about monthly self-exams.

How to Examine Your Testicles

The best time for you to examine your testicles is during or after a shower, when the skin of the scrotum is relaxed.

- Hold the penis out of the way and examine each testicle separately.

- Hold the testicle between your thumbs and fingers with both hands and roll it gently between the fingers.

- Look and feel for any hard lumps or nodules (smooth, rounded masses) or any change in the size, shape, or consistency of the testes.

You should be aware that each normal testis has an epididymis, which can feel like a small bump on the upper or middle outer side of the testis. If you have any concerns, ask your doctor. Note that the ACS recommends a testicular exam as part of a routine cancer-related check-up.

Source: American Cancer Society, "Do I Have Testicular Cancer? Testicular Self-Exam," Revised January 2010, www.cancer.org/Cancer/TesticularCancer /MoreInformation/DoIHaveTesticularCancer/do-i-have-testicular-cancer-self-exam. Reprinted by the permission of the American Cancer Society, Inc. from www.cancer.org. All rights reserved.

---

intercourse and no later than age 21 and continue annually until age 30. If a woman then has three normal Pap tests in a row, she may opt for less frequent tests. For endometrial cancer, women at menopause and of average risk should report unexpected bleeding to their physician.

Male Reproductive Tract Cancers

Male reproductive tract cancers include those of the prostate and testicles.

Prostate Cancer Prostate cancer is the most common cancer in men and the second-most frequent cause of male cancer deaths. Symptoms may include weak or interrupted urine flow, difficulty starting or stopping urination, feeling the urge to urinate frequently, pain upon urination, blood in the urine, or pain in the low back, pelvis, or thighs. Prostate cancer can be slow-growing and symptom-free in the early stages, making testing and early diagnosis important.

Prostate cancer risk increases with age; 97 percent of cases occur in men over the age of 50.[27] Race is also a significant factor: African American men and Jamaican men of African descent have the highest rates of prostate cancer in the world. Other risk factors include family history of prostate cancer, high BMI, and a diet high in saturated fats and low in fiber, fruits, and vegetables.[28] The American Cancer Society recommends that starting at age 50, men at average risk talk with their doctor to determine whether to have a *prostate-specific antigen test* with or without a digital rectal exam.

Testicular Cancer Unlike prostate cancer, testicular cancer tends to be diagnosed in younger men, mostly between the ages of 20 and 34.[29] It is also much less common than prostate cancer. Tour de France champion Lance Armstrong developed metastatic testicular cancer in his 20s and survived it through surgery, chemotherapy, and lifestyle changes. Genetic predisposition may increase the risk of testicular cancer, as does having undescended testicles. The box Testicular Self-Exam explains how to perform a testicular self-examination to check for early symptoms.

Colon and Rectal Cancers

Cancers of the colon and rectum are the third most common cancer in both men and women.[30] In the early stages, colorectal cancer has no symptoms. Bleeding from the rectum, blood in the stool, and changes in bowel habits can signal later-stage colorectal cancer. Risk factors include being over age 50, race (African Americans appear to have the highest risk of colorectal cancer), obesity, a personal or family history of polyps (benign growths) in the colon or rectum, or bowel problems such as colitis. Research suggests that the risk of developing colorectal cancer can be lowered significantly by eating a low-fat, high-fiber diet rich in fruits and vegetables; exercising regularly; and getting regular colorectal screening—a simple blood test (*fecal occult blood test*) and *colonoscopy* after age 50. Polyp removal during these procedures can prevent a growth from progressing to cancer later. Treatment of a colorectal cancer often requires radiation or surgery. Medical researchers are currently developing a simple urine test for colon cancer that could one day replace the more invasive tests.[31]

Pancreatic Cancer and Leukemia

Two additional cancers are among the most-often diagnosed: pancreatic cancer and leukemia. Risk factors for pancreatic cancer include being male, being over age 45, smoking, eating a high-fat diet, having diabetes, and having a family history of cancer.[32]

Leukemia is a cancer of the blood-forming tissues, particularly the soft, spongy marrow of the bones. There are several types of leukemia; these can be acute or chronic and can strike both sexes and all age groups. Although it is the most common childhood cancer, over 90 percent of all leukemia cases occur in adults aged 20 and over.[33] Symptoms may include frequent infections, flu-like symptoms, headaches, vomiting, anemia, and pain or swelling in the joints.

How Can I Reduce My Risk of Cancer?

Lab 12.1 will help you to assess yourself for risk factors associated with many common cancers, and the box Reduce Your Cancer Risk summarizes wellness behaviors that can lower your cancer risk. Completing **Lab 12.2** can help you plan for cancer prevention.

LIVE IT! ONLINE

Worksheet 40
Cancer Risk
Assessment

DO IT! ONLINE

TOOLS FOR **CHANGE** •

Reduce Your Cancer Risk

Here is a checklist of wellness behaviors that can lower your risk of developing cancer:

☐ Don't smoke or use tobacco.

☐ Limit alcohol consumption to one drink per day or less for women, and two drinks a day or less for men.

☐ Limit consumption of grilled meats, blackened meats, and processed meats.

☐ Limit intake of saturated and *trans* fats.

☐ Eat at least five servings per day or more of fruits and vegetables.

☐ Eat several servings per day of whole-grain foods.

☐ Engage in regular physical activity and exercise.

☐ Maintain your BMI within recommended levels (18.5 to 24.9).

☐ Practice stress management techniques.

☐ Limit environmental exposures to carcinogens including infectious agents, radiation, and chemicals.

☐ Limit sun exposure by using sunscreen (SPF 15 or higher) and protective clothing and by staying out of the sun during the brightest midday hours.

☐ Learn to do regular self-exams for breast cancer, skin cancer, and testicular cancer.

☐ Get regular medical check-ups and the professional screenings recommended for your sex and age group

In addition to assessing and reducing your risks, being "in touch" with your body, and seeking medical attention when suspicious changes occur, can be critical to increasing the chances of successful intervention and treatment. There are seven general early warning signs of cancer, summarized by the acronym CAUTION:

Change in bowel or bladder habits

A sore that does not heal

Unusual bleeding or discharge

Thickening or lump in breast or elsewhere

Indigestion or difficulty in swallowing

Obvious change in a wart or mole

Nagging cough or hoarseness

If you have what may be a warning sign of cancer, make an appointment with your doctor. If it is an indicator of cancer, your chances of full recovery are higher the earlier you detect it. If it isn't cancer, you can rest easier that much sooner.

Lifestyle Choices Can Reduce Your Cancer Risk

Your lifestyle choices can substantially affect your risk of developing cancer (Figure 12.5). **Lifetime risk** refers to the probability that you will develop cancer at some point during your life. **Relative risk** is a measure of how likely you are to develop

lifetime risk The probability that a person will develop cancer at some point during his or her lifetime

relative risk A measure of how likely a person is to develop cancer while engaging in known risk behaviors compared to people who abstain from these behaviors

cancer while engaging in a known risk behavior, compared to people who abstain from that behavior.

Quit Smoking, Drink Less, Avoid Drugs Smoking, excessive alcohol use, or illegal drug use can increase cancer risk. If you are a smoker, your relative risk of developing lung cancer is about 18 to 20 times higher

Being overweight or obese → **Increases susceptibility to**

Breast, colon, thyroid, ovarian, cervical, prostate, endometrial, pancreatic, gallbladder, and kidney cancers; multiple myeloma; Hodgkin's disease; adenocarcinomas of the esophagus

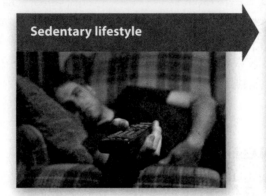

Sedentary lifestyle → **Increases susceptibility to**

Colon cancer, breast cancer

Smoking, tobacco use → **Increases susceptibility to**

Lung, esophageal, pancreatic, uterine, cervical, kidney, bladder, stomach, and nasopharyngeal cancers; cancers of the nasal cavity, lip, and oral cavity

Alcohol → **Increases susceptibility to**

Liver, esophageal, and breast cancers; cancers of the mouth, pharynx, and larynx

FIGURE **12.5** Lifestyle factors such as smoking, drinking alcohol, overeating, and too little physical activity can increase the risk of cancer.

than that of a nonsmoker.[34] Drinking alcohol, especially in combination with smoking, increases the risk of oral and pancreatic cancers. Drinking more than one glass of alcohol daily is also associated with an increased risk of breast cancer among women.[35] Hepatitis, which can be contracted from contaminated needles, increases the risk of liver cancer, as does the use of anabolic steroids.[36]

Watch Your Weight, Move More, and Eat Right

Scientific evidence suggests that about one-third of cancer deaths are related to overweight or obesity, poor nutritional habits, and lack of exercise.[37] This means that people could prevent a significant number of cancer deaths through their own weight control, healthier eating, and increased physical activity.

Several studies have shown reductions in cancer risk through physical exercise: in one study, the most physically active women had a 20 percent lower risk of breast cancer;[38] in another study, leisure-time physical activity appeared to reduce the risk of colon cancer by 20 percent in men and women.[39] Physical activity also seems to lower a man's risk for the more aggressive forms of prostate cancer.[40]

Certain food additives are suspected of causing cancer, particularly *sodium nitrate,* a chemical used to preserve and give color to red meat. There is also evidence that consumption of grilled meats and processed lunch meats can increase the risk of some types of cancer.[41]

Manage Stress Stress has been implicated in increased susceptibility to several types of cancers.[42] People who are under chronic, severe stress or who suffer from depression or other persistent psychological disorders

show higher rates of cancer than their healthy counterparts. Sleep disturbances, diet, or a combination of factors may weaken the body's immune system, increasing susceptibility to cancer.

Biological Factors Play a Role in Cancer Risk

Our genes, our internal hormonal environments, and our exposures to biological agents such as viruses can increase our risk of cancer.

Genetics Cancers of the breast, stomach, colon, prostate, uterus, ovaries, and lungs appear to run in families.[43] For example, a woman runs a much higher risk of breast cancer if her mother or sisters have had the disease. Hodgkin's lymphoma and certain leukemias also seem to be hereditary.

Reproductive Hormones The effect estrogen has on breast cancer risk is well documented. A woman's risk of breast cancer increases a small but statistically significant amount if she begins menstruation early (before age 12), has no children or has her first child after age 30, or uses hormone replacement therapy after menopause—all of which increase the amount of estrogen a woman is exposed to over a lifetime. Conversely, the risk of breast cancer decreases slightly in women who experience late menstruation (after age 14), have their first child at a young age, have many children, breast feed, or experience early menopause (before age 45), all circumstances that reduce the amount of estrogen a woman is exposed to in her lifetime.[44]

Infectious Agents According to recent estimates, microbes and their by-products cause some 20 percent of new cancers worldwide.[45] Hepatitis B virus (HBV) and hepatitis C virus (HCV), for example, can cause DNA damage that leads to liver cancer. Meanwhile, virtually all women with cervical cancer have evidence of infection from certain strains of human papillomavirus (HPV), which also causes genital warts.[46]

Environmental Factors Can Increase Cancer Risk

Exposure to radiation, chemicals, and other carcinogens in the environment can increase your cancer risk. Limiting your exposure to such environmental factors can decrease the risk.

Radiation *Ionizing radiation (IR)*—such as radiation from X rays, radioactive material, radon gas, cosmic rays, and ultraviolet radiation (UV) from sunlight—can cause cancer. IR can promote cancer in virtually any part of the body, but bone marrow and the thyroid gland are particularly susceptible. Routine diagnostic medical and dental X rays are usually set at the lowest possible levels of radiation in order to minimize such risk. Radon, both in industrial settings and in homes, is the leading cause of lung cancer in non-smokers and the second leading cause of lung cancer overall.[47] Exposure to ultraviolet radiation through sun-tanning and the use of tanning booths is a well-known risk for skin cancers.

Occupational Exposures Certain occupations expose workers to known carcinogens at a much higher level than the average person would ever encounter. For example, uranium miners, sewage workers, and petroleum refinery workers tend to encounter high levels of radon gas and have higher-than-average rates of lung cancer.[48]

What If I or Someone I Know Is Facing Cancer?

radiation Powerful, targeted beams of ionizing energy that can kill cancerous cells

chemotherapy The use of drugs to kill cancerous cells

The emotional distress of facing cancer can cloud a person's critical health-care decision-making. Find a close friend or family member who will support you.

casestudy

TIM

"I don't smoke, so that's one huge risk factor for cancer that I don't have to worry about. But I do spend a lot of time out in the sun without sunscreen—which I see now is a risk. I just didn't think much about it. Seeing what Kevin is going through with his cancer treatment was a wake-up call. Now that I know my 'base tan' won't protect me, I put on sunscreen before I head outdoors."

THINK! Do you know anyone who is being treated for cancer? Do any of your behaviors increase your risk of cancer?

ACT! Examine your own life. Write down one behavior you could change that would reduce your risk for cancer.

HEAR IT! ONLINE

After any cancer diagnosis, find out the type and stage of the cancer and the prognosis for recovery. Ask about the benefits, risks, and possible side effects of each treatment option. Seek out well-established hospitals and treatment centers that specialize in your kind of cancer and interview cancer specialists, surgeons, and chemo and radiation therapists. Surgical removal of tumors, radiation, chemotherapy, immunotherapies, and gene therapies are all possible treatment avenues.

Radiation and Chemotherapy Radiation, targeted beams of ionizing energy, works by destroying malignant cells or stopping cell growth. It is most effective in treating localized cancers. Unfortunately, radiation also destroys some healthy cells and increases the risk of other types of cancers. Nonetheless, radiation continues to be one of the most common and effective forms of treatment.

During **chemotherapy**, the patient receives intravenous doses of drugs capable of targeting and killing fast-growing cells throughout the body, including metastasized cancer cells. Because chemotherapy also kills the fast-dividing cells in normal hair follicles, it tends to cause hair loss. Damage to rapidly dividing digestive-tract cells explains the nausea and nutritional deficiencies so common to patients undergoing chemotherapy.

Radiation and chemotherapy can cause long-term damage to the heart, brain, and other organs, so the decision to undergo either treatment is a serious one. However, millions of people have gone on to live productive lives for years or decades after radiation or chemotherapy treatment.

New Approaches to Treatment Today, researchers are exploring treatments that target cancer as a genetic disease that is brought on by a mutation, either inherited or acquired. Potential treatments include *immunotherapies*, such as those that enhance the body's immune system to help control cancer, and *gene therapies*, such as those that manipulate genes to increase the patient's immune response to a cancerous tumor or that allow the patients' bone marrow to withstand stronger doses of chemotherapeutic drugs. Stem-cell research, though controversial, may also yield promising new cancer treatments.

SEE IT! ONLINE

Treating Cancer with Bone Drugs

SEE IT! ONLINE

Possible Melanoma Treatment

chapterin**review**

videos

Log on to **www.pearsonhighered.com/hopson** or MyFitnessLab to view these chapter-related videos.

Mammogram Controversy
Tanning Beds

Treating Cancer with Bone Drugs
Alcohol and Cancer

Possible Melanoma Treatment

onlineresources

Log on to **www.pearsonhighered.com/hopson** or MyFitnessLab for access to these book-related resources, and for links to other useful websites.

 Audio case study and
Audio PowerPoint lecture

 Lab 12.1 Assess Your Personal Risk
of Cancer
Lab 12.2 Plan for Cancer Prevention

 Take Charge of Your Health! Worksheets:
Worksheet 40 Cancer Risk Assessment
Behavior Change Log Book and Wellness
Journal

 Pre- and post-quizzes
Glossary flashcards

reviewquestions

1. Which of the following can help you decrease your risk of developing cancer?
   a. Smoking only a few cigarettes per day
   b. Drinking one to two drinks per day
   c. Maintaining a BMI over 25
   d. Getting 60 to 90 minutes of exercise per day

2. The difference between a benign tumor and a malignant tumor is that
   a. a benign tumor is cancerous; a malignant tumor is noncancerous.
   b. a benign tumor is inherited; a malignant tumor is caused by lifestyle factors.
   c. a benign tumor is noncancerous; a malignant tumor is cancerous.
   d. a benign tumor is caused by lifestyle factors; a malignant tumor is inherited.

3. Suspected cancer-causing genes are called
   a. carcinogens.
   b. oncogenes.
   c. phytochemicals.
   d. metastases.

4. A physician who specializes in cancer is an
   a. internist.
   b. oncologist.
   c. endocrinologist.
   d. epidemiologist.

5. Cancers characterized by an increased number of white blood cells are classified as
   a. leukemias.
   b. lymphomas.
   c. sarcomas.
   d. carcinomas.

6. You can lower your risk of lung cancer by reducing your exposure to
   a. UV radiation from sunlight.
   b. asbestos.
   c. radon gas.
   d. oncogenes.

7. In the "ABCD" warning signs of melanoma, the "A" stands for
   a. asymmetry.
   b. asbestos.
   c. angiogenesis.
   d. alcohol use.

8. Angiogenesis is
   a. a method of treating cancer.
   b. the process by which malignant cells induce new blood vessel growth.
   c. the spread of cancer cells throughout the body.
   d. a synonym for metastasis.

9. The leading cancer killer for both men and women in the United States is
   a. breast cancer.
   b. lung cancer.
   c. skin cancer.
   d. pancreatic cancer.

10. Testicular cancer tends to strike
    a. men in their 70s.
    b. men between the ages of 20 to 34.
    c. teenage males.
    d. boys under age 10.

critical**thinking**questions

REVIEW IT! ONLINE

1. What is cancer? How does it spread? What is the difference between a benign and a malignant tumor?

2. What are the differences among carcinomas, sarcomas, lymphomas, and leukemia?

3. What are five controllable risk factors for developing cancer?

references

1–4. American *Cancer Society, Cancer Facts and Figures 2011* (Atlanta: American Cancer Society, 2011).

5. National Cancer Institute, "Understanding Cancer Series: Angiogenesis," www.cancer.gov/cancertopics/understandingcancer/angiogenesis (reviewed September 2006).

6. National Cancer Institute, "Fact Sheet: Angiogenesis Inhibitors Therapy," www.cancer.gov/cancertopics/factsheet/Therapy/angiogenesis-inhibitors (reviewed November 2008).

7. American Cancer Society, *Cancer Facts and Figures* 2011, 2011.

8. Ibid.

9–11. L. C. Brody and B. B. Biesecker, "Breast Cancer Susceptibility Genes BRCA1 and BRCA2," *Medicine* (Baltimore) 77, no. 3 (1998): 208–26,

12. Colette Coyne Melanoma Awareness Campaign, "Statistics," www.ccmac.org/index.php?option=com_content&view=article&id=27&Itemid=6 (accessed October 2011).

13. Ibid.

14. American Cancer Society, *Cancer Facts and Figures 2011*, 2011.

15. S. A. Kenfield and others, "Smoking and Smoking Cessation in Relation to Mortality in Women," *Journal of the American Medical Association* 299, no. 17 (2008): 2037–47.

16. J. Samet and others, "Lung Cancer in Never Smokers: Clinical Epidemiology and Environmental Risk Factors," *Clinical Cancer Research* 15, no. 18 (2009): 5626–45.

17. American Cancer Society, *Cancer Facts and Figures* 2011, 2011.

18. American Cancer Society, "American Cancer Society Guidelines for the Early Detection of Cancer," www.cancer.org/Healthy/FindCancerEarly/CancerScreeningGuidelines/american-cancer-society-guidelines-for-the-early-detection-of-cancer (revised June 2011).

19. U.S. Preventive Services Task Force, "Screening for Breast Cancer," www.uspreventiveservicestaskforce.org/uspstf/uspsbrca.htm (reviewed July 2010).

20–22. National Cancer Institute, "Ovarian Cancer Screening (PDQ)," www.cancer.gov/cancertopics/pdq/screening/ovarian/Patient (modified September 2011).

23. National Cancer Institute, "Endometrial Cancer," www.cancer.gov/cancertopics/types/endometrial (accessed October 2011).

24–26. Centers for Disease Control and Prevention, "Human Papillomavirus (HPV): HPV Vaccines," www.cdc.gov/hpv/vaccine.html (updated September 2011).

27. American Cancer Society, "Prostate Cancer Overview: What Causes Prostate Cancer?" www.cancer.org/Cancer/ProstateCancer/OverviewGuide/prostate-cancer-overview-what-causes (revised June 2011).

28. American Cancer Society, *Cancer Facts and Figures* 2011, 2011.

29. National Cancer Institute, "SEER Stat Fact Sheet: Testis," http://seer.cancer.gov/statfacts/html/testis.html (accessed October 2011).

30. American Cancer Society, *Cancer Facts and Figures 2011*, 2011.

31. Y. Qiu and others, "Urinary Metabonomic Study on Colorectal Cancer," *Journal of Proteome Research* 9, no. 3 (2010): 1627–34.

32–36. American Cancer Society, *Cancer Facts and Figures 2011*, 2011.

37. T. J. Key, E. A. Spencer, and G. K. Reeves, "Symposium 1: Overnutrition: Consequences and Solutions, Obesity and Cancer Risk," *The Proceedings of the Nutrition Society* 69, no. 1 (2010): 86–90.

38. L. A. Healy and others, "Obesity Increases the Risk of Postmenopausal Breast Cancer and Is Associated with More Advanced Stage at Presentation But No Impact on Survival," *The Breast Journal* 16, no. 1 (2010): 95–7.

39. R. F. Zoeller, Jr., "Lifestyle in the Prevention and Management of Cancer: Physical Activity," *American Journal of Lifestyle Medicine* 3, no. 5 (2009): 353–61.

40. Ibid.

41. National Cancer Institute, "Fact Sheet: Chemicals in Meat Cooked at High Temperatures and Cancer Risk," www.cancer.gov/cancertopics/factsheet/Risk/cooked-meats (reviewed October 2010).

42. K. Ross, "Mapping Pathways from Stress to Cancer Progression," *Journal of the National Cancer Institute* 100, no. 13 (2008): 914–5, 917.

43. National Cancer Institute, "Cancer Genetics Risk Assessment and Counseling (PDQ)," www.cancer.gov/cancertopics/pdq/genetics/risk-assessment-and-counseling/HealthProfessional (modified September 2011).

44. American Cancer Society, "Breast Cancer Overview: What Causes Breast Cancer?" www.cancer.org/Cancer/BreastCancer/OverviewGuide/breast-cancer-overview-what-causes (revised June 2011).

45. National Institute of Allergy and Infectious Diseases, "Viral Infections: Treating Cancer as an Infectious Disease," www.niaid.nih.gov/topics/viral/Pages/cancerInfectiousDisease.aspx (updated March 2009).

46. National Cancer Institute, "Fact Sheet: Human Papillomaviruses and Cancer," www.cancer.gov/cancertopics/factsheet/Risk/HPV (reviewed September 2011).

47. U.S. Environmental Protection Agency, "Radon (Rn): Health Risks: Exposure to Radon Causes Lung Cancer in Non-Smokers and Smokers Alike," www.epa.gov/radon/healthrisks.html (updated February 2011).

48. R. J. Roscoe and others, "Lung Cancer Mortality among Nonsmoking Uranium Miners Exposed to Radon Daughters," *JAMA* 262, no. 5 (1989): 629–33.

ASSESS YOURSELF

LAB 12.1 • ASSESS YOUR PERSONAL RISK OF CANCER

Name: _____ Date: _____

Instructor: _____ Section: _____

Purpose: To assess your personal risk of common cancers.

Directions: Read each question and select the number corresponding to your Yes or No answer. Be honest and accurate in order to get the most complete understanding of your cancer risks.

Section I: Breast Cancer	Yes	No
1. Do you check your breasts at least monthly using breast self-examination (BSE) procedures?	1	2
2. Do you look at your breasts in the mirror regularly, checking for any irregular indentations/lumps, discharge from the nipples, or other noticeable changes?	1	2
3. Has your mother, sister, or daughter been diagnosed with breast cancer?	2	1
4. Have you ever been pregnant?	1	2
5. Have you had a history of lumps or cysts in your breasts or underarm?	2	1
Total Section I (Breast Cancer) Points	_____	_____
Section II: Skin Cancer	**Yes**	**No**
1. Do you spend a lot of time in the sun, either at work or at play?	2	1
2. Do you use sunscreens with an SPF rating of 15 or more when you are in the sun?	1	2
3. Do you use tanning beds or sun booths regularly to maintain a tan?	2	1
4. Do you examine your skin once a month, checking any moles or other irregularities, particularly in hard-to-see areas?	1	2
5. Do you purchase and wear sunglasses that adequately filter out harmful sun rays?	1	2
Total Section II (Skin Cancer) Points	_____	_____
Section III: Cancers of the Reproductive System—Men	**Yes**	**No**
1. Do you examine your penis regularly for unusual bumps or growths?	1	2
2. Do you perform regular testicular self-examination?	1	2
3. Do you have a family history of prostate or testicular cancer?	2	1
4. Do you practice safer sex and wear condoms with every sexual encounter?	1	2
5. Do you avoid exposure to harmful environmental hazards such as mercury, coal tars, benzene, chromate, and vinyl chloride?	1	2
Total Section III (Reproductive Cancer) Points—MEN	_____	_____

Section III: Cancers of the Reproductive System—Women	Yes	No
1. Do you have a regularly scheduled Pap smear?	1	2
2. Have you been infected with the human papillomavirus, Epstein-Barr virus, or other viruses believed to increase cancer risk?	2	1
3. Has your mother, sister, or daughter been diagnosed with breast, cervical, endometrial, or ovarian cancer (particularly at a young age)?	2	1
4. Do you practice safe sex and use condoms with every sexual encounter?	1	2
5. Are you obese, taking estrogen, and/or consuming a diet that is very high in saturated fats?	2	1
Total Section III (Reproductive Cancer) Points—Women	_____	_____
Section IV: Cancers in General	Yes	No
1. Do you smoke cigarettes on most days of the week?	2	1
2. Do you consume a diet that is rich in fruits and vegetables?	1	2
3. Are you obese and/or do you lead a primarily sedentary lifestyle?	2	1
4. Do you live in an area with high air pollution levels or work in a job where you are exposed to several chemicals on a regular basis?	2	1
5. Are you careful about the amount of animal fat in your diet, substituting olive oil or canola oil for animal fat whenever possible?	1	2
6. Do you limit your overall consumption of alcohol?	1	2
7. Do you eat foods rich in lycopenes (such as tomatoes) and antioxidants?	1	2
8. Are you "body aware" and alert for changes in your body?	1	2
9. Do you have a family history of ulcers or of colorectal, stomach, or other digestive system cancers?	2	1
10. Do you avoid unnecessary exposure to ionizing radiation such as X rays, radon, and ultraviolet radiation?	1	2
Total Section IV (General Cancer) Points	_____	_____

REFLECTING ON YOUR SCORES

Take a careful look at each question where you marked a "2" and any areas in which you marked mostly 2s. Did you receive total points of six or higher in Sections I through III? Did you receive at least 11 total points in Section IV? If so, you have at least one identifiable risk, and a higher score indicates a higher risk level.

Name: _____ Date: _____

Instructor: _____ Section: _____

Purpose: To develop a plan to change risky behaviors and employ healthy behaviors for cancer prevention.

Directions: Complete Sections I and II below, outlining your behavior, goals, and plan for cancer prevention.

SECTION I: BEHAVIOR EVALUATION

After reviewing the chapter and completing Lab 12.1, evaluate your behavior and identify patterns and specific things you are doing that may be risky for cancer.

1. What behaviors could you change now?

_____

_____

2. What behaviors will take longer to change?

_____

_____

SECTION II: CANCER PREVENTION GOALS

Create goals for cancer prevention. Be sure to use SMART (*specific, measurable, action-oriented, realistic, time-oriented*) goal-setting guidelines. Select appropriate target dates and rewards for completing your goals.

Behavior Change Goal #1: _____

Target Date: _____ Reward: _____

Behavior Change Goal #2: _____

Target Date: _____ Reward: _____

Behavior Change Goal #3: _____

Target Date: _____ Reward: _____

13 Avoiding Substance Use, Abuse, and Addiction

Learning Outcomes

1. Define *addiction* and list four of its symptoms.   Audio case study and audio Power Point lecture

2. Describe the short-term and long-term health effects of alcohol use.

3. Identify the characteristics of a "problem drinker" and describe strategies for treatment.   Hidden Addictions Spring Break Nightmare

4. Discuss strategies for avoiding alcohol abuse. Lab 13.1 Assessing Your Alcohol Use and Risk of Abuse

5. Describe the short-term and long-term health effects of tobacco use.

6. Define *secondhand smoke* and discuss the health risks associated with it.   Secondhand Smoke Smash the Ash

7. Discuss strategies for avoiding tobacco use. Lab 13.2 Identify Smoking Behaviors and Create a Plan to Quit

8. Explain *drug use* and *drug abuse*.   Campus Drug Dealers

9. List several common types of drugs and their effects on the body.   Heroin in Suburbia Eliminating Meth

10. Discuss strategies for avoiding drug abuse. Lab 13.3 Learn to Recognize Drug Use and Potential Abuse

Pre- and post-quizzes and glossary flashcards

405

casestudy

NATHAN

"My name is Nathan. I'm like most people: I experimented with alcohol in high school. But I never smoked or did drugs because I was on sports teams and frankly, I didn't want to get caught and lose my chance at a scholarship. Now that I'm in college, I am constantly exposed to drinking. I've seen some of my friends and fraternity brothers get in big trouble with it, too. I also have friends who have started smoking and some who grow marijuana in their dorm rooms or go clubbing and do Ecstasy. People make it seem like it's no big deal. So how dangerous are drugs like these? When do people cross the line between having fun and getting in trouble?"

HEAR IT! ONLINE

FIGURE **13.1** Singer Amy Winehouse, who died of alcohol poisoning in 2011 at the age of 27, is one of many performers who earned notoriety for struggling with substance abuse.

These days, it is easy to find high-profile cases of compulsive and destructive behavior. Stories of celebrities and politicians struggling with drug and alcohol addictions are splashed in the headlines and profiled on television news programs (Figure 13.1). But millions of "everyday" people throughout the world are battle addiction as well. In this chapter, we will focus on the health risks of alcohol, tobacco, and other types of drug use. We will cover the short-term and long-term effects of substance use, discuss ways to identify patterns of addiction, and describe treatment options for those struggling with substance abuse.

What Is Addiction?

LIVE IT! ONLINE

Worksheet 30
Are You
Addicted?

Addiction is a persistent, compulsive dependence on a behavior or substance, including mood-altering behaviors or activities, despite ongoing negative

> **addiction** Persistent, compulsive dependence on a behavior or substance, despite ongoing negative consequences

consequences. Although the mechanism is not well understood, all forms of addiction probably reflect dysfunction of certain biochemical systems in the brain.[1]

Addictions are characterized by four common symptoms:

- *Compulsion,* or excessive preoccupation with the behavior (drinking, drug use, gambling, etc.) and an overwhelming need to perform it

- *Loss of control,* or the inability to reliably predict whether any isolated occurrence of the behavior will be healthy or damaging

- *Negative consequences,* such as physical damage, legal trouble, financial problems, academic failure, or family problems caused by the behavior

- *Denial,* or the inability to perceive that the behavior is self-destructive

These four components are present in all addictions, whether chemical or behavioral.[2]

Addictive substances or behaviors initially provide a sense of pleasure or stability that the addict cannot achieve in other ways. To be addictive, a substance or behavior must have the potential to produce a positive mood change. Chemicals are responsible for the most profound addictions; they produce dramatic mood changes and cause cellular changes to which the body adapts so well that it eventually requires the chemical to function normally. *Withdrawal* is the variety of symptoms that occur after use of some addictive drugs is reduced or stopped. Other behaviors, such as gambling, spending money, working, and sex, create somewhat milder changes at the cellular level, along with elevating mood—which explains why these behaviors can also be addictive.

What Are the Health Risks of Alcohol Use and Abuse?

Alcohol is the most widely used (and abused) recreational drug in our society. An estimated 52 percent of Americans consume alcoholic beverages regularly. Of them, about seven percent are heavy drinkers, defined as those who habitually consume more than five drinks in one sitting.[4] Nearly half of Americans, however, are light drinkers or non-drinkers: About 13 percent drink fewer than a dozen drinks per year. About 35 percent don't drink at all.

Alcohol on Campus

Alcohol is also the most popular drug on college campuses, where approximately 60 percent of students report having consumed alcoholic beverages in the last 30 days.[5] Students have more freedom, and more social pressures and opportunities to drink than do other young people. A higher percentage of full-time college students drink more heavily than do same-aged peers who aren't in school (Figure 13.2).[6] About 43 percent of all college students engage in **heavy episodic (binge) drinking**; this usually involves drinking five or more drinks in a row (men) or four or more in a row (women) in about 2 hours.[7] Students who engage in **pre-gaming** (also called pre-loading or front-loading) are binge drinking: They gather to drink heavily before going to a bar, nightclub, or sporting event where the drinks might be expensive or drinking might be prohibited. Binge drinking is dangerous because it poses high risk for alcohol-related injuries and death, the number-one cause of preventable death among undergraduate college students in the United States today.[8]

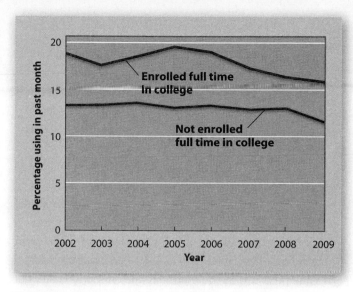

FIGURE **13.2** A higher percentage of college students engage in heavy alcohol use than do their 18- to 22-year-old peers who are not enrolled in school.

Source: Substance Abuse and Mental Health Services Administration, *Results from the 2009 National Survey on Drug Use and Health: Volume I, Summary of National Findings*, NSDUH Series H-38A, HHS Publication No. SMA 10-4856 Findings (Rockville, MD: Office of Applied Studies, 2010).

Alcohol Profoundly Affects Your Body

Alcoholic beverages contain **ethyl alcohol** or **ethanol**. Unlike the molecules found in most foods and drugs, ethanol molecules are sufficiently small and fat soluble to be absorbed throughout the entire gastrointestinal system. A negligible amount of alcohol is absorbed through the lining of the mouth. Approximately 20 percent of ingested alcohol diffuses through the stomach lining into the bloodstream, and nearly 80 percent passes through the lining of the upper third of the small intestine.

Several factors influence how quickly your body absorbs alcohol, including the alcohol concentration in your drink, the amount of alcohol you consume, the amount of food in your stomach, your metabolism, your weight and body mass index, and your mood. The higher the concentration

heavy episodic (binge) drinking Drinking for the express purpose of becoming intoxicated; five drinks or more at one sitting for men; four drinks or more at one sitting for women

pre-gaming A form of binge drinking during which people gather to drink heavily before going to a bar, nightclub, or sporting event

ethanol (ethyl alcohol) An addictive drug produced by fermentation and found in many beverages

blood alcohol concentration (BAC) The ratio of alcohol to blood volume; used as a measure of intoxication

proof A measure of the percentage of alcohol in a beverage

of alcohol in your drink, the more rapidly it will be absorbed in your digestive tract. For example, your body would absorb the alcohol in a one-ounce shot of tequila more rapidly than the alcohol in one ounce of beer because the beer is less concentrated. Carbonated alcoholic beverages, such as champagne and mixed drinks made with soda, are absorbed more rapidly than noncarbonated drinks because the carbonation raises the gas pressure in the stomach and this drives alcohol molecules through the stomach wall more quickly. If your stomach is full of food, alcoholic beverages empty more slowly into the small intestine, slowing absorption. Mood affects absorption as well; powerful moods, such as stress and tension, are likely to cause the stomach to dump its contents into the small intestine, speeding absorption.

Blood alcohol concentration (BAC) is the ratio of alcohol to total blood volume. A drinker's BAC depends on weight and body fat, the water content in body tissues, the concentration of alcohol in the beverage consumed, the rate of consumption, and the volume of alcohol consumed. Figure 13.3 shows approximate blood alcohol concentrations based on body weight and number of drinks consumed. The liver can

metabolize (break down) about one ounce of alcohol per hour. If you drink more than that, the excess alcohol remains in your bloodstream, increasing your BAC.[9]

The **proof** of an alcoholic drink represents the percentage of alcohol in the beverage—the drink's strength. Alcohol percentage is half of the given proof. For example, 80-proof whiskey is 40 percent alcohol by volume. Lower-proof drinks will produce fewer effects than the same amount of higher-proof drinks. Most beers are between 2 to 5 percent alcohol, and most wines are about 12 percent alcohol (see Figure 13.4).

Short-Term Effects of Alcohol Use
Alcohol has numerous intertwined short-term effects on the body that occur within minutes or hours of taking a drink. Figure 13.5 on page 410 summarizes both the short- and long-term effects of alcohol on the body.

Nervous System Effects In the central nervous system, alcohol depresses the functioning of nerve and brain tissue. It slows your reaction time and impairs your judgment and motor coordination. This is why it is so dangerous to drink and drive. Alcohol also decreases vital functions controlled by the brain including your respiratory rate, pulse rate, and blood pressure. The more you drink, the more pronounced are these effects. Very high blood alcohol concentrations can lead to coma and death.

FIGURE **13.3** These charts show the approximate blood alcohol concentration (BAC) for women and men, based on body weight and number of drinks consumed.

Alcoholic beverage	Percentage of alcohol by volume	Amount of alcohol per serving
Light beer (12-oz. can)	2.4–4.8%	0.29–0.58 oz.
Regular beer (12-oz. can)	3.2–5.0%	0.38–0.60 oz.
Wine (4-oz. glass)	12%	0.48 oz.
Cocktail (mixed drinks)	40–50%	1 oz.

FIGURE **13.4** This chart shows the approximate amount of alcohol typically contained in four common alcoholic beverages.

Cardiovascular System Effects Slowed breathing, decreased pulse rate, and lowered blood pressure are all short-term cardiovascular effects. Binge drinkers put themselves at risk for irregular heartbeat or even total loss of heart rhythm, which can disrupt blood flow and damage the heart muscle.

Urinary and Gastrointestinal System Effects Alcohol is a diuretic that causes increased urinary output. The resulting imbalance in body fluids can cause sluggish activity in your brain and nervous system and the fierce headache and sensory overload that typically accompany a hangover. Alcohol also irritates and inflames the gastrointestinal system. If taken in large quantities or ingested on an empty stomach, it may cause indigestion, heartburn, and nausea.

Sexual Impairment Drinking alcohol can lower your sexual inhibitions. This can result in poor choices such as having sex with someone you might not choose if you were sober and exposing yourself to greater risk for a sexually transmitted infection. Drinking alcohol can also lead to less satisfying sex. Because it's a diuretic and depresses nerve function, alcohol decreases vaginal lubrication in women and can lead to erectile dysfunction in men.

Hangover Drinkers often experience a **hangover** the morning after a night of heavy consumption. The symptoms of a hangover include headache, muscle aches, upset stomach, anxiety, depression, diarrhea, and thirst. It usually takes 12 hours to recover from a hangover. Bed rest, solid food, fluid intake, and aspirin may help relieve its discomforts, but the only real cure for a hangover is to avoid one by abstaining from excessive alcohol use.[10]

Long-Term Effects of Alcohol Use

Long-term use of alcohol can cause problems in addition to the ones above, including chronic diseases of the nervous system, cardiovascular system, and liver, as well as some cancers.

Nervous System Effects Even people who drink moderately may, over time, experience shrinkage in brain size and weight.[11] Recent research suggests that in adolescents alcohol may damage the frontal areas of the brain (crucial for controlling impulses and thinking through consequences), and that these areas are much more prone to damage than was previously thought.[12] In addition, research shows that 47 percent of those who begin drinking alcohol before age 14 become *alcohol dependent* at some time in their lives, compared to 9 percent of those who wait until at least age 21.[13]

Cardiovascular System Effects The effects of alcohol on the cardiovascular system are complex. Numerous studies have associated light to moderate alcohol consumption (no more than two drinks a day) with a reduced risk of coronary artery disease. However, this does not mean that alcohol consumption is recommended as a preventive measure against heart disease. Alcohol contributes to high blood pressure and slightly increased heart rate and cardiac output. People who drink regularly have higher systolic blood pressure than people who do not.[14]

Liver Effects Heavy drinking causes the liver to deposit and store fat—a condition

hangover A physiological reaction to excessive drinking, including symptoms such as headache, upset stomach, anxiety, depression, diarrhea, and thirst

Short-term effects

- Impaired judgment/reaction time, impaired motor coordination, headache
- Decreased respiratory rate
- Decreased pulse rate and blood pressure; high amounts of alcohol can cause irregular heartbeat
- Irritation of gastrointestinal system, indigestion, heartburn, nausea
- Reduced sexual responsiveness
- Increased urination
- Muscle ache

Long-term effects

- Reduced brain size, damaged brain cells, dependency
- Increased risk of cancers of the mouth and tongue
- High blood pressure, increased heart rate
- Increased risk of breast cancer
- Fatty liver, alcoholic hepatitis, cirrhosis, increased risk of liver cancer
- Increased risk of cancers of the esophagus and stomach
- Chronic inflammation of pancreas, increased risk of pancreatic cancer
- Impaired nutrient absorption
- Increased risk of osteoporosis
- Risk of giving birth to babies with fetal alcohol syndrome

FIGURE **13.5** The short-term and long-term effects of alcohol on the body.

known as *fatty liver.* Over time, fat-filled liver cells can stop functioning. Prolonged heavy drinking can also cause **alcoholic hepatitis**, another alcohol-related liver disease in which the liver becomes inflamed. Alcoholic hepatitis may itself be fatal or it may progress to **cirrhosis**, a condition in which the liver cells are damaged and scarring occurs. Eventually, the liver cells die, damage becomes permanent, and the liver can no longer carry out its functions in the body. Among moderate to heavy drinkers, this damage may begin in the teens and progress rapidly in early adulthood. By middle-age (45 to 65 years old) cirrhosis is the most common cause of death in Americans after heart disease, cancer, accidents, and suicide.[15]

alcoholic hepatitis A condition resulting from prolonged use of alcohol in which the liver is inflamed

cirrhosis The last stage of liver disease associated with chronic heavy use of alcohol, during which liver cells die and damage becomes permanent

Cancer Alcohol is considered a *carcinogen* (cancer-causing agent). The repeated irritation caused by long-term alcohol use has been linked to cancers of the esophagus, stomach, mouth, tongue, and liver. There is also substantial evidence that even light drinkers (those who consume one drink per day) have a slightly increased risk for breast cancer. Women who drink two to five drinks per day have 150 percent greater risk of developing breast cancer than women who abstain from drinking altogether.[16]

Other Effects Alcohol abuse is a major cause of chronic inflammation of the pancreas, the organ that produces digestive enzymes and insulin. Chronic alcohol abuse inhibits enzyme production, which further inhibits the absorption of nutrients. Drinking alcohol can block the absorption of calcium, which may contribute to a woman's risk of developing *osteoporosis*, a disease characterized by bone thinning due to calcium loss.

Women who are pregnant should avoid alcohol altogether.[17] Alcohol ingested by the mom passes through the placenta, enters the growing baby's bloodstream, and can cause **fetal alcohol syndrome (FAS)**.

Drinking and Driving

In 2009, approximately 32 percent of all traffic fatalities in the United States were alcohol related.[18] Over two-thirds of those killed were driving with BAC levels above 0.08, the legal limit in most states. Of those drunk drivers, 60 percent were aged 21 to 34.[19] Laboratory and test-track research shows that the vast majority of drivers are impaired even at the legal limit of 0.08 BAC, showing decreased ability in braking, steering, and lane changing.[20]

Alcohol Use Can Lead to Alcoholism

Alcohol use becomes **alcohol abuse** when it interferes with work, school, or social and family relationships—or when it entails any violation of the law, including driving under the influence (DUI).[21] **Alcoholism**, or **alcohol dependence**, is suspected when personal and health problems related to alcohol use are severe and when stopping alcohol use results in withdrawal symptoms. The four symptoms of alcoholism include craving—a strong urge to drink; loss of control—not being able to

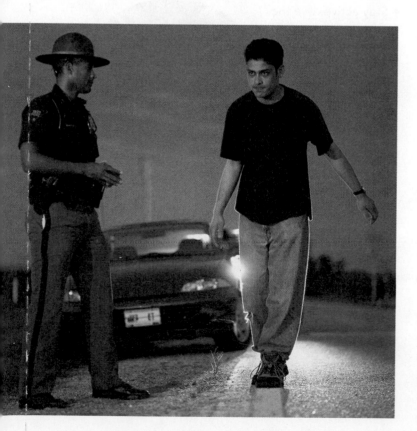

stop drinking once started; physical dependence—withdrawal symptoms such as nausea, sweating and shaking after stopping drinking; and the need to drink ever more alcohol to feel drunk due to tolerance—a physiological phenomenon in which the body requires larger and larger doses of a drug or an addictive behavior in order to produce an effect.

Identifying a Problem Drinker Recognizing and admitting the existence of an alcohol problem is often extremely difficult. Alcoholics deny their problem, often making statements such as, "I can stop any time I want to. I just don't want to right now." Their families also tend to deny the problem, making excuses like "He really has been under a lot of stress lately. Besides, he only drinks beer." The fear of being labelled a "problem drinker" often prevents people from seeking help. **Lab 13.1** provides a questionnaire for assessing your risk of alcohol abuse.

SEE IT! ONLINE
Hidden Addictions

DO IT! ONLINE

Recovery from Alcohol Addiction

Many alcoholics and problem drinkers who seek help have experienced a turning point: flunking out of school, getting arrested for drunk driving, being fired from a job, or having a spouse walk out. He or she has, in many cases, reached a low point and finally recognized that alcohol controls his or her life. The first step on the road to recovery is assuming responsibility for personal actions.

Treatment Programs The alcoholic who is ready for help has several avenues of treatment: psychologists and psychiatrists specializing in the treatment of alcoholism, private treatment centers, hospitals specifically designed to treat alcoholics, community mental health facilities, and support groups such as Alcoholics Anonymous.

On some college campuses, the problems associated with alcohol abuse are so great that schools are instituting strong policies

fetal alcohol syndrome (FAS) A disorder that may affect the fetus when the mother consumes alcohol during pregnancy; among its effects are mental retardation, small head, tremors, and physical abnormalities

alcohol abuse Use of alcohol that interferes with work, school, or personal relationships or that entails violations of the law

alcoholism (alcohol dependence) A condition in which personal and health problems related to alcohol use are severe and stopping alcohol use results in withdrawal symptoms against drinking and programs to help students dealing with alcohol-related problems: University presidents have formed a leadership group to help curb the problem of alcohol abuse; many fraternities and sororities have elected to have "dry" houses; and student health centers are opening their own treatment programs. For example, the University of Texas sponsors a center where students in recovery can get support services and hang out together. And at over a dozen schools including Rutgers University, Case Western Reserve University, Columbia University and others, students in recovery can live together in "clean and sober" housing.[22] It can be difficult to recover from an alcohol abuse problem in college, and programs such as these provide the support and comfortable environment recovering students need.

The Family's Role Members of an alcoholic's family sometimes take action before the alcoholic does. They may seek help from an organization or a treatment facility for themselves and their relative. *Intervention*—a planned confrontation with the alcoholic that involves friends, family members, and professional counselors—is an effective method of helping an alcoholic recognize they have a problem.

Learning to Drink Responsibly

The social atmosphere on college campuses encourages drinking in many ways. College students, both men and women, seek peer approval; and drinking is part of many college traditions such as Greek rush and football games. Advertising for the alcoholic beverage industry targets college students. Students believe alcohol will make them feel less stressed, more sociable, and less self-conscious. Many turn 21 while at

SEE IT! ONLINE

Spring Break Nightmare

LIVE IT! ONLINE

Worksheet 32 A Dozen Drinking Dilemmas

TOOLS FOR **CHANGE** •

How to Cut Down on Your Drinking

If you think you drink too much, you may want to cut down or abstain. If you have a severe drinking problem, alcoholism in your family, or other medical problems, you should stop drinking completely. Talk to a counselor or clinician who can advise you how to do that safely.

If you need to cut down on your drinking, these steps can help you:

• Write down your reasons for cutting down or stopping.

• Determine a limit for how much you will drink. You may choose to cut down or to not drink at all. If you aren't sure what is healthy for you, talk with your counselor. Write down your drinking goal and post it where you'll see it.

• Keep a diary of your drinking. For three or four weeks, write down every time you have a drink. You may be surprised how much you drink and when. How different is your limit from the amount you drink now?

• Keep little or no alcohol at home. You don't need the temptation.

• Take a break from alcohol. Pick a day or two each week when you will not drink at all. Then try to stop drinking for one week. Think about how you feel physically and emotionally on these days. When you succeed and feel better, you may find it easier to cut down for good.

• Learn to say "no, thank you." You do not have to drink when other people are, or take a drink when offered one. Stay away from people who give you a hard time about not drinking.

• Stay active. Use the time and money once spent on drinking to do something fun with your family or friends. Go out to eat, see a movie, or play sports or a game.

• Get support. Ask your family and friends to help you reach your goal. Talk to your counselor if you are having trouble cutting down. Get the help you need.

• Avoid people, places, or events that tempt you to drink. Plan ahead of time what you will do to avoid drinking when you are tempted.

• Don't give up! Most people don't cut down or give up drinking all at once. If you don't reach your goal the first time, try again.

• •

college and celebrate by getting drunk. In addition, campus communities often have a large number of bars and liquor stores with relatively low prices.

How can you drink responsibly in an atmosphere with so many pressures to drink? Here are some tips:

- Eat before and while you drink.
- Don't drink before a party or event.
- Avoid drinking if you are angry, anxious, depressed, or taking any medication.
- Pace yourself. Drink one alcoholic drink or less per hour.
- Alternate alcoholic and non-alcoholic drinks.
- Determine ahead of time the number of drinks you will have for the evening.
- Avoid drinking games.
- Don't drink and drive. Volunteer to be the sober driver.
- Avoid parties where you expect heavy drinking.

If you have trouble doing any of the above and suspect that you may have a drinking problem, try using the information in the box How to Cut Down on Your Drinking.

casestudy

NATHAN

"At some parties, they'll card you to make sure you're over 21, but a lot of the time they don't. I'm underage, but it's easy to get a fake ID. When we go out to parties on weekends, or when we have one here at the fraternity house, I usually have three or four drinks a night. After three drinks, I definitely feel drunk, but I'm pretty moderate compared to other people I know. My friend Chris usually has six or more drinks in a night and I've seen him pass out from it."

THINK! Would you consider Nathan a heavy drinker? What about Chris? Explain. How many times per week do you drink alcohol? Are you a binge drinker?

ACT! Calculate what your BAC would have been toward the end of the most recent party you attended. Have you ever drunk more than you wanted to because of social pressure? Write down three things you could have said or done to avoid this.

What Are the Health Risks of Tobacco Use?

Every puff of tobacco smoke causes harm, according to a recent report from the U.S. Surgeon General's office.[23] There is no safe level of tobacco use. Yet, despite the health risks, an estimated 46 million people in the United States, or 20.6% of all adults (aged 18 years and older) smoke cigarettes. Cigarette smoking is more common among men (23.5%) than women (17.9%).[24] In addition to the dangers, tobacco use is expensive. The average base cost of a pack of cigarettes is $4.63; however, with state taxes pushing prices as high as $11.90 per pack, the average actual cost is $6.50. At those prices, a pack-a-day smoker can spend more than $2300 per year on cigarettes. This does not include the costs of higher health care bills and higher insurance premiums for the smoker and those exposed to his or her secondhand smoke. The long-term health consequences are incalculably higher.

LIVE IT! ONLINE

Worksheet 34
Smoke
and Snuff
Stumpers

Smoking on Campus

Smoking among today's college students appears to be lower than it's been in decades: 16.4 percent in 2010 compared to 30.6 percent in 1999, and 24.4 percent in 1982.[25] College-educated people are less likely to smoke than other people, but still more than 1 in 6 students do. Why? The largest group, 38 percent, say it helps them control stress. Other less common reasons are social pressure, experimentation, weight control, and addiction.

An important reason that students may not be aware of is advertising. With the number of smokers declining by about one million each year, the tobacco industry tries to recruit new smokers by aiming 90 percent of its advertising budget at children and teenagers. The tobacco industry targets young women with pictures of svelte models smoking "slim or light" brands to promote a belief that smoking can help with weight loss. The industry recruits minorities using targeted print ads and neighborhood billboards. It sponsors concerts, races, and other popular events to try to equate social fun with smoking.

Tobacco Products and Tobacco Smoke Contain Many Harmful Substances

The chemical stimulant **nicotine** is the major psychoactive substance in all tobacco products. In its natural form, nicotine is a colorless

> **nicotine** The primary stimulant chemical in tobacco products

liquid that turns brown upon exposure to air. When smokers burn tobacco leaves in a cigarette, pipe, or cigar, nicotine is released and inhaled into the lungs. Chewing tobacco releases nicotine into the saliva, and the nicotine is then absorbed through the mucous membranes of the mouth.

Smoking is the most common form of tobacco use and delivers a strong dose of nicotine to the user. Tobacco smoke also contains over 4,000 other chemical compounds, including arsenic, formaldehyde, and ammonia. More than 60 of the chemicals in tobacco smoke are known or suspected to cause cancer. Particulate matter from smoke condenses in the lungs to form a thick, brownish sludge called *tar,* which contains at least 69 known cancer-causing chemicals.[26] Also among the many chemicals in tobacco smoke are various gases and vapors that may have significant effects on the heart and circulatory system. Even exposure to the secondhand smoke from just one cigarette per day accelerates the progression of atherosclerosis,[27] suggesting that even low doses of tobacco smoke exposure could negatively impact heart function.[28]

Of the toxic gases in cigarette smoke, the most dangerous is **carbon monoxide**. The concentration of carbon monoxide is 800 times higher than the level considered safe by the U.S. Environmental Protection Agency (EPA). In the human body, carbon monoxide reduces the oxygen-carrying capacity of the red blood cells by binding with the receptor sites for oxygen, causing oxygen deprivation in body tissues.

The heat from tobacco smoke is also harmful. Inhaling hot gases exposes sensitive mucous membranes to irritating chemicals that weaken tissues and contribute to cancers of the mouth, larynx, and throat.

Main Types of Tobacco Use

Tobacco comes in several forms. Cigarettes, cigars, pipes, and bidis are used for burning and inhaling tobacco. Smokeless tobacco is sniffed or placed in the mouth.

Cigarettes Filtered cigarettes designed to reduce levels of gases such as hydrogen cyanide and hydrocarbons may actually deliver *more* hazardous carbon monoxide to the user than non-filtered brands. Even the use of low-tar and low-nicotine products is self-defeating: Users wind up exposing themselves to the same harmful

carbon monoxide A gas found in cigarette smoke that binds at oxygen receptor sites in the blood

substances they would with regular-strength cigarettes. Clove cigarettes contain about 40 percent ground cloves (a spice), about 60 percent tobacco, and higher levels of tar, nicotine, and carbon monoxide than regular cigarettes.

Cigars Cigars are no safer than cigarettes.[29] Cigar smoke contains 23 poisons and 43 carcinogens. Smoking as little as one cigar per day can double the risk of several cancers. Daily cigar smoking also increases the risk of heart and lung diseases.

Bidis These small hand-rolled flavored cigarettes are generally made in India or Southeast Asia. They are far more toxic than cigarettes. Research clearly indicates that bidi smokers are at the same, if not higher, risk for coronary heart disease and cancer as smokers of regular cigarettes.[30]

Hookahs A *hookah* is a pipe that draws smoke from burning substances through water. It does not, however, filter out toxins. Hookah smoking is just as dangerous as cigarette smoking.[31]

Smokeless Tobacco Approximately five million U.S. adults use smokeless tobacco. *Chewing tobacco* contains tobacco leaves treated with flavorings; it is placed between the gums and teeth. Another type of smokeless tobacco is *snuff*, a fine ground form of tobacco that can be inhaled, chewed, or placed against the gums.

A major risk of chewing tobacco use is *leukoplakia*, a condition characterized by leathery white patches inside the mouth. Three to 17 percent of diagnosed leukoplakia cases develop into oral cancer. It is estimated that 75 percent of the more than 30,000 cases of oral cancer diagnosed in the United States each year result from either smokeless tobacco or cigarette use.[32]

Short-Term Effects of Tobacco Use

In healthy lungs, millions of tiny hair-like projections called *cilia* line the respiratory passageways and sweep away foreign matter, which is expelled from the lungs by coughing. Nicotine paralyzes the cilia for up to an hour following the smoking of a single cigarette. This allows tar and other solids in tobacco smoke to accumulate and irritate sensitive tissue.

Nicotine is also a powerful central nervous system stimulant that produces a variety of physiological effects. In the cerebral cortex, it produces an aroused, alert mental state. Nicotine also stimulates the adrenal glands, which increase the production of adrenaline. Nicotine stimulation increases heart and respiratory rates, constricts blood vessels, and, in turn, increases blood pressure because the heart must work harder to pump blood through the narrowed vessels.

nicotine poisoning Symptoms often experienced by beginning smokers, including dizziness, diarrhea, light-headedness, rapid and erratic pulse, clammy skin, nausea, and vomiting

Nicotine raises blood sugar levels and decreases the stomach contractions that signal hunger. These factors, along with decreased sensation in the taste buds, reduce appetite. Beginning smokers usually feel some or all of the effects of **nicotine poisoning**— including dizziness, light-headedness, rapid and erratic pulse, clammy skin, nausea, vomiting, and diarrhea— with their first puff. The effects cease as tolerance to the chemical develops. Tolerance develops almost immediately in new users, perhaps after the second or third cigarette. Tolerance to most other drugs, such as alcohol, develops over a period of months or years. Regular smokers often do not feel the "buzz" of smoking. They continue to smoke because stopping is too difficult.

Figure 13.6 summarizes both the short- and long-term health effects of smoking.

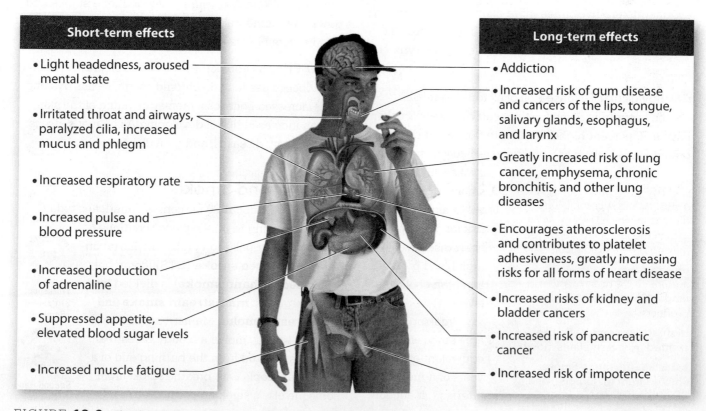

Short-term effects

- Light headedness, aroused mental state
- Irritated throat and airways, paralyzed cilia, increased mucus and phlegm
- Increased respiratory rate
- Increased pulse and blood pressure
- Increased production of adrenaline
- Suppressed appetite, elevated blood sugar levels
- Increased muscle fatigue

Long-term effects

- Addiction
- Increased risk of gum disease and cancers of the lips, tongue, salivary glands, esophagus, and larynx
- Greatly increased risk of lung cancer, emphysema, chronic bronchitis, and other lung diseases
- Encourages atherosclerosis and contributes to platelet adhesiveness, greatly increasing risks for all forms of heart disease
- Increased risks of kidney and bladder cancers
- Increased risk of pancreatic cancer
- Increased risk of impotence

FIGURE **13.6** The short-term and long-term effects of smoking on the body.

Long-Term Effects of Tobacco Use

With its long list of chronic health effects, cigarette smoking adversely affects the well-being of smokers, as well as the health of everyone nearby. Each day, cigarettes contribute to more than 1,000 deaths from cancer, cardiovascular disease, and respiratory disorders. In the United States, tobacco use is the single most preventable cause of death. It kills more Americans than alcohol, car accidents, suicide, AIDS, homicide, and illegal drugs combined.[33]

Cancer The American Cancer Society estimates that smoking causes 85 to 90 percent of all cases of lung cancer. Fewer than 10 percent of cases occur among nonsmokers.[34] Lung cancer can take 10 to 30 years to develop, and the outlook for its victims is poor. Most lung cancer is not diagnosed until it is fairly widespread in the body; at that point, the five-year survival rate is only 15 percent. By comparison, the five-year survival rate for breast cancer is 87 percent, for colon cancer 59–62 percent, and for prostate cancer 92.5 percent.[35]

Tobacco is linked to other cancers as well. The rate of pancreatic cancer is more than twice as high for smokers as nonsmokers. The five-year survival rate for pancreatic cancer is less than five percent. Cancers of the lips, tongue, salivary glands, and esophagus are five times more likely to occur among smokers than among nonsmokers. Smokers are also more likely to develop kidney, bladder, and larynx cancers.[36]

Cardiovascular Disease Half of all tobacco-related deaths occur from some form of heart disease.[37] Smokers have a 70 percent higher death rate from heart disease than do nonsmokers and are twice as likely to suffer strokes. In fact, smoking cigarettes poses as great a risk for developing heart disease as do high blood pressure and high cholesterol levels.

Smoking also appears to add the equivalent of 10 years of aging to the arteries.[38] It encourages the build up of fatty deposits in the heart and major blood vessels (atherosclerosis) and it contributes to *platelet adhesiveness,* the sticking together of red blood cells that is associated with blood clots. Smoking decreases the oxygen supplied to the heart and can weaken tissues. It also contributes to irregular heart rhythms, which can trigger a heart attack. Both carbon monoxide and nicotine in cigarette smoke can precipitate angina attacks (pain spasms in the chest when the heart muscle does not get the blood supply it needs).

Respiratory Diseases Smokers may develop *chronic bronchitis* because their inflamed lungs produce more mucus and constantly try to rid themselves of this mucus and foreign particles. The effort to do so results in "smoker's hack," the persistent cough that most smokers experience. Smokers are also more prone to respiratory ailments such as influenza, pneumonia, and colds.

Emphysema is a chronic disease in which breathing becomes difficult because the alveoli (the tiny air sacs in the lungs) are destroyed, impairing the lungs' ability to obtain oxygen and remove carbon dioxide. There is no known cure for emphysema, and once the damage is done, it is irreversible. Smoking is the major cause of emphysema and smokers are 12 to 15 times more likely to die of emphysema than are non-smokers. Exposure to secondhand smoke and other environmental exposures also increase risks for this irreversible disease.[39]

Other Effects Other long-term health effects of smoking and tobacco use include chronic cough, sexual dysfunction, increased bone loss, premature aging of the skin, and an increased risk of developing Alzheimer's disease, inflammatory diseases, and gum disease.

Secondhand Smoke

Although only about 20 percent of Americans today smoke, smoking in public places continues to cause an air pollution problem.[40] **Environmental tobacco smoke (ETS)** (commonly called **secondhand smoke**) is divided into two categories: **mainstream smoke** and **sidestream smoke**. Mainstream smoke is emitted from a smoker's mouth. Sidestream smoke is emitted from the burning end of a cigarette. People who breathe smoke from someone else's smoking product are said to be *involuntary* or *passive* smokers.

emphysema A chronic lung disease in which the tiny air sacs in the lungs are destroyed, making breathing difficult

environmental tobacco smoke (ETS) or **secondhand smoke** Smoke from tobacco products

mainstream smoke Smoke emitted from a smoker's mouth

sidestream smoke Smoke emitted from the burning end of a cigarette

LIVE IT! ONLINE
Worksheet 31 Passive Smoking

SEE IT! ONLINE
Second Hand Smoke

Although involuntary smokers breathe less tobacco than active smokers do, they still face risks from the exposure. About 85 percent of secondhand smoke is sidestream smoke, which contains five times more carbon monoxide and 50 times more ammonia than mainstream smoke (which has already been partially filtered by the lungs of the smoker who exhaled it).[41] The U.S. Surgeon General and the Centers for Disease Control and Prevention estimate that 126 million Americans breathe in secondhand smoke each year and about 50,000 die from it: 3,400 from lung cancer, 46,000 from cardiovascular disease, and 430 newborns from sudden infant death syndrome.[42]

Children, especially those under five, are vulnerable to secondhand smoke and show a greater chance of developing pneumonia, bronchitis, and other infections of the lower respiratory tract as a result of exposure. Additionally, children exposed to secondhand smoke are twice as likely to become smokers during adolescence than children who are not exposed to it.[43] Because of these increased risks, many states have enacted or are considering legislation that prohibits smoking in vehicles when children are present.

Quitting Smoking

Smash the Ash

About 70 percent of adult smokers want to quit and up to 44 percent make a serious attempt to quit each year, but only four to seven percent succeed.[44] College students who begin smoking regularly want to stop, but only 13 percent are able to.[45] Most daily smokers continue throughout college.

Smokers must break both the physical addiction to nicotine and the habit of lighting up at certain times of day. The box Why Is It So Hard to Quit Smoking? investigates some of the reasons why quitting smoking is so challenging—and why the best strategy is never to start. New federally mandated cigarette packaging is aimed at discouraging smoking and encouraging quitting (Figure 13.7).

Breaking Nicotine Addiction Withdrawing from nicotine can cause irritability, restlessness, nausea, vomiting, and intense cravings for tobacco. Several non-tobacco products that replace depleted levels of nicotine in the bloodstream, such as nicotine gum, the nicotine patch, prescription nasal sprays, and the nicotine inhaler have helped some people wean themselves off tobacco.

Non-nicotine strategies for breaking addiction include the prescription drugs Zyban and Chantix. Zyban

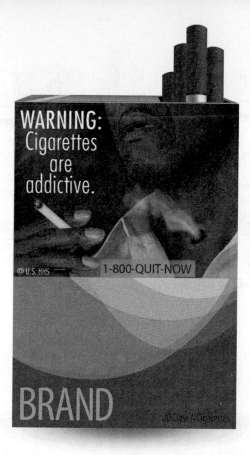

FIGURE **13.7** This label is one of nine designed by the FDA to cover most of a cigarette package and motivate people to think about health risks before they light up. The labels are scheduled to appear on packages by September 2012; however, pending lawsuits by tobacco companies may delay or cancel their implementation.

is thought to work on dopamine and norepinephrine receptors in the brain to decrease craving and withdrawal symptoms. Chantix may help smokers quit by providing nicotine-like effects to ease withdrawal symptoms and blocking the effects of nicotine if the patient resumes smoking.[46] A relatively new approach is an anti-nicotine vaccine now in early testing. The drug stimulates the immune system to generate antibodies that prevent nicotine from entering or acting upon the brain.[47]

How effective are these therapies? The evidence is strong that consistent pharmacological treatments can help a smoker quit, with estimated abstinence after use ranging from 16 to 30 percent.[48] Those who cannot quit with drug therapies alone may benefit from antismoking behavioral therapy. Self-control strategies such as those described in **Lab 13.2** help people resist the temptation to smoke by identifying the specific situations in which they reach for a cigarette.

Benefits of Quitting Many tissues damaged by smoking can repair themselves. As soon as smokers stop, the body begins the repair process (Figure 13.8).[49] Within

Why Is It So Hard to Quit Smoking?

After just two to three cigarettes, the immediate side effects of nicotine subside and the craving begins. Once fully addicted to nicotine, nine out of ten people who try to stop smoking fail. Why is this?

The way cigarettes taste while being inhaled (and feel while being exhaled) appears to be as important to some smokers as the actual craving for nicotine—and it's a clue to why nicotine replacement therapy works poorly for some.[1] What's more, some people fail to use nicotine patches, gum, and inhalers as directed—stopping too soon or using too little—which also contributes to the failure to quit smoking.[2]

Researchers at the University of Southern California recently discovered that a brain region called the *insula* seems to be involved in nicotine's powerful addictiveness.[3] Patients who have suffered injury to this region appear able to quit smoking easily. This discovery may someday allow doctors to manipulate the insula with drugs or biofeedback to help block addiction.

Several smoking-cessation research groups are working on new methods to help people stop. One is non-nicotine cigarettes that would provide all the sensory gratification of smoking but without the nicotine (unfortunately still including the cancer-causing tars and other toxins). Another is a drug to block the effects of nicotine while allowing people to smoke regular cigarettes. The best way to avoid cigarette addiction? Don't start smoking in the first place.

Sources:
1. J. E. Rose, "Nicotine and Nonnicotine Factors in Cigarette Addiction," *Psychopharmacology* 184, nos. 3–4 (2006): 274–85.
2. S. Shiffman and others, "Reduction of Abstinence-Induced Withdrawal and Craving Using High Dose Nicotine Replacement Therapy," *Psychopharmacology* 184, nos. 3–4 (2006): 637–44.
3. N. H. Naqvi and others, "Damage to the Insula Disrupts Addiction to Cigarette Smoking," *Science* 315, no. 5811 (2007): 531–4.

START HERE

8 hours
- Carbon monoxide level in blood drops to normal.
- Oxygen level in blood increases to normal.

48 hours
- Nerve endings start regrowing.
- Ability to smell and taste is enhanced.

1 to 9 months
- Coughing, sinus congestion, fatigue, shortness of breath decreases.
- Cilia regrow in lungs, which increases ability to handle mucus, clean the lungs, reduce infection.
- Body's overall energy increases.

5 years
- Lung cancer death rate for average former smoker (one pack a day) decreases by almost half.

15 years
- Risk of coronary heart disease is that of a nonsmoker.

20 minutes
- Blood pressure drops to normal.
- Pulse rate drops to normal.
- Body temperature of hands and feet increases to normal.

24 hours
- Chance of heart attack decreases.

2 weeks to 3 months
- Circulation improves.
- Walking becomes easier.
- Lung function increases up to 30%.

1 year
- Excess risk of coronary disease is half that of a smoker.

10 years
- Lung cancer death rate similar to that of nonsmokers.
- Precancerous cells are replaced.
- Risk of cancer of the mouth, throat, esophagus, bladder, kidney, and pancreas decreases.

FIGURE **13.8** The benefits of quitting smoking begin 20 minutes after smoking cessation and continue for years.

casestudy

NATHAN

"I went through a phase where I tried smoking clove cigarettes. My friends told me they weren't as bad as regular cigarettes, and I liked the way they tasted. I stopped, though, because the next morning I always woke up coughing and hacking up phlegm and my clothes were starting to smell. My roommate Kevin is still a smoker. He's not allowed to smoke inside the fraternity house, but he does it anyway. He tries to do it when I'm not there, but sometimes when I walk in, I can still see smoke hanging in the air. So my clothes still smell!"

THINK! Is Nathan correct that clove cigarettes "aren't as bad" as regular cigarettes? Explain your answer. What hazard is Nathan's roommate exposing him to? What are the dangers involved?

ACT! Do you smoke? If so, list three strategies you could employ to limit or eventually stop your tobacco use. If you are around others who smoke, name two things you can do to limit your exposure to secondhand smoke.

HEAR IT! ONLINE

TABLE 13.1 Annual Prevalence of Use for Various Types of Drugs among Full-Time College Students	
Drug	% of College Students Reporting Use
Alcohol	78.6
Cigarettes	28.1
Any illicit drug	35.0
Any illicit drug other than marijuana	17.1
Marijuana	32.7
Inhalants	1.7
Hallucinogens	4.9
Cocaine	3.5
Heroin	0.2
Narcotics other than heroin	7.2
Amphetamines, adjusted	9.0
Sedatives (Barbiturates)	2.5
Tranquilizers	4.9
Steroids	0.3

Source: L. D. Johnston and others, *Monitoring the Future, National Survey Results on Drug Use, 1975–2010: Volume II, College Students and Adults Ages 19–50* (Ann Arbor: Institute for Social Research, The University of Michigan, 2011).

eight hours "smoker's breath" disappears. Often, the mucus that clogs airways is broken up and eliminated within a month of quitting. Many ex-smokers say they have more energy, sleep better, and feel more alert.

What Are the Health Risks of Drug Use and Abuse?

Drug misuse and abuse are huge problems in our society. **Drug misuse** involves using a drug for a purpose for which it was not intended, while **drug abuse** is defined as excessive use of any drug. Each year, such abuse and misuse of drugs contributes to tens of thousands of deaths and costs taxpayers hundreds of billions of dollars in preventable health care costs, extra law enforcement, auto crashes, crime, and lost productivity.[50] Drug use is still on the rise: In the most recent National Survey on Drug Use and Health, 10 percent of Americans aged 12 to 17 reported having used illicit drugs during the past month, compared to 9.3 percent reporting past-month use in the previous year's survey.[51] For Americans aged 18 to 25, reported use of illicit drugs during the past month rose from 19.6 percent to 21.2 percent.

Drug Use among College Students

Marijuana is the most commonly used illegal drug on college campuses, and the use of club drugs such as Ecstasy and prescription narcotics, stimulants, tranquilizers, and sedatives has been on the rise. A recent Columbia University study showed that student use of stimulants such as Ritalin is up 93 percent; the use of opioids such as OxyContin has risen 343 percent; and the use of tranquilizers such as Valium has risen 450 percent in recent years.[52] Students use these drugs under the mistaken impression that they are a safe way to stay awake for studying, to alleviate anxiety or depression, or to increase their stamina for sports.[53] Table 13.1 shows annual drug use among full-time college students.

SEE IT! ONLINE
Campus Drug Dealers

> **drug misuse** Use of a drug for a purpose for which it was not intended
>
> **drug abuse** Excessive use of a drug

Commonly Used Drugs

In this section, we discuss the health risks of various drugs, including marijuana, so-called club drugs, stimulants, depressants, hallucinogens, inhalants, and steroids.

Marijuana Marijuana is the most popular illicit drug used by college students and the third most popular drug (after alcohol and tobacco) used by students overall. Users usually smoke marijuana in a cigarette, called a *joint,* or in a pipe or bong. The psychoactive substance *tetrahydrocannabinol* (THC) causes the high that marijuana users experience. THC's most noticeable effect is the dilation of the eyes' blood vessels, which produces characteristic bloodshot eyes. Users can also experience coughing, dry mouth and throat, increased thirst and appetite, lowered blood pressure, mild muscular weakness, severe anxiety, panic, paranoia, psychosis, sensory alterations and slowed reaction time that lead to an impaired ability to drive.[54]

Studies of long-term marijuana users indicate that marijuana causes lung damage comparable to that caused by tobacco smoking.[55] Other risks associated with long-term marijuana use may include diminished oxygen-carrying capacity of the blood, suppression of the immune system, blood pressure changes, and impaired memory function.[56] Pregnant women who smoke marijuana are at higher risk for stillbirth or miscarriage and for delivering low-birth-weight babies with abnormalities of the nervous system.

Designer or "Club" Drugs

Designer (club) drugs are produced in chemical laboratories, often in homes, and are sold illegally. They include Ecstasy, GHB, Special K, and Rohypnol. Research has shown that club drugs can produce a range of unwanted side effects, including hallucinations, paranoia, amnesia, and in some cases death. Some club drugs work on the same brain mechanisms as alcohol and using them together can dangerously boost the effects of both substances.

Ecstasy Ecstasy (methylene dioxy-methylamphet-amine, or MDMA) has had a resurgence of popularity on college campuses. Young people may initially use Ecstasy

to improve mood or get energized; it also increases heart rate and blood pressure and may raise body temperature to the point of kidney or cardiovascular failure. Chronic use of this hallucinogen appears to damage the brain's ability to think and to regulate emotion, memory, sleep, and pain. Combined with alcohol, Ecstasy can be extremely dangerous and sometimes fatal.[57]

Rohypnol and GHB The tranquilizers Rohypnol (the brand name of the prescription drug flunitrazepam) and gamma-hydroxybutyrate (GHB) are a growing problem on college campuses. Sometimes called the "date rape" drug, Rohypnol has been slipped into the drinks of victims in hopes of lowering their inhibitions and facilitating sexual conquest.[58] Like Rohypnol, GHB may be slipped into drinks undetected, resulting in memory loss, unconsciousness, amnesia, and even death for the victim. Other side effects include nausea, vomiting, seizures, hallucinations, coma, and respiratory distress.

Ketamine Ketamine, or "Special K," is used legitimately as an anesthetic in many hospital and veterinary clinics. On the street, liquid Special K is cooked and dried by dealers and ground into powder. Special K is classed as a hallucinogen. The drug inhibits the relay of sensory input, and the brain fills the resulting void with visions, dreams, memories, and intense sensory distortions that can mimic schizophrenia.

Stimulants Stimulants generally improve mood and decrease fatigue. Illegal stimulants include cocaine and

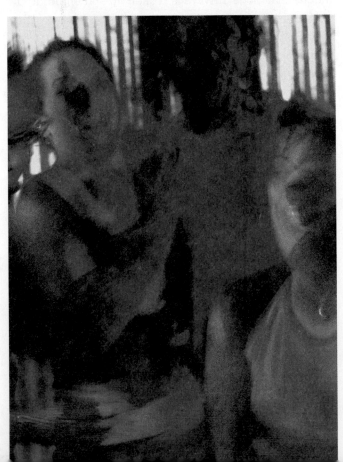

---

marijuana Chopped leaves and flowers of a *Cannabis* plant; a psychoactive stimulant

designer (club) drugs Synthetic versions of existing illicit drugs; includes Ecstasy, Rohypnol, GHB, and Special K methamphetamine. Legal stimulants include prescribed Ritalin and Adderall and caffeine.

Cocaine Cocaine is a powerful and addictive stimulant. Snorted cocaine enters the bloodstream through the mucus membranes and binds to receptor sites in the central nervous system, where it produces intense pleasure. This feeling quickly disappears, however, and the desire to regain the initial high makes the user crave more cocaine.

Cocaine is both an anesthetic and a central nervous system stimulant. In tiny doses, it can slow the heart rate. In larger doses, it increases heart rate and blood pressure, decreases appetite, and causes convulsions, muscle twitching, irregular heartbeat, and eventual death. Other effects include temporary relief of depression, decreased fatigue, talkativeness, increased alertness, and heightened self-confidence. As the dose increases, users become irritable and apprehensive, and their behavior may turn paranoid or violent.

Amphetamines Amphetamines include a large and varied group of synthetic agents that stimulate the central nervous system. Small doses of physician-prescribed amphetamines can improve alertness, lessen fatigue, and elevate mood. With repeated use, however, physical and psychological dependency develops. Amphetamine users may experience insomnia; increases in heart rate, breathing rate, and blood pressure; restlessness; anxiety; appetite suppression; and vision problems.

SEE IT! ONLINE
Eliminating Meth

One type of illegal amphetamine called *methamphetamine* (also known as meth or crystal meth) is an increasingly serious problem. Its use began primarily in the western U.S. The problem has spread to all states now, but continues to be highest in California, Nevada, Wyoming, and Montana.[59] Methamphetamine is a potent, long-acting, addictive drug that strongly activates the brain's reward center by producing a sense of euphoria. It can cause brain damage that results in impaired motor skills and cognitive functions, as well as psychosis and increased risk for heart attack and stroke.

Certain types of amphetamines are legal when used as prescribed. Physicians prescribe drugs such as Ritalin and Adderall to treat children with attention deficit/hyperactive disorder. However, in recent years these drugs have been increasingly misused by students to stay awake for all-night cramming sessions. There is also a false perception that these drugs improve academic performance.[60]

Caffeine While legal, the stimulant caffeine can be abused if consumed to excess. One caffeine pill, such as No-Doz, has about as much caffeine as a cup of caffeinated coffee. An overdose of caffeine can produce confusion, convulsions, breathing problems, sweating, and irregular heartbeat.[61] Too, the caffeine in energy drinks can mask your level of intoxication if you combine them with alcohol.

LIVE IT! ONLINE
Worksheet 33 Caffeine Countdown

Depressants Depressants include opiates, sedatives and tranquilizers. Among the oldest pain relievers known to humans, **opiates** are derived from the parent drug *opium*, made from the opium poppy seed pod. Illegal opiate drugs (also referred to as *narcotics*) include opium, heroin, and black tar heroin. Morphine and codeine, and the synthetic opiates Vicodin, Oxycontin, and Percocet may be prescribed legally as painkillers, but are also frequently abused. All opiates are highly addictive.

SEE IT! ONLINE
Heroin in Suburbia

Opiates are powerful depressants of the central nervous system. In addition to relieving pain, these drugs lower heart rate, respiration, and blood pressure. Side effects include weakness, dizziness, nausea, vomiting, euphoria, decreased sex drive, visual disturbances, and lack of coordination. Of all opiates, *heroin* has the greatest notoriety as being addictive.

stimulants An agent, especially a chemical one, that temporarily arouses or accelerates physiological activity

opiates A class of drugs derived from the parent drug opium, characterized by the ability to relieve pain, induce drowsiness, and cause euphoria

Tranquilizers and sedatives, such as Valium, Ativan, Xanax, and barbiturates, are also nervous system depressants. These drugs may be prescribed legally to reduce anxiety or promote sleep, and they may also be abused. As with the opiates, the depressant effects of tranquilizers and sedatives are increased when taken in conjunction with other depressants, including alcohol. Combining these drugs with alcohol can lead to respiratory failure and death.

Hallucinogens (psychedelics) **Hallucinogenic** or **psychedelic** drugs include *lysergic acid diethylamide (LSD)*, *mescaline* (derived from the peyote cactus), *psilocybin* (one of the active chemicals in mushrooms consumed for their hallucinogenic side effects), and *phencyclidine (PCP)*. The primary pharmacological effect of these drugs is to alter feelings, perceptions, and thoughts. All of them are illegal and carry severe penalties for manufacture, possession, transportation, or sale.

Ketamine and Ecstasy (both discussed above) are technically classed as hallucinogens, as is the most commonly abused over-the-counter drug, *dextromethorphan* (DXM), an ingredient in cough and cold medicines.[62] Often referred to as "robo-tripping," "skittling," or "dexing," the misuse of DXM can cause effects similar to PCP and ketamine, including impaired motor functioning, numbness, nausea and increased heart rate and blood pressure. It can also lead to brain damage and death.[63]

Inhalants **Inhalants** are legal products, such as rubber cement and model glue, that can be purchased in many stores but are dangerous when misused for mind-altering effects. They contain vapor-producing chemicals that, when sniffed, can cause dizziness, lack of coordination, hallucinations, and euphoria. Their effects usually last for fewer than 15 minutes and users often overlap several "hits." This can create an overdose of fumes that can, in turn, cause unconsciousness. If the user's oxygen intake is reduced during the inhaling process, death can result within five minutes.[64]

Anabolic steroids **Anabolic steroids** are artificial forms of the male hormone testosterone that promote muscle growth and strength but also cause depression,

hallucinogenic (psychedelic) Refers to substances capable of creating auditory or visual distortions and heightened states

inhalants Products that are sniffed or inhaled in order to produce a high

anabolic steroids Artificial forms of the hormone testosterone that promote muscle growth and strength

hostility, and aggression and acne, stunted height, and increased risk of heart disease and cancer.[65] (The box on page 150 in Chapter 4 discusses the health consequences of anabolic steroid use in more detail.)

Overcoming Drug Abuse

Alan Leshner, the former director of the National Institute of Drug Abuse, has called addiction the "oops phenomenon." All drug users start out making voluntary, controllable decisions to try drugs just a few times for the experience. The "oops," writes Leshner, "is how easily and often quickly the brain adapts to habit-forming drugs so use becomes compulsive and uncontrollable." A vast body of hard evidence, he concludes, "shows that it is virtually inevitable that prolonged drug use will lead to addiction."[66] Once people become addicted, the chance of quitting on their own is very low. Nearly all addicted persons need specialized medical and psychological treatment to recover. However, of the 23.2 million Americans who needed treatment for addiction to alcohol or illicit drugs in 2007, only 2.4 million received it.[67]

LIVE IT! ONLINE

Worksheet 36
What Is Substance Abuse

Worksheet 37
Substance Use Log

SEE IT! ONLINE

Treating Ad-
dictions with
Virtual Reality

Drug programs are designed to help people safely withdraw from chemical dependency, to improve their day-to-day functioning, to avoid future **relapse**, to understand why they became addicted, to return to abstinence after relapses, and ultimately to achieve long-term abstinence and successful functioning in society. Drug treatment usually includes medications (such as the methadone used to block addiction to heroin or morphine) and behavioral therapy involving individuals, groups, or families and led by drug counselors, psychologists, or psychiatrists. Community-based 12-step programs such as Narcotics Anonymous also include a spiritual component.

Because prolonged drug use can ultimately lead to tolerance and dependence, it is vitally important to educate people about drug experimentation and use. Past antidrug strategies have featured total prohibition (as in the alcohol prohibition during the 1920s) and "scare tactics," but both approaches have proven ineffective. Researchers in the field of drug education agree that students should be taught the difference between drug use and abuse, how to handle social situations where drugs are present, and how to recognize signs of drug dependence in themselves and their friends. Completing Labs 13.1– 13.3 can help you assess your use of alcohol, tobacco, and drugs and determine your potential risk of abuse. Reading the box If Someone Offers You Drugs can prepare you in advance to handle social pressure.

> **relapse** Resumption of behavior that one is attempting to cease

TOOLS FOR **CHANGE** ●

If Someone Offers You Drugs

It is likely that you will be invited to use drugs at some point in your life. Here are some questions to consider before you find yourself presented with the opportunity to use illegal drugs or feel pressure to do so:

- Why am I considering trying drugs?

- Am I using this drug to cope? Am I depressed?

- What could taking drugs cost me? Could this cost me my job or career?

- What are the long-term consequences of using this drug?

- What will this cost me in terms of my friendships and family? How would my close family and friends respond if they knew I was using drugs?

Even when you make the decision not to use drugs, it can be difficult to say no gracefully. Some good ways to turn down an offer:

- "Thanks, but I've got a big test (game, meeting) tomorrow morning."

- "I've already got a great buzz right now. I really don't need anything more."

- "I don't like how (insert drug name here) makes me feel."

- "I'm driving tonight."

- "I want to go for a run in the morning."

- "No thanks."

chapterin**review** ....

videos

SEE IT! ONLINE

Log on to **www.pearsonhighered.com/hopson** or MyFitnessLab to view these chapter-related videos.

Hidden Addictions
Alcohol and Cancer
Spring Break Nightmare

Secondhand Smoke
Smash the Ash
Heroin in Suburbia

Eliminating Meth
Campus Drug Dealers
Treating Addictions with Virtual Reality

onlineresources

Log on to **www.pearsonhighered.com/hopson** or MyFitnessLab for access to these book-related resources, and for links to other useful websites.

Audio case study
Audio PowerPoint lecture

Lab 13.1 Assess Your Alcohol Use and Risk of Abuse
Lab 13.2 Identify Smoking Behaviors and Create a Plan to Quit
Lab 13.3 Learn to Recognize Drug Use and Potential Abuse

Take Charge of Your Health! Worksheets:
Worksheet 30 Are You Addicted?
Worksheet 31 Passive Smoking
Worksheet 32 A Dozen Drinking Dilemmas
Worksheet 33 Caffeine Countdown
Worksheet 34 Smoke and Snuff Stumpers
Worksheet 35 Test Your Drug I.Q.
Worksheet 36 What Is Substance Abuse?
Worksheet 37 Substance Use Log
Behavior Change Log Book and Wellness Journal

Pre- and post-quizzes
Glossary flashcards

reviewquestions

1. Which of the following characterizes addiction?
   a. Compulsion
   b. Ability to control the addictive behavior
   c. Positive consequences
   d. Acceptance and admittance of a problem

2. Consuming five or more drinks in a row (for a male) or four or more drinks in a row (for a female) is called
   a. gorging.
   b. pre-loading.
   c. periodic drinking.
   d. binge drinking.

3. Blood alcohol concentration (BAC) is
   a. the "proof" value of an alcoholic beverage.
   b. the percentage of alcohol in a beverage.
   c. the level of alcohol in the blood before becoming drunk.
   d. the ratio of alcohol to total blood volume.

4. That last stage of liver disease, which involves the formation of scar tissue, is called
   a. alcoholic hepatitis
   b. leukoplakia.
   c. fatty liver.
   d. cirrhosis.

5. Smoke emitted from a smoker's mouth is called
   a. mainstream smoke.
   b. sidestream smoke.
   c. active smoke.
   d. chronic smoke.

6. About 85 percent of secondhand smoke is
   a. mainstream smoke.
   b. sidestream smoke.
   c. harmless.
   d. partially filtered by smokers' lungs.

7. The main reason college students cite for smoking is to
   a. stay awake.
   b. control stress.
   c. look cool.
   d. improve academic performance.

8. What is the major psychoactive ingredient in tobacco products?
   a. Carbon monoxide
   b. Tar
   c. Formaldehyde
   d. Nicotine

9. Ecstasy, GHB, and Rohypnol are examples of
   a. inhalants.
   b. "club" drugs.
   c. marijuana.
   d. prescription drugs.

10. Heroin is a type of
    a. stimulant.
    b. opiate.
    c. "club" drug.
    d. steroid.

critical**thinking**questions

REVIEW IT! ONLINE

1. Why is quitting an addictive behavior so difficult?
2. How would you design alcohol and smoking prevention strategies targeted at college students?
3. Discuss how addiction affects family and friends. What role do they play in helping the addict get help and maintain recovery, whether from alcohol or other drugs?

references

1. R. Goldberg, *Drugs Across the Spectrum*, 6th ed. (Belmont, CA: Thomson/Brooks-Cole, 2010).
2. C. Nakken, *The Addictive Personality: Understanding the Addictive Process and Compulsive Behavior*, 2nd ed. (Center City, MN: Hazelden, 2000).
3. R. Goldberg, *Drugs Across the Spectrum*, 2010.
4. J. R. Pleis, B. W. Ward, and J. W Lucas, "Summary Health Statistics for U.S. Adults, National Health Interview Survey 2009," *Vital Health Stat* 10, no. 249 (2010).
5. American College Health Association, *American College Health Association-National College Health Assessment II: Reference Group Executive Summary Fall 2010* (Linthicum, MD: American College Health Association, 2011).
6. Substance Abuse and Mental Health Services Administration (SAMHSA), *Results from the 2009 National Survey on Drug Use and Health: Volume I, Summary of National Findings*, NSDUH Series H-38A, HHS Publication No. SMA 10-4856 (Rockville, MD: Office of Applied Studies, 2010).
7. National Institute on Alcohol Abuse and Alcoholism (NIAAA), "What Colleges Need to Know: An Update on College Drinking Research," NIH Publication no. 07-5010, www.collegedrinkingprevention.gov/1College_Bulletin-508_361C4E.pdf (2007).
8. NIAAA, "As College Drinking Problems Rise, New Studies Identify Effective Prevention Strategies," NIH News, www.niaaa.nih.gov/NewsEvents/NewsReleases/Pages/college_drinking_strategies.aspx (2009).
9. Princeton University Health Services, " Alcohol: Effects of Alcohol on Your Body," www.princeton.edu/uhs/healthy-living/hot-topics/alcohol (updated August 2011).
10. R. Swift and D. Davidson, "Alcohol Hangover: Mechanisms and Mediators," *Alcohol Health and Research World* 22, no. 1, (1998): 54–60.
11. J. Ding and others, "Alcohol Intake and Cerebral Abnormalities on Magnetic Resonance Imaging in a Community-Based Population of Middle-Aged Adults," *Stroke* 35, no. 1 (2004): 16–21.
12. K. Butler, "The Grim Neurology of Teenage Drinking," *New York Times* (July 4, 2006).
13. R. W. Hingson and others, "Age at Drinking Onset and Alcohol Dependence," *Archives of Pediatric and Adolescent Medicine* 160, no. 7 (2006): 739–46.
14. L. Chen and others, "Alcohol Intake and Blood Pressure," A Systematic Review Implementing a Mendelian Randomization

Approach," *PLoS Medicine* 5, no. 3 (2008): e52.
15. National Center for Health Statistics, "FastStats: Leading Causes of Death," www.cdc.gov/nchs/fastats/lcod.htm (reviewed May 2011).
16. American Cancer Society, "What Are the Risk Factors for Breast Cancer?" www.cancer.org/cancer/breastcancer/detailedguide/breast-cancer-risk-factors (revised September 2011).
17. National Organization on Fetal Alcohol Syndrome, "FASD: What Everyone Should Know," www.nofas.org/MediaFiles/PDFs/factsheets/everyone.pdf (2006).
18. National Center for Injury Prevention and Control, "Impaired Driving: Get the Facts," www.cdc.gov/MotorVehicleSafety/Impaired_Driving/impaired-drv_factsheet.html (updated February 2011).
19. National Highway Traffic Safety Administration (NHTSA), *Traffic Safety Facts 2009 Data: Alcohol-Impaired Driving* (Washington, DC: NHTSA, 2010).
20. Insurance Institute for Highway Safety, "Fatality Facts 2009: Alcohol," www.iihs.org/research/fatality_facts_2009/alcohol.html (2010).
21. Medline Plus, "Alcoholism and Alcohol Abuse," www.nlm.nih.gov/medlineplus/ency/article/000944.htm (updated March 2011).
22. Association of Recovery Schools, "College Members," www.recoveryschools.org/schools_college.html (accessed October 2011).
23. Office of the Surgeon General, "A Report of the Surgeon General: How Tobacco Smoke Causes Disease—The Biology and Behavioral Basis for Smoking-Attributable Disease Fact Sheet," www.surgeongeneral.gov/library/tobaccosmoke/factsheet.html (December 2010).
24. Centers for Disease Control and Prevention (CDC), "Vital Signs: Current Cigarette Smoking Among Adults Aged ≥18 Years—United States, 2005–2010," *Morbidity and Mortality Weekly Report* 60, no. 35 (2011): 1135–40.
25. L. D. Johnston and others, *Monitoring the Future National Survey Results on Drug Use, 1975–2010: Volume II, College Students and Adults Ages 19–50* (Ann Arbor: Institute for Social Research, The University of Michigan, 2011).
26. Office of the Surgeon General, "A Report of the Surgeon General: How Tobacco Smoke Causes Disease," 2010.
27. Ibid.
28. American Heart Association (AHA), "Air Pollution, Heart Disease and Stroke," http://stoptitan.com/resources

/documents/handouts/American-Heart-Assoc-Air-Pollution-study%202011.pdf (February 2011).
29. American Cancer Society (ACS), "Cigars: Still Tobacco, Still Dangerous to Your Health," www.cancer.org/Cancer/CancerCauses/TobaccoCancer/CigarSmoking/cigar-smoking-intro (revised November 2010).
30. ACS, "What about More Exotic Forms of Smoking Tobacco, Such as Clove Cigarettes, Bidis, and Hookahs?" www.cancer.org/Cancer/CancerCauses/TobaccoCancer/QuestionsaboutSmokingTobaccoandHealth/questions-about-smoking-tobacco-and-health-other-forms-of-smoking (revised June 2011).
31. Ibid.
32. PubMedHealth, "Leukoplakia," www.ncbi.nlm.nih.gov/pubmedhealth/PMH0002041 (reviewed July 2011).
33–36. American Cancer Society, "Cigarette Smoking," www.cancer.org/Cancer/CancerCauses/TobaccoCancer/CigaretteSmoking/cigarette-smoking-who-and-how-affects-health (revised June 2011).
37. CDC, "Smoking and Tobacco Use: Tobacco-Related Mortality," www.cdc.gov/tobacco/data_statistics/fact_sheets/health_effects/tobacco_related_mortality (updated March 2011).
38. AHA, "Heart Disease and Stroke Statistics 2011 Update: A Report from the American Heart Association," *Circulation* 123, no. 4 (2011): e18–209.
39. CDC, "Smoking and Tobacco Use: Health Effects of Cigarette Smoking," www.cdc.gov/tobacco/data_statistics/fact_sheets/health_effects/effects_cig_smoking (updated March 2011).
40. CDC, "Smoking and Tobacco Use: Secondhand Smoke (SHS) Facts," www.cdc.gov/tobacco/data_statistics/fact_sheets/secondhand_smoke/general_facts/index.htm (updated March 2011).
41. Office on Smoking and Health, *The Health Consequences of Involuntary Exposure to Tobacco Smoke: A Report of the Surgeon General—Executive Summary* (Washington, DC: U.S. Department of Health and Human Services, 2006).
42. CDC, "Smoking and Tobacco Use: Health Effects of Secondhand Smoke," www.cdc.gov/tobacco/data_statistics/fact_sheets/secondhand_smoke/health_effects/index.htm (updated March 2011).
43. O. Shafey and others, "Chapter 9: Secondhand Smoking," *The Tobacco Atlas*, 3d ed. (Atlanta: American Cancer Society, 2009).
44. M. C. Fiore and others, *Treating Tobacco Use and Dependence: 2008 Update*,

Clinical Practice Guideline (Rockville, MD: U.S. Department of Health and Human Services, 2008).

45. National Center on Addiction and Substance Abuse at Columbia University (CASA), *Wasting the Best and the Brightest: Substance Abuse at America's Colleges and Universities* (New York: CASA, 2007).

46. M. C. Fiore and others, *Treating Tobacco Use and Dependence*, 2008.

47. V. Willingham, "Nicotine Vaccine Effective in Early Tests," CNN Health, www.cnn.com/2010/HEALTH/04/21/nicotine.vaccine.nicvax/index.html (April 22, 2010).

48. ACS, *Cancer Facts and Figures 2011* (Atlanta: American Cancer Society, 2011).

49. American Lung Association, "Benefits of Quitting," www.lungusa.org/stop-smoking/how-to-quit/why-quit/benefits-of-quitting (accessed October 2011).

50. SAMHSA, *Results from the 2009 National Survey on Drug Use and Health*, 2010.

51. Ibid.

52. CASA, *Wasting the Best and the Brightest*, 2007.

53. CDC, "CDC Statement Regarding the Misuse of Prescription Drugs," CDC Online Newsroom, www.cdc.gov/media/pressrel/2010/s100603.htm (June 3, 2010).

54. National Institute on Drug Abuse (NIDA), "NIDA InfoFacts: Drugged Driving," www.nida.nih.gov/infofacts/driving.html (revised December 2010).

55. D. P. Tashkin, "Smoked Marijuana as a Cause of Lung Injury," *Monaldi Archives for Chest Disease* 63, no. 2 (2005): 93–100.

56. NIDA, *Research Report: Marijuana Abuse*, NIH Publication no. 10-3859, www.drugabuse.gov/ResearchReports/Marijuana/marijuana3.html (revised September 2010).

57. NIDA, "NIDA InfoFacts: MDMA (Ecstasy)," www.drugabuse.gov/infofacts/ecstasy.html (revised March 2010).

58. NIDA, "NIDA InfoFacts: Club Drugs (GHB, Ketamine, and Rohypnol)," www.drugabuse.gov/infofacts/clubdrugs.html (revised July 2010).

59. CDC, "Methamphetamine Use and Risk for HIV/AIDS," www.cdc.gov/hiv/resources/factsheets/meth.htm (modified May 2007).

60. D. L. Rabiner and others, "Motives and Perceived Consequences of Nonmedical ADHD Medication Use by College Students: Are Students Treating Themselves for Attention Problems?" *Journal of Attention Disorders* 13, no. 3 (2009): 259–70.

61. Medline Plus, "Caffeine Overdose," www.nlm.nih.gov/medlineplus/ency/article/002579.htm (updated January 2010).

62. NIDA, "InfoFacts: Prescription and Over-the-Counter Medications," www.nida.nih.gov/infofacts/painmed.html (revised July 2009).

63. NIDA, "Facts on Dextromethorphan (DXM)," http://teens.drugabuse.gov/peerx/pdf/PEERx_Toolkit_FactSheets_DXM.pdf (August 2011).

64. NIDA, "InfoFacts: Inhalants," www.drugabuse.gov/infofacts/inhalants.html (revised March 2010).

65. NIDA for Teens, "Anabolic Steroids," http://teens.drugabuse.gov/drnida/drnida_ster1.php (accessed October 2011).

66. A. I. Leshner, "Oops: How Casual Drug Use Leads to Addiction," NIDA, www.nida.nih.gov/Published_Articles/Oops.html (accessed October 2011).

67. NIDA, "InfoFacts: Treatment Approaches for Drug Addiction," www.drugabuse.gov/infofacts/treatmeth.html (revised September 2009).

LAB 13.1 • ASSESS YOUR ALCOHOL USE AND RISK OF ABUSE

Name: _____ Date: _____

Instructor: _____ Section: _____

Purpose: To assess your patterns of alcohol use and your risk for alcohol abuse, and to explore the possibilities for positive behavior changes.

Directions: Complete Sections I and II below.

SECTION I: EVALUATING YOUR DRINKING PATTERNS AND ABUSE RISK

Select the answer that reflects the best choice for you and add up the points:

	0 points	1 point	2 points	3 points	4 points
1. How often do you have a drink containing alcohol?	Never (skip to #9–10)	Monthly or less	2–4 times a month	2–3 times a week	4 or more times a week
2. How many alcoholic drinks do you have on a typical day when you are drinking?	1 or 2	3 or 4	5 or 6	7 to 9	10 or more
3. How often do you have six drinks or more on one occasion?	Never	Less than monthly	Monthly	Weekly	Daily or almost daily
4. How often during the last year have you been unable to stop drinking once you had started?	Never	Less than monthly	Monthly	Weekly	Daily or almost daily
5. How often during the last year have you failed to do what was normally expected from you because of drinking?	Never	Less than monthly	Monthly	Weekly	Daily or almost daily
6. How often during the last year have you needed a drink in the morning to get yourself going after a heavy drinking session?	Never	Less than monthly	Monthly	Weekly	Daily or almost daily
7. How often during the last year have you had a feeling of guilt or remorse after drinking?	Never	Less than monthly	Monthly	Weekly	Daily or almost daily
8. How often during the last year have you been unable to remember what happened the night before because you had been drinking?	Never	Less than monthly	Monthly	Weekly	Daily or almost daily
9. Have you or has someone else been injured as a result of your drinking?	No		Yes, but not in the last year		Yes, during the last year
10. Has a relative, friend, doctor, or other health worker been concerned about your drinking or suggested you cut down?	No		Yes, but not in the last year		Yes, during the last year

Total for Section I = _____16_____

Analyzing Your Answers

Scores below 6: Congratulations! You are in control of your drinking behaviors and do a good job of consuming alcohol responsibly and in moderation.

Scores between 6 and 8: Your alcohol consumption is possibly risky. Try taking steps to change your drinking behavior. It might be hard when you are surrounded by friends who participate in the same risky actions, but try to make some positive changes for your health and safety.

Scores above 8: Your drinking patterns are putting you at high risk for illness, unsafe sexual situations, or alcohol-related injuries and may even affect your academic performance. Look back at how you answered each question and identify some changes you can make to reduce your risk.

Source: "Assess Your Alcohol Use and Risk of Abuse" from AUDIT Manual, box 4, p. 17, World Health Organization, Division of Mental Health and Prevention of Substance Abuse, http://whqlibdoc.who.int/hq/2001/WHO_MSD_MSB_01.6apdf. Used by permission of the World Health Organization.

SECTION II: REFLECTION

If you were surprised when evaluating your alcohol consumption behaviors or were not sure how to answer some of the questions, you may want to take steps to change your behavior.

1. Which of your drinking behaviors and patterns are most worrisome to you?

_____

_____

2. Select one drinking behavior that you can change right away and describe it below. What is one drinking behavior that may take a while to change?

_____

_____

3. What are some reasons why you would like to stop or cut down on your drinking?

_____

_____

4. Write a specific short-term goal for your drinking behaviors using the SMART goal-setting guidelines. Set a target date and reward for meeting your goal.

_____

_____

5. Chart your progress in a behavior log or journal. At the end of a week, month, or school session, consider how successful you were in following your plan. What helped you be successful? What made change more difficult? What will you do differently next week?

6. Revise your plan as needed: Are your goals attainable? Are the target dates realistic and the rewards satisfying?

LAB 13.2 • IDENTIFY SMOKING BEHAVIORS AND CREATE A PLAN TO QUIT

Name: _____ Date: _____

Instructor: _____ Section: _____

Purpose: To identify smoking behavior patterns and develop a plan to quit smoking.

Directions: Complete Sections I–III, outlining your current and past behaviors, and a plan for smoking cessation.

SECTION I: BEHAVIOR EVALUATION—WHY DO YOU SMOKE?

Identifying why you smoke can help you develop a plan to quit.

	Often	Sometimes	Never
Reason #1: Smoking gives me more energy.			
I smoke to keep from slowing down.	☐	☐	☐
I reach for a cigarette when I need a lift.	☐	☐	☐
When I'm tired, smoking perks me up.	☐	☐	☐
Reason #2: I like to touch and handle cigarettes.			
I feel more comfortable with a cigarette in my hand.	☐	☐	☐
I enjoy getting a cigarette out of the pack and lighting up.	☐	☐	☐
I like to watch the smoke when I exhale.	☐	☐	☐
Reason #3: Smoking is a pleasure.			
Smoking is pleasant and enjoyable.	☐	☐	☐
Smoking makes good times better.	☐	☐	☐
I want a cigarette most when I am comfortable and relaxed.	☐	☐	☐
Reason #4: Smoking helps me relax when I'm tense or upset.			
I light up a cigarette when something makes me angry.	☐	☐	☐
Smoking relaxes me in a stressful situation.	☐	☐	☐
When I'm depressed, I reach for a cigarette to feel better.	☐	☐	☐
Reason #5: I crave cigarettes; I'm addicted to smoking.			
If I run out of cigarettes, it's almost unbearable until I get more.	☐	☐	☐
I am very aware of not smoking if I have no cigarette in my hand.	☐	☐	☐
If I haven't smoked in a while, I get a gnawing hunger for a cigarette.	☐	☐	☐
Reason #6: Smoking is a habit.			
I smoke cigarettes automatically without even being aware of it.	☐	☐	☐
I light up without realizing I have a cigarette burning in the ashtray.	☐	☐	☐
I find a cigarette in my mouth I don't remember putting there.	☐	☐	☐

Adapted from: National Institutes of Health, 1990. *Why Do You Smoke?* NIH Pub. No. 93–1822. U.S. Department of Health and Human Services.

SECTION II: MOTIVATION AND PAST BEHAVIORS

1. Why do you want to quit smoking?_____

_____

2. Have you tried to quit smoking in the past? What worked and what did not?

_____

_____

SECTION III: SMOKING CESSATION PLAN

Answer the following questions to create a plan for quitting smoking.

1. Quit smoking date:_____

2. What family members and friends will you tell of your goal? How can they support you?

_____

_____

3. What health care provider, counseling program, or support groups are available to you?

_____

_____

4. What times in your daily routine do you smoke? What activities can you do instead at those times?

_____

_____

5. What medications have you considered using to help you quit smoking? Make a plan for getting and using the right medications appropriately.

_____

_____

6. What barriers, obstacles, or difficult situations might hinder your smoking cessation goal? Write out specific strategies that you will use with each barrier, obstacle, or difficult situation that may arise.

_____

_____

For tips on quitting smoking, check out the CDC resources at www.cdc.gov/tobacco/quit_smoking/how_to_quit.

Name: _____ Date: _____

Instructor: _____ Section: _____

Purpose: To learn the skills necessary to recognize drug use and potential abuse or addiction.

Directions: Review the information and complete the questionnaires in Sections I and II below.

SECTION I: SELF-ASSESSMENT

How do you know whether you are chemically dependent? Take the following assessment. The more "yes" checks you make, the more likely it is that you have a problem.

Are You Controlled By Drugs?	Yes	No
1. Do you use drugs to handle stress or escape from life's problems?	☐	☐
2. Have you unsuccessfully tried to cut down on or quit using your drug?	☐	☐
3. Have you ever been in trouble with the law or been arrested because of your drug use?	☐	☐
4. Do you think a party or social gathering isn't fun unless drugs are available?	☐	☐
5. Do you avoid people or places that do not support your drug use?	☐	☐
6. Do you neglect your responsibilities because you'd rather use your drug?	☐	☐
7. Have your friends, family, or employer expressed concern about your drug use?	☐	☐
8. Do you do things under the influence of drugs that you would not normally do?	☐	☐
9. Have you seriously thought that you might have a chemical dependency problem?	☐	☐

SECTION II: ASSESSMENT OF OTHERS

Is your life controlled by a chemical abuser? Try this assessment; the more "yes" checks you make, the more likely it is that there's a problem.

Are You Controlled by a Drug User?	Yes	No
1. Do you often have to lie or cover up for the chemical abuser?	☐	☐
2. Do you spend time counseling the person about the problem?	☐	☐
3. Have you taken on additional financial or family responsibilities?	☐	☐
4. Do you feel that you have to control the chemical abuser's behavior?	☐	☐
5. At the office, have you done work or attended meetings for the abuser?	☐	☐

(Continued)

Are You Controlled by a Drug User?	Yes	No
6. Do you often put your own needs and desires after the user's?	☐	☐
7. Do you spend time each day worrying about your situation?	☐	☐
8. Do you analyze your behavior to figure out how it might affect the chemical abuser?	☐	☐
9. Do you feel powerless and at your wit's end about the abuser's problem?	☐	☐

Source: Learn to Recognize Drug Use and Potential Abuse used by permission of Krames StayWell, LLC.

14

Reducing Your Risk of Sexually Transmitted Infections

Learning Outcomes

1. Discuss how sexually transmitted infections (STIs) spread.

 HEAR IT! ONLINE — Audio case study and audio PowerPoint lecture

DO IT! ONLINE — Lab 14.1 Assess Your Attitudes and Beliefs about STIs

2. Name several of the major bacteria-caused STIs, as well as their symptoms, risk factors, and typical treatments.

3. List several of the major viral-based STIs, as well as their symptoms, risk factors, and typical treatments.

 SEE IT! ONLINE — Human Papillo-mavirus Vaccine Mandatory

4. Describe the transmission of the human immuno-deficiency virus (HIV), as well as the infection, treatment, and prevention of AIDS.

5. Itemize and discuss other major types of STIs caused by fungi, protozoans, and other agents.

6. Identify strategies to protect yourself from STIs.

 DO IT! ONLINE — Lab 14.2 Effectively Communicating Sexual Information, Boundaries, and Preferences

Lab 14.3 Preventing Sexually Transmitted Infections

LIVE IT! ONLINE — Take Charge of Your Health worksheets and Behavior Change Logs for assessing your STI risk and creating a change plan

Pre- and post-quizzes and glossary flashcards REVIEW IT! ONLINE

433

casestudy

JASON

"Hi, I'm Jason. I have slept with
only one person in my life—my
girlfriend, Sara. We use condoms most of the time, but I'll
admit that once in a while, we
drink a few too many at a party and get careless.
We've known each other since freshman year
in high school, though, so we trust each other
completely. I don't consider myself at risk
for getting a sexually transmitted
infection. Am I wrong not to worry?"

HEAR IT! ONLINE

FIGURE **14.1** People between ages 15 and 24 contract
nearly half of all sexually transmitted infections. Protecting oneself
begins with learning about risky behaviors.

Each year, nearly 19 million Americans contract a **sexually transmitted infection
(STI)**, an infection (usually caused by viruses
or bacteria) spread through intimate contact.[1] If you
live in the United States, you have a 50-50 chance of
getting an STI by age 25.[2] Some STIs, such as chlamydia, are relatively mild and treatable and some,
such as genital herpes, are relatively mild but incurable. Others, including HIV/AIDS, are incurable and
fatal. The most recent statistics suggest that more
than 65 million Americans are currently living with
an incurable STI, most of them with herpes.[3]

Although people between ages 15 and 24 represent
only 25 percent of the sexually active population,
they contract nearly half of the new cases of STIs
reported in the United States each year (Figure 14.1).[4]
Teenagers and young adults are more likely to have
three or more sexual partners, to have sex partners
who have or had an
STI, and to engage
in **unprotected
sex**, that is, sexual
intercourse without
a condom or other
method of protec-
tion.[5] The frequency
of STIs in young
people makes them an important concern for college
students.

In this chapter, we cover the major
types of STIs, discuss behaviors that put
you at risk, and present strategies for
protecting yourself from these potentially
harmful infections. You can assess your
attitudes and beliefs about them in **Lab
14.1**. To check your knowledge about STIs
right now, take the quiz in the box What
Do You Know about STIs?

LIVE IT! ONLINE

Worksheet 41
Myths about
Sexually
Transmitted
Infections

DO IT! ONLINE

Early symptoms of an STI are often mild and un-
recognizable. Some STIs have no symptoms in
one or both sexes. For other STIs, men and women
share certain symptoms, but based on anatomy, have
some unique indicators of sexually transmitted infection (Figure 14.2). It's important to get checked out
if you have any of these symptoms. Left untreated,
some STIs can have tragic consequences: sterility,
blindness, central nervous system destruction, disfig-
urement, and even death.

How Do STIs Spread?

Sexually transmitted infections are generally spread
through some form of intimate sexual contact. Sexual
intercourse is the most common mode of transmission, regardless of whether it's oral-to-genital contact,
hand-to-genital contact, or anal intercourse. Less likely
modes of transmission include mouth-to-mouth contact
or contact with fluids from body sores that may

**sexually transmitted
infection (STI)** An infection
spread through intimate contact
with another person's skin or
body fluids

unprotected sex Sexual intercourse (vaginal, oral, or anal)
without a condom or other
method of protection

What Do You Know about STIs?

Here are several common beliefs about sexually transmitted infections. Consider each one and then answer: Is it Fact or Fallacy?

1. **Some STIs can be passed on by skin-to-skin contact in the genital area.** ☐ Fact ☐ Fallacy

2. **Herpes can be transmitted only when a person has visible sores on his or her genitals.** ☐ Fact ☐ Fallacy

3. **Oral sex is safe sex.** ☐ Fact ☐ Fallacy

4. **Condoms reduce your risk of both pregnancy and STIs.** ☐ Fact ☐ Fallacy

5. **As long as you don't have anal intercourse, you can't get HIV.** ☐ Fact ☐ Fallacy

6. **All sexually active females should have a regular Pap smear.** ☐ Fact ☐ Fallacy

7. **Once genital warts have been removed, there is no risk of passing on the virus.** ☐ Fact ☐ Fallacy

8. **You can get several STIs at one time.** ☐ Fact ☐ Fallacy

9. **You can get an STI more than once.** ☐ Fact ☐ Fallacy

Now read the answers and see if you were right!

1. **Fact.** Some viruses, including herpes simplex virus and human papillomavirus are present on the skin around the genital area.

2. **Fallacy.** Herpes is most easily passed on when the sores and blisters are present, but the virus is also found on the skin around the genital area.

3. **Fallacy.** Oral sex is not safe sex. Herpes, genital warts, and chlamydia can all be passed on through oral sex. Condoms should be used on the penis, and dental dams over the female genitals during oral sex.

4. **Fact.** Condoms significantly reduce the risk of pregnancy when used correctly. Only abstinence provides complete protection against pregnancy and STIs.

5. **Fallacy.** HIV is present in blood, semen, and vaginal fluid. Any activity that allows the transfer of these fluids is risky. Anal intercourse is a high-risk activity, but other sexual activity is also a risk.

6. **Fact.** All sexually active women should have regular Pap smears.

7. **Fallacy.** Genital warts can be removed, but the virus that caused the warts will always be present in the body and can be passed on to a sexual partner.

8. **Fact.** It is possible to have many STIs at one time. In fact, having one STI may make it more likely that a person will acquire more STIs. For example, the open sore from herpes creates a place for HIV to be transmitted.

9. **Fact.** A person can be reinfected many times with the same STI. This is especially true if a person does not get treated for the STI and thus re-infects his or her partner with the same STI.

Source: Adapted from Family Planning Victoria, "Play Safe" Updated 2005, www.fpv.org.au. © Family Planning Victoria; also adapted from "STD Quiz," modified March 2009, from Jefferson County Public Health, Colorado, www.jeffco.us. Used with permission.

Men only
- A drip or drainage from penis

Men and Women
- Sore bumps or blisters near sex organs or mouth
- Burning or pain when urinating
- Swelling or redness in throat
- Fever, chills, aches
- Swelling of lymph nodes near genitals or swelling of genitals
- Feeling the need to urinate frequently

Women only
- Vaginal discharge or odor from the vagina
- Pain in the lower pelvis or deep in the vagina during sex
- Burning or itching around the vagina
- Bleeding from the vagina at times other than the regular menstrual periods

FIGURE **14.2** Men and women share certain STI symptoms but have separate ones, as well. Many are mild and easy to overlook.

be spread by the hands. Although each type of STI involves a specific disease-producing agent or *pathogen* with its own mode of infection, all STI pathogens prefer dark, warm, moist places, especially the mucous membranes lining the reproductive organs. Most of these disease agents are susceptible to light and excess heat, cold, and dryness, and many die quickly on exposure to air.

What Are the Major Types of Bacterial STIs?

chlamydia The most common bacterial STI in the United States, caused by the bacterium *Chlamydia trachomatis*

pelvic inflammatory disease (PID) An infection of the female reproductive tract that can result from an untreated sexually transmitted infection

gonorrhea The second most common bacterial STI in the United States, caused by the bacterium *Neisseria gonorrhoeae*

Avoiding sexually transmitted diseases begins with knowing the common types of STIs and how to identify their characteristic symptoms. Let's start by discussing three common STIs—chlamydia, gonorrhea, and syphilis—that are caused by simple, single-celled, microscopic bacteria.

Chlamydia

Chlamydia is the most common bacterial STI in the United States (Figure 14.3) and reported cases are on the rise, due, in part, to more vigorous screening campaigns. The bacterium *Chlamydia trachomatis* infects an estimated 2.8 million people in the United States each year, mostly women.[6] Chlamydia often presents no symptoms and most cases continue to go unreported; thus, people can transmit chlamydia to sexual partners without realizing they have it.[7]

Symptoms and Complications Most people infected with chlamydia display no symptoms. In women who do experience symptoms, early signs (which usually appear within one to three weeks after infection) include abnormal vaginal discharge or a burning sensation while urinating. Later symptoms may include abdominal pain, lower back pain, and bleeding between periods. In men, early symptoms include painful urination and a watery, pus-like discharge from the penis.

In women, an untreated chlamydia infection can spread to the uterus or fallopian tubes, causing **pelvic inflammatory disease (PID)**. PID can permanently damage reproductive organs and cause infertility. A pregnant woman infected with chlamydia has a high risk for miscarriage and stillbirth. She can also pass the bacteria to her newborn. Long-term complications for men are uncommon, though in rare cases can result in sterility.[8]

Treatment Chlamydia is treatable with antibiotics if detected early. Sexually active young people, particularly women, should request chlamydia screening every six months to a year as part of their regular gynecological exam.

Gonorrhea

Gonorrhea is the second most common bacterial STI in the United States (see Figure 14.3). Cases peaked in the mid 1970s and stabilized at the current high levels. The Centers of Disease Contol and Prevention (CDC) estimates that more than 700,000 persons in the U.S. get new gonorrheal infections each year.

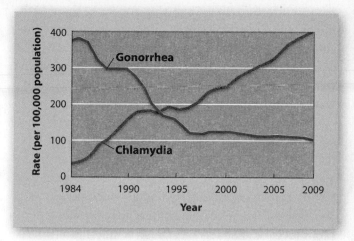

FIGURE **14.3** Chlamydia and gonorrhea are the most common bacterial STIs. Chlamydia rates have been rising for more than 20 years, while gonorrhea rates have been on the decline.

Data from the CDC, Sexually Transmitted Disease Surveillance Report, 2010

Physicians and clinics report fewer than half of these infections to the CDC, however, and in 2009, reported cases totalled about 301,000 cases.[9]

Symptoms and Complications Men usually notice a white, milky discharge from the penis accompanied by painful, burning urination two to nine days after intimate contact with an infected partner. As a result, men are more likely to seek medical attention and receive an early diagnosis (Figure 14.4). Only about 20 percent of males with gonorrhea show no symptoms.

Gonorrhea symptoms in women are often mild, absent, or so non-specific they are mistaken for a bladder or vaginal infection. Initial signs and symptoms in women may include a painful or burning sensation when urinating, increased vaginal discharge, or vaginal bleeding between periods. About 20 percent of infected women experience a yellowish or bloody discharge or a burning sensation during urination.[10] Most women experience no noticeable symptoms aside from an occasional low-grade fever. A woman could thus be unaware she is carrying the disease and risk infecting sexual partners.

The bacterium *Neisseria gonorrhoeae* primarily infects the linings of the urethra, genital tract, pharynx, and rectum, but it may spread to the eyes or other body regions via the hands or body fluids, typically during vaginal, oral, or anal sex. Undetected, untreated gonorrhea can spread to a man's reproductive and urinary organs where it can cause sterility and

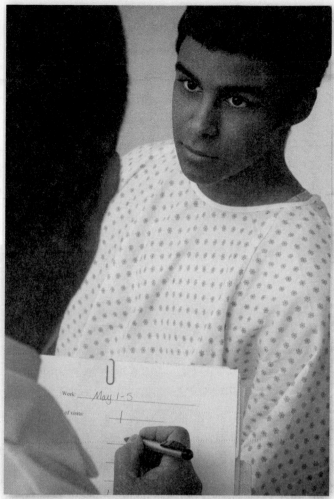

FIGURE **14.4** Bacterial STIs such as chlamydia, gonorrhea, and syphilis can be treated with antibiotics if they are diagnosed early enough, but people with early stage STIs have no symptoms. However, 80% of men with gonorrhea have a burning sensation when urinating and discharge from the penis.

in some cases induce a painful curvature of the penis during erection. In a woman, untreated gonorrhea can spread to the reproductive organs, causing PID and potential infertility. In rare cases, gonorrhea bacteria can enter the bloodstream and infect the joints, heart valves, or brain. As with chlamydia, gonorrhea can pass from a woman to her newborn and infect its eyes.

Treatment Antibiotics are usually effective in treating gonorrhea when it is detected early. It is recommended that people at risk for gonorrhea—for example, sexual partners of people with gonorrhea, sex workers, and people with multiple sex partners—be screened yearly for the disease.

Syphilis

Syphilis is caused by the bacterium *Treponema pallidum*. It is generally transmitted via direct contact with a syphilis sore on a partner's sexual organs during intercourse. However, it can also be transmitted via a break in the skin or through deep kissing in which partners exchange body fluids. After declining for many years, the rate of primary and secondary syphilis infections levelled off and then began to rise again, slightly for women and more dramatically for men. Between 2006 and 2007, syphilis infections increased 15.2 percent, with the number of cases growing from 9,756 to 11,466 in the United States (Figure 14.5).[11] The fastest growing rates were among men and women in their 20s. The steepest incline has been among young homosexual and bisexual men, with African and Hispanic men in these groups experiencing the highest rates of infection.[12]

Symptoms and Complications Untreated, syphilis generally progresses through several distinct stages. At the first stage, *primary syphilis,* a **chancre** (pronounced "SHANK-er") may develop. This is a sore most frequently located at the site of initial infection.[13] It usually appears three to four weeks after infection, and although it is painless, the chancre oozes infectious bacteria. Men tend to develop a chancre on the penis or scrotum, but it can also appear in the mouth, throat, or other site of initial infection. In women, the site of infection is often internal, on the vaginal wall or on the cervix, and may go unnoticed. In both men and women, the chancre disappears within three to six weeks, whether or not it is detected and treated.

Symptoms of the second stage, *secondary syphilis,* usually appear one month to a year after the chancre disappears. These include a skin rash and lesions or sores on the mucous membranes of the mouth, throat, or genitals; enlarged lymph nodes; and occasionally hair loss. The sufferer may develop a slight fever or headache. Because symptoms vary so much and appear so much later than the initial sexual contact that caused them, people rarely think to connect them. The underlying infection thus often goes undetected even at the secondary stage.

In the third stage, the *T. pallidum* begins to invade body organs and can cause lesions called "gummas." This stage is called *latent syphilis.* People rarely transmit latent syphilis to others except during pregnancy, when the mother can pass the infection to the fetus, potentially causing death or severe birth defects. If latent syphilis remains unrecognized and untreated for years, it becomes *late-stage syphilis.* Signs of late-stage syphilis include heart and central nervous system damage, blindness, deafness, paralysis, premature senility, and ultimately dementia.

Treatment With early diagnosis, syphilis can be cured with antibiotics. However, misdiagnosis and lack of access to health care can be obstacles to the successful treatment of syphilis.

What Are the Major Types of Viral STIs?

In the next section, we discuss STIs caused by viruses, including herpes, human papillomavirus (HPV), hepatitis B, and the human immunodeficiency virus (HIV).

Herpes

An estimated 16.2 percent of the American population (or about one out of every six people between ages 14 and 49) is infected with a genital *herpes simplex virus.*[14] There are two types of herpes simplex virus: *herpes simplex virus 1 (HSV-1)* and *herpes simplex virus 2 (HSV-2).*

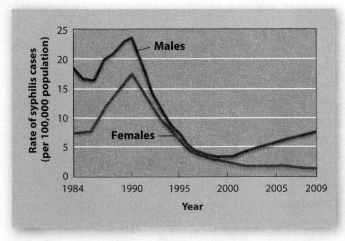

FIGURE **14.5** Cases of syphilis, while less common than either gonorrhea or Chlamydia in the United States, have been increasing in recent years.

Data from the CDC, Sexually Transmitted Disease Surveillance Report, 2010

casestudy

JASON

"After sitting through a lecture about STIs, I started thinking about Sara and me. The summer after high school, we broke up for a while. She went away to Spain, and I spent the summer hanging out at the beach. We got back together when college started, but we never talked much about that summer. Like I said, I completely trust Sara. I think she would tell me if anything had happened in Spain. And she's completely healthy. If she had an infection, I'd know it."

THINK! Can Jason be sure that he and Sara are both free of STIs? If you are sexually active, do you really know everything about your sexual partner(s)? Are you certain?

ACT! Find out the STI status of partners before becoming exposed. Identify all of your own risk behaviors for STIs and come up with a plan to correct them.

HEAR IT! ONLINE

• •

Women are more likely to have genital HSV-2 (one in five women ages 14 to 49 compared to one in nine men), but men are more likely to transmit the virus to their partners.[15] Racial disparities are also striking in the incidence of herpes: African Americans are three times more likely than Caucasians to contract genital **herpes**.[16] Although HSV-1 is generally associated with "cold sores" around the mouth area and HSV-2 is generally associated with genital herpes sores, both HSV-1 and HSV-2 can infect and cause sores on any area of the body. A person with a cold sore caused by HSV-1, for example, can transmit that virus to a partner's genitals during oral sex.

Symptoms and Complications After the herpes virus has been transmitted but before blisters or sores appear, a tingling or burning sensation and redness at the site of infection may occur. This *prodromal* stage lasts only a day or two and is followed by a second phase in which one or more blisters form, each filled with a clear fluid containing the virus. These crust over, dry up, and disappear within a few days. Whether treated with drugs or not, once a herpes virus becomes established, it remains in the body for life. It typically becomes *dormant*, lurking in nerve roots near the site of infection, until emotional or physical stress triggers the blistering cycle to begin all over again.

Herpes sores can shed highly infectious virus particles even before any blisters show. A person may contract genital herpes through oral or sexual contact with another person who has no awareness of being infected or who shows no outward signs of infection. A pregnant woman can pass genital herpes on to her baby as the baby moves through the birth canal. Genital herpes may also increase the chances of developing cervical cancer.

Treatment There is no cure for herpes. During the prodromal period, taking prescription medications such as acyclovir and over-the-counter medications can lessen the severity of the outbreak. Other drugs, such as famciclovir (FAMVIR), may reduce viral shedding between outbreaks, lessening the chance that a herpes sufferer will infect a partner.

Human Papillomavirus (HPV) and Genital Warts

Genital warts are caused by a small group of viruses known as **human papillomaviruses (HPV)**. An estimated 20 million Americans are infected with HPV, and about one percent of sexually active Americans have genital warts.[17] HPV infection occurs during sexual contact, when virus particles penetrate the skin and mucous membranes of the genitals or anus. After six to eight weeks, a person may notice itchy bumps on the cervix, vagina, vulva, penis, scrotum, or anus. However, only some forms of the HPV virus cause "warts;" most people with HPV have no symptoms and have no idea they are infected.

Symptoms and Complications Most HPV infections cause no symptoms at all. Others can cause two types of genital warts, either full-blown warts that are noticeable as tiny bumps or growths, or flat warts that are not usually visible to the naked eye. Either can develop inside the reproductive tract, where they are difficult to see or feel.

> **herpes** A condition characterized by sores or eruptions on the skin, caused by *herpes simplex virus 1* (HSV-1) or *herpes simplex virus 2* (HSV-2)
>
> **genital warts** Small, fleshy growths on the cervix, vagina, vulva, penis, scrotum, or anus; also called *venereal wart* or *condyloma*
>
> **human papillomaviruses (HPV)** A group of viruses, some of which are linked to cervical cancer, and some of which cause *genital warts*

The greatest threat from genital warts lies in the apparent correlation between certain HPV strains and cancer. No one is sure how, but HPV infection can lead to cervical cancer; within five years of initial infection, 30 percent of HPV cases in women will lead to precancerous changes in cervical cells. Pap smears and newer kinds of screening can detect these altered cells. Although details are just emerging, oral sex with a partner who carries the HPV virus also appears to pose a risk for oral HPV infection and cancer of the mouth or throat.[18]

Treatment A vaccine against a common strain of HPV is highly effective at preventing cervical cancer. The vaccine, which is administered via a series of three shots, is recommended for females ages 9 to 26 (Figure 14.6).[19] The U.S. Centers for Disease Control and Prevention have also approved the vaccine for use in boys and men to help prevent genital warts.[20]

SEE IT! ONLINE

Human Papillomavirus Vaccine Mandatory

Many genital warts eventually disappear on their own, although the virus remains in the body. Physicians can usually treat small genital warts with topical drugs and can remove large ones by surgical excision or *cryosurgery* (freezing the tissue with liquid nitrogen).

Hepatitis B

Hepatitis B virus (HBV) is one of seven forms of the hepatitis virus that can inflame and damage the liver. Of the 200,000 new cases of hepatitis B in the United States each year, approximately half are transmitted via sexual contact.[21] Hepatitis B is also transmitted by the sharing of infected drug needles or from an infected mother to her infant.

Symptoms and Complications

Many people infected with hepatitis B have no symptoms.[22] Others may experience jaundice, fatigue, abdominal pain, loss of appetite, nausea, vomiting, and joint pain. Over time, hepatitis B can lead to cirrhosis or liver cancer.

hepatitis B virus (HBV) One of seven forms of the hepatitis virus, which infects the liver; hepatitis B is the most common sexually transmitted form

human immunodeficiency virus (HIV) The virus that causes AIDS, transmissible through direct sexual contact or exchange of saliva, semen, vaginal fluid, blood, or other bodily fluids

acquired immunodeficiency syndrome (AIDS) A disease of the immune system caused by human immunodeficiency virus (HIV); characterized by extremely low CD4 counts or susceptibility to opportunistic infections or illnesses

FIGURE **14.6** A vaccine against several common strains of HPV can help prevent cervical cancer.

Treatment There is no cure for hepatitis B infection. A preventive vaccine is now available, which can protect people from new infections but cannot treat existing ones.

HIV and AIDS

Since 1981, more than 65 million people worldwide have become infected with the **human immunodeficiency virus (HIV)**, the virus that causes **AIDS**, or **acquired immunodeficiency syndrome**.[23] Today, an estimated 33.3 million people around the world are living with HIV or AIDS, and it is a significant global health threat.[24] In 2009 alone, 1.8 million people died of AIDS. Most cases and deaths occur in sub-Saharan Africa. In the United States, about one million people are currently infected with HIV, and 21 percent of them are unaware of their infection.[25] More than 576,000 Americans have died of AIDS since the disease was first identified, with 18,000 dying each year.[26]

HIV Transmission and Progression HIV typically enters a person's body when the semen, vaginal secretions, or blood of an infected individual gain entry through a break in the recipient's body surface. Breaks in the mucous membranes of the genital organs and anus—as can occur during sexual intercourse, particularly anal intercourse—provide the

LIVE IT! ONLINE

Worksheet 42 Should You Have the HIV Test?

easiest route of entry. The virus can also be transmitted through contaminated needles. Some people became infected with HIV through blood transfusions before 1985, when blood donation programs began testing all donated blood products for the virus. An infected mother can pass the virus through the placenta to her unborn baby, and rarely, in breast milk. Antiretroviral drug treatment can prevent this transmission in most cases.

During *primary infection*, HIV multiplication is rapid, and the virus invades the bloodstream and destroys immune cells called *CD4 cells*. In response to this invasion, the body produces antibodies. Within one to three months of infection, mild symptoms of illness occur, including night sweats, fatigue, weight loss, skin rashes, mouth ulcers, persistent cold sores, fevers, and fungal infections.

After the primary stage, HIV-infected individuals typically enter an *asymptomatic stage* during which they may look and feel healthy and experience no symptoms of illness. This stage may last for several years. Infected individuals may not know they have the virus and may unknowingly transmit HIV to others.[27]

Without treatment, nearly all HIV-positive individuals will progress to full-blown AIDS. HIV-infected individuals are considered to have AIDS when their CD4 levels fall below 200 per cubic millimeter of blood or when they experience illnesses that are considered markers for AIDS, such as the blood cancer *Kaposi's sarcoma* or recurrent opportunistic infections.

With treatment, the asymptomatic phase of HIV can be extended, allowing the person to survive several years with the infection "in check." Throughout all phases, the HIV virus remains transmissible. However, the virus is not highly contagious. Studies of people living in households with an AIDS patient have shown no documented cases of HIV infection due to casual contact. In addition, HIV does not appear to be transmissible by insects.[28]

High-Risk Behaviors The following behaviors put you at high risk of contracting HIV:

- *Unprotected sexual intercourse.* The exchange of HIV-infected body fluids (such as blood, semen, or vaginal secretions) during vaginal or anal intercourse is the greatest risk factor. In rare instances, the virus has been found in saliva, but most health officials state that saliva poses a less significant risk than other shared body fluids.

- *Injecting drugs or sharing needles.* An estimated 15 to 25 percent of AIDS cases in the United States result from sharing or using HIV-contaminated needles and syringes.[29] Anyone who shares needles, whether to use illegal drugs or in tattooing and piercing, is at risk.

Although AIDS strikes some minority populations disproportionately, it is not a disease limited to homosexuals or minority groups. People who engage in high-risk behaviors increase their chances of contracting the disease. People who do not engage in these behaviors have minimal risk. Figure 14.7 illustrates the sources of HIV infection for men and women in the United States.

Drugs and Treatments There is no cure for HIV or AIDS, but drugs can slow the progression from HIV

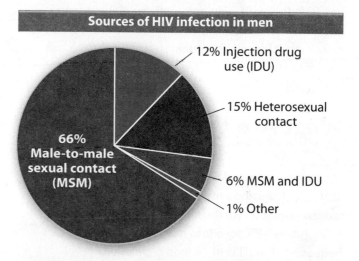

Sources of HIV infection in men

- 12% Injection drug use (IDU)
- 15% Heterosexual contact
- 6% MSM and IDU
- 1% Other
- 66% Male-to-male sexual contact (MSM)

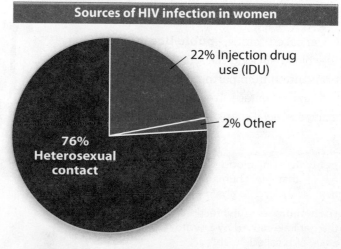

Sources of HIV infection in women

- 22% Injection drug use (IDU)
- 2% Other
- 76% Heterosexual contact

FIGURE **14.7** Sources of HIV infection in men and women with an AIDS diagnosis in the United States.

Data from the CDC, HIV/AIDS Surveillance Report, 2011 (Vol. 21).

to AIDS and prolong the lives of most HIV patients. Current treatments combine several specific types of drugs, especially *protease inhibitors* and *reverse transcriptase inhibitors*. The protease drugs seem to work best in combination with other therapies, but the combinations (sometimes called "cocktails") are still experimental, and no combination has proven to be effective for all patients.

Medical researchers around the world are searching for new drugs and treatment approaches for HIV/AIDS. Two separate studies, one international study based in San Francisco and another in South Africa, found that taking antiretroviral drugs before exposure significantly protects a person from HIV infection.[30] Researchers are also working hard to create a vaccine against the HIV virus, but most of the vaccines tested have as yet been ineffective.[31]

The only sure way to prevent HIV infection is to avoid risky behaviors such as those described in the box Safe Is Sexy. If you are concerned about your risk or the risk of a close friend, arrange a confidential meeting with a health educator or other health professional at your college health service, local public health department, or community STI clinic.

What Are the Other Major Types of STIs?

In addition to bacterial and viral infections, a variety of other parasites and pathogens cause sexually transmitted infections, as we discuss below. The box Who Gets STIs? (page 445) goes into more detail about the frequency of all STIs in various populations.

Pubic Lice

Often called "crabs," **pubic lice** are tiny blood-sucking insects that can be transmitted from partner to partner during sexual contact. Treatment includes using a special soap to kill lice on the

> **pubic lice** Tiny blood-sucking insects that infest human pubic hair; also called "crabs"
>
> **trichomoniasis** An infection of the genitals caused by a protozoan; also called "trich"
>
> **candidiasis** A fungal infection often transmitted sexually; also called "yeast infection"

body, and washing clothing, furniture, and linens that may harbor lice. Avoid pubic lice by staying away from sexual partners with pubic itching or obvious insect bites and sores in the pubic hair region. Avoid sharing bed sheets, towels, and other linens and clothing. When trying on bathing suits in a store, wear underwear.[32]

Trichomoniasis

Trichomoniasis, or "trich," is caused by a parasitic protozoan. Symptoms include a foamy, yellowish, unpleasant-smelling discharge accompanied by a burning sensation, itching, and painful urination. Trichomoniasis is usually transmitted by direct sexual contact, and can be prevented by using condoms. Trichomoniasis is often treated in both sexual partners with oral metronidazole to avoid the "ping-pong" effect of repeated cross-infection.

Candidiasis

Candidiasis, or a "yeast infection" can occur when the normal chemical balance of the vagina is disturbed, leading to an overgrowth of the fungus *Candida*. Symptoms can include itching, burning and a clumpy white discharge. Over-the-counter creams and suppositories are usually effective in killing the fungi and restoring the normal balance.

Urinary Tract Infections

Some infections of the urethra or bladder can be sexually transmitted when organisms from one partner's genital area or rectum move across and travel up

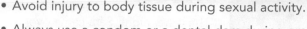

TOOLS FOR **CHANGE**

Safe Is Sexy

In a world with serious and potentially deadly sexually transmitted infections, caution is important. Consider this list of protections, always use common sense, and remember this simple phrase: When in doubt, don't!

- Avoid casual sexual partners. Ideally, sex should be limited to long-term, mutually monogamous relationships in which both partners have tested negative for HIV and other STIs.

- Avoid unprotected sexual activity that involves the exchange of blood, semen, or vaginal secretions with people at risk for infection. Ask intimate questions about your partner's sexual past, and postpone sexual involvement until you know, through testing, that he or she is not infected.

- If you are not in a lifelong monogamous relationship, practice safer sex by using latex condoms. Always use them properly and remember, condoms can fail. Spermicidal and germicidal products are a second line of defense.

- Never share any instruments through which the exchange of blood could occur, including needles, razors, tattoo instruments, and body-piercing instruments.

- Avoid injury to body tissue during sexual activity.

- Always use a condom or a dental dam during oral sex to prevent the entry of saliva, semen, blood, or vaginal secretions through breaks in mucous membranes.

- Drink responsibly and avoid drug use. Drugs or alcohol can cloud your judgment and impair your ability to make responsible decisions about potential sex partners and activities.

- Wash your hands before and after sexual encounters. Urinate after sexual relations and, if possible, wash your genitals.

- Total abstinence is the only absolute means of preventing the sexual transmission of HIV and other STIs. If you are in doubt about a partner's sexual history or infection status, use other means of intimacy such as closed-mouth kissing, hugging, or massage until test results can assure safety.

- Don't risk infecting others: If you are worried about your own status, get tested for STIs.

- Remember that you have a responsibility to your partner to disclose your own status and find out your partner's history and status. Be direct, honest, and determined in talking about sex before you become involved. A person who will not communicate openly and honestly with you may very well fail to take responsibility for his or her actions, as well.

- Decide what you will do if your partner does not agree with you. Anticipate potential objections or excuses, and prepare your responses accordingly.

another's urinary tract. Women are more likely than men to contract **urinary tract infections (UTIs)**. Bathing and handwashing with soap and water before sexual intimacy can help prevent some UTIs. Treatment depends on the organism transmitted.

How Can I Decrease My Risk of STIs?

Nineteen million Americans contract an STI each year. To avoid becoming one of them, learn about STIs and how to prevent them, choose a partner wisely, avoid

mixing sex with drinking and drugs, and be prepared before challenging situations arise.

Learn about STIs

Reading this chapter is a good step toward educating yourself about STIs. Recognizing the signs and symptoms of STIs can help you identify an infection early on—and prevent transmission to a partner. Evaluate your own beliefs and

urinary tract infections (UTI) Infections of the urethra or bladder caused by microorganisms; can be sexually transmitted or autoinoculated

casestudy

JASON

"The other night, Sara came over and we had a long, awkward conversation. It turns out that there *was* someone else while she was on vacation that summer. She says they slept together only once, and she felt awful about it, but after all, we were broken up. This was more than two years ago, and she says she's only been with me since then. I insisted that we both go to the student health center and get tested for STIs. She thinks I'm crazy—she feels perfectly healthy and says I am being paranoid. But she did agree to go."

THINK! Name three STIs that often show no symptoms in either men or women.

ACT! If you are sexually active, learn about the STI screening available on campus. Get screened yourself and make sure your partners have been, too.

attitudes toward sexual health by completing Lab 14.1. Part of getting fit and staying well is being aware of your sexual wellness. Consider being screened for STIs, especially if you have any of the risk factors discussed in this chapter. If you choose to be sexually active, know your risk and protect yourself (Figure 14.8).

Choose Your Partner Wisely

Choose someone who is willing to engage in low-risk behaviors and is willing to wait for more intimate contact until both partners have been tested for STIs. Keep in mind that a partner with other recent sexual partners

or multiple sexual partners represents a high risk. The same is true for a partner with blisters, sores, vaginal or penile discharge, or any other physical signs of an STI, regardless of how recently they may have been tested.

Stay Sober for Sex

Recent research confirms that drinking is a major factor in high-risk sex. When they are drinking heavily, males are less likely to use a condom, females are less likely to insist on it, and both show poorer judgment in choosing sexual partners and adhering to safe sex practices. As a result, both sexes are more likely to contract STIs, and women are more likely to experience date rape and/or have unintended pregnancies.[33]

Be Prepared

It can be difficult to make good decisions "in the heat of the moment." Before you encounter a potentially risky situation, follow these steps:

- Make decisions about what you will say and do if, for example, you and your partner want to have sex, but neither of you has a condom.

- Rehearse with a friend what you will say and do before such a situation arises (see **Lab 14.2**).

- If your decision involves using condoms or other barriers, learn how to use them properly. Practice using the products by following the instructions on the packaging *prior* to engaging in sexual activity. Have the supplies when and where you need them. If you have questions, get help from a physician or counselor at the student health service or a community STI clinic. For more information about condom effectiveness, see the box How Reliable Are Condoms?

High-risk behaviors	Moderate-risk behaviors	Low-risk behaviors	No-risk behaviors
Unprotected vaginal, anal, and oral sex—any activity that involves direct contact with bodily fluids, such as ejaculate, vaginal secretions, or blood—are high-risk behaviors.	Vaginal, anal, or oral sex with a latex or polyurethane condom and a water-based lubricant used properly and consistently can greatly reduce the risk of STI transmission. Dental dams used during oral sex can also greatly reduce the risk of STI transmission.	Mutual masturbation, if there are no cuts on the hand, penis, or vagina, is very low risk. Rubbing, kissing, and massaging carry low risk, but herpes can be spread by skin-to-skin contact from an infected partner.	Abstinence, phone sex, talking, and fantasy are all no-risk behaviors.

FIGURE **14.8** Sexual behaviors fall on a continuum from high risk to no risk, depending on the level of direct contact with blood, semen, or vaginal secretions.

DIVERSITY

Who Gets STIs?

People of both sexes and of all ages, races, and socioeconomic groups contract STIs. Some populations, however, experience higher rates of certain STIs than others.

- **HIV/AIDS.** Three-quarters of the more than one million Americans living with HIV or AIDS are male. Men who have sex with men make up the majority of all new HIV infections and about half of all on-going infections.[1] Individuals who contract HIV through heterosexual contact account for 31 percent of new cases and 28 percent of on-going infections. Women account for 27 percent of new infections and 25 percent of on-going ones. Injection drug users make up 12 percent of new infections, 19 percent of on-going ones. African Americans make up about 12 percent of the U.S. population but comprise 46 percent of the HIV/AIDS cases.[2] Caucasian Americans account for 31 percent of the cases, Hispanics 18 percent, and all other groups just two percent. The incidence of HIV infection among black women is 15 times higher than among white women and four times higher than among Hispanic women.[3]

- **Chlamydia.** Women are diagnosed with chlamydia three times more often than men. African American women have rates eight times higher than Caucasian American women; African American men have rates almost 12 times higher than white men.[4] Female Hispanics, Native Americans, and Alaskan

natives have rates from three to four times higher than whites.

- **Gonorrhea.** Men and women are diagnosed with gonorrhea about equally, but African Americans accounted for 71 percent of all cases in 2009. Hispanics, Native Americans, and Alaskan natives have rates two to four times higher than Caucasians, while Asian Americans and Pacific Islanders have half as many cases of gonorrhea.[5]

- **Syphilis.** Men are three to ten times more likely than women to be diagnosed with primary or secondary syphilis, depending on race. Rates have been highest in African American and Hispanic males compared to other groups, but have risen rapidly among African American teenaged girls in recent years.[6]

- **Hepatitis B virus.** In the United States, Asian Americans and Pacific Islanders are more likely than other ethnic groups to contract HBV.[7]

Understanding STI Disparities

Public health researchers have identified many factors in an attempt to understand the racial disparities in HIV infection and other STIs.[8] They include poverty, discrimination, and lack of insurance leading to lower quality health care; younger age at the time sexual activity begins; use of illicit drugs; greater numbers of sexual partners; living in communities where STIs are common; higher rates of incarceration leading to a greatly increased risk of STI exposure; and lower rates of circumcision.[9]

Sources:
1. Centers for Disease Control and Prevention, "HIV/AIDS Fact Sheet: HIV in the United States," www.cdc.gov/hiv/resources/factsheets/us.htm (June 2010).
2. Ibid.
3. Ibid.
4. Centers for Disease Control and Prevention, "2009 Sexually Transmitted Diseases Surveillance: STDs in Racial and Ethnic Minorities," www.cdc.gov/std/stats09/minorities.htm (November 2010).
5. Ibid.
6. Ibid.
7. Ibid.
8. Centers for Disease Control and Prevention, Sexually Transmitted Disease Surveillance 2009 (Atlanta: U.S. Department of Health and Human Services, 2010); J. Kraut-Becher and others, "Examining Racial Disparities in HIV: Lessons from Sexually Transmitted Infections Research," Journal of Acquired Immune Deficiency Syndromes 47, Suppl 1 (2008): S20–7.
9. CDC, Sexually Transmitted Disease Surveillance 2009 (2010); A. Tobian and others, "Male Circumcision for the Prevention of HSV-2 and HPV Infections and Syphilis," New England Journal of Medicine 360, no. 13 (2009): 1298–1309.

How Reliable Are Condoms?

In her well-received book *Condom Sense*, New York physician Monica Sweeney called condoms her "candidate for the greatest technological invention of the past 2,000 years."[1] Used consistently and correctly, condoms do provide protection from AIDS and other STIs, as well as prevent pregnancies. But how reliable are they?

Consistent use of latex condoms helps protect against STIs that involve mainly skin-to-skin contact with sores or ulcers (or infected skin that appears norma), including herpes genital warts (HPV), and skin-to-skin transmission of syphilis. Some skin contact is still possible above and near the condom, however, and these diseases can cause infection in areas not covered by condoms, so the CDC does not consider condoms completely effective in preventing such STIs.[2]

Condoms are better at preventing STIs such as HIV, gonorrhea, chlamydia, and trichomoniasis, which are typically transmitted via semen, vaginal fluid, or other body fluids. The CDC considers condoms "highly effective" at preventing fluid contact, since careful, consistent use can block virtually all fluid exchange. Nevertheless, they warn that no protective method is 100 percent effective against STIs.[3] In addition, statistics suggest that the best available degrees of protection require a consistency of use that many people can't manage. Explanations for inconsistent condom use include thinking that pregnancy or an STI wasn't a risk at the time, running out of condoms, disliking them, forgetting to use them, getting coerced into unprotected sex by one's partner, not expecting to have sex on that occasion, drinking too much, or being overtaken by passion.

Health experts offer the following warnings about condoms:

- Lambskin and other "real-skin" condoms are not effective in protecting against STIs, as they have pores that can allow the passage of virus-sized particles.

- Storage of latex condoms in warm places (such as wallets and glove compartments) can lead to deterioration and breakage.

- Condoms lubricated with spermicides give no extra protection against STIs, and some studies suggest that nonoxynol-9 spermicides may facilitate the passage of virus particles through microscopic holes in the latex created during manufacture.

- Oil-based lubricants (petroleum jelly, mineral oil, or lotions containing oils) make condoms quickly lose up to 90 percent of their strength and easily tear.

- The time to practice proper condom use is before you get into a sexually charged situation.

The bottom line: Condoms aren't perfect but they can help protect you from a serious—even deadly—STI.

Sources:
1. M. Sweeney and R. Kirwan Grisman, *Condom Sense: A Guide to Sexual Survival in the New Millennium* (New York: Lantern Books, 2004).
2. Centers for Disease Control, "Male Latex Condoms and Sexually Transmitted Diseases: Condom Fact Sheet in Brief," www.cdc.gov/condomeffectiveness /brief.html (updated April 2011).
3. Ibid.

chapterin**review**

videos

Log on to **www.pearsonhighered.com/hopson** or MyFitnessLab to view these chapter-related videos.

Human Papillomavirus Vaccine Mandatory

onlineresources

Log on to **www.pearsonhighered.com/hopson** or MyFitnessLab for access to these book-related resources, and for links to other useful websites.

 Audio case study
Audio PowerPoint lecture

 Lab 14.1 Assess Your Attitudes and Beliefs about STIs
Lab 14.2 Effectively Communicating Sexual Information, Boundaries, and Preferences
Lab 14.3 Preventing Sexually Transmitted Infections

 Take Charge of Your Health! Worksheets:
  Worksheet 41 Myths about Sexually Transmitted Infections
  Worksheet 42 Should You Have the HIV Test?
Behavior Change Log Book and Wellness Journal

 Pre- and post-quizzes
Glossary flashcards

reviewquestions

1. Each year, the number of Americans who contract an STI is about
   a. 190,000.
   b. 1,900,000.
   c. 19,000,000.
   d. 190,000,000.

2. Young people aged 15 to 24 make up approximately what percentage of STI cases?
   a. 5 to 10 percent
   b. 10 to 15 percent
   c. 15 to 20 percent
   d. Nearly 50 percent

3. Which of the following is a recommended strategy for preventing STIs?
   a. Intermittent abstinence
   b. Occasional condom use
   c. Mutual monogamy with a medically-cleared partner
   d. A partner's assurance of infection-free status

4. Chlamydia is a threat to wellness because
   a. it is the most common viral STI.
   b. a small percentage of the afflicted have no symptoms.
   c. there are currently no effective drug treatments.
   d. chlamydia infection can lead to pelvic inflammatory disease.

5. Gonorrhea is a threat to wellness because
   a. about 80 percent of males with gonorrhea show no symptoms.
   b. about 20 percent of females with gonorrhea show no symptoms.
   c. it is the most common STI caused by a protozoan.
   d. untreated gonorrhea can cause scarring and potential sterility in either sex.

6. In what stage of syphilis does a chancre develop?
   a. Primary syphilis
   b. Secondary syphilis
   c. Latent syphilis
   d. Late-stage syphilis

7. Which of these can lead to liver cancer?
   a. Hepatitis B
   b. Syphilis
   c. Chlamydia
   d. HIV antibodies

8. Which of these is a low-risk activity for HIV infection?
   a. Unprotected vaginal intercourse
   b. Unprotected anal intercourse
   c. Sharing needles with another person
   d. Living in the same household as an AIDS patient

9. Chlamydia, gonorrhea, and syphilis are caused by
   a. viruses.
   • b. bacteria.
   c. protozoans.
   d. yeast.

10. Herpes, genital warts, hepatitis B, and HIV are all STIs caused by
   • a. viruses.
   b. bacteria.
   c. protozoans.
   d. yeast.

critical**thinking**questions

REVIEW IT! ONLINE

1. Is chlamydia a more serious health concern for men or for women? Explain your answer. *both*

2. Compare the symptoms of three major bacterial STIs and the long-term problems they can cause.

3. Does a person who has HIV automatically have AIDS? Explain your answer. *NO*

references

1. Centers for Disease Control and Prevention (CDC), "Trends in Sexually Transmitted Diseases in the United States: 2009 National Data for Gonorrhea, Chlamydia, and Syphilis," www.cdc.gov/std/stats09/trends.htm (updated November 2010).

2. CDC, *Sexually Transmitted Diseases Surveillance, 2009* (Atlanta: U.S. Department of Health and Human Services, 2010).

3. Guttmacher Institute, "In Brief: Fact Sheet—Facts on Sexually Transmitted Infections in the United States," www.guttmacher.org/pubs/FIB_STI_US.html (June 2009).

5. E. Wildsmith and others, "Sexually Transmitted Diseases among Young Adults: Prevalence, Perceived Risk, and Risk-Taking Behaviors," *Child Trends Research Brief* #2010-10 (May 2010).

6–8. CDC, "Chlamydia—CDC Fact Sheet," www.cdc.gov/std/chlamydia/STDFact-Chlamydia.htm (updated August 2011).

9. CDC, "Gonorrhea—CDC Fact Sheet," www.cdc.gov/std/gonorrhea/STDFact-gonorrhea.htm (updated April 2011).

10. Ibid.

11. CDC, *Sexually Transmitted Diseases Surveillance, 2010.*

12. J. R. Su and others, "Primary and Secondary Syphilis among Black and Hispanic Men Who Have Sex with Men: Case Report Data from 27 States," *Annals of Internal Medicine* 155, no. 3 (2011): 145–51.

13. National Institute of Allergy and Infectious Diseases (NIAID), "Syphilis: Symptoms," www.niaid.nih.gov/topics/syphilis/understanding/Pages/symptoms.aspx (updated December 2010).

14. CDC, "Genital Herpes—CDC Fact Sheet," www.cdc.gov/std/herpes/stdfact-herpes.htm (updated July 2010).

15. Ibid.

16. CDC, "CDC Analysis of National Herpes Prevalence," www.cdc.gov/std/herpes/herpes-NHANES-2010.htm (updated April 2010).

17. CDC, "Genital HPV Infection—CDC Fact Sheet," www.cdc.gov/std/HPV/STDFact-HPV.htm (updated August 2011).

18. M. L. Gillison, "Oral Sex and Risk for Oral HPV Infection and Oropharyngeal Cancer," AAAS 2011 Annual Meeting, Presentation 2872, http://aaas.confex.com/aaas/2011/webprogram/Paper2872.html (February 2011); AAAS symposium, "Oral Sex Is Sex and Can Lead to Cancer," AAAS 2011 Annual Meeting, http://aaas.confex.com/aaas/2011/webprogram/Session2736.html (February 2011).

19. CDC, "Genital HPV Infection—CDC Fact Sheet," 2011.

20. CDC, "FDA Licensure of Quadrivalent Human Papillomavirus Vaccine (HPV4, Gardasil) for Use in Males and Guidance from the Advisory Committee on Immunization Practices (ACIP)," *Morbidity and Mortality Weekly Report* 59, no. 20 (2010): 630–2.

21. CDC, "Hepatitis B: General Information," Publication 21-1073. www.cdc.gov/hepatitis/HBV/PDFs/HepBGeneralFactSheet.pdf (June 2010).

22. CDC, "Hepatitis B FAQs for the Public," www.cdc.gov/hepatitis/B/bFAQ.htm (updated June 2009).

23. UNAIDS, "Global Summary of the AIDS Epidemic, 2009," www.who.int/hiv/data/2009_global_summary.png (accessed May 2011).

24. Joint United Nations Programme on HIV/AIDS (UNAIDS) and World Health Organization (WHO), *Global Report: UNAIDS Report on the Global AIDS Epidemic 2010* (Geneva: UNAIDS, 2010).

25. CDC, "HIV in the United States," www.cdc.gov/hiv/resources/factsheets/us.htm (reviewed July 2010).

26. Ibid.

27. Medline Plus, "Acute HIV Infection," www.nlm.nih.gov/medlineplus/ency/article/000604.htm (updated December 2009).

28. San Francisco AIDS Foundation, "HIV Basics," www.sfaf.org/hiv-info/basics (2010).

29. CDC, "Cases of HIV Infection and AIDS in the United States and Dependent Areas, 2005," *HIV/AIDS Surveillance Report* 17, Table 17 (updated June 2010).

30. R. Grant and others, "Preexposure Chemoprophylaxis for HIV Prevention in Men Who Have Sex with Men," *New England Journal of Medicine* 363, no. 27 (2010): 2587–99; K. Q. Abdool and others, "Effectiveness and Safety of Tenofovir Gel, an Antiretroviral Microbicide, for the Prevention of HIV Infection in Women," *Science* 329, no. 5996 (2010): 1168–74.

31. S. Rerks-Ngarm and others, "Vaccination with ALVAC and AIDSVAX to Prevent HIV-1 Infection in Thailand," *New England Journal of Medicine* 361, no. 23 (2009): 2209–20.

32. Medline Plus, "Pubic Lice," www.nlm.nih.gov/medlineplus/ency/article/000841.htm (updated October 2010).

33. J. Griffin, "Alcohol Use and High-Risk Sexual Behavior among Collegiate Women: A Review of Research on Alcohol Myopia Theory," *Journal of American College Health* 58, no. 6 (2010): 523–32.

LAB 14.1 • ASSESSING YOUR ATTITUDES AND BELIEFS ABOUT STIs

Name: _____ **Date:** _____

Instructor: _____ **Section:** _____

Purpose: To assess whether your attitudes and beliefs may lead you to behaviors that increase your risk of STIs.

Directions: Complete the questionnaire below, indicating whether you believe the statement to be TRUE or FALSE. Score your responses and analyze your score after completing the questionnaire.

STI Attitude and Belief Scale	True	False
1. You can usually tell whether someone is infected with an STI, especially HIV.	☐	☐
2. Chances are that if you haven't caught an STI by now, you probably have a natural immunity and won't get infected in the future.	☐	☐
3. A person who is successfully treated for an STI needn't worry about getting it again.	☐	☐
4. As long as you keep yourself fit and healthy, you needn't worry about STIs.	☐	☐
5. The best way for sexually active people to protect against STIs is to practice safer sex.	☐	☐
6. The only way to catch an STI is to have sex with someone who has one.	☐	☐
7. Talking about STIs with a partner is so embarrassing that it's better not to raise the subject and instead hope the other person will.	☐	☐
8. STIs are mostly a problem for people who have numerous sex partners.	☐	☐
9. You don't need to worry about contracting an STI so long as you wash yourself thoroughly with soap and hot water immediately after sex.	☐	☐
10. You don't need to worry about AIDS if no one you know has ever come down with it.	☐	☐
11. When it comes to STIs, it's all in the cards—either you're lucky or you're not.	☐	☐
12. The time to start worrying about STIs is when you come down with one.	☐	☐
13. As long as you avoid risky sexual practices such as anal intercourse, you're safe from STIs.	☐	☐
14. The time to talk about safer sex is before any sexual contact occurs.	☐	☐
15. A person needn't be concerned about an STI if the symptoms clear up in a few weeks without treatment.	☐	☐

SCORING

All questions are FALSE except numbers 5 and 14, which are TRUE. Give yourself one point for each right answer.

Total correct: _____

A higher correct score indicates a lower risk of contracting an STI. A lower correct score indicates an increased risk. A score of 13 or more means that your attitudes may lower your risk level. However, even one wrong response on this scale can increase your risk of an STI.

Source: From Nevid, Jeffrey S., Gotfried, Fern, CHOICES: SEX IN THE AGE OF STDS, 2nd Edition, © 1998. Reprinted and Electronically reproduced by permission of Pearson Education, Inc., Upper Saddle River, New Jersey.

LAB 14.2 • EFFECTIVELY COMMUNICATING SEXUAL INFORMATION, BOUNDARIES, AND PREFERENCES

Name: _____ Date: _____

Instructor: _____ Section: _____

Purpose: To learn and practice the skills necessary to communicate effectively to a potential sexual partner.

Background: To protect yourself from STIs such as HIV and to honor your own needs and wishes, you must be able to communicate clearly and directly with any potential sexual partner. If you are uncomfortable with anything a partner is proposing, you must be able to say "No," firmly and without hesitation. You must also be able to state what you want and need, whether it is more time to get to know someone, more proof of non–infectious status, a desire for less intimacy at the present, or a different way of being held or touched. *Before* placing yourself in a situation that could escalate beyond your level of safety or comfort, you should practice communicating.

Directions: Choose a trusted, nonsexual partner with whom you can communicate fully and freely. Imagine it is 10 p.m. and you are in a parked car with a potential sexual partner. He or she moves closer to you and puts an arm around your shoulder. In your own words, practice verbalizing the following:

- I don't want intimate contact right now.

- I'm worried about STIs.

- I want to make sure neither of us has an STI before getting intimate, even kissing.

- No matter what, no condom, no sexual activity.

- Hugs are OK now.

- I need to know someone pretty well before getting intimate with them.

- My sexual preference is _____.

- I'm OK with _____ but not _____.

- I like my partner to _____.

Name: _____ Date: _____

Instructor: _____ Section: _____

Materials: None

Purpose: Develop a plan to prevent getting a sexually transmitted infection.

Directions: Answer the questions below.

1. Do you consider yourself knowledgeable about sexually transmitted infections? Why or why not?

_____

_____

2. Think about three to five behaviors that you can minimize or eliminate in order to reduce your risk of an STI. Write those behaviors here:

_____

_____

_____

3. Think about three to five behaviors that you can add to your lifestyle in order to reduce your risk of an STI. Write those behaviors here:

_____

_____

_____

4. Identify three small action steps that you can take immediately to reduce your risk of an STI:

1. _____

2. _____

3. _____

5. What barriers or obstacles might hinder your STI prevention plan? Indicate your top three obstacles below:

1. _____

2. _____

3. _____

6. Write out three strategies for overcoming the obstacles listed above:

1. _____

2. _____

3. _____

7. List resources you will use to get more information or to help you reduce your risk of an STI:

Friend/partner/relative: _____

School-based resource: _____

Community-based resource: _____

Other: _____

15 Maintaining Lifelong Fitness and Wellness

Learning Outcomes

1. Describe three theories of aging.

 HEAR IT! ONLINE Audio case study and audio PowerPoint lecture

 SEE IT! ONLINE Seniors Saying No to Retirement

2. Identify the skills that promote successful communication and healthy relationships.

 DO IT! ONLINE Lab 15.1 Being an Assertive Communicator

3. Discuss strategies for becoming an informed health consumer.

 DO IT! ONLINE Lab 15.2 Being a Better Health Consumer

 SEE IT! ONLINE What Health Care's Passage Means for You
Holistic Health Care
Dr. Web's Credentials

4. List things you can do to live in an environmentally conscious way.

 SEE IT! ONLINE Crack Those Recycling Codes
Power of 2: Get an Energy Audit

5. Lay out a detailed plan for lifelong fitness and wellness.

 LIVE IT! ONLINE Take Charge of Your Health worksheets for assessing your communication skills and health care savvy, and for creating a plan for healthy aging.

 SEE IT! ONLINE Vitality Project

Pre- and post-quizzes and glossary flashcards REVIEW IT! ONLINE

casestudy

LYNN

"Hi, I'm Lynn. I'm 44 and just recently returned to college for the BA that I always meant to finish. I definitely stand out in my classes, but not as much as I thought I would! I've always been athletic— I used to run marathons—but I had foot surgery for an injury last year, and my running days are over. I'm not good at sitting still, though. What can I do to stay active and healthy as I get older?"

HEAR IT! ONLINE

• •

How do some people stay active and healthy even after age 80, while others begin to decline much earlier? There is no single answer, but establishing positive habits in all the dimensions of wellness—physical, social, intellectual, emotional, spiritual, and environmental—while you are young can go a long way toward increasing your chances of "aging gracefully." A lifelong fit-and-well lifestyle can reduce your risk of chronic illness. Moreover, it can allow you greater physical mobility, sharper mental acuity, and additional years of independence as you grow older.

This chapter focuses on how to maintain wellness over the course of a lifetime. It integrates fitness and personal health topics from earlier chapters and emphasizes specific long-term wellness strategies including skills that promote successful communication and relationships; tips for becoming a smart and informed health consumer; and strategies for dealing with the environmental challenges that face our world today.

What Happens as We Age?

As we enter and move through the later part of the life cycle, our bodies typically begin experiencing some degree of **aging**— a slow, progressive decline in the maximum functional level of individual cells,

> **aging** A progressive decline in the maximum functional level of individual cells, whole organs, and entire organisms

whole organs, and entire organisms (in this case, you). Researchers are still debating the underlying reasons why our bodies begin to decline after they have reached their physical peak in our 20s or 30s. One theory is the *wear and tear theory*—the idea that over time, an accumulation of damage from internal processes and environmental stress eventually wears the body out. Another theory, the *cellular theory*, posits that from birth, our cells are genetically programmed to divide or reproduce a limited number of times. Once these cells reach the end of their reproductive cycle, they die, and the organs they make up begin to deteriorate. A third theory, the *genetic mutation theory*, proposes that the number of cells exhibiting unusual or different characteristics increases with age. Proponents of this theory believe that aging is related to mutational damage within genes.

The exterior signs of aging are familiar to most of us. They include the onset of wrinkles, baldness, and gray hair; sensory deficits such as farsightedness and hearing loss; neurological changes that lead to slower reflexes and memory lapses; hormonal changes leading to menopause; weight gain and energy declines; and shifts in the sleep/wake cycle. Other common changes include mineral loss from bones that can lead to osteoporosis; declining flexibility in tendons and ligaments; declines in the healthy functioning of the heart, lungs, and other organs; and the onset of chronic diseases such as type 2 diabetes, cardiovascular diseases, diseases of the lungs, liver, or kidneys, and cancer.

Aging and Wellness

By 2009, 39.6 million Americans were age 65 or older— more than 12.9 percent of the population—and more than 5.7 million had reached age 85 by 2010—a 36 percent increase in the past decade (Figure 15.1).[1] As the Baby Boom generation ages, the number of Americans over 65 is predicted to reach 72.1 million by 2030, nearly double the number of seniors in 2008 and representing almost 20 percent of the population.[2]

Society will face issues of caring for these aging citizens: rising health costs, Social Security, and the need for appropriate housing and transport. At the same time, the demographics of Americans over 65 have improved steadily. In 1965, for instance, only one quarter of retirees had high school diplomas and just five percent had a college degree. By 2009, however, more than three-quarters were high school graduates and 21.7 percent had at least a bachelor's degree. With increasing education has come greater financial

FIGURE **15.1** The number of Americans aged 65 or older has grown from 3.1 million in 1900 to about 40.2 million in 2010, and is projected to grow to 72.1 million by the year 2030.

Source: Administration on Aging, *A Profile of Older Americans: 2010.*

well-being: The net worth of this age group has risen by 80 percent in the past 20 years.[3]

Overall Happiness and Well-Being What some may dread as a sad and limited time of life is actually, for most people, a period of happiness and satisfaction. A telephone survey of more than 340,000 people in 2008 reported that while people experienced the highest levels of anger in their 20s and while worry increases after age 18 and remains high throughout middle age, both happiness (mood) and satisfaction (life appraisal) rose steadily after age 50.[4] The survey conductors are unsure why, but overall, people in their 80s are happier than people in their 20s.[5]

Worksheet 6
Satisfaction with Life/ Happiness Inventory

A long-term Harvard University study that examined which factors correlated best with healthy aging found that not smoking was the single most significant one.[6] Other factors included independence; emotional maturity; financial security (including good health insurance); a stable marriage or partnership; strong social contacts; good coping skills; a positive attitude; not abusing alcohol; regular exercise; good nutrition; and maintaining a healthy-range BMI. The study also found that education was correlated with healthy aging: People with more years of education were healthier at age 70 than those with fewer years.[7]

Physical Wellness It is both possible and desirable to stay fit as we age (Figure 15.2). Efforts to maintain fitness throughout life contribute to all aspects of well-

ness, increasing longevity and reducing disability.[8] Regular stretching, strength training, and aerobics in later years can help preserve muscle and bone mass, reduce muscle wasting, help prevent falls, maintain higher metabolic rate, and reduce rates of cancer, osteoporosis, cardiovascular disease, and diabetes.[9]

Intellectual and Emotional Wellness As we've discussed throughout this book, the dimensions of wellness are interrelated, and that is equally true for older adults. Staying physically, socially, and occupationally active are all related to better mental functioning and improved mood. In a recent large German study, moderately to highly active people over 55 were significantly less likely to develop dementia than sedentary people.[10] Although demographic factors play a significant role in aging, a research team recently deduced from a survey of more than 22,000 Americans over 50 that retiring is more often accompanied by declines in memory and mental functioning than is continuing to work throughout one's 60s and beyond.[11]

Worksheet 5
Emotional Intelligence Assessment

Seniors Saying No to Retirement

How Do Relationships Contribute to Lifelong Wellness?

Social and emotional support can affect your health almost as strongly as can exercise and good nutrition. Living alone, having few friends or social

FIGURE **15.2** Born in 1910, Kozo Haraguchi began competing in track-and-field events at age 65. In 2005, at age 95, he set a world record for the 100 m dash for men aged 95 to 99.

acquaintances, doing few things socially, and feeling lonely are all associated with the risk of poorer physical and mental health, especially in older adults.[12] The key to the social dimension of wellness is to maintain strong friendships, healthy relationships with family members, and other types of long-term, committed relationships.[13]

Healthy Relationships Rely on Effective Communication

LIVE IT! ONLINE

Worksheet 12 How Healthy Is Your Relationship?

Common to all healthy relationships is an important trait: effective communication. The essence of good communication is a willingness to acknowledge and accept differences while actively exchanging ideas, thoughts, and feelings with others. If we are positive, assertive, and open with others (rather than cynical, distrustful, or guarded), we promote two-way communication and understanding. A willingness to reveal your inner states and past experiences through **self-disclosure** encourages others to share their thoughts and experiences with you.[14]

Active listening is an important skill for communication. This includes nodding, smiling, saying yes, and asking questions; using positive body language and an encouraging tone of voice; showing empathy and sympathy; and controlling the urge to interrupt, react defensively, or correct what you perceive to be the speaker's errors. If another person gives you the same considerations, the exchange can foster true understanding and communication. The following guidelines can help:

- Try to be specific about how you feel. State what is upsetting you and why.

- Begin statements using the word "I" rather than "You." "I" statements communicate in a direct, clear, and effective way and are less likely to put the listener on the defensive.

self-disclosure The process of revealing one's inner thoughts, feelings, and beliefs to another person

active listening Attentive and engaged listening that includes giving positive cues to the speaker

family of origin The people present in one's household during the first years of life

- If you have mixed feelings, say so. Express each feeling, and then explain what each is about.

You can assess your communication style in **Lab 15.1**.

DO IT! ONLINE

Relationships Provide Support

Relationships can provide practical, spiritual, and psychological support in the form of intimacy, social integration, and reassurance of our own worth.

Families A family is a recognizable group of people with roles, tasks, boundaries, and personalities whose central focus is to protect, care for, love, and socialize with one another. Healthy families foster a sense of security and feelings of belonging that are central to growth and development. It is from our **family of origin**, the people present in our household during our first years of life, that we initially learn about feelings, problem-solving, love, intimacy, and gender roles. We rely on these initial experiences and skills modeled by our family of origin as we establish relationships outside of the family.

Friendships Good friends can make a boring day fun or a gut-wrenching worry disappear. They can make us feel that we matter and that we have the strength to get through just about anything. They can also anger us, disappoint us, or jolt our comfortable ideas about right and wrong. Psychologists Jeffrey Turner and Laurna Rubinson summarized the consensus among experts on characteristics that make a good friendship: enjoyment of each other's company, acceptance of differences, mutual trust, respect, assistance, confiding, understanding, and the freedom to "be themselves."[15]

Friendships contribute significantly to both fitness and wellness throughout our lives. In a surprising study that supports the theme of interrelated wellness dimensions, a team of medical researchers from Chicago found that socializing with friends is associated with retaining better motor skills.[16] Following a large group of older adults over a period of five years, Aron Buchman and colleagues found that seniors with the most friends and social activities kept their mobility longer and more completely than did people with smaller social circles. An Australian study also found that, with all other factors held constant, older people who had large social networks were less likely to die during their 10-year study period.[17]

Love Relationships *Love relationships* typically include all the traits of friendship, as well as the following characteristics: a fascination or a healthy preoccupation with the other; exclusiveness or a special relationship that takes priority and excludes others of the same type; sexual desire; a willingness to sacrifice for the other; and being a champion or advocate for the other's interests and successes. Such relationships include married heterosexual couples, gay/lesbian couples, and unmarried cohabiting couples.

Commitment within long-term relationships means making choices and taking actions over time

that perpetuate the well-being of oneself, one's partner, and the relationship. Most adults want intimate, committed relationships, whether they are gay or straight, men or women. Lesbians and gay men seek the same things in primary relationships that heterosexual partners do—friendship, communication, validation, companionship, and a sense of stability—and many states are beginning to recognize and validate these relationships through legislation. The U.S. Census Bureau reported 741,000 same-sex couple households in their 2010 Community Population Survey. This is more than three and a half times the total reported in the 1990 Census.[18]

Marriage can provide emotional support by combining the benefits of friendship and a loving committed relationship. Healthy marriages contribute to lower levels of stress in three important ways: financial stability, expanded support networks, and improved personal behaviors. Married adults are about half as likely to be smokers as single, divorced, or separated adults. They are also less likely to be heavy drinkers or to engage in risky sexual behavior. They do, however, tend to weigh more than single adults.[19]

Although a successful marriage can bring much satisfaction, traditional marriage does not work for everyone. **Cohabitation**—two unmarried people with an intimate connection residing in the same household—has increased dramatically in the United States over the past few decades.[20] These relationships can be stable and happy,

casestudy

LYNN

"After finding out I couldn't run anymore, I decided to go back to something I haven't done in years: rowing! A friend of mine was on a recreational rowing team that needed more people, so I volunteered. We row three times a week, and there are so many great things about it. It's a terrific workout, it's easier on my foot, and I really like the other members of the team. There is nothing like being on the water at 6:00 AM and watching the sun come up with good friends."

THINK! How are the wellness practices that Lynn is using beneficial to her lifelong wellness? What are the benefits of strong social networks for physical fitness?

ACT! Choose someone to share your fitness plan and work together on mutual goals. List other ways that socializing can benefit your fitness plan.

HEAR IT! ONLINE

commitment In the context of a relationship, making choices and taking actions over time that perpetuate the well-being of the other person, oneself, and the relationship

cohabitation Living intimately together without being married

self-care Knowing your body and taking appropriate action to stop progression of illness or injury

with a high level of commitment between partners. Cohabitation can offer many of the same benefits as marriage: love, sex, companionship, and the ongoing opportunity to know a partner better over time. It can serve as a prelude to marriage, although current data do not support the idea that living together before marriage is a good way to find out whether a marriage will be successful. However, cohabitation can have its drawbacks, including lack of societal and legal validation for the relationship.

How Can I Be a Smart Health Consumer?

Perhaps the single greatest difficulty that we face as health consumers is the sheer magnitude of choices. **Lab 15.2** allows you to identify areas in which you can improve your effectiveness as a health consumer.

Worksheet 48
Advertisement
Claims for
Health Care
Products

Take Responsibility for Your Own Health Care

Our health care system is massive, and it can be overwhelming. However, you can learn how, when, and where to enter the system without incurring unnecessary risk and expense.

Self-Care and Seeking Medical Advice If you are not feeling well, you must first decide whether to seek professional medical advice. **Self-care** consists of knowing your body, paying attention to its signals, and taking appropriate action to stop the progression of illness or injury. Effective self-care also means understanding when to seek professional medical attention rather than treating a condition yourself. Table 15.1 lists several forms of self-care, as well as situations that require medical attention.

Assessing Health Professionals When you decide you do need medical help and you're selecting a physician from a network of providers, make sure you understand your coverage options and gather some background information on the physicians you are considering. Two of the most important things to find out are what

TABLE **15.1** When to Practice Self-Care and When to Seek Medical Advice	
Common forms of self-care include the following:	Consult a physician if you experience any of the following:
Diagnosing minor symptoms or conditions (for example, colds, minor abrasions	A serious accident or injury
	Sudden or severe chest pains
	Breathing difficulties
Performing monthly breast and testicular self-examinations	Trauma to the head or spine
Learning first aid for common, uncomplicated injuries and conditions	Tingling sensation in an arm accompanied by slurred speech or impaired thoughts
	Adverse reactions to a drug or insect bite
Learning to check your blood pressure, pulse, and body temperature	Unexplained bleeding or loss of body fluid from any body opening
Using home pregnancy and ovulation kits and HIV test kits	Sudden high fever or recurring high temperature (102°F for children and 103°F for adults) and/or sweating
	Unexplained sudden weight loss
Using reliable self-help books, tapes, software, websites, and videos	Persistent or recurring diarrhea or vomiting
	Any lump, swelling, thickness, or sore that does not subside or that grows for over a month
Using relaxation techniques including meditation, nutrition, rest, exercise, and stress management	Any marked change or pain in bowel or bladder habits
	Yellowing of the skin or the whites of the eyes
	Any symptom that is unusual and recurs over time
	You think you are pregnant

DIVERSITY

What Is Complementary and Alternative Medicine?

Complementary and alternative medicine (CAM), as defined by the National Center for Complementary and Alternative Medicine (NCCAM), is a group of diverse medical and health care systems, practices, and products that are not presently considered part of conventional medicine. *Complementary medicine* is used together with conventional medicine; for example, an aromatherapist might work with a cancer specialist to reduce a patient's nausea during chemotherapy. *Alternative medicine* has traditionally been used *in place of* conventional medicine; for example, someone suffering from allergies might use acupuncture instead of allergy medicine to relieve his or her symptoms.

A few of the better-known CAM practices are *traditional Chinese medicine*, with its emphasis on *qi* (pronounced "chi"), or vital energy, in health and disease; *acupuncture* and *acupressure*, which use needles and pressure points to balance the body's "energy flow" and are components of traditional Chinese medicine; Indian traditional medicine, or *ayurveda*. which aims to integrate and balance body, mind, and spirit; *homeopathic medicine*, which employs herbal medicine, minerals, and chemicals in extremely diluted forms to treat disease; and *chiropractic medicine*, which employs the manipulation of body structures (primarily the spine) to preserve and restore health.

Research CAM practitioners as carefully as you would a conventional physician. Ask your doctor or other health professional to recommend or refer you to a CAM therapist. If your insurance covers CAM therapies, ask your carrier for a list of approved providers. A good place to learn more about CAM is at the NCCAM website at http://nccam.nih.gov.

LIVE IT! ONLINE

Worksheet 49
Researching
Complementary
and Alternative
Medicine

SEE IT! ONLINE

Holistic Health
Care

---

professional educational training they had and what license or board certification they hold. *Board certified* indicates that the physician has passed the national board examination for their specialty. *Board eligible* merely means they are eligible to take the exam but have not necessarily passed it. Find out whether the physicians you are considering are affiliated with an accredited medical facility or institution, and whether they are open to complementary medicine or alternative medicine. (This is described in the box What Is Complementary and Alternative Medicine?)

When you speak to a new physician, pay attention to how they communicate. Do they listen to you, respect you as an individual, and give you time to ask questions? Do they indicate clearly how long a given treatment may last, what side effects you might expect, and what problems you should watch for? When

a doctor orders a test or suggests a procedure, you might ask questions such as these:

- Why has this test been ordered? What is the doctor trying to find or exclude?

- How often has the doctor performed this test or procedure, and with what proportion of successful outcomes?

- What are the side effects, and can these side effects be treated or reduced?

- Does this procedure require an overnight stay at a hospital, or can it be performed in a doctor's office?

Many patients find that writing their questions down before an appointment helps them get answers. You should not accept a defensive or hostile response: Asking questions is your right as a patient.

casestudy

LYNN

"I have a family history of breast cancer, so I do breast self-exams pretty regularly. I had a slight scare last month when I found a small lump in my right breast. I went to my doctor to have it checked out. They did a mammogram, an ultrasound, and a needle biopsy—all of which came back negative for cancer. My doctor told me that the lump is most likely normal breast tissue responding to hormonal changes but that I should continue to monitor the lump for any changes."

THINK! What kinds of questions should Lynn ask her doctor about the diagnostic tests being performed? Lynn's self-care includes regular breast exams. What kinds of self-care do you practice in your own life?

ACT! Make a list of wellness practices for daily, weekly, monthly, and yearly effort. Set up checklists for each level until they become habit.

- -

Being Proactive in Your Own Health Care The more

Worksheet 50 Risky Business: Let the Buyer Beware

Dr. Web's Credentials

you know about your own body and your personal and family health history, the better you will be at communicating with health providers. Use reputable sources to research any health condition you may have rather than relying solely on your doctor, and ask for a written summary of the results of your visit and any lab tests. Ask your doctor or practitioner to explain any problems and possible treatments, tests, and drugs in a clear and understandable way. If you have any doubt about the doctor's recommended treatment, seek a second opinion. Be sure to inform your primary health care provider about all of the therapies you are pursuing, including CAM.

Ask whether prescribed medications have generic equivalents that cost less. If you need to take a prescription medication for an extended time, ask for the maximum number of

sustainable choices Lifestyle choices that preserve and protect the planet's resources

doses allowed by your plan. Remember that "natural" and "safe" are not necessarily the same. Be cautious about combining herbal medications with any other medications.

Paying for Health Care At some point in your life, you'll probably use insurance to pay for your health care. The idea behind insurance is that you pay affordable premiums so that you never have to face overwhelming bills. In 2009, approximately 20 percent of college students reported not having health insurance.[21] The Patient Protection and Affordable Care Act of 2010 extended to age 26 the time students can remain on their parents' health plan.[22] It also removed lifetime caps on benefit payouts for student health coverage, and will make campus health plans more affordable.

What Health Care's Passage Means for You

If you are a college student and are not already covered under your parents' insurance, ask your student health center if your school has a program you can enroll in (or if they can recommend third-party providers). The box Understanding Health Insurance can help you decide what kind of insurance to buy in the future.

Environment and Wellness: What Are the Links?

Today, the natural world is under siege from a burgeoning population that consumes massive amounts of natural resources while producing millions of tons of pollution.[23] Crowding and pollution not only harm Earth but affect your own wellness directly in many ways. Learning how to make **sustainable choices** can improve both Earth's wellness and your own.

Overconsumption of Natural Resources

Americans consume far more energy and raw materials per person than do citizens of other countries. For example, although Americans comprise only five percent of the world's population, we consume one-quarter of the oil used globally each year.[24]

Pollution

Air pollution is altering our atmosphere and climate, while water pollution is reducing the viability of saltwater and freshwater bodies. Solid waste is filling up usable land and sometimes poisoning it for future uses.

Chemical compounds produced by automobile engines and industry contribute to the formation of smog

Understanding Health Insurance

Health insurance is a necessary part of maintaining life-long fitness and wellness. The information listed here can help you make decisions about the right kind and level to choose for your current situation.

Private health insurance may cover hospital costs and/or routine physicians' treatment and other areas such as dental services and pharmaceuticals. *Preexisting condition clauses* limit the insurance company's liability for medical conditions that a consumer had before obtaining coverage. All insurers set some limits on the types of services they cover (e.g., most exclude cosmetic surgery, private rooms, and experimental procedures). Private insurance companies increasingly employ several mechanisms to limit their losses. *Deductibles*, for example, are front-end payments (commonly $250 to $1,000) that you must make to your provider before your insurance company will start paying for any services you use. *Copayments* are set amounts that you pay per service received, regardless of the cost of the service (e.g., $20 per doctor visit or per prescription). *Coinsurance* is the percentage of the bill that you must pay.

Managed care describes a health care delivery system consisting of a network of physicians, hospitals, and other providers and facilities linked contractually to deliver comprehensive health benefits within a predetermined budget. Types of managed care plans include health maintenance organizations (HMOs), preferred provider organizations (PPOs), and point of service (POS). Doctors in managed care networks are given incentives to keep their patient pool healthy and avoid preventable ailments. As such, prevention and health education to reduce risk are often capstone components of such plans.

Health maintenance organizations (HMOs) provide a wide range of covered health benefits for a fixed amount prepaid by the patient, the employer, Medicaid, or Medicare. Usually, HMOs are the least expensive form of managed care, but also are the most restrictive. The downside of HMOs is that patients are typically required to use the plan's doctors and hospitals and to get approval from a primary care physician for treatment and referrals.

Preferred provider organizations (PPOs) are networks of independent doctors and hospitals that contract to provide care at discounted rates. Although they offer greater choice in doctors than HMOs do, they are less likely to coordinate a patient's care. Members do have a choice of seeing doctors who are not on the preferred list, but this choice may come at considerable cost.

Point of service (POS) plans—offered by many HMOs—are among the fastest growing of the managed care plans. Under POS plans, the patient selects a primary care physician from a list of participating providers, and this physician becomes the patient's "point of service." If referrals are made outside of the network, then the patient is still partially covered.

• •

and act as respiratory irritants and in some cases, carcinogens. The Environmental Protection Agency publishes a color-coded air quality index (AQI) that shows current air quality levels (Figure 15.3).[25] The higher the AQI value is, the greater the level of air pollution and associated health risks will be. When AQI values rise above 100, air quality is considered unhealthy, at first for certain groups of people, then for everyone.

Water pollution presents another major health challenge. According to a World Health Organization/UNICEF report, almost half the world's population faces chronic

When the AQI is in this range:	... air quality conditions are	... as symbolized by this color:
0 to 50	Good	Green
51 to 100	Moderate	Yellow
101 to 150	Unhealthy for sensitive groups	Orange
151 to 200	Unhealthy	Red
201 to 300	Very unhealthy	Purple
301 to 500	Hazardous	Maroon

FIGURE **15.3** The EPA's Air Quality Index shows air quality levels.

shortages of clean, safe water.[26] Globally, diarrhea from polluted water sources is the second leading cause of death in children under age five, and half of all hospital beds on the planet are filled with people whose diseases stem from poor sanitation, poor hygiene, and polluted drinking water.[27]

Each day, the average person in the U.S. generates 4.34 pounds of **municipal solid waste**—containers and packaging, discarded food, yard debris, hazardous waste (such as paints, oils, and solvents), and other refuse.[28] About three-fourths of this waste is buried in rapidly expanding landfills near urban

areas, dumped at sea, or shipped to landfills in developing countries. Solid waste can impact human health by leaking toxins and pathogenic organisms into groundwater and by emitting methane during decomposition and particulates and **greenhouse gases** during burning that contribute to **global warming**. Although experts believe that up to 90 percent of our trash is recyclable, we currently recycle only about 34 percent (Figure 15.4).[29]

> **municipal solid waste** Solid wastes from residential, commercial, institutional, and industrial sources
>
> **greenhouse gases** Gases that contribute to global warming by trapping heat near the Earth's surface
>
> **global warming** An increase in Earth's overall temperature

SEE IT! ONLINE
Crack Those Recycling Codes

Living in an Environmentally Conscious Way

What can you, as an individual, do to protect your own health and that of the planet? Here are a few ideas:

- Minimize pollution by using public transportation or a bicycle, driving only when necessary, keeping your car well-tuned, and choosing a fuel-efficient car.

- Conserve water, energy, paper, and other resources, and recycle the materials that you do use.

LIVE IT! ONLINE
Worksheet 47 Living in an Environmentally Conscious Way

What's in our trash?

- Food waste 14.1%
- Yard waste 13.7%
- Wood 6.5%
- Rubber, leather and textiles 8.3%
- Plastic 12.3%
- Paper 28.2%
- Other 3.5%
- Glass 4.8%
- Metal 8.6%

What happens to what we put in the trash?

- 54.3% Landfill
- 33.8% Recycled
- 11.9% Incinerated

FIGURE **15.4** The composition and disposal of trash in the United States.

Source: U.S. Environmental Protection Agency, *Municipal Solid Waste Generation, Recycling, and Disposal in the United States: Facts and Figures for 2009* (Washington, DC: U.S. Environmental Protection Agency, 2010).

- Avoid environmentally harmful products such as caustic cleaners, flushable cleaning cloths, and laundry soaps with fragrances or dyes.

- Learn how food cultivation, harvesting, and consumption impact ecosystems, and seek ways to minimize your impact through your food buying choices.

- Be eco-politically active: Write e-mails and letters, attend lectures and events, volunteer for community projects, and vote for alternative energy sources.

SEE IT! ONLINE

The Power of 2: Get an Energy Audit

How Can I Plan for Lifelong Fitness and Wellness?

We have emphasized throughout this book that fitness and wellness must be lifelong pursuits. The box Does Exercise Help Achieve Brain Fitness? underscores the importance of lifelong physical activity. One of the best ways to maintain healthy exercise habits as well as wellness efforts in other dimensions is to examine your motivations and work with them. Let's use exercise as an example of wellness motivation.

SEE IT! ONLINE

Vitality Project

Understand Your Lifelong Fitness Motivations

What motivates you in the long term? Health benefits? The thrill of competition? The pleasure of being in nature? Thinking about your motivations can help you stick with fitness activities for the long haul:

- *I want to gain health benefits.* Try to design a program centered on physical activities that you find enjoyable and easy to incorporate in your day-to-day life.

- *I want to have fun.* Join an intramural sports team that interests you, or go on regular outdoor trips with friends. Seek out activities that, first and foremost, you know you will enjoy—for instance, a day hike in a beautiful spot—and that have the beneficial "side effect" of fitness.

- *I want to meet new people or exercise with friends.* Participate in a fitness program—it's a great way to socialize and it can be a strong motivator for continued participation! Join a gym, club, or

team that meets regularly for workout sessions or games.

- *I like the challenge of setting goals and doing well in competition.* You may find a clearly defined target—such as an upcoming 5K race—to be just what you need to get started. Find a fun, competitive, active event happening in your area, and sign up!

- *I really want to lose some weight.* Be sure to include long-term nutrition and diet plans along with your plan for enjoyable calorie-burning activities.

- *I would like to have a stronger, more toned body.* Select your favorite aerobic activity, begin strength training, or take a sport-specific class regularly.

Make a Personal Commitment to Regular Exercise

Deciding to be more physically active is a good first step; the next and harder step is committing to that decision. Examine what a more active lifestyle would mean to you and write out a *personal commitment statement:* a list of reasons to commit to fitness for life. Review that statement regularly, especially if your commitment flags, until your new behaviors become routine.

Continually Reassess Your Fitness and Wellness

Review your pre-course assessment. Now that you've completed the course, fill out the post-course part of it. Reassess your plans for change and your progress in making it. In which areas have you made greatest progress? In which areas do you need continued improvement? Consider drafting a new behavior change contract to continue to improve your lifestyle habits.

Your body and lifestyle will change as you age, and you may need to adjust your fitness program accordingly over time. With the multiple demands of career, home, and family, personal health is too often forgotten until something goes wrong—you start feeling sick, have signs of a chronic disease, or have a doctor advising you to lose weight. Remember that your overall health and wellness is one of the most important things to attend to. Over time and with continued practice, your efforts to get fit and stay well will increase your chances of living a longer, happier, healthier life!

Does Exercise Help Achieve Brain Fitness?

Resistance exercise benefits the adult body at every age, increasing lean body mass and reducing fat tissue, but what about the brain? Does resistance exercise stimulate brain fitness as well as physical fitness?

A recent review of studies relating exercise to brain function confirmed a positive association between physical activity and brain function in both children and older adults.[1] Researchers have found that older adults who exercise regularly and have the greatest aerobic fitness also tend to have greater brain volume, better responses to sensory stimuli, and higher levels of growth factors that promote a better blood supply to the brain and better growth of nerve and brain tissue.

While health experts predict that the number of adults with Alzheimer's disease could triple from 4.5 million to 13.2 million over the next 50 years, a group of San Francisco researchers reports that physical activity could prevent half of those additional cases or delay them by five years or more.[2] Staying active throughout life and into the later years, they explain, reduces the risk of cardiovascular diseases, diabetes, and high blood pressure; it reduces obesity; it enhances the function of the brain and nervous system; and it lowers levels of inflammatory markers such as interleukin 6 and C-reactive protein.[3] Resistance training, in particular, lowers one's risk of metabolic syndrome, reduces inflammatory markers, improves blood sugar metabolism, lowers hypertension, lowers body fat, strengthens bones, and speeds the resting metabolic rate![4]

Sources:
1. R. F. Zoeller, "Exercise and Cognitive Function: Can Working Out Train the Brain, Too?" *American Journal of Lifestyle Medicine* 4, no. 5 (2010): 397–409 .
2. D. E. Barnes and others, "Physical Activity and Dementia: The Need for Prevention Trials," *Exercise and Sport Sciences Reviews* 35, no. 1 (2007): 24–9.
3. Ibid.
4. M. Phillips and others, "Resistance Training at Eight-Repetition Maximum Reduces the Inflammatory Milieu in Elderly Women," *Medicine and Science in Sports and Exercise* 42, no. 2 (2010): 314–25.

chapterin**review**

videos

Log on to **www.pearsonhighered.com/hopson** or MyFitnessLab to view these chapter-related videos.

Seniors Saying No to Retirement
What Health Care's Passage Means for You

Holistic Health Care
Dr. Web's Credentials
Crack Those Recycling Codes

Power of 2: Get an Energy Audit
Vitality Project

onlineresources

Log on to **www.pearsonhighered.com/hopson** or MyFitnessLab for access to these book-related resources, and for links to other useful websites.

 Audio case study
Audio PowerPoint lecture

 Lab 15.1 Being an Assertive Communicator
Lab 15.2 Being a Better Health Consumer

 Take Charge of Your Health! Worksheets:
Worksheet 5 Emotional Intelligence Assessment
Worksheet 6 Satisfaction with Life/Happiness
 Inventory
Worksheet 12 How Healthy Is Your Relationship?
Worksheet 47 Living Simply
Worksheet 48 Advertisement Claims for
 Health Care Products
Worksheet 49 Researching Complementary
 and Alternative Medicine
Worksheet 50 Risky Business: Let the Buyer
 Beware
Behavior Change Log Book and Wellness Journal

 Pre- and post-quizzes
Glossary flashcards

reviewquestions

1. The *wear and tear* theory of aging is the idea that
   a. over time, an accumulation of damage from internal processes and environmental stress eventually wears the body out.
   b. our cells are genetically programmed to divide or reproduce a limited number of times.
   c. mutational damage in genes causes aging.
   d. science can stop the aging process.

2. Which is a characteristic of *active listening*?
   a. Reading a magazine and occasionally nodding at the speaker
   b. Asking questions
   c. Correcting a speaker's errors immediately
   d. Looking away while the speaker is making a point so they feel less self-conscious.

3. Relationships contribute to wellness by
   a. decreasing intimacy.
   b. allowing you to share worries and concerns.
   c. requiring you to build your own self-worth.
   d. increasing your BMI.

4. By the formal definition of friendship, a good friend is likely to
   a. borrow your possessions.
   b. point out differences between your attitudes, beliefs, and habits.
   c. trust you.
   d. offer helpful ways to change your personality.

5. Healthy marriages provide emotional support by
   a. allowing you to combine incomes.
   b. expanding social networks.
   c. improving personal habits.
   d. requiring effort toward commitment.

6. Which of the following is an example of self-care?
   a. Performing yearly breast or testicular self-exams
   b. Administering first aid
   c. Taking a home-pregnancy test
   d. Self-diagnosing and treating chest pains

7. Which of the following is true about student health care coverage in America?
   a. Fifty percent of students lack coverage.
   b. Students can remain on their parents' health plan until age 26.
   c. Few student health plans provide complete coverage.
   d. Your student health policy will have a lifetime cap on benefit payments.

8. According to experts, what percentage of our trash is recyclable?
   a. 70
   b. 80
   c. 90
   d. 100

9. You can increase your carbon footprint by
   a. riding a bicycle.
   b. setting your thermostat at 65 in winter.
   c. keeping your car tires inflated.
   d. choosing a six- or seven-passenger vehicle.

10. Which of the following would contribute to lifelong fitness and wellness?
    a. Looking for physical activities that you find fun
    b. Setting up a permanent dietary plan
    c. Creating an exercise plan after you notice middle aged weight gain
    d. Cutting back on physical activity as you get older to get enough rest

critical**thinking**questions

REVIEW IT! ONLINE

1. Which of the biological theories of aging do you find most compelling? Why?
2. How do effective communication and healthy relationships contribute to wellness?
3. What are some of the traits of a good health care provider?
4. What does it mean to live in an environmentally conscious way?

references

1–3. U.S. Department of Health and Human Services, Administration on Aging, *Profile of Older Americans: 2010* www.aoa.gov /aoaroot/aging_statistics/Profile/2010 /docs/2010profile.pdf (2011).

4. A. A. Stone and others, "A Snapshot of the Age Distribution of Psychological Well-Being in the United States," *Proceedings of the National Academy of Sciences* 107, no. 22 (2010): 9985–90.

5. N. Bakalar, "Happiness May Come with Age, Study Says," *New York Times*, June 1, 2010.

6. G. E. Vaillant, *Aging Well* (New York: Little Brown and Company, 2002).

7. Ibid.

8. C. Christmas and R. A. Andersen, "Exercise and Older Patients: Guidelines for the Clinician," *Journal of the American Geriatrics Society* 48, no. 3 (2000): 318–24.

9. W. J. Vans, "Effects of Aging and Exercise on Nutrition Needs of the Elderly," *Nutrition Reviews* 54, no. 1 pt. 2 (1996): S35–9; A. Bauman and T. J. Campbell, "Heart Week 2001: 'Get Active'! A Call to Action," *Medical Journal of Australia* 174, no. 8 (2001): 381–2.

10. T. Etgen and others, "Physical Activity and Incident Cognitive Impairment in Elderly Persons: The INVADE Study," *Archives of Internal Medicine* 170, no. 2 (2010): 186–93.

11. R. Willis and S. Rohwedder, "Mental Retirement," RAND Working Paper Series WR-711, October 2009; G. Kolata, "Taking Early Retirement May Retire Memory, Too," *New York Times*, October 11, 2010.

12. E.Y. Cornwell and L. J. Waite, "Social Disconnectedness, Perceived Isolation, and Health among Older Adults," *Journal of Health and Social Behavior* 50, no. 1 (2009): 31–48.

13. C. J. Hale, J. W. Hannum, and D. L. Espelage, "Social Support and Physical Health: The Importance of Belonging," *Journal of American College Health* 53, no. 6 (2005): 276–84.

14. J. Caputo, H. C. Hazel, and C. McMahon *Interpersonal Communication* (Boston: Allyn & Bacon, 1994): 224.

15. J. Turner and L. Robinson, *Contemporary Human Sexuality* (Englewood Cliffs, NJ: Prentice Hall, 1993): 457.

16. A. Buchman and others, "Association between Late-Life Social Activity and Motor Decline in Older Adults," *Archives of Internal Medicine* 169, no. 12 (2009): 1139–46.

17. T. Parker-Pope, "What Are Friends For? A Longer Life," *New York Times*, April 20, 2009.

18. U.S. Census Bureau, "Families and Living Arrangements: Current Population Survey (CPS) Reports," www.census.gov/population /www/socdemo/hh-fam.html (2010).

19. P. Gordon-Larsen, "Determinants of Obesity," presented at The Obesity Society 2007 Annual Scientific Meeting, New Orleans, Oct. 20–24, 2007.

20. U.S. Census Bureau, "Families and Living Arrangements," 2010.

21. Lookout Mountain Group, "Analysis and Policy Recommendations for Providing Health Insurance and Health Care for the College Student Population," www .hbc-slba.com/LMG/LMG_abstract_3.5.pdf (June 2009).

22. B. Burnsed, "5 Ways Health Reform Affects College Students," *U.S. News and World Report*, September 9, 2010.

23. C. Flavin and others, *State of the World 2008: Innovations for a Sustainable Economy* (Washington, DC: Worldwatch Institute, 2008).

24. CIA World Factbook 2011, "Country Comparison: Oil—Consumption," https://www .cia.gov/library/publications/the-world-factbook/rankorder/2174rank.html (accessed October 2011).

25. AirNow, "Air Quality Index (AQI)—A Guide to Air Quality and Your Health," www .airnow.gov/index.cfm?action=aqibasics .aqi (September 2010).

26. World Health Organization/UNICEF Joint Monitoring Programme for Water Supply and Sanitation, *Progress on Drinking Water and Sanitation: Special Focus on Sanitation* (New York: UNICEF; and Geneva: WHO, 2008).

27. Water.org, "Water Facts," water.org /learn-about-the-water-crisis/facts (accessed May 2011).

28. U.S. Environmental Protection Agency, *Municipal Solid Waste Generation, Recycling, and Disposal in the United States: Facts and Figures for 2009* (Washington, DC: U.S. Environmental Protection Agency, 2010).

29. Ibid.

LAB 15.1 • BEING AN ASSERTIVE COMMUNICATOR

Name: _____ **Date:** _____

Instructor: _____ **Section:** _____

Purpose: To evaluate your ability to communicate assertively, and to identify ways to improve your communication skills.

Directions: Read the following situations and assess your response according to the following five-point scale:

	Never	Seldom	Sometimes	Frequently	Always
1. Friends ask you to ride home with them after they've all been drinking. You know you shouldn't, but you don't want to seem like a prude. You take the ride.	1	2	3	4	5
2. Your decisions can be easily swayed by a strong argument from someone else pushing you in the opposite direction.	1	2	3	4	5
3. You feel strongly about a political issue, but it is the opposite of the opinion your parents hold. You remain silent rather than getting into an argument.	1	2	3	4	5
4. You start out by saying no to something but get talked into doing it after a short time.	1	2	3	4	5
5. You're stressed out with too much to do and too little time, but you can't say no when someone asks a favor.	1	2	3	4	5
6. Someone says something really nasty about a person you like. You jump to the defense of the person being criticized, even though you are in the minority opinion.	1	2	3	4	5
7. You would describe yourself as assertive and tend to quickly let others know your thoughts about certain issues.	1	2	3	4	5
8. Someone is critical of something you do. You quickly defend your actions by explaining why you did what you did.	1	2	3	4	5

INTERPRETING YOUR SCORE

Think about your responses to each statement. Do your responses indicate an assertive communication style in which you stand up for your feelings or beliefs? What factors cause you to hold back when you should probably speak up? How can you work to improve your communication behaviors in this area? Make a list of skills you could develop to help you communicate more assertively. It is important to know your own likes and dislikes and put them forward in a tactful but forthright way to avoid conflicts later.

Name: _____ Date: _____

Instructor: _____ Section: _____

Purpose: To assess your savvy as a health care consumer

Directions: Answer the following questions, and determine what you might do to become a better health care consumer.

1. Do you have a physician? ___ Yes ___ No

2. Do you have health insurance? ___ Yes ___ No

3. Have you determined which health care services are available free or at a reduced cost in your area? ___ Yes ___ No If so, what are they?

4. When you receive a prescription, do you ask the pharmacist if a generic brand could be substituted? ___ Yes ___ No

5. Do you ask the pharmacist about potential side effects before or after the prescription is filled, including possible food and drug interactions? ___ Yes ___ No

6. Do you take medication as directed? ___ Yes ___ No

7. Do you report any unusual side effects to your doctor? ___ Yes ___ No

8. When you receive a diagnosis, do you seek more information about the diagnosis and treatment? ___ Yes ___ No

9. If surgery or an invasive type of treatment is indicated by your doctor, do you seek a second opinion? ___ Yes ___ No

10. Where do you find most health information? _____

11. How do you know this source of information is a reliable and credible source?

_____

12. When you purchase an over-the-counter (OTC) medication, do you read the label? ___ Yes ___ No

13. What attracts you most to a new product? (check all that apply)

_____ price   _____ savings or coupons

_____ promises of a new lifestyle   _____ spokesperson

_____ appears to meet a need   _____ testing for product safety

_____ positive testimonials

14. How much of a role do you think advertising plays in your decision to purchase a new health care product?

_____

Photo Credits

Chapter 1

Chapter Opener p. 1 moodboard/Alamy; 1.1 Ale Ventura/Jupiter Images; p. 2 Image Source/Jupiter Images Royalty Free; 1.2 Irreversible damage: ImageState Royalty Free/Alamy; Chronic illness: MBI/Alamy; Signs of illness: Ariel Skelley/Alamy; Average wellness: Fancy/Alamy; Increased wellness: Tetra Images/Alamy; Optimum wellness: Blend Images/Alamy; 1.3 Alamy; p. 4 Corbis RF; p. 6 Thinkstock; 1.4 iStock; 1.7 Goodshoot/Jupiter Images Royalty Free; p. 9 Masterfile Royalty Free Division; p. 11 Corbis RF; p. 12 Masterfile Royalty Free Division; p. 13 Alamy; p. 15 Andrew Manley/iStockphoto.com; p. 17 Edyta Pawlowska/Shutterstock.

Chapter 2

Chapter Opener p. 31: Nicole Hill/RubberBall/Alamy; p. 32 Ryan McVay/Getty Images Inc. - PhotoDisc; 2.1a Light physical activity: Ken Gillespie Photography/Alamy; 2.1b Moderate physical activity: Doug Menuez/Getty Images Inc.-PhotoDisc; 2.1c Vigorous physical activity: Getty Images - Stockbyte; p. 34 Denkou Images/AGE Fotostock America, Inc - Royalty-free; p. 37 George Doyle/Getty Images, Inc - Stockbyte Royalty Free; 2.4a cardiorespiratory endurance: Dan Dalton/Getty Images/Digital Vision; 2.4b muscular fitness: MIXA/Getty Images Inc. RF; 2.4c flexibility: Daniel Grill/Alamy; p. 41 Alamy; p. 43 Dreamstime; p. 44 Alamy; p. 45 Shutterstock; p. 46 Paul Burns/Jupiter Images Royalty Free; p. 48 Alamy; p. 50 Dreamstime.

Chapter 3

Chapter Opener p. 67: Franck Camhi/Alamy; 3.1 rubberball/Getty Images Inc - Rubberball Royalty Free; p. 68 Jupiter Images - Thinkstock Images Royalty Free; 3.2 Radius Images/Jupiter Images Royalty Free; p. 73 Alamy Images Royalty Free; 3.5 Andres Rodriguez/Alamy; p. 75 Dennis Welsh/AGE Fotostock America, Inc - Royalty-free; 3.6a Elena Dorfman/Elena Dorfman; 3.6b Elena Dorfman/Elena Dorfman; 3.7 Thinkstock; p. 78 PhotoLibrary; p. 82 Eric Fowke/PhotoEdit Inc.; p. 85 iStock; p. 86 Thinkstock; p. 87 iStock; p. 89 Rob Melnychuk/Getty Images/Digital Vision; Table 3.4 Alamy; p. 97 Elena Dorfman/Pearson Education/Pearson Science; p. 112 Asia Images Group/PhotoLibrary.

Chapter 4

Chapter Opener p. 115 Tero Sivula/Alamy; p. 116 Comstock Images/Jupiter Images PictureArts Corporation/Brand X Royalty Free; 4.4 Alamy; p. 122 Masterfile Royalty Free Division; 4.5a, b U.S. Department of Agriculture; Table 4.1 p. (both) Elena Dorfman/Pearson Education/Pearson Science; p. 128 Alamy; p. 130 Masterfile Royalty Free Division; 4.9.1-4.9.3 (all) Elena Dorfman/Pearson Education/Pearson Science; 4.9.4-4.9.5 (all) Rolland Renaud/Pearson Education/Pearson Science; 4.9.5a Rolland Renaud/Pearson Education/Pearson Science; 4.9.5b Jac Mat/Pearson Education/Pearson Science; 4.9.6a (both) Rolland Renaud/Pearson Education/Pearson Science; 4.9.6b (both) Elena Dorfman/Pearson Education/Pearson Science; 4.9.7a (both) Rolland Renaud/Pearson Education/Pearson Science; 4.9.7b (both) Elena Dorfman/Pearson Education/Pearson Science; 4.9.7c hip adduction with ball: Jac Mat/Pearson Education/Pearson Science; 4.9.8a, b (both) Elena Dorfman/Pearson Education/Pearson Science; 4.9.9 (both) Jac Mat/Pearson Education/Pearson Science; 4.9.10 (both) Rolland Renaud/Pearson Education/Pearson Science; 4.9.11a (both) Elena Dorfman/Pearson Education/Pearson Science; 4.9.11b (both) Creative Digital Visions/Pearson Education/Pearson Science; 4.9.12a, b (both) Elena Dorfman/Pearson Education/Pearson Science; 4.9.13a (both) Elena Dorfman/Pearson Education/Pearson Science; 4.9.13b (both) Jac Mat/Pearson Education/Pearson Science; 4.9.14-4.9.18 (all) Elena Dorfman/Pearson Education/Pearson Science; 4.9.19a (both) Rolland Renaud/Pearson Education/Pearson Science; 4.9.19b (both) Elena Dorfman/Pearson Education/Pearson Science; 4.9.20a, b Elena Dorfman/Pearson Education/Pearson Science; 4.9.20c (both) Jac Mat/Pearson Education/Pearson Science; 4.9.20d Elena Dorfman/Pearson Education/Pearson Science; 4.9.20e Jac Mat/Pearson Education/Pearson Science; 4.9.21a (both) Elena Dorfman/Pearson Education/Pearson Science; 4.9.21b (both) Creative Digital Solutions/Pearson Education/Pearson Science; 4.9.22a, b Elena Dorfman/Pearson Education/Pearson Science; 4.9.22c p. 143 triceps extension with resistance band: Jac Mat/Pearson Education/Pearson Science; 4.9.23a, b Elena Dorfman/Pearson Education/Pearson Science; 4.9.23c (both) Jac Mat/Pearson Education/Pearson Science; 4.9.24a (both) Elena Dorfman/Pearson Education/Pearson Science; 4.9.24b (both) Jac Mat/Pearson Education/Pearson Science; 4.9.25-4.9.28 (both) Elena Dorfman/Pearson Education/Pearson Science; p. 150 (left) Shutterstock; p. 150 (right) Superstock; p. 150 (bottom) Ralph Kerpa/PhotoLibrary; p. 152 Shutterstock; p. 161 (all) Elena Dorfman/Pearson Education/Pearson Science; p. 162 (both) Elena Dorfman/Pearson Education/Pearson Science; p. 169: GoGo Images Corporation/Alamy.

Chapter 5

Chapter Opener p. 173 Superstock Royalty Free; p. 174 Alamy; p. 174 Plush Studios/Getty Images Inc. - PhotoDisc; p. 177 Tetra Images/Getty Images, Inc/Tetra Images Royalty Free; p. 179 John Cumming/Getty Images/Digital Vision; 5.2a, b Elena Dorfman/Pearson Education/Pearson Science; 5.3.2 Jac Mat/Pearson Education/Pearson Science; 5.3.3-5.312 (all) Elena Dorfman/Pearson Education/Pearson Science; 5.3.10a Elena Dorfman/Pearson Education/Pearson Science; 5.3.10b Rolland Renaud/Pearson Education/Pearson Science; 5.3.11-5.3.14 Elena Dorfman/Pearson Education/Pearson Science; 5.3.16 Jac Mat/Pearson

Education/Pearson Science; 5.3.15a-c Jac Mat/Pearson Education/Pearson Science; p. 188 Photo Library; p. 189 Newscom; 5.4 Compiled from above images; 5.7.1-5.7.4 Elena Dorfman/Pearson Education/Pearson Science; p. 197 iStock; p. 200 (both) Elena Dorfman/Pearson Education/Pearson Science; p. 210 istockphoto; p. 213 Alamy.

Chapter 6

Chapter Opener p. 215 stockphoto4u/istockphoto; p. 216 Pixland/Jupiter Images - Pixland Royalty Free; 6.1 Thinkstock; p. 218 iStockphoto; p. 220 Getty Images Inc. - PhotoDisc; 6.5 Newscom; 6.6 PhotoEdit Inc.; 6.7 Newscom; 6.8 Kristin Piljay/Pearson Education/Pearson Science; p. 225 Shutterstock; p. 226 Thinkstock; p. 230 (both) Kristin Piljay/Pearson Education/Pearson Science; p. 232 (both) Elena Dorfman/Pearson Education/Pearson Science; p. 233 (all) Elena Dorfman/Pearson Education/Pearson Science.

Chapter 7

Chapter Opener p. 237: Jerzyworks/Masterfile Corporation; p. 238 Ryan McVay/Getty Images Inc. - PhotoDisc; 7.1 (left) Alamy; 7.1 (right) PhotoLibrary; p. 241 Thinkstock; 7.3 (all) Pearson Learning Photo Studio; 7.5a BrandX/AGE Fotostock America, Inc - Royalty-free; 7.5b Corbis RF; p. 246 iStock; Table 7.1 (left) Smileus/Shutterstock; (right) Shutterstock; p. 248 Bora Ucak/iStockphoto.com; p. 253 Shutterstock; Table 7.2 peas: Brand Pictures/AGE Fotostock America, Inc - Royalty-free; spinach: Corbis RF; eggs: Corbis RF; strawberries: Corbis RF; mangos: BrandPictures/AGE Fotostock America, Inc - Royalty-free; milk: Corbis RF; almonds: Corbis RF; p. 256 Dorling Kindersley/Dorling Kindersley Media Library; Table 7.3 cheese: Corbis RF; kale: Brand Pictures/AGE Fotostock America, Inc - Royalty-free; pinto beans: Pearson Learning Photo Studio; beans: Brand Pictures/AGE Fotostock America, Inc - Royalty-free; Table 7.3 fish: Corbis RF; meat: Corbis RF; p. 260 Alamy; p. 262 Shutterstock; 7.8 ConAgra Foods Inc.; 7.9 GMA; p. 267 Alamy; 7.12a Kristin Piljay/Pearson Education/Pearson Science; 7.12b Norman Hollands/Dorling Kindersley Media Library; 7.13 Stuart Monk/Shutterstock; Table 7.5 brown rice: Alamy; hot dog: Alamy; Table 7.5 celery iStock; p. 274: Olga Shelego/iStockphoto.com;

Chapter 8

Chapter Opener p. 283 Alamy; p. 284 Ryan McVay/Getty Images Inc. - PhotoDisc; 8.2 Lose Luis Pelaez Inc./Getty Images, Inc. - Blend Images Royalty Free; 8.4 (all) Brand X Pictures/Getty Images Royalty Free; p. 287 Alamy; p. 288 John Giustina/Getty Images/Digital Vision; p. 288 Shutterstock; p. 289 Cusp/Photolibrary Royalty Free; 8.5 Big Cheese Photo LLC/Alamy Images Royalty Free; 8.6 PhotoLibrary; 8.7a p. 292 Newscom; 8.7b p. 292 Newscom; p. 293 Getty Images; 8.9 p. 296 PhotoLibrary; p. 298 Dreamstime; p. 299 Alamy; p. 313 iStock.

Chapter 9

Chapter Opener p. 317 Dreamstime; p. 318 iStock; 9.1 Moodboard/Corbis RF; p. 323 Shutterstock; p. 324 Bridget Montgomery/AP Wide World Photos; 9.3 Thinkstock; 9.4 Alamy; p. 327 Getty Images, Inc - Stockbyte Royalty Free; p. 328 Photo Library; p. 330 Alamy Images Royalty Free; p. 331 Laura Doss/Photolibrary Royalty Free; p. 332 John Dowland/Photolibrary.com - Royalty Free; p. 344 Science Photo Library/Alamy.

Chapter 10

Chapter Opener p. 347 iStockphoto; p. 348 Thinkstock; p. 350 Alamy; p. 352 Irina Iglina/iStockphoto; p. 353 Alamy; p. 355 Shutterstock; p. 357 Dreamstime; p. 358 Rayman/Getty Images - Digital Vision; 10.3 Radius Images/Alamy Images; p. 362 Alamy; p. 363 Suzannah Skelton/iStockphoto.com.

Chapter 11

Chapter Opener p. 369: UpperCut Images/Superstock Royalty Free; 11.1 all Over Photography/Alamy Images; p. 370: Jack Hollingsworth/Getty Images Inc. - PhotoDisc; p. 371 Alamy; 11.2 Dreamstime; p. 374 Photo Library; 11.3 PhotoAlto/Alamy Images; 11.4a SPL/Photo Researchers, Inc.; 11.4b Professor Pietro M. Motta/Photo Researchers, Inc.; 11.6 Alamy.

Chapter 12

Chapter Opener p. 385 iStockphoto; p. 386 Stockbyte/Getty Images, Inc - Stockbyte Royalty Free; 12.3a Dr. P. Marazzi/Photo Researchers, Inc.; 12.3b Dr. P. Marazzi/SPL/Photo Researchers, Inc.; 12.3c James Stevenson/SPL/Photo Researchers, Inc.; p. 390 Rick Gomez/Masterfile Corporation; p. 392 Don Farrall/Getty Images Inc. - PhotoDisc; p. 395 Eric Fowke/PhotoEdit Inc.; 12.6a Alamy; 12.6b iStockphoto.com; 12.6c Photolibrary Royalty Free; 12.6d iStockphoto.com; p. 397 Getty Images, Inc-Purestock Royalty Free.

Chapter 13

Chapter Opener Shutterstock; 13.1 Newscom; p. 406 Image Source/Jupiter Images Royalty Free; 13.5 Shutterstock; p. 411 William Fritsch/Jupiter Images PictureArts Corporation/Brand X Royalty Free; p. 412 PhotoLibrary; p. 414 chewing tobacco: iStock; cigarettes: iStock; iStock; p. 415: Dorling Kindersley/Dorling Kindersley Media Library; 13.7 FDA; p. 418: Blend Images/SuperStock; p. 420 Alamy; p. 421 Alamy; p. 423 iStock.

Chapter 14

Chapter Opener Orenstein/Photodisc/Getty Images, Inc. - PhotoDisc; 14.1 Alamy; p. 434 Rob Melnychuk/Jupiter Images PictureArts Corporation/Brand X Royalty Free; p. 435 Tomas Rodriguez/Corbis/Corbis; p. 435 Tomas Rodriguez/Corbis; 14.4 Corbis; 14.6 John Amis/AP Wide World Photos; p. 442 Dreamstime; p. 443 Alamy; p. 445 Alamy.

Chapter 15

Chapter Opener Sam Edwards/Alamy; p. 454 Alamy; 15.1 Rolf Bruderer/Jupiter Images Royalty Free; 15.2 Newscom; p. 456 Masterfile Royalty Free Division; p. 457 Digital Vision/Getty Images/Digital Vision; p. 458 Jiang Jin/SuperStock, Inc.; p. 460 fStop/Alamy Images; p. 461 Shutterstock; p. 463 Jupiter Images PictureArts Corporation/Brand X Royalty Free; p. 464 PhotoLibrary.

Index

Note: page numbers followed by f or t refer to Figures or Tables

PRE-COURSE/POST-COURSE ASSESSMENT

Name: _____ **Date:** _____

As you complete the key fitness/wellness lab assessments in this course, record your results in the "Pre-Course Assessment" column. At the end of the course, re-do the labs, record your results in the "Post-Course Assessment" column, and see the progress you have made!

Lab	Pre-Course Assessment	Post-Course Assessment

Lab 3.2: Assessing Your Cardiorespiratory Fitness Level	**3-minute step test**
	  1 minute recovery HR: _____ (bpm)
	  Fitness rating: _____
	1-mile walk test
	  VO$_2$ max: _____ Fitness rating: _____
	1.5-mile run test
	  VO$_2$ max: _____ Fitness rating: _____
		3-minute step test
		  1 minute recovery HR: _____ (bpm)
		  Fitness rating: _____
		1-mile walk test
		  VO$_2$ max: _____ Fitness rating: _____
		1.5-mile run test
		  VO$_2$ max: _____ Fitness rating: _____

Lab 4.1: Assessing Your Muscular Strength	**Chest press**
	  S/BW ratio: _____ Rating: _____
	Leg press
	  S/BW ratio: _____ Rating: _____
		Chest press
		  S/BW ratio: _____ Rating: _____
		Leg press
		  S/BW ratio: _____ Rating: _____

Lab 4.2: Assessing Your Muscular Endurance	**20RM assessment**
	  Chest press 20RM weight lifted: _____
	  Leg press 20RM weight lifted: _____
	Push-up assessment
	  Repetitions: _____ Rating: _____
	Curl-up assessment
	  Repetitions: _____ Rating: _____
		20RM assessment
		  Chest press 20RM weight lifted: _____
		  Leg press 20RM weight lifted: _____
		Push-up assessment
		  Repetitions: _____ Rating: _____
		Curl-up assessment
		  Repetitions: _____ Rating: _____

Lab 5.1: Assessing Your Flexibility	**Sit-and-reach test**
	  Reach distance (in or cm): _____
	  Rating: _____
		Sit-and-reach test
		  Reach distance (in or cm): _____
		  Rating: _____

Lab 6.1: How to Calculate Your BMI	BMI: _____ kg/m^2 Weight classification: _____	BMI: _____ kg/m^2 Weight classification: _____
Lab 6.2: Measure and Evaluate Your Body Circumferences	Waist: _____ Hip: _____ WHR Ratio: _____ Upper arm: _____ (right) _____ (left) Forearm: _____ (right) _____ (left) Thigh: _____ (right) _____ (left) Calf: _____ (right) _____ (left) Neck: _____ Disease risk rating for WHR: _____ Disease risk rating for WC: _____	Waist: _____ Hip: _____ WHR Ratio: _____ Upper arm: _____ (right) _____ (left) Forearm: _____ (right) _____ (left) Thigh: _____ (right) _____ (left) Calf: _____ (right) _____ (left) Neck: _____ Disease risk rating for WHR: _____ Disease risk rating for WC: _____
Lab 6.3: Estimate Your Percent Body Fat (Skinfold Test)	Sum of 3 skinfolds: _____ % body fat estimate: _____ Rating: _____	Sum of 3 skinfolds: _____ % body fat estimate: _____ Rating: _____
Lab 7.2: Keeping a Food Diary and Analyzing Your Daily Nutrition **Lab 7.3:** Improving Your Nutrition	Milk intake: _____ cups Meat and beans intake: _____ oz. Vegetables intake: _____ cups Fruits intake: _____ cups Grains intake: _____ oz.	Milk intake: _____ cups Meat and beans intake: _____ oz. Vegetables intake: _____ cups Fruits intake: _____ cups Grains intake: _____ oz.
Lab 8.1: Calculating Energy Balance and Setting Energy Balance Goals	Estimated calorie intake: _____ Estimated calorie expenditure: _____ Calorie balance (intake minus expenditure): _____	Estimated calorie intake: _____ Estimated calorie expenditure: _____ Calorie balance (intake minus expenditure): _____
Lab 8.2: Your Weight Management Plan	% body fat: _____ Weight: _____ lb. BMI: _____ kg/m^2	% body fat: _____ Weight: _____ lb. BMI: _____ kg/m^2
Lab 9.1: How Stressed Are You?	Sum of negative scores: _____ Interpretation: _____	Sum of negative scores: _____ Interpretation: _____
Lab 10.1: Understanding Your CVD Risk	Family risk for CVD, total points: _____ Lifestyle risk for CVD, total points: _____ Additional risks for CVD, total points: _____	Family risk for CVD, total points: _____ Lifestyle risk for CVD, total points: _____ Additional risks for CVD, total points: _____
Lab 12.1: Assessing Your Personal Risk of Cancer	Breast cancer risk, total points: _____ Skin cancer risk, total points: _____ Reproductive cancer risk, total points: _____ General cancer risk, total points: _____	Breast cancer risk, total points: _____ Skin cancer risk, total points: _____ Reproductive cancer risk, total points: _____ General cancer risk, total points: _____
Lab 13.1: Assessing Your Alcohol Use and Risk of Abuse	Drinking patterns and abuse risk score: _____ How risky is your alcohol use? _____	Drinking patterns and abuse risk score: _____ How risky is your alcohol use? _____

Answers to End-of-Chapter Questions

Chapter 1
1.b; 2.b; 3.d; 4.a; 5.a; 6.b; 7.b; 8.d; 9.a; 10.d

Chapter 2
1.b; 2.c; 3.d; 4.a; 5.b; 6.d; 7.d; 8.b; 9.d; 10.a

Chapter 3
1.c; 2.a; 3.a; 4.d; 5.c; 6.b; 7.d; 8.c; 9.a; 10.c

Chapter 4
1.d; 2.c; 3.a; 4.d; 5.a; 6.b; 7.c; 8.b; 9.a; 10.c

Chapter 5
1.a; 2.c; 3.b; 4.d; 5.d; 6.b; 7.c; 8.b; 9.c; 10.a

Chapter 6
1.c; 2.d; 3.c; 4.b; 5.b; 6.b; 7.a; 8.c; 9.a; 10.a

Chapter 7
1.d; 2.d; 3.d; 4.c; 5.d; 6.d; 7.d; 8.a; 9.c; 10.d

Chapter 8
1.d; 2.d; 3.b; 4.b; 5.c; 6.a; 7.a; 8.b; 9.a; 10.d

Chapter 9
1.c; 2.b; 3.a; 4.d; 5.d; 6.a; 7.b; 8.d; 9.a; 10.d

Chapter 10
1.d; 2.d; 3.c; 4.a; 5.c; 6.b; 7.d; 8.a; 9.a; 10.b

Chapter 11
1.d; 2.d; 3.d; 4.a; 5.c; 6.d; 7.b; 8.a; 9.d; 10.d

Chapter 12
1.d; 2.c; 3.b; 4.b; 5.a; 6.c; 7.a; 8.b; 9.b; 10.b

Chapter 13
1.a; 2.d; 3.d; 4.d; 5.a; 6.b; 7.b; 8.d; 9.b; 10.b

Chapter 14
1.c; 2.d; 3.c; 4.d; 5.d; 6.a; 7.a; 8.d; 9.b; 10.a

Chapter 15
1.a; 2.b; 3.b; 4.c; 5.d; 6.c; 7.b; 8.c; 9.d; 10.a

Coaching for Your Students 24/7

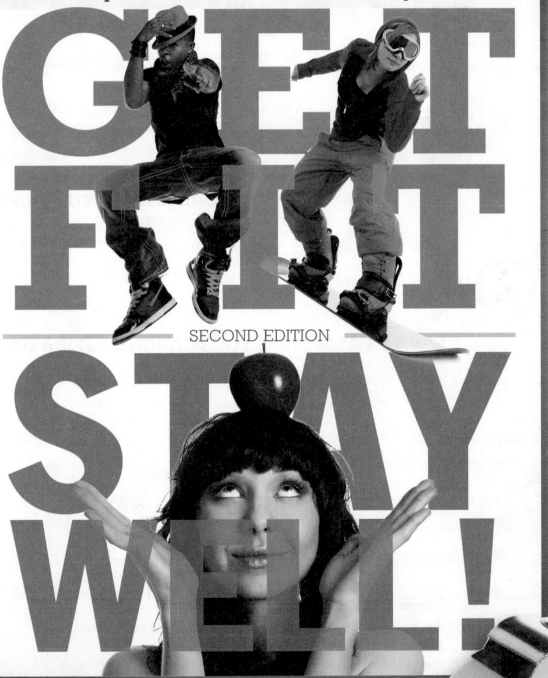

Janet L. Hopson · Rebecca J. Donatelle · Tanya R. Littrell

GET FIT

SECOND EDITION

STAY WELL!

Student Coaching for the Gym

Labs employ a unique three-pronged approach.
The book includes three types of labs:

1 **Skill-acquisition labs**

LEARN A SKILL
LAB 3.1 • MONITORING INTENSITY DURING A WORKOUT

2 **Self-assessment labs**

ASSESS YOURSELF
LAB 3.2 • ASSESSING YOUR CARDIORESPIRATORY FITNESS LEVEL

3 **Action-plan labs**

DO IT! ONLINE PLAN FOR CHANGE
LAB 3.3 • PLAN YOUR CARDIORESPIRATORY FITNESS GOALS AND PROGRAM

Three-pronged Approach to Labs

The labs not only measure a student's current level of fitness/wellness, but also teach practical lifelong skills and encourage real behavior change. All labs are also available in an online interactive PDF format.

PROGRAM A ♥ GOAL: Increase cycling minutes while maintaining a moderate intensity level three to four days a week, building to 100 total minutes by week four.

	Mon			Tue			Wed			Thu		Fri		Sat		Sun	
	T*	I*	T	I	T	I	T	I	T	I	T	I	T	I	T	I	T	I
Week 1	20	L					20	L					20	L–M				
Week 2	25	M					25	M					25	M				
Week 3	20	M					25	M					15	M	30	L–M		
Week 4	25	M					25	M					25	M	25	L–M		

T*: Time. Total time is listed in minutes.
I*: Intensity. Intensity is listed as Light/Lifestyle (L), Moderate (M), or Vigorous (V). (See Table 3.3.)
** Workouts do not include warm-up or cool-down time.

INTENSITY LEVEL **L** **M** **V**
Light Moderate Vigorous

PROGRAM B ♥ GOAL: Cycle at a moderate intensity level three to five days a week, build to a 40-minute ride, and incorporate vigorous interval training sessions each week.

	Mon			Tue			Wed			Thu			Fri		Sat		Sun	
	T*	I*	T	I	T	I	T	I	T	I	T	I	T	I	T	I	T	I
Week 1	25	L–M 3–5					25	L–M 3–5					25	M 5–6	25	M 5–6		
Week 2	25	L–M 3–5			30	M 5–6							25	L–M 3–5	35	M 5–6		
Week 3	30	M 5–6	Interval	L–M–V	20	L–M 3–5	Interval	L–M–V	30	M 5–6								
Week 4	30	M 5–6	Interval	L–M–V	25	L–M			30	M 5–6					40	L–M 3–5		

T*: Time. Total time is listed in minutes.
I*: Intensity. Intensity is listed as Light/Lifestyle (L), Moderate (M), or Vigorous (V), and the OMNI scale of 0–10. (See Figure 3.8, and Table 3.3.)

INTENSITY LEVEL **L** **M** **V**
Light Moderate Vigorous

PROGRAM C ♥ GOAL: Ride 20k/12.4mi in ≤ 60 minutes (indoors or out)!

	Mon		Tue		Wed		Thu		Fri		Sat		Sun	
	T/D*	I*	T/D	I	T/D	I	T/D	I	T/D	I	T/D	I	T/D	I
Week 1	25	L–M 62–70	35	M 3–5 65–85	25	L–M 62–70	25	M 5–6 65–85			35	M 5–6 65–85		
Week 2	30	M 5–6 62–70	20	M 7–8 80–94	6 miles	L–M 3–5 62–70	30	M 5–6 65–85			40	M 5–6 65–85		
Week 3	35	M 5–6 65–85	Interval	L–M–V		Interval	L–M–V	35	L–M 5–6 62–70			45	M 5–6 65–85		
Week 4	40	M 5–6 62–70	20	L–M 3–5	40	M 5–6 62–70	Interval	L–M–V			Goal: 20k Ride!	M 5–6 65–85		

T/D*: Time/Distance. Total time/distance is listed in minutes or miles.
I*: Intensity. Intensity is listed as Light/Lifestyle (L), Moderate (M), or Vigorous (V), the OMNI scale of 0–10, and % of HRmax. (See Figure 3.8 and Table 3.3.)
** Workouts do not include warm-up or cool-down time

INTENSITY LEVEL **L** **M** **V**
Light Moderate Vigorous

activate, motivate, & ADVANCE YOUR FITNESS

A CYCLING PROGRAM ♥ LIVE IT! ONLINE

ACTIVATE!

Whether you cycle indoors or take your bike out on the road or trail, you can get a fun and amazing workout.

Cycling Program Preparation & Safety

Sure, cycling can be an intense, calorie-burning workout, but it can also be a simple way to take care of errands, commute, meet up with friends, or just enjoy the great outdoors. Follow the programs below to get started. As you get stronger, you can increase your mileage and speed.

What Do I need for Cycling?

GEAR: Safe cycling requires quite a bit of equipment (helmet, padded cycling shorts, gloves, shoes, reflective gear, racks) and, of course, the bike. You can start on almost any style of bicycle, but most importantly, you need a bike that fits. Visit your local bike shop to get the right bike for you. When indoor cycling, adjust both seat and handlebar height to create a comfortable and safe fit. If you are new to indoor cycling or unfamiliar with the stationary bikes at your facility, be sure to ask a trained instructor to assist you with proper bike setup.

How Do I Start a Cycling Program?

TECHNIQUE: Work on developing a smooth and efficient pedaling technique. Lighten up, pedal in a smooth circle, and pull through the back of the stroke. *Cadence* is pedaling speed in revolutions per minute (RPM). A cadence of 60 RPM means that one pedal makes a complete revolution 60 times in one minute. Monitor your cadence with periodic cadence checks. Count the revolution of one leg for 15 seconds and then multiply by four. The cadence range is 80–110 RPM for cycling on a flat road and 60–80 RPM for climbing hills.

ETIQUETTE: Participating in group rides will teach you the etiquette for road cycling and mountain biking. Inquire about weekly rides or a beginners' cycling group at your local bike shop.

Cycling Tips

INDOOR CYCLING: Weather, traffic, flat tires ... with indoor cycling you won't have these excuses for missing your workout. Indoor cycling also allows you to precisely control your workout and mix periods of higher-intensity cycling with resting pedal strokes.

OUTDOOR CYCLING: Whether you choose streets, bike paths, or trails, plan safe routes that take into consideration

CHAPTER 3 CONDITIONING YOUR CARDIORESPIRATORY SYSTEM **109**

NEW! Activate/Motivate/Advance Sample Fitness Programs

These new programs, appearing at the ends of Chapters 2–5 and 8–9, are like having a personal trainer built into the book. Each program contains guidance on three parts of a fitness or wellness program: getting started, motivating to continue, and modifying/taking to the next level. The customizable "pre-fab" programs and the related tracking features and technique videos on the website make it easy to jump into a fitness behavior change project. These sample fitness programs are also accessible by mobile phone.

Exercise Videos

More than 100 videos of exercises are available on the Companion Website at www.pearsonhighered.com/hopson—allowing students access to additional instruction on their own time, and giving them the ability to exercise from the comfort of their own homes. Selected videos with assignable quiz questions that report to the gradebook are available in MyFitnessLab.™

Pearson Video Player - Mozilla Firefox

http://media.pearsoncmg.com/bc/bc_0media_hk/exercisevideos/media/lowbackkneetocheststretch.html

Low Back Knee-to-Chest Stretch PEARSON

Lie on your back and lift one knee toward your chest, grasping behind the thigh for support. Hold for 8-10 seconds. Return to the start position. Repeat with the other leg. Hold for 8-10 seconds. Now lift both knees toward your chest. Hold for 8-10 seconds.

00:13 Hide Text

Transferring data from media.pearsoncmg.com...

Students can pace themselves when studying

New Media Callouts in the chapter openers, end-of-chapter material, and throughout the text direct students to the extensive supporting electronic media, including videos, audio files, assignments, and review materials.

casestudy

CARLOS

"I know that my life is pretty good. I'm in college, studying what interests me, and I'm excited about the future. I just constantly feel behind. I fall asleep in class sometimes, eat a lot of junk food, and I'm not exercising—who has time? Then I got this cold, partly because I have been stressed out and not sleeping much. I've made some friends in my dorm, and it helps to know that a lot of them are going through the same thing. Talking to Liz every night on the phone helps, too."

THINK! In which dimensions of wellness could Carlos be stronger? Where would you place him on the wellness continuum? How do you compare to Carlos?

ACT! Identify your strongest wellness dimensions as well as the ones you could improve. Create a wellness balance chart and plan the balance you would like to achieve (Lab 1.2).

spectrum of existence; and promote feelings of love, joy, peace, contentment, and wonder over life's experiences.

Environmental Wellness

Our home, work, community, and school environments can be relaxing, safe havens or toxic, threatening, and stressful places to be. **Environmental wellness** entails understanding how the environment can positively or negatively affect you; the role you play in preserving, protecting, and improving the world around you; and what you can do to conserve dwindling resources for future generations.

Related Dimensions of Wellness

Occupational and financial wellness overlap with other wellness areas, and are sometimes considered their own dimensions. Your wellness in these areas can dramatically affect your overall wellness and add to your life's balance (or lack thereof). If you ask family members and friends about their current problems, many will identify their jobs or finances as the top stressors in their lives.

Occupational Wellness Occupational wellness is the level of happiness and fulfillment you experience in

your work. An important component of occupational wellness is finding a non-toxic, hazard-free work environment that provides contact with managers and co-workers who value your skills and opinions. Contrary to what people often think, job satisfaction is not closely tied to high wages.[2] You can reach optimal occupational wellness when your personal goals align closely with those of your employer, and when you feel that you are making significant contributions to both sets of goals.

Financial Wellness Financial wellness is the ability to successfully balance and manage your financial needs and wants with your income, debts, savings, and investments. If you cannot pay your bills, it can be hard to think of much else and this dimension can overshadow and unbalance the others. People who are managing their finances but just breaking even will still need to make wise consumer choices, carefully control debt, and continually prioritize expenses (see the box How Can I Handle My Finances Better?).

Balancing Your Wellness Dimensions

You may have healthy relationships, but no fondness for exercise. Perhaps your spiritual life is rich, but you have trouble juggling academic demands. Virtually everyone is stronger in some dimensions of wellness than others. Striving for improvement in all six wellness dimensions is a lifelong process. One good approach is to concentrate on those dimensions that present the most pressing need, while working on the others in a steady but relaxed and motivated way. Over time, a balance of work on all the dimensions—one or two now, others later—will eventually promote overall wellness. Your brain and body, your thoughts and emotions, your actions and reactions, your relationship to yourself and others—all are interconnected and integrated. Likewise, the dimensions of wellness are interrelated. For example, increasing your exercise and general activity will also help you manage stress, mood, body composition, and so on.

environmental wellness An appreciation of how the external environment can affect oneself, and an understanding of the role one plays in preserving, protecting, and improving it

occupational wellness A level of happiness and fulfillment in work, including harmony with personal goals, appreciation from bosses and co-workers, and a safe workplace

financial wellness The ability to balance and manage financial needs and wants with income, debts, savings, and investments

CHAPTER 1 CHANGING PERSONAL BEHAVIORS FOR OPTIMAL WELLNESS **5**

Good Wellness Habits Benefit Society as a Whole

The higher a population's levels of wellness, the happier and more productive are its people and the less money it spends on health care. Accordingly, achieving better wellness and combating today's chronic diseases are important national priorities.

National public health priorities cited by the Office of the Surgeon General of the United States are summarized in a set of objectives titled *Healthy People 2020*, which has four broad goals: 1) attain high-quality, longer lives free of preventable disease, disability, injury, and premature death; 2) achieve health equity, eliminate disparities, and improve the health of all groups; 3) create social and physical environments that promote good health for all; and 4) promote quality of life, healthy development, and healthy behaviors across all life stages.[13] In order to address some of these major public health priorities, the Surgeon General advises Americans to eat healthier, be more physically active, not smoke, limit alcohol, and avoid drugs—all of which are wellness behaviors.[14]

The high cost of health care and health insurance is a major concern for Americans. In 2009, Americans spent $2.5 trillion on health care, or 17.6 percent of the gross domestic product (GDP).[15] Employer health insurance premiums increased by 131 percent between 1999 and 2009 at four times the rate of inflation.[16] Nearly 49 million Americans lack health insurance, largely due to the high cost of coverage.[17] This makes them less likely to seek preventive care and adopt wellness behaviors early enough to prevent illness down the line. Such concerns led to sweeping new health legislation in 2010 to increase the percentage of Americans with health coverage.[18]

How Can I Change My Behavior to Increase My Wellness?

New Years' Resolutions

If you are like most people, you have made a New Year's resolution on January 1, have worked hard to adopt some new behavior until about the 10th, have started slipping back to your old habits by the 15th, and have forgotten about the whole thing by the 31st. Your resolution may well have been a new wellness behavior—lots of resolutions are. Perhaps it was an easy one, such as "eat more fruit," and you

succeeded. More likely, it was a harder one—"start lifting weights three times a week," or "lose 20 pounds," or "give up junk food"—and despite your good intentions, it just didn't stick.

People often see change as a singular event instead of a process that requires preparation, has several stages, and takes time to succeed. Classic research shows that we must go through a series of mental and emotional stages over a period of months to adequately prepare ourselves for **behavior change**. The rest of this chapter takes you through a series of practical steps inspired by a blueprint for change called the *transtheoretical model of behavior change* developed by psychologists James Prochaska and Carlo DiClemente.[19]

Step One: Understand the Stages of Behavior Change

The transtheoretical model of behavior change delineates six **stages of behavior change**: precontemplation, contemplation, preparation, action, maintenance, and termination. The model shows that changing behaviors usually involves a gradual process of awareness, preparation, and then action. Understanding this process can help you proceed more deliberately to identify and successfully change a problem behavior. Keep in mind that the steps of this model are general and people often backtrack as they work on them.

behavior change An organized, deliberate effort to alter or replace an existing habit or pattern of activity

stages of behavior change From the transtheoretical model, a set of states most people pass through in their awareness of, determination to alter, and efforts to replace existing habits or actions

CHAPTER 1 CHANGING PERSONAL BEHAVIORS FOR OPTIMAL WELLNESS

PAY OFF CREDIT CARDS

NEW! Media Callouts in Book

The printed text shows you exactly where the associated media is.

Active Media Callouts—Pearson eText Version

In the eText version, media callouts provide direct links to the media resources.

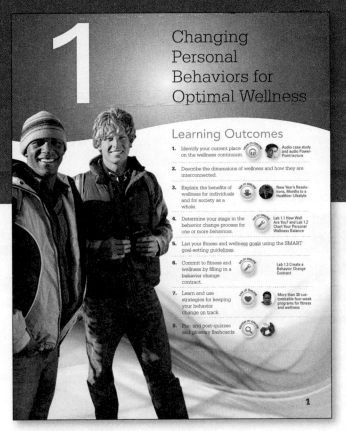

The **Second Edition** better addresses student questions and needs within the course through learning outcomes, and in their fitness/wellness behavior choices through the Question Boxes and Think!/Act! features.

NEW! Learning Outcomes

Learning Outcomes replace Chapter Objectives In the chapter openers.

Question Boxes

These boxes investigate common questions and concerns students may have about applying chapter topics to improve their own fitness & wellness.

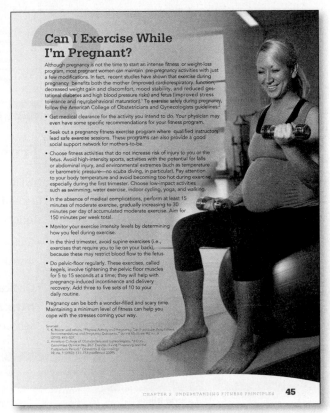

Can I Exercise While I'm Pregnant?

Although pregnancy is not the time to start an intense fitness or weight-loss program, most pregnant women can maintain pre-pregnancy activities with just a few modifications. In fact, recent studies have shown that exercise during pregnancy benefits both the mother (improved cardiorespiratory function, decreased weight gain and discomfort, mood stability, and reduced gestational diabetes and high blood pressure risks) and fetus (improved stress tolerance and neurobehavioral maturation). To exercise safely during pregnancy, follow the American College of Obstetricians and Gynecologists guidelines:

- Get medical clearance for the activity you intend to do. Your physician may even have some specific recommendations for your fitness program.

- Seek out a pregnancy fitness exercise program where qualified instructors lead safe exercise sessions. These programs can also provide a good social support network for mothers-to-be.

- Choose fitness activities that do not increase risk of injury to you or the fetus. Avoid high-intensity sports, activities with the potential for falls or abdominal injury, and environmental extremes (such as temperature or barometric pressure—no scuba diving, in particular). Pay attention to your body temperature and avoid becoming too hot during exercise, especially during the first trimester. Choose low-impact activities such as swimming, water exercise, indoor cycling, yoga, and walking.

- In the absence of medical complications, perform at least 15 minutes of moderate exercise, gradually increasing to 30 minutes per day of accumulated moderate exercise. Aim for 150 minutes per week total.

- Monitor your exercise intensity levels by determining how you feel during exercise.

- In the third trimester, avoid supine exercises (i.e., exercises that require you to lie on your back), because these may restrict blood flow to the fetus.

- Do pelvic-floor regularly. These exercises, called kegels, involve tightening the pelvic floor muscles for 5 to 15 seconds at a time; they will help with pregnancy-induced incontinence and delivery recovery. Add three to five sets of 10 to your daily routine.

Pregnancy can be both a wonder-filled and scary time. Maintaining a minimum level of fitness can help you cope with the stresses coming your way.

Sources:
1. K. Melzer and others, "Physical Activity and Pregnancy: Cardiovascular Adaptations, Recommendations and Pregnancy Outcomes," *Sports Medicine* 40, no. 6 (2010): 493–507.
2. American College of Obstetricians and Gynecologists, "ACOG Committee Opinion No. 267: Exercise During Pregnancy and the Postpartum Period," *Obstetrics & Gynecology* 99, no. 1 (2002): 171–173 (reaffirmed 2009).

CHAPTER 2 UNDERSTANDING FITNESS PRINCIPLES **45**

caseStudy

ANGELA

"I thought I would kick-start my plan to get back into shape by doing one of the workouts my tennis coach had us do in high school. I jogged for a mile, did some calisthenics on the court, and then played two sets of tennis with a friend. That was a mistake. My friend has a killer serve—it's like a bullet coming at you. She won every point she served because I couldn't move fast enough to return the ball. Also, I was surprised at how much that jog tired me out. I used to run a mile with no problem at all! By the end of the first set, I was completely exhausted. My friend won 6-1, 6-1."

THINK! Which energy system do you think Angela's friend relied on most while hitting her explosive serves?

ACT! Write out activities you would do for a 10-minute cardiorespiratory warm-up. Now, try your 10-minute warm up and think about how the three energy systems are providing fuel to keep your muscles moving.

NEW! Think!/Act!

These questions at the end of the case studies and other points within the chapters are designed to encourage critical thinking and to help students reflect on how the material applies to their own lives.

Add an assistant coach to your line up

Engaging experience

MyFitnessLab™ provides a one-stop spot for accessing a wealth of preloaded content and tools, while giving you the ability to customize your course as much (or as little) as you'd like.

NEW! *ABC News* Videos

These videos bring fitness & wellness topics to life and are available on the Instructor Resource DVD, MyFitnessLab, and the Companion Website.

Trusted partner

MyFitnessLab delivers engaging, dynamic learning opportunities—focused on instructor learning objectives and responsive to each student's progress—with improved registration and instructor support.

• Quick Start Videos demonstrate MyFitnessLab basics for instructors giving just-in-time help.

• Dedicated instructor and student support via internet chat at **http://247pearsoned.custhelp.com** or dedicated customer service line at 800-677-6337.

Exercise Videos

More than 100 videos of exercises are available; selected videos with assignable, gradable quiz questions make assigning homework on proper forms, technique, and safety easy to do.

MyFitnessLab™

www.myfitnesslab.com

The new MyFinessLab from Pearson has been designed and refined with a single purpose in mind: to help educators create that moment of understanding with their students. The MyFitnessLab system helps instructors maximize class time with customizable, easy-to-assign, and automatically graded assignments that motivate students to learn outside of class and arrive prepared for lecture. By complementing your teaching with our engaging technology and content, you can be confident your students will arrive at that moment—the moment of true understanding.

NEW! Active Media Callouts on Pearson eText

New media callouts in the chapter openers, end-of-chapter material, and throughout the text, provide direct links to the extensive supporting electronic media, including videos, audio files, assignments, and review materials.

Proven Results

MyFitnessLab has a consistently positive impact on the quality of learning in higher education fitness & wellness instruction. MyFitnessLab can be successfully implemented in any environment—lab-based, hybrid, fully online, traditional—and demonstrates the quantifiable difference that integrated usage of these products has on student retention, subsequent success, and overall achievement.

NEW! Pre- and Post-Evaluations

You can now easily measure before and after results for both Student Learning Outcomes and Fitness Evaluations. A 50-question exam can be assigned at the start of the course, and again at the end, to effectively measure Student Learning Outcomes. Additionally, an editable version of the Pre-/Post-Fitness assessment from the beginning of the book is available so students can track before and after results.

NEW! Over 180 Pre-built Assignments

Instructors can lessen their prep time and simplify their lives with preloaded quiz and test questions (specific to the textbook) that they can assign and/ or edit, a gradebook that automatically records student results from assigned tests, and the ability to customize the course as much (or as little) as desired.

Tools to Help You Coach Better

Teaching Tool Box

978-0-321-78043-0 • 0-321-78043-4

Save hours of valuable planning time with one comprehensive course planning kit. In one handy box, adjuncts, part-time, and full-time faculty will find a wealth of supplements and resources that reinforce key learning from the text and suit virtually any teaching style.

The Teaching Tool Box includes:

• Instructor Resource DVD

• Instructor Resource and Support Manual

• Test Bank

• User's Quick Guide reference guide

• Access to MyFitnessLab™ course management website

• *Great Ideas: Active Ways to Teach Health and Wellness*

• *Behavior Change Log Book and Wellness Journal*

• *Eat Right! Healthy Eating in College and Beyond*

• *Live Right! Beating Stress in College and Beyond*

• *Take Charge of Your Health!* Worksheets

• *Teaching with Student Learning Outcomes*

• *Teaching with Web 2.0*

• *Food Composition Table*

Health & Wellness Teaching Community

www.pearsonhighered.com/healthcommunity

Connect with other health instructors! The Health & Wellness Teaching Community website serves instructors like you by offering teaching tips and ideas, and by providing a forum for you to discuss health-related issues with your peers.

Student Supplements

MyFitnessLab
www.myfitnesslab.com

Behavior Change Log Book and Wellness Journal
978-0-321-80317-7 • 0-321-80317-5

Live Right! Beating Stress in College and Beyond
978-0-321-49149-7 • 0-321-49149-1

Eat Right! Healthy Eating in College and Beyond
978-0-8053-8288-4 • 0-8053-8288-7

Take Charge of Your Health! Worksheets
978-0-321-49942-4 • 0-321-49942-5

Food Composition Table
978-0-321-66793-9 • 0-321-66793-X

Companion Website
www.pearsonhighered.com/hopson

BEHAVIOR CHANGE CONTRACT

Choose a health behavior that you would like to change, starting this quarter or semester. Sign the contract at the bottom to affirm your commitment to making a healthy change and ask a friend to witness it.

My behavior change will be:

_____

My long-term goal for this behavior change is:

_____

Barriers I must overcome to make this behavior change are (things I am currently doing or situations that contribute to this behavior or make it harder to change):

1. _____

2. _____

3. _____

The strategies I will use to overcome these barriers are:

1. _____

2. _____

3. _____

Resources I will use to help me change this behavior include:

A friend/partner/relative _____

A school-based resource _____

A community-based resource _____

A book or reputable website _____

In order to make my goal more attainable, I have devised these short-term goals:

Short-Term Goal _____ **Target Date**_____ **Reward** _____

Short-Term Goal _____ **Target Date**_____ **Reward** _____

Short-Term Goal _____ **Target Date**_____ **Reward** _____

When I make the long-term behavior change described above, my reward will be:

Short-Term Goal _____ **Target Date**_____ **Reward** _____

I intend to make the behavior change described above, I will use the strategies and rewards to achieve the goals that will contribute to a healthy behavior change.

Signed _____ **Date**_____

Witness _____ **Date**_____